Volume 13
CHEMISTRY AND BRAIN DEVELOPMENT
Edited by R. Paoletti and A. N. Davison • 1971

Volume 14
MEMBRANE-BOUND ENZYMES
Edited by G. Porcellati and F. di Jeso • 1971

Volume 15
THE RETICULOENDOTHELIAL SYSTEM AND IMMUNE PHENOMENA
Edited by N. R. Di Luzio and K. Flemming • 1971

Volume 16A
THE ARTERY AND THE PROCESS OF ARTERIOSCLEROSIS: Pathogenesis
Edited by Stewart Wolf • 1971

Volume 16B
THE ARTERY AND THE PROCESS OF ARTERIOSCLEROSIS: Measurement and
Modification
Edited by Stewart Wolf • 1971

Volume 17
CONTROL OF RENIN SECRETION
Edited by Tatiana A. Assaykeen • 1972

Volume 18
THE DYNAMICS OF MERISTEM CELL POPULATIONS
Edited by Morton W. Miller and Charles C. Kuehnert • 1972

Volume 19
SPHINGOLIPIDS, SPHINGOLIPIDOSES AND ALLIED DISORDERS
Edited by Bruno W. Volk and Stanley M. Aronson • 1972

Volume 20
DRUG ABUSE: Nonmedical Use of Dependence-Producing Drugs
Edited by Simon Btesh • 1972

Volume 21
VASOPEPTIDES: Chemistry, Pharmacology, and Pathophysiology
Edited by N. Back and F. Sicuteri • 1972

Volume 22
COMPARATIVE PATHOPHYSIOLOGY OF CIRCULATORY DISTURBANCES
Edited by Colin M. Bloor • 1972

Volume 23
THE FUNDAMENTAL MECHANISMS OF SHOCK
Edited by Lerner B. Hinshaw and Barbara G. Cox • 1972

Volume 24
THE VISUAL SYSTEM: Neurophysiology, Biophysics, and Their Clinical Applications
Edited by G. B. Arden • 1972

Volume 25
GLYCOLIPIDS, GLYCOPROTEINS, AND MUCOPOLYSACCHARIDES
OF THE NERVOUS SYSTEM
Edited by Vittorio Zambotti, Guido Tettamanti, and Mariagrazia Arrigoni • 1972

Volume 26
PHARMACOLOGICAL CONTROL OF LIPID METABOLISM
Edited by William L. Holmes, Rodolfo Paoletti,
and David Kritchevsky • 1972

Volume 27
DRUGS AND FETAL DEVELOPMENT
Edited by M. A. Klingberg, A. Abramovici, and J. Chemke • 1973

Volume 28
HEMOGLOBIN AND RED CELL STRUCTURE AND FUNCTION
Edited by George J. Brewer • 1972

Volume 29
MICROENVIRONMENTAL ASPECTS OF IMMUNITY
Edited by Branislav D. Janković and Katarina Isaković • 1972

Volume 30
HUMAN DEVELOPMENT AND THE THYROID GLAND: Relation to Endemic Cretinism
Edited by J. B. Stanbury and R. L. Kroc • 1972

Volume 31
IMMUNITY IN VIRAL AND RICKETTSIAL DISEASES
Edited by A. Kohn and M. A. Klingberg • 1973

Volume 32
FUNCTIONAL AND STRUCTURAL PROTEINS OF THE NERVOUS SYSTEM
Edited by A. N. Davison, P. Mandel, and I. G. Morgan • 1972

Volume 33
NEUROHUMORAL AND METABOLIC ASPECTS OF INJURY
Edited by A. G. B. Kovach, H. B. Stoner, and J. J. Spitzer • 1972

Volume 34
PLATELET FUNCTION AND THROMBOSIS: A Review of Methods
Edited by P. M. Mannucci and S. Gorini • 1972

Volume 35
ALCOHOL INTOXICATION AND WITHDRAWAL: Experimental Studies
Edited by Milton M. Gross • 1973

Volume 36
RECEPTORS FOR REPRODUCTIVE HORMONES
Edited by Bert W. O'Malley and Anthony R. Means • 1973

Volume 37A
OXYGEN TRANSPORT TO TISSUE: Instrumentation, Methods, and Physiology
Edited by Haim I. Bicher and Duane F. Bruley • 1973

Volume 37B
OXYGEN TRANSPORT TO TISSUE: Pharmacology, Mathematical Studies, and Neonatology
Edited by Duane F. Bruley and Haim I. Bicher • 1973

Volume 38
HUMAN HYPERLIPOPROTEINEMIAS: Principles and Methods
Edited by R. Fumagalli, G. Ricci, and S. Gorini • 1973

Volume 39
CURRENT TOPICS IN CORONARY RESEARCH
Edited by Colin M. Bloor and Ray A. Olsson • 1973

Volume 40
METAL IONS IN BIOLOGICAL SYSTEMS: Studies of Some Biochemical and Environmental Problems
Edited by Sanat K. Dhar • 1973

Volume 41A
PURINE METABOLISM IN MAN: Enzymes and Metabolic Pathways
Edited by O. Sperling, A. De Vries, and J. B. Wyngaarden • 1973

Volume 41B
PURINE METABOLISM IN MAN: Biochemistry and Pharmacology of Uric Acid Metabolism
Edited by O. Sperling, A. De Vries, and J. B. Wyngaarden • 1973

OXYGEN TRANSPORT TO TISSUE

Instrumentation, Methods, and Physiology

Edited by

Haim I. Bicher

Associate Professor of Pharmacology
University of Arkansas Medical Center
Little Rock, Arkansas

and

Duane F. Bruley

Professor of Chemical Engineering
Clemson University
Clemson, South Carolina

SPRINGER SCIENCE+BUSINESS MEDIA, LLC

Library of Congress Cataloging in Publication Data

International Symposium on Oxygen Transport to Tissue, Medical University of South Carolina and Clemson University, 1973.
   Oxygen transport to tissue.

   (Advances in experimental medicine and biology, v. 37A-B)
   Editors' names in reverse order in v. 2.
   Sponsored by American Microcirculation Society and European Microcirculation Society.
   Includes bibliographies.
   CONTENTS: [1] Instrumentation, methods, and physiology.—[2] Pharmacology, mathematical studies, and neonatology.
   1. Tissue respiration—Congresses. 2. Biological transport—Congresses. 3. Microcirculation—Congresses. I. Bicher, Haim I., ed. II. Bruley, Duane F., ed. III. American Microcirculation Society. IV. European Microcirculation Society. V. Title. VI. Series. [DNLM: 1. Biological transport—Congresses. 2. Oxygen—Blood—Congresses. W1 AD599 v. 37 1973 / QV312 I613o 1973]
QP121.A1I56   1973   599'.01'24   73-13821
ISBN 978-1-4684-3290-9   ISBN 978-1-4684-3288-6 (eBook)
DOI 10.1007/978-1-4684-3288-6

The first half of the International Symposium on Oxygen
Transport to Tissue held in Charleston—Clemson, South Carolina,
April 22-28, 1973

© 1973 Springer Science+Business Media New York
Originally published by Plenum Press, New York in 1973
Softcover reprint of the hardcover 1st edition 1973

INTERNATIONAL SYMPOSIUM ON

OXYGEN TRANSPORT TO TISSUE

HOSTS   MEDICAL UNIVERSITY OF SOUTH CAROLINA
                    Charleston, South Carolina

                        CLEMSON UNIVERSITY
                    Clemson, South Carolina

SPONSORS   AMERICAN MICROCIRCULATION SOCIETY

               EUROPEAN MICROCIRCULATION SOCIETY

SUPPORT   MEDICAL UNIVERSITY OF SOUTH CAROLINA
                        CLEMSON UNIVERSITY
                       SCHERING CORPORATION
                           CIBA-GEIGY
               INTERNATIONAL BIOPHYSICS CORPORATION
               MEDISCIENCE TECHNOLOGY CORPORATION
                        BRISTOL LABORATORIES
                         BURROUGHS WELCOME
                  TRANSIDYNE GENERAL CORPORATION
                  SCIENTIFIC RESEARCH INSTRUMENTS
               DAAD and DFG (GERMAN SCIENTIFIC AGENCIES)

INTERNATIONAL SOCIETY

OF

OXYGEN TRANSPORT TO TISSUE

PAST PRESIDENT - DR. MELVIN H. KNISELY, CHARLESTON, U.S.A.
PRESIDENT-ELECT - DR. GERHARD THEWS, MAINZ, GERMANY
SECRETARY - DR. HAIM I. BICHER, LITTLE ROCK, U.S.A.
TREASURER - DR. IAN A. SILVER, BRISTOL, ENGLAND

MEMBERS - INTERNATIONAL COMMITTEE

DR. HERBERT J. BERMAN, BOSTON, U.S.A.

DR. DUANE F. BRULEY, CLEMSON, U.S.A.

DR. BRITTON CHANCE, PHILADELPHIA, U.S.A.

DR. LELAND C. CLARK, JR., CINCINNATI, U.S.A.

DR. LARS-ERIK GELIN, GOTEBORG, SWEDEN

DR. JÜRGEN GROTE, MAINZ, GERMANY

DR. MANFRED KESSLER, DORTMUND, GERMANY

DR. DIETRICH W. LÜBBERS, DORTMUND, GERMANY

DR. DANIEL D. RENEAU, RUSTON, U.S.A.

DR. JOSE STRAUSS, MIAMI, U.S.A.

DR. WILLIAM J. WHALEN, CLEVELAND, U.S.A.

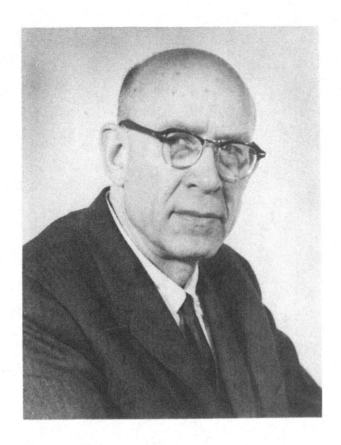

Dr. Melvin H. Knisely

DEDICATION

It is with sincere gratitude that we would like to dedicate this
book and meeting to Dr. Melvin H. Knisely for his important contribution to the world of science in the area of microcirculation. His
hard and productive work over a number of years prior to our association has been the foundation of everything that we have accomplished
as an interdisciplinary team. Dr. Knisely is a tireless researcher
for the benefit of mankind. His willingness to work with profound
interest, at any hour of the day or night, has stimulated our group
effort more than any other single factor. Ideas and enthusiasm flow
from Dr. Knisely and his ability to transform them into simple terms
has to be appreciated by even the most sophisticated. We are greatly
honored to have the opportunity to work with Dr. Knisely.

PREFACE

It can honestly be said that the scope and magnitude of this meeting surpassed initial expectations with respect to the number and quality of the papers presented. Our group has grown since we last met in Dortmund in 1971. This is a good indication that a spiraling of our interests has taken place with the effects of the initial good work felt, not just in one corner of the globe, but in all four. With such a start, it was only appropriate that an international society was formed at the meeting to further coordinate our mutual undertaking. Henceforth it shall be known as the International Society of Oxygen Transport to Tissue.

A final note of acknowledgement should be made to those who were in the supporting cast, not only in making the meeting in Charleston and Clemson a success, but also in the compiling of this book. Gratitude is due to Dr. Daniel H. Hunt for his efforts, the end product of which you have in your hands. Considerable service was rendered by Mr. Robert J. Adams, Mr. Buddy Bell and Mr. Nathan Kaufman during the symposium itself. Much typing, organizing and record keeping was done by our lovely secretaries, Laura B. Grove, Muff Graham and Kaye Y. Zook.

Haim I. Bicher, MD, PhD

Duane F. Bruley, PhD

June, 1973

CONTRIBUTORS

Dr. H. Acker
Max-Planck-Institut für Systemphysiologie (formerly Arbeitsphysiologie), Dortmund, West Germany

Mr. Robert J. Adams
Department of Anatomy, Medical University of South Carolina,
Charleston, South Carolina, U.S.A.

Dr. Trenton Allison
Department of Internal Medicine, University of Nebraska Medical
Center, Omaha, Nebraska, U.S.A.

Dr. William Baetz
Case Western Reserve University School of Medicine, Cleveland, Ohio,
U.S.A.

Dr. Rex Baker
Department of Pediatrics, University of Miami School of Medicine,
Miami, Florida, U.S.A.

Dr. J. Douglas Balentine
Department of Pathology, Medical University of South Carolina,
Charleston, South Carolina, U.S.A.

Dr. Wolfgang Barnikol
Physiologisches Institut der Universität, Mainz, West Germany

Dr. Ronald E. Barr
Department of Ophthalmology, University of Missouri-Columbia,
Columbia, Missouri, U.S.A.

Dr. Fernando Becattini
The Children's Hospital Research Foundation, Children's Hospital
Medical Center, Cincinnati, Ohio, U.S.A.

Dr. Hartmut Benzing
Physiologisches Institut der Universität, Tübingen, West Germany

Dr. Anthony V. Beran
Department of Pediatrics, University of California, Irvine,
California, U.S.A.

Dr. Maurice Berard
New York University Medical Center, Institute of Rehabilitation
Medicine, 400 East 34th Street, New York, New York, U.S.A.

Dr. Herbert J. Berman
Department of Biology, Boston University, Boston, Massachusetts, U.S.A.

Dr. E. Betz
Physiologisches Institut der Universität, Tübingen, West Germany

Dr. Haim I. Bicher
Department of Pharmacology, University of Arkansas Medical Center,
Little Rock, Arkansas, U.S.A.

Dr. Dieter Bingmann
Physiologisches Institut der Universität, Münster/Westf.,
West Germany

Dr. Edward H. Bloch
Department of Anatomy, Case Western Reserve University, Cleveland,
Ohio, U.S.A.

Mr. Beauford A. Bogue
Engineering Center, Arizona State University, Temple, Arizona, U.S.A.

Dr. B. Bölling
Max-Planck-Institut für Systemphysiologie, Dortmund, West Germany

Dr. Jeannine Bordeau-Martini
University of Paris, Paris, France

Dr. Joseph Bratton
U.S. Army Medical Research Laboratory, Fort Knox, Kentucky, U.S.A.

Dr. W. Braunbeck
Physiologisches Institut der Universität Johannes Gutenberg,
Mainz, West Germany

Dr. George J. Brewer
Department of Human Genetics, University of Michigan, Ann Arbor,
Michigan, U.S.A.

Dr. Daniel Brooks
U.S. Army Medical Research Laboratory, Fort Knox, Kentucky, U.S.A.

Dr. Edwin G. Brown
Department of Pediatrics, Cleveland Metropolitan General Hospital,
Cleveland, Ohio, U.S.A.

Dr. Duane F. Bruley
Department of Chemical Engineering, Clemson University, Clemson,
South Carolina, U.S.A.

Dr. S. P. Bruttig
Department of Biochemistry and Medicine, University of Nebraska
College of Medicine, Omaha, Nebraska, U.S.A.

Dr. T. F. Burks
Program in Physiology, The University of Texas Medical School at
Houston, Texas Medical Center, Houston, Texas, U.S.A.

Dr. Mark G. Burns
U.S. Army Medical Research Laboratory, Fort Knox, Kentucky, U.S.A.

Dr. Raul Busto
Department of Neurology, University of Miami School of Medicine,
Miami, Florida, U.S.A.

Dr. Bruce F. Cameron
Papanicolaou Cancer Research Institute, 1155 North West 14th Street,
Miami, Florida, U.S.A.

Dr. J. Carey
Thoracic and Cardiovascular Surgery Department, Veterans Administration Hospital, Los Angeles, California, U.S.A.

Dr. H. Caspers
Physiologisches Institut der Universität, Münster/Westf.,
West Germany

Dr. John Cassell
Department of Neurology, University of Miami School of Medicine,
Miami, Florida, U.S.A.

Dr. Britton Chance
Johnson Research Foundation, Department of Biophysics and Physical
Biochemistry, University of Pennsylvania, Philadelphia, Pennsylvania,
U.S.A.

Mr. Bong H. Chang
Department of Chemical Engineering, University of Louisville,
Louisville, Kentucky, U.S.A.

Dr. Hsin-kang Chang
Department of Civil Engineering, State University of New York at
Buffalo, Buffalo, New York, U.S.A.

Dr. Guy M. Chisolm, III
Department of Chemical Engineering, University of Virginia,
Charlottesville, Virginia, U.S.A.

Dr. Eleanor W. Clark
Division of Cardiology and Neurophysiology, Children's Hospital
Research Foundation, Children's Hospital, Cincinnati, Ohio, U.S.A.

Dr. Howard G. Clark
Department of Biomedical Engineering, Duke University, Durham,
North Carolina, U.S.A.

Dr. Leland C. Clark, Jr.
Division of Cardiology and Neurophysiology, Children's Hospital
Research Foundation, Children's Hospital, Cincinnati, Ohio, U.S.A.

Dr. Ronald F. Coburn
Department of Physiology, University of Pennsylvania School of
Medicine, Philadelphia, Pennsylvania, U.S.A.

Dr. Clark K. Colton
Department of Chemical Engineering, Massachusetts Institute of
Technology, Cambridge, Massachusetts, U.S.A.

Dr. R. S. Comline
Physiological Laboratory, Cambridge CB2 3 EG, Cambridge, England

Dr. John E. Connolly
Department of Surgery, University of California, Irvine,
California, U.S.A.

Dr. M. F. Crass, III
Department of Medicine, University of Nebraska Medical Center,
Omaha, Nebraska, U.S.A.

Dr. R. L. Curl
Department of Chemical Engineering, University of Michigan, Ann
Arbor, Michigan, U.S.A.

Dr. J. W. Dalton
Thoracic and Cardiovascular Surgery Department, Veterans Administration Hospital, Los Angeles, California, U.S.A.

Dr. W. Dempsey
Institut für Anaesthesiologie, Physiologisches Institut und
Universitatsfrauenklinik der Universität Mainz, Germany

Dr. R. Dieterle
Max-Planck-Institut für Systemphysiologie, Dortmund, West Germany

Dr. Jørn Ditzel
Department of Medicine, Aalborg Kommunehospital, Aalborg, Denmark

Mr. William E. Donovan
Department of Surgery, Veterans Administration Hospital, New
Orleans, Louisiana, U.S.A.

Dr. William J. Dorson, Jr.
Engineering Center, Arizona State University, Tempe, Arizona, U.S.A.

Dr. Jochen Duhm
Department of Physiology, Medical Faculty, Technical University,
D 51 Aachen, West Germany

Dr. Brian R. Duling
Department of Physiology, University of Virginia School of Medicine,
Charlottesville, Virginia, U.S.A.

Dr. Patrick Eberhard
Department of Bioelectronics, Hoffmann-La Roche & Company,
Grenzacherstr. 124, CH 4002, Basle, Switzerland

Dr. Robert S. Eliot
Division of Cardiology, University of Nebraska Medical Center,
Omaha, Nebraska, U.S.A.

Dr. Wilhelm Erdmann
Institute for Anesthesiology, Johannes Gutenberg University,
Mainz, West Germany

Dr. Edward A. Ernst
Department of Anesthesiology, University Hospitals, Case Western
Reserve University, Cleveland, Ohio, U.S.A.

Dr. Kevin D. Fallon
Instrumentation Laboratory, 113 Hartwell Avenue, Lexington,
Massachusetts, U.S.A.

Dr. H. Fehlau
Max-Planck-Institut für Systemphysiologie, Dortmund, West Germany

Dr. Charles T. Fitts
Department of Surgery, Medical University of South Carolina,
Charleston, South Carolina, U.S.A.

Dr. Marvin Fleischman
Department of Chemical Engineering, University of Louisville,
Louisville, Kentucky, U.S.A.

Dr. John E. Fletcher
Laboratory of Applied Studies, Division of Computer Research and
Technology, Building 12A, Room 2041, Bethesda, Maryland, U.S.A.

Dr. George C. Frazier
Department of Chemical Engineering, University of Tennessee,
Knoxville, Tennessee, U.S.A.

Dr. Uwe E. Freese
Department of Obstetrics and Gynecology, Chicago Lying In Hospital,
5841 Maryland Avenue, Chicago, Illinois, U.S.A.

Dr. Robert L. Fuhro
Department of Biology, Boston University, Boston, Massachusetts,
U.S.A.

Dr. John L. Gainer
Department of Chemical Engineering, University of Virginia,
Charlottesville, Virginia, U.S.A.

Dr. E. Gärtner
Physiologisches Institut der Universität, Tübingen, West Germany

Dr. Randall N. Gatz
Department of Physiology, Max-Plank Institut für Experimentelle
Medizin, Gottingen, West Germany

Dr. Lars-Eric Gelin
Surgical Department I, University of Goteborg, Goteborg, Sweden

Dr. Joe D. Goddard
Department of Chemical Engineering, University of Michigan, Ann
Arbor, Michigan, U.S.A.

Dr. Lothar Goernandt
Max-Planck-Institut für Systemphysiologie, Dortmund, West Germany

Dr. Harry L. Goldsmith
McGill University Medical Clinic, Montreal General Hospital,
Montreal, Quebec, Canada

Dr. Thomas K. Goldstick
Department of Applied Mechanics and Engineering Sciences, University
of California at San Diego, LaJolla, California, U.S.A.

Dr. Anthony H. Goodman
Department of Physiology and Biophysics, University of Mississippi
Medical Center, Jackson, Mississippi, U.S.A.

Dr. R. J. Gordon
Department of Chemical Engineering, University of Florida,
Gainesville, Florida, U.S.A.

Dr. Carl A. Goresky
Montreal General Hospital, Medicine Department, University Medical
Clinic, Montreal, Quebec, Canada

Dr. Lothar Görnandt
Max-Planck-Institut für Systemphysiologie, Dortmund, West Germany

Dr. D. Neil Granger
Department of Physiology and Biophysics, University of Mississippi
Medical Center, Jackson, Mississippi, U.S.A.

Dr. Harris J. Granger
Department of Physiology and Biophysics, University of Mississippi
Medical Center, Jackson, Mississippi, U.S.A.

Dr. Alan C. Groom
Department of Biophysics, University of Western Ontario, London,
Ontario, Canada

Professor Jürgen Grote
Physiologisches Institut, Universität Mainz, Mainz, West Germany

Dr. Dr. Wolfgang Grunewald
Max-Planck-Institut für Systemphysiologie, Dortmund, West Germany

Dr. Eric J. Guilbeau
Department of Biomedical Engineering, Louisiana Technical University,
Ruston, Louisiana, U.S.A.

Dr. Heinz Günther
Johannes Gutenberg Universität, Mainz, West Germany

Dr. K. Hájek
Max-Planck-Institut für Systemphysiologie, Dortmund, West Germany

Dr. Denis F. J. Halmagyi
Department of Surgery PH 12-124, College of Physicians and Surgeons,
Columbia University, New York, New York, U.S.A.

Dr. H. Hamelmann
Laboratory for Cytology and Histology, R. K. University, Nijmegen,
Netherlands

Dr. Konrad Hammacher
Universitätsfrauenklinik, Basle, Switzerland

Dr. Donald R. Harkness
Department of Neurology, University of Miami School of Medicine,
Miami, Florida, U.S.A.

Dr. Thomas R. Harris
Department of Pediatrics, University of Arizona College of Medicine,
Tucson, Arizona, U.S.A.

Dr. Herbert B. Hechtman
Boston University Medical Center, Boston, Massachusetts, U.S.A.

Dr. J. Heidenreich
Institut für Anaesthesiologie, Physiologisches Institut und
Universitätsfrauenklinik der Universität Mainz, Mainz, West Germany

Dr. F. Hess
Laboratory for Cytology and Histology, R. K. University, Nijmegen,
Netherlands

Dr. Robert A. B. Holland
The University of New South Wales, Kensington N.S.W. 2033, Australia

Dr. Donald E. Holness
Defense and Civil Institute of Environmental Medicine, Box 2000, S.T.K.
Downsview, Ontario, Canada

Dr. James W. Holsinger, Jr.
Division of Cardiology, University of Nebraska Medical Center, Omaha,
Nebraska, U.S.A.

Dr. Carl R. Honig
Department of Physiology, University of Rochester, Rochester, New
York, U.S.A.

Dr. Jens Höper
Max-Planck-Institut für Systemphysiologie, Dortmund, West Germany

Dr. K. Horak
Max-Planck-Institut für Systemphysiologie, Dortmund, West Germany

Dr. Albert Huch
Universitäts-Frauenklinik, Marburg (Lahn), West Germany

Dr. Renate Huch
Universitäts-Frauenklinik, Marburg (Lahn), West Germany

Dr. Daniel H. Hunt
Department of Anatomy, Medical University of South Carolina,
Charleston, South Carolina, U.S.A.

Professor Dr. H. Hutten
Johannes Gutenberg Universität, Mainz, West Germany

Dr. William A. Hyman
Rioengineering Program, Teague Research Center, Texas A and M
University, College Station, Texas, U.S.A.

Dr. John W. Irwin
Eaton-Peabody Laboratory, Massachusetts Eye and Ear Infirmary,
243 Charles Street, Boston, Massachusetts, U.S.A.

Dr. Franz Jann
Universitätsfrauenklinik, Basle, Switzerland

Dr. C. R. Jerusalem
Laboratory for Cytology and Histology, R. K. University, Nijmegen,
Netherlands

Dr. Franz Jesch
Thoracic and Cardiovascular Surgery Department, Veterans Administration Hospital, Los Angeles, California, U.S.A.

Dr. Samuel Kaplan
Division of Cardiology and Neurophysiology, Children's Hospital
Research Foundation, Children's Hospital, Cincinnati, Ohio, U.S.A.

Professor Dr. Manfred Kessler
Max-Planck-Institut für Systemphysiologie, Dortmund, West Germany

Dr. Chang Yong Kim
Department of Neurology, University of Miami School of Medicine,
Miami, Florida, U.S.A.

Dr. Peter Kiwull
Arbeitsgruppe Regulationsphysiologie, Institut Physiologie,
Ruhr-Universität, Bochum, West Germany

Dr. Melvin H. Knisely
Department of Anatomy, Medical University of South Carolina,
Charleston, South Carolina, U.S.A.

Dr. J. A. Knopp
Department of Biochemistry, North Carolina State University,
Raleigh, North Carolina, U.S.A.

Dr. Kyuya Kogure
Department of Neurology, University of Miami School of Medicine
Miami, Florida, U.S.A.

Dr. Stefan Kunke
Department of Anesthesiology and Physiology, University of Mainz,
Mainz, West Germany

Professor Dr. Klaus Kunz
Department of Clinical Neurophysiology, University of Giessen,
West Germany

Dr. L. L. Lafitte
Department of Biomedical Engineering, Louisiana Technical University,
Ruston, Louisiana, U.S.A.

Dr. Helmut Lang
Max-Planck-Institut für Systemphysiologie, Dortmund, West Germany

Dr. J. Leigh
Department of Surgery, Gordon Craig Research Laboratory, University
of Sydney, Sydney, N.S.W., Australia

Dr. E. N. Lightfoot
Department of Chemical Engineering, University of Wisconsin, Madison,
Wisconsin, U.S.A.

Professor Chung-Chiun Liu
Chemical and Petroleum Engineering Department, School of Engineering,
University of Pittsburgh, Pittsburgh, Pennsylvania, U.S.A.

Dr. Wolfgang Lixfeld
Cardiovascular Laboratory, Banting Institute, University of Toronto
Toronto, Ontario, Canada

Dr. B. Isabel Lockard
Department of Anatomy, Medical University of South Carolina,
Charleston, South Carolina, U.S.A.

Dr. Ian S. Longmuir
Department of Biochemistry, North Carolina State University,
Raleigh, North Carolina, U.S.A.

Dr. B. Lösse
Physiologisches Institut der Universität, Tübingen, West Germany

Dr. Edward W. Lowman
Laboratory of Biochemical Pharmacology, Institute of Rehabilitation
Medicine, New York University Medical Center, New York, New York, U.S.A.

Professor Dr. Dietrich W. Lübbers
Max-Planck-Institut für Systemphysiologie, Dortmund, West Germany

Dr. David C. MacGregor
Director, Cardiovascular Laboratories, First Floor, University
Wing, Toronto General Hospital, Toronto, Ontario, Canada

Dr. D. Mailman
Programs in Physiology and Pharmacology, University of Texas Medical
School at Houston, Texas Medical Center, Houston, Texas, U.S.A.

Dr. A. L. Malenfant
Instrumentation Laboratory, 113 Hartwell Avenue, Lexington,
Massachusetts, U.S.A.

Dr. K. Mandalenaki
Department of Pediatrics, St. Sophia Hospital, Athens University
Medical School, Athens, Greece

Dr. A. Mayevsky
Johnson Research Foundation, University of Pennsylvania, Philadelphia,
Pennsylvania, U.S.A.

Dr. Francis E. McDonnell
Department of Pediatrics and the Preinatal Clinical Research Center,
Case Western Reserve University at Cleveland Metropolitan General
Hospital, Cleveland, Ohio, U.S.A.

Dr. David Meixner
U.S. Army Medical Research Laboratory, Fort Knox, Kentucky, U.S.A.

Mr. Jerry H. Meldon
Department of Chemical Engineering, Massachusetts Institute of
Technology, Cambridge, Massachusetts, U.S.A.

Dr. M. Mendlowitz
Department of Medicine, Mt. Sinai School of Medicine, New York,
New York, U.S.A.

Dr. Konrad Messmer
Institute of Surgical Research, University of Munich, Munich,
West Germany

Dr. Hermann Metzger
Johannes Gutenberg Universität, Mainz, West Germany

Dr. C. Eugene Miller
Department of Civil Engineering, University of Louisville,
Louisville, Kentucky, U.S.A.

Dr. James A. Miller, Jr.
Tulane University School of Medicine, New Orleans, Louisiana, U.S.A.

Dr. Wolfgang Mindt
Basle and Universitätsfrauenklinik, Basle, Switzerland

Dr. Masaji Mochizuki
Research Institute of Applied Electricity, Hokkaido University,
Sapporo, Japan

Professor Dr. Waldemar Moll
Physiologisches Institut der Universität Regensburg, Regensburg,
West Germany

Dr. Lorna G. Moore
Department of Human Genetics, University of Michigan, Ann Arbor,
Michigan, U.S.A.

Dr. Catherine A. Morrazzi
Department of Chemical Engineering, Northeastern University,
Boston, Massachusetts, U.S.A.

Dr. L. G. Morphis
Department of Pediatrics, St. Sophia Hospital, Athens University
Medical School, Athens, Greece

Dr. M. Bert Myers
Department of Surgery, Veterans Administration Hospital, New Orleans,
Louisiana, U.S.A.

Dr. Ronald E. Myers
NINDS LPP, Auburn Building, Room 106, National Institutes of
Health, Bethesda, Maryland, U.S.A.

Dr. N. Eric Naftchi
Laboratory of Biochemistry and Pharmacology, Institute for Rehabil-
itation Medicine, New York University Medical Center, New York,
New York, U.S.A.

Mr. Dennis Nelson
Case Western Reserve University School of Medicine, Cleveland, Ohio,
U.S.A.

Dr. Michael R. Neuman
Department of Pediatrics, Cleveland Metropolitan General Hospital,
Cleveland, Ohio, U.S.A.

Dr. N. Niederle
Max-Planck-Institut für Systemphysiologie, Dortmund, West Germany

Dr. Michael Nugent
Department of Pediatrics, University of Arizona College of Medicine,
Tucson, Arizona, U.S.A.

Dr. Virginia Obrock
Division of Cardiology and Neurophysiology, Children's Hospital
Research Foundation, Children's Hospital, Cincinnati, Ohio, U.S.A.

Dr. Fred J. Oelshlegel, Jr.
Department of Human Genetics, University of Michigan, Ann Arbor,
Michigan, U.S.A.

Dr. Robert W. Ogilvie
Department of Anatomy, Medical University of South Carolina,
Charleston, South Carolina, U.S.A.

Dr. Larry O'Maley
U.S. Army Medical Research Laboratory, Fort Knox, Kentucky, U.S.A.

Dr. Tsukasa Ono
Research Institute of Applied Electricity, Hokkaido University,
Sapporo, Japan

Dr. N. Oshino
Johnson Research Foundation, Department of Biophysics and Physical
Biochemistry, University of Pennsylvania, Philadelphia, Pennsylvania,
U.S.A.

Dr. Lee E. Ostrander
Department of Biomedical Engineering, Case Western Reserve University,
Cleveland, Ohio, U.S.A.

Professeur Maurice Panigel
Biologie de la Reproduction, Université de Paris, Paris, France

Dr. Douglas J. Pappajohn
Department of Medicine, Hahnemann Hospital, 230 North Broad Street
Philadelphia, Pennsylvania, U.S.A.

Dr. Raymond Penneys
Department of Medicine, Hahnemann Hospital, 230 North Broad Street,
Philadelphia, Pennsylvania, U.S.A.

Dr. Garry Phillips
U.S. Army Medical Research Laboratory, Fort Knox, Kentucky, U.S.A.

Dr. Johannes Piiper
Abteilung Physiologie, Max-Planck-Institut für Experimentelle Medizine,
Göttingen, West Germany

Mr. Michael J. Plyley
Department of Biophysics, University of Western Ontario, London,
Ontario, Canada

Dr. Stefan Racoceanu
Department of Medicine, Mt. Sinai School of Medicine, New York,
New York, U.S.A.

Dr. Herbert Rahmer
Chirurgische Universitätsklinik, Tübingen, West Germany

Dr. John H. G. Rankin
Department of Obstetrics, Madison General Hospital, 202 South Park
Street, Madison, Wisconsin, U.S.A.

Dr. Theobald Reich
Laboratory of Biochemistry and Pharmacology, Institute for Rehabil-
itation Medicine, New York University Medical Center, New York,
New York, U.S.A.

Dr. Daniel D. Reneau
Department of Biomedical Engineering, Louisiana Technical University,
Ruston, Louisiana, U.S.A.

Dr. Richard D. Rink
Max-Planck Institut für Systemphysiologie, Dortmund, West Germany

Dr. Ernest L. Roetman
Department of Mathematics, Mathematical Sciences Building, University
of Missouri, Columbia, Missouri, U.S.A.

Dr. Andrew M. Rose
Department of Human Genetics, University of Michigan, Ann Arbor,
Michigan, U.S.A.

Dr. Theodore Rosett
Department of Biochemistry, Temple University School of Dentistry,
Philadelphia, Pennsylvania, U.S.A.

Dr. Joseph W. Rubin
Department of Thoracic Surgery, Medical University of South
Carolina, Charleston, South Carolina, U.S.A.

Professor Boris Rybak
Zoophysiologie, Université de Caen, Caen, France

Dr. R. E. Safford
Department of Chemical Engineering, University of Wisconsin,
Madison, Wisconsin, U.S.A.

Dr. J. M. Salhany
Department of Biophysics, University of Chicago, Chicago, Illinois,
U.S.A.

Dr. Stanley H. Saulson
Cordis Corporation, P. O. Box 428, Miami, Florida, U.S.A.

Dr. Hans Schäfer
Johannes Gutenberg University, Mainz, West Germany

Dr. Peter D. Schäfer
Max-Planck-Institut für Systemphysiologie, Dortmund, West Germany

Dipl. Biochem. Ursala Schindler
Physiologisches Institut der Universität Tübingen, Tübingen, West
Germany

Dr. Dietgard Schmeling
Max-Planck-Institut für Systemphysiologie, Dortmund, West Germany

Dr. Heidrun Schöne
Physiologisches Institut der Ruhr Universität, Bochum, West Germany

Dr. Sebastian Schuchhardt
Max-Planck-Institut für Systemphysiologie, Dortmund, West Germany

Dr. Jerome S. Schultz
Department of Chemical Engineering, University of Michigan, Ann
Arbor, Michigan, U.S.A.

Dr. H. Schulze
Max-Planck-Institut für Systemphysiologie, Dortmund, West Germany

Dr. Stuart J. Segall
Department of Biology, Boston University, Boston, Massachusetts, U.S.A.

Dr. E. Seidl
Max-Planck-Institut für Systemphysiologie, Dortmund, West Germany

Dr. Heiner Sell
Laboratory of Biochemistry and Pharmacology, Institute for Rehabil-
itation Medicine, New York University Medical Center, New York,
New York, U.S.A.

Dr. V. L. Shah
Department of Energetics, College of Engineering and Applied
Science, University of Wisconsin, Milwaukee, Wisconsin

Dr. A. P. Shepherd
Program in Physiology, The University of Texas Medical School at
Houston, Texas Medical Center, Houston, Texas, U.S.A.

Dr. Charles E. Shields
Blood Research Division, U.S. Army Medical Research Laboratory,
Fort Knox, Kentucky, U.S.A.

Dr. J. C. Shipp
Departments of Biochemistry and Medicine, University of Nebraska
College of Medicine, Omaha, Nebraska, U.S.A.

Dr. S. E. Shumate, II
Department of Chemical Engineering, University of Tennessee,
Knoxville, Tennessee, U.S.A.

Dr. John S. Sierocki
Department of Biochemistry, Temple University School of Dentistry,
Philadelphia, Pennsylvania, U.S.A.

Dr. Ian A. Silver
Department of Pathology, Medical School, Bristol BS8 T.T.D. England

Dr. Marian Silver
Physiological Laboratory, Cambridge CB2 3 EG, Cambridge, England

Dr. Ekkehardt Sinagowitz
Department of Pediatrics, University of Miami School of Medicine,
Miami, Florida, U.S.A.

Dr. Durwood J. Smith
Department of Pharmacology, Given Medical Building, The University
of Vermont College of Medicine, Burlington, Vermont, U.S.A.

Professor Kenneth A. Smith
Department of Chemical Engineering, Massachusetts Institute of
Technology, Cambridge, Massachusetts, U.S.A.

Dr. W. Don Smith
Department of Biomedical Engineering, Duke University, Durham,
North Carolina, U.S.A.

Dr. S. H. Song
Department of Biophysics, University of Western Ontario, London,
Ontario, Canada

Dr. R. Soto
Department of Environmental Medicine, Medical College of Wisconsin,
Milwaukee, Wisconsin, U.S.A.

Dr. E.-J. Speckmann
Physiologisches Institut der Universität, Münster/Westf.,West Germany

Dr. Donald R. Sperling
Department of Pediatrics, University of California, Irvine,
California, U.S.A.

Dr. Hilde Starlinger
Max-Planck-Instut für Systemphysiologie, Dortmund, West Germany

Dr. Richard R. Stewart
Department of Chemical Engineering, College of Engineering, Northeastern University, Boston, Massachusetts, U.S.A.

Dr. Jose Strauss
Department of Pediatrics, University of Miami Medical School,
Miami, Florida, U.S.A.

Dr. R. Strehlau
Max-Planck-Institut für Systemphysiologie, Dortmund, West Germany

Dr. Shyam R. Suchdeo
Department of Chemical Engineering, University of Michigan, Ann
Arbor, Michigan, U.S.A.

Dr. T. Sugano
Johnson Research Foundation, Department of Biophysics and Physical
Biochemistry, University of Pennsylvania, Philadelphia, Pennsylvania,
U.S.A.

Dr. Ludger Sunder-Plassmann
Institute of Surgical Research, University of Munich, Munich, West
Germany

Dr. Avron Y. Sweet
Department of Pediatrics and the Perinatal Clinical Research Center,
Case Western Reserve University at Cleveland Metropolitan General
Hospital, Cleveland, Ohio, U.S.A.

Dr. Ronald C. Tai
Department of Civil Engineering, State University of New York at
Buffalo, Buffalo, New York, U.S.A.

Mrs. Yasar Tanrikut
Department of Chemical Engineering, University of Florida,
Gainesville, Florida, U.S.A.

Dr. Paul M. Taylor
Department of Pediatrics, Magee-Womens Hospital, University of
Pittsburgh School of Medicine, Pittsburgh, Pennsylvania, U.S.A.

Dr. W. J. Taylor
Department of Medicine, Division of Cardiology, University of
Florida, Gainesville, Florida, U.S.A.

Dr. Hiroshi Tazawa
Research Institute of Applied Electricity, Hokkaido University
Sapporo, Japan

Dr. R. S. Tepper
Department of Physiology, University of Wisconsin, Madison,
Wisconsin, U.S.A.

Dr. M. Thermann
Chirurgische Universitäts-Klinik und Poliklinik, Marburg (Lahn),
West Germany

Dr. Gerhard Thews
Physiologisches Institut der Universität Mainz, Mainz, West Germany

Dr. Volker Thiemann
Physiologisches Institut der Universität Kiel, Kiel, West Germany

Dr. U. Tlolka
Max-Planck-Institut für Systemphysiologie, Dortmund, West Germany

Dr. Harvey Tritel
Department of Medicine, Division of Cardiology, University of Florida,
Gainesville, Florida, U.S.A.

Dr. Hugh D. Van Liew
Department of Physiology, State University of New York at Buffalo,
Buffalo, New York, U.S.A.

Dr. D. Varga
Gordon Craig Research Laboratory, Department of Surgery, University
of Sydney, Sydney, N.S.W., Australia

Dr. Peter Vaupel
Physiologisches Institut der Universität Johannes Gutenberg, Mainz,
West Germany

Dr. Waltraud Wahler
Physiologisches Insititut der Universität Mainz, Mainz, West Germany

Dr. Akio Wakabayashi
Department of Surgery, University of California, Irvine,
California, U.S.A.

Dr. Robert D. Walker, Jr.
Department of Chemical Engineering, University of Florida,
Gainesville, Florida, U.S.A.

Dr. L. M. Webber
Thoracic and Cardiovascular Surgery Department, Veterans Administration Hospital, Los Angeles, California, U.S.A.

Dr. Hartmut Weigelt
Max-Planck-Institut für Systemphysiologie, Dortmund, West Germany

Dr. Richard D. Weisel
Instrumentation Laboratory, Inc., Lexington, Massachusetts, U.S.A.

Professor Dr. Christoph Weiss
Physiologisches Institut der Universität Kiel, Kiel, West Germany

Dr. Harvey R. Weiss
Department of Physiology, College of Medicine and Dentistry of
New Jersey, Rutgers Medical School, Piscataway, New Jersey, U.S.A.

Dr. William J. Whalen
St. Vincent Charity Hospital, 2351 North Broad Street, Philadelphia,
Pennsylvania, U.S.A.

Dr. J. D. Whiffen
Department of Chemical Engineering, University of Wisconsin,
Madison, Wisconsin, U.S.A.

Dr. Mary P. Wiedeman
Temple Medical School, Philadelphia, Pennsylvania, U.S.A.

Professor Dr. Wolfgang Wiemer
Institut für Physiologie, Arbeitsgruppe Regulationsphysiologie der
Rurh-Universität Bochum, Bochum, West Germany

Mr. Gregory John Wilson
125 Forest Avenue, Apt. 601, Hamilton, Ontario, Canada

Dr. P. David Wilson
Center for Study of Trauma, University of Maryland Medical School,
22 South Greene Street, Baltimore, Maryland, U.S.A.

Dr. Eugene H. Wissler
College of Engineering, University of Texas at Austin, Austin,
Texas, U.S.A.

Dr. Dr. Reinhard Wodick
Max-Planck-Institut für Systemphysiologie, Dortmund, West Germany

Dr. Dabney R. Yarbrough, III
Department of Surgery, Medical University of South Carolina,
Charleston, South Carolina, U.S.A.

Dr. Histaka Yasui
Defence and Civil Institute of Environmental Medicine, Toronto,
Ontario, Canada

Dr. Angelo Zegna
U.S. Army Medical Research Laboratory, Fort Knox, Kentucky, U.S.A.

Dr. O. Zelder
Laboratory for Cytology and Histology, R. K. University, Nijmegen,
Netherlands

DISCUSSION PARTICIPANTS

Dr. C. P. Boyan
Department of Anesthesiology, Medical College of Virginia, 1200
Broad Street, Richmond, Virginia, U.S.A.

Dr. Justin Clark
Biophysics Research, Primary Children's Hospital, Salt Lake City,
Utah, U.S.A.

Dr. Vin Cuiryla
Department of Chemical Engineering, Northwestern University,
Evanston, Illinois, U.S.A.

Dr. R. W. Flower
8621 Georgia Avenue, Silver Spring, Maryland, U.S.A.

Dr. William J. Gibson
Department of Surgery, Royal Alexandra Hospital, Edmonton,
Alberta, Canada

Dr. A. S. Iberall
General Technical Services, Inc., 8794 West Chester Pike, Upper
Darby, Pennsylvania, U.S.A.

Dr. Goran Kolmodin
Department of Neurology, Karolinska Sjunkhuset, Stockholm, Sweden

Professor Arisztide Kovach
Experimentelles Forschungs-laboratorium der Med., Universität,
Budapest, Hungary

Dr. Vincent B. Murthy
Department of Radiology, University Medical Center, University of
Missouri, Columbia, Missouri, U.S.A.

Dr. Edwin M. Nemoto
Department of Anesthesiology, University of Pittsburgh Medical
School, Pittsburgh, Pennsylvania, U.S.A.

Dr. Paul A. Nicoll
Bloomington, Indiana, U.S.A.

Dr. David H. Pearce
Department of Physiology, University of Mississippi Medical Center,
Jackson, Mississippi, U.S.A.

Dr. H. W. Puffer
Box 599, 1200 N. State Street, Los Angeles, California, U.S.A.

Dr. Karel Rakusan
Department of Physiology, Faculty of Medicine, University of Ottawa,
Ottawa, Canada

Dr. Andrew Zielinski
Bloomfield, Michigan, U.S.A.

CONTENTS OF VOLUME 1   (VOLUME 37A)

Contents of Volume 2 xlv

Welcome! 1
  Melvin H. Knisely

Session I - INSTRUMENTATION AND METHODS

The Oxygen Micro-Electrode 7
  I. A. Silver

Intracellular Oxygen Microelectrodes 17
  William J. Whalen

Standardization of Producing Needle Electrodes 23
  E. Sinagowitz and M. Kessler

High Speed Pulsatile Operation of Miniature
        Oxygen Electrodes . . . . , ... 29
  Stanley H. Saulson

Absolute PO$_2$-Measurements with Pt-Electrodes
        Applying Polarizing Voltage Pulsing 35
  K. Kunze and D. W. Lübbers

Spectrophotometric Examination of Tissue
        Oxygenation 45
  D. W. Lübbers

A New Histochemical Stain for Intracellular
        Oxygen 55
  I. S. Longmuir and J. A. Knopp

Analysis of Gas Transport in Lungless and
        Gill-less Salamanders Using Inert
        Gas Washout Techniques   59
    Randall Neal Gatz and Johannes Piiper

Measurement of Tissue Gas Levels with a Mass
        Spectrometer   67
    William E. Donovan and Bert Myers

Analysis of Diffusion Limitations on a
        Catheter Imbedded in Body Tissues   73
    Robert D. Walker, Jr. and Yasar Tanrikut

Dual Wavelength Micro-oximeter of Hamster Whole
        Blood In Vitro   83
    Herbert J. Berman, Stuart J. Segall, and
    Robert L. Fuhro

P50 Determinations: Techniques and Clinical
        Importance   93
    K. D. Fallon, A. L. Malenfant, R. D. Weisel,
    and H. B. Hechtman

Catheterizable Absolute Photometer   99
    B. Rybak

Clinical Use of a New Intra-arterial Catheter
        Electrode System   107
    Haim I. Bicher, Joseph W. Rubin, and
    Robert J. Adams

Problems of Transcutaneous Measurement of
        Arterial Blood Gases   115
    D. W. Lübbers, R. Huch, and A. Huch

Flow Limited Properties of Teflon and Silicone
        Diffusion Membranes   121
    D. Nelson, L. Ostrander, E. Ernst, and
    W. Baetz

Differential Anodic Enzyme Polarography for the
        Measurement of Glucose   127
    Leland C. Clark, Jr. and Eleanor W. Clark

Problems Involved in the Measurement of
        Microcirculation by Means of
        Microelectrodes   135
    H. Hutten, M. Kessler, and M. Thermann

Discussion of Session I   141

Session II - PHYSIOLOGY OF OXYGEN TRANSPORT TO TISSUE

Subsession: D P G

Effect of Plasma Inorganic Phosphate on Tissue
        Oxygenation During Recovery from
        Diabetic Ketoacidosis 163
    Jørn Ditzel

Effects of Reduced 2,3 Diphosphoglycerate on
        Oxygen Release from Blood of Alloxan
        Diabetic Rats: Myocardial Cellular
        Hypoxia 173
    T. B. Allison, S. P. Bruttig, J. C. Shipp,
    R. S. Eliot, and M. F. Crass III

2,3-DPG-Induced Displacements of the Oxyhemoglobin
        Dissociation Curve of Blood: Mechanisms
        and Consequences 179
    Jochen Duhm

Evidence for a Relationship between 2,3-
        Diphosphoglycerate-Depleted Red
        Blood Cells, Slow Oxygen Release and
        Myocardial Ischemia 187
    J. W. Holsinger, Jr., J. M. Salhany, and
    R. S. Eliot

The Oxygen-Affinity of Hemoglobin: Influence of
        Blood Replacement and Hemodilution after
        Cardiac Surgery 193
    F. Jesch, L. M. Webber, J. W. Dalton, and
    J. S. Carey

Analysis of 2,3 Diphosphoglycerate-Mediated,
        Hemoglobin-Facilitated Oxygen
        Transport in Terms of the Adair
        Reaction Mechanism 199
    Jerry H. Meldon, Kenneth A. Smith, and
    Clark K. Colton

Discussion of Subsession: DPG   207

Subsession: Brain

Autoregulation of Oxygen Supply to Brain Tissue
        (Introductory Paper) 215
    Haim I. Bicher

Local PO_2 in Relation to Intracellular pH,
        Cell Membrane Potential and Potassium
        Leakage in Hypoxia and Shock 223
    I. A. Silver

Energy-Rich Metabolites and EEG in Hypoxia
        and in Hypercapnia 233
    Ursula Schindler, E. Gärtner, and E. Betz

A New Long-Term Method for the Measurement of
        NADH Fluorescence in Intact Rat Brain
        with Chronically Implanted Cannula 239
    A. Mayevsky and B. Chance

Actions of Hypoxia and Hypercapnia on Single
        Mammalian Neurons 245
    E.-J. Speckmann, H. Caspers, and D. Bingmann

Response of Feline Brain Tissue to Oscillating
        Arterial pO_2 251
    W. J. Dorson and B. A. Bogue

Changes of Oxygen Supply to the Tissue Following
        Intravenous Application of Anesthetic
        Drugs 261
    Wilhelm Erdmann and Stefan Kunke

Local PO_2 and O_2-Consumption in the Isolated
        Sciatic Nerve 271
    K. Kunze

Basic Principles of Tissue Oxygen Determination
        from Mitochondrial Signals 277
    B. Chance, N. Oshino, T. Sugano, and
    A. Mayevsky

Selective Vulnerability of the Central Nervous
        System to Hyperbaric Oxygen 293
    J. Douglas Balentine

Oxygen Tensions in the Deep Gray Matter of Rats
        Exposed to Hyperbaric Oxygen 299
    Robert W. Ogilvie and J. Douglas Balentine

The Interdependence of Respiratory Gas Values and
        pH as a Function of Base Excess in Human
        Blood at 37°C 305
    Jürgen Grote and Gerhard Thews

Regulatory Dysfunction of Microvasculature
and Catecholamine Metabolism in
Spinal Cord Injury 311
N. Eric Naftchi, Edward W. Lowman,
Maurice Berard, G. Heiner Sell, and
Theobald Reich

The Effect on Cerebral Energy Metabolites
of the Cyanate Produced Shift of
the Oxygen Saturation Curve 319
John Cassel, Kyuya Kogure, Raul Busto,
Chang Yong Kim, and Donald R. Harkness

On the Accuracy of an Improved Method for
the Measurement of O_2-Dissociation-
Curves According to Niesel and
Thews, 1961 325
Wolfgang Barnikol and Waltraud Wahler

Discussion of Subsession: Brain 333

Subsession: Abdominal Organs

Homeostasis of Oxygen Supply in Liver
and Kidney 351
M. Kessler, H. Lang, E. Sinagowitz,
R. Rink, and J. Höper

Tissue PO_2 Levels in the Liver of Warm and
Cold Rats Artificially Respired
with Different Mixtures of O_2 and CO_2 361
James A. Miller, Jr. and Manfred Kessler

Preservation of ATP in the Perfused Liver 371
Jens Höper, Manfred Kessler, and
Hilde Starlinger

Influence of Hemoglobin Concentration in
Perfusate and in Blood on Fluorescence
of Pyridine Nucleotides (NADH and
NADPH) of Rat Liver 377
Herbert Rahmer and Manfred Kessler

Studies of Oxygen Supply of Liver Grafts 383
M. Thermann, O. Zelder, F. Hess,
C. R. Jerusalem, and M. Hamelmann

A Contribution Concerning the Unsettled Problem
of Intrasplenic Microcirculation 389
W. Braunbeck, H. Hutten, and P. Vaupel

The Local Oxygen Supply in Tissue of
          Abdominal Viscera and of Skeletal
          Muscle in Extreme Hemodilution
          with Stromafree Hemoglobin Solution 395
   L. Sunder-Plassmann, E. Sinagowitz, R. Rink,
   R. Dieterle, K. Messmer, and M. Kessler

Respiratory Gas Exchange and pO_2- Distribution
          in Splenic Tissue 401
   P. Vaupel, W. Braunbeck, and G. Thews

Renal Tissue Oxygenation During Pulsatile and
          Nonpulsatile Left Heart Bypass 407
   A. V. Beran, D. R. Sperling, A. Wakabayashi,
   and J. E. Connolly

New Aspects on the Mechanism of Autoregulation
          of Blood Flow 417
   Christoph Weiss and Volker Thiemann

Sympathetic Nervous Control of Intestinal
          O_2 Extraction 423
   A. P. Shepherd, D. Mailman, T. F. Burks,
   and H. J. Granger

Discussion of Subsession: Abdominal Organs 429

                    Subsession: Muscle

Oxygen Autoregulation in Skeletal Muscle 441
   Thomas K. Goldstick

Intrinsic Metabolic Regulation of Blood Flow,
          O_2 Extraction and Tissue O_2 Delivery
          in Dog Skeletal Muscle 451
   Harris J. Granger, Anthony H. Goodman,
   and D. N. Granger

Regional Heterogeneity of P_{CO_2} and P_{O_2}
          in Skeletal Muscle 457
   Hugh D. Van Liew

Discussion of Subsession: Muscle 463

                    Subsession: Shock

Signs of Hypoxia in the Small Intestine of
          the Rat During Hemorrhagic Shock 469
   R. Rink and M. Kessler

Blood and Tissue Oxygenation During
        Hemorrhagic Shock as Determined
        with Ultramicro Oxygen Electrodes 477
  Charles T. Fitts, Haim I. Bicher, and
  Dabney R. Yarbrough III

Local and Whole Organ Renal Oxygenation
        under Hemorrhagic Shock 485
  J. Strauss, R. Baker, A. V. Beran,
  and E. Sinagowitz

Factors Determining Total Body and Hind
        Limb Oxygen Consumption in
        Normal and Shocked Dogs 491
  D. F. J. Halmagyi, J. Leigh, A. H. Goodman,
  and D. Varga

Oxygen Transport Changes after Transfusion
        with Stored Blood in a Hemorrhagic
        Canine Model 499
  C. E. Shields, M. G. Burns, A. Zegna,
  D. Meixner, J. Bratton, D. Brooks,
  L. O'Malley, and G. Phillips

Local Oxygen Supply in Intra-Abdominal Organs
        and in Skeletal Muscle During
        Hemorrhagic Shock 505
  E. Sinagowitz, H. Rahmer, R. Rink,
  L. Görnandt, and M. Kessler

Discussion of Subsession: Shock 513

Subsession: Heart

O_2 and the Number and Arrangement of Coronary
        Capillaries: Effect on Calculated
        Tissue PO_2 519
  Carl R. Honig and Jeannine Bourdeau-Martini

Respiratory Gas Transport in Heart 525
  Jürgen Grote and Gerhard Thews

The Histogram of Local Oxygen Pressure
        (PO_2) in the Dog Myocardium and
        the PO_2 Behavior During Transitory
        Changes of Oxygen Administration 535
  B. Lösse, S. Schuchhardt, N. Niederle,
  and H. Benzing

Simultaneous Measurement of Regional Blood
        Flow and Oxygen Pressure in the
        Dog Myocardium During Coronary
        Occlusion or Hypoxic Hypoxia 541
    H. Benzing, B. Lösse, S. Schuchhardt,
    and N. Niederle

Mass Spectrometry for Measuring Changes in
        Intramyocardial pO_2 and pCO_2 547
    G. J. Wilson, D. C. MacGregor,
    D. E. Holness, W. Lixfeld, and H. Yasui

Effect of Increasing Heart Rate by Atrial
        Pacing on Myocardial Tissue Oxygen
        Tension 553
    Harvey R. Weiss

Oxygen Consumption and Convective Transport
        During Cardio-pulmonary Bypass 561
    R. E. Safford, J. D. Whiffen, E. N. Lightfoot,
    R. S. Tepper, and J. H. G. Rankin

Red Cell Washout from the Coronary Vessels of
        Isolated Feline Hearts 567
    S. H. Song

Mean Myoglobin Oxygen Tension in Skeletal
        and Cardiac Muscle 571
    R. F. Coburn

Discussion of Subsession: Heart 579

        Subsession: Vascular Chemoreceptors and
                     Oxygen Barrier

Microvascular Diameter Changes During Local
        Blood Flow Regulation: Independence
        of Changes in PO_2 591
    Brian R. Duling

Activity of Chemoreceptor Fibers in the Sinus
        Nerve and Tissue PO_2 in the Carotid
        Body of the Cat 597
    D. Bingmann, H. Acker, and H. Schulze

Role of the Carotid Chemoreflexes in the
        Regulation of Arterial Oxygen
        Pressure 603
    Heidrun Schöne, Wolfgang Wiemer, and
    Peter Kiwull

The Oxygen Barrier in the Carotid Body of
        Cat and Rabbit   609
    H. Acker, D. W. Lübbers, H. Weigelt,
    D. Bingmann, D. Schäfer, and E. Seidl

Role of the Carotid Chemoreceptors in the
        Adjustment of Arterial Blood
        Pressure to Hypoxia   617
    Wolfgang Wiemer, Heidrun Schöne, and
    Peter Kiwull

Discussion of Subsession: Vascular
        Chemoreceptors and Oxygen Barrier   623

Summary - Sessions I and II   627
    I. A. Silver

General Discussion of Session II   631

CONTENTS OF VOLUME 2   (VOLUME 37B)

Contents of Volume 1 xix

Session III - THE PHARMACOLOGY OF IMPROVING

OXYGEN TRANSPORT TO TISSUE

Blood Cell Aggregation and Pulmonary
        Embolism 637
  John W. Irwin

Sludged Blood, Human Disease and Chemotherapy 641
  Edward H. Bloch

Intravascular Aggregation of Blood Cells
        and Tissue Metabolic Defects 647
  Lars-Erik Gelin

Anti-Adhesive Drugs and Tissue Oxygenation 657
  H. I. Bicher, D. F. Bruley, and
  M. H. Knisely

Oxygen Transport and Tissue Oxygenation
        During Hemodilution with Dextran 669
  K. Messmer, L. Görnandt, F. Jesch,
  E. Sinagowitz, L. Sunder-Plassmann,
  and M. Kessler

Platelet Aggregates Induced by Red Blood
        Cell Injury 681
  Mary P. Wiedeman

Recent Advances in the Preparation and Use
        of Perfluorodecalin Emulsions for
        Tissue Perfusion 687
  Leland C. Clark, Jr., Samuel Kaplan,
  Fernando Becattini, and Virginia Obrock

Pharmacological Stimulation of Red Blood Cell
        Metabolism for High Altitude
        Preadaptation 693
    Lorna Grindlay Moore, George J. Brewer,
    Fred J. Oelshlegel, Jr., and Andrew M. Rose

Catecholamine Metabolism and Digital
        Circulation after Histamine
        and Its Analogue 699
    Nosrat Eric Naftchi, Milton Mendlowitz,
    Stefan Racoceanu, and Edward W. Lowman

Augmentation of Tissue Oxygen by Dimethyl
        Sulfoxide and Hydrogen Peroxide 713
    Bert Myers and William Donovan

In Vitro Respiration of Ischemic Skin from
        Amputated Human Legs 717
    John S. Sierocki, Theodore Rosett,
    Raymond Penneys, and Douglas J. Pappajohn

Altering Diffusion Rates 729
    John L. Gainer and Guy M. Chisolm III

Discussion of Session III 733

Session IV - MATHEMATICAL STUDIES OF TISSUE OXYGENATION

PART A

Mathematical Considerations for Oxygen
        Transport to Tissue: Introductory Paper 749
    Duane F. Bruley

Geometric Considerations in Modeling
        Oxygen Transport Processes
        in Tissue 761
    Hermann Metzger

Capillary-Tissue Exchange Kinetics:
        Diffusional Interactions between
        Adjacent Capillaries 773
    Carl A. Goresky and Harry L. Goldsmith

Computer Calculation for Tissue Oxygenation and
        the Meaningful Presentation of the
        Results 783
    W. Grunewald

Stochastic versus Deterministic Models
        of Oxygen Transport in the
        Tissue 793
    R. Wodick

Existing Anatomical Parameters and
        the Need for Further Determinations
        for Various Tissue Structures 803
    Isabel Lockard

Mathematical Analysis of Oxygen Transport
        to Tissue in the Human 813
    Eugene H. Wissler

A Mathematical Model of the Unsteady
        Transport of Oxygen to
        Tissues in the Microcirculation 819
    John E. Fletcher

Simplifying the Description of Tissue
        Oxygenation 827
    E. N. Lightfoot

A Simplified Model of the Oxygen
        Supply Function of Capillary
        Blood Flow 835
    William A. Hyman

Oxygen Transport in the Human Brain -
        Analytical Solutions 843
    Richard R. Stewart and Catherine A. Morrazzi

Calculation of Concentration Profiles of
        Excess Acid in Human Brain Tissue
        During Conditions of Partial
        Anoxia 849
    Daniel D. Reneau and Larry L. Lafitte

Simulating Myocardium Oxygen Dynamics 859
    Duane F. Bruley, Daniel H. Hunt,
    Haim I. Bicher, and Melvin H. Knisely

Numerical Solutions of Blood Flow in the
        Entrance of a Tube 867
    V. L. Shah and R. Soto

Discussion of Session IV -
        Part A 873

Session IV - MATHEMATICAL STUDIES OF TISSUE OXYGENATION

PART B

Distributed Model Solution Techniques
        for Capillary-Tissue Systems 887
    Daniel H. Hunt, Duane F. Bruley,
    Haim I. Bicher, and Melvin H. Knisely

Heterogeneous Models of Oxygen Transport
        in Tissue Slices 891
    Ronald C. Tai and Hsin-kang Chang

Mathematical Modelling of the Cornea and
        an Experimental Application 897
    Ernest L. Roetman and Ronald E. Barr

Instrumentation and Control Techniques
        for Dynamic Response Experiments
        in Living Tissue 903
    B. A. Bogue and W. J. Dorson, Jr.

Oxygen Transport in Skeletal Muscle: How
        Many Blood Capillaries Surround
        Each Fibre? 911
    A. C. Groom and M. J. Plyley

Filtering and Prediction of Blood Flow
        and Oxygen Consumption for
        Patient Monitoring 917
    P. David Wilson

Computer Analysis of Automatically Recorded
        Oxygen Dissociation Curves 923
    Bruce F. Cameron

A Polygonal Approximation for Unsteady State
        Diffusion of Oxygen into Hemoglobin
        Solutions 929
    R. L. Curl and J. S. Schultz

Gaseous Transport in Hemoglobin Solutions 937
    George C. Frazier and S. E. Shumate II

Mechanochemical Pumping as an Adjunct to Diffusion
        in Oxygen Transport 945
    H. G. Clark and W. D. Smith

An Analysis of the Competitive Diffusion
        of O_2 and CO through Hemoglobin
        Solutions 951
   S. R. Suchdeo, J. D. Goddard, and
   J. S. Schultz

Oxygen Mass Transfer Rates in Intact
        Red Blood Cells 963
   B. H. Chang, M. Fleischman, and
   C. E. Miller

Effect of Carbonic Anhydrase on the
        Facilitated Diffusion of CO_2
        through Bicarbonate Solutions 969
   Shyam Suchdeo and Jerome S. Schultz

Modeling the Coronary Circulation:
        Implications in the Pathogenesis
        of Sudden Death 975
   R. J. Gordon, W. Jape Taylor, and
   Harvey Tritel

Discussion of Session IV -
        Part B 983

Session V - OXYGEN TRANSPORT PROBLEMS IN NEONATOLOGY

Subsession: *Placental Oxygen Transfer*

Experimental and Theoretical Investigations
        of Oxygen Transport Problems in
        Fetal Systems: Introductory Paper 995
   Daniel D. Reneau

Microphotometry for Determining the
        Reaction Rate of O_2 and CO
        with Red Blood Cells in the
        Chorioallantoic Capillary 997
   Masaji Mochizuki, Hiroshi Tazawa, and
   Tsukasa Ono

Mathematical Analysis of Combined
        Placental-Fetal Oxygen
        Transport 1007
   Eric J. Guilbeau and Daniel D. Reneau

Placental Function and Oxygenation in
        the Fetus 1017
   Waldemar Moll

Morphological Determinants in O_2-Transfer
  across the Human and Rhesus
  Hemochorial Placenta 1027
  Uwe E. Freese

Umbilical and Uterine Venous PO_2 in
  Different Species During
  Late Gestation and Parturition 1041
  M. Silver and R. S. Comline

Threshold Values of Oxygen Deficiency
  Leading to Cardiovascular
  and Brain Pathological Changes
  in Term Monkey Fetuses 1047
  Ronald E. Myers

Placental Oxygen Gradients Due to
  Diffusion and Chemical Reaction 1055
  Robert A. B. Holland

Experimental Models for in vivo and
  in vitro Investigations on
  Placental Hemodynamics and
  Oxygen Supply to the Fetus 1061
  Maurice Panigel

Material Alkalosis and Fetal Oxygenation 1067
  John H. G. Rankin

Hemoglobin Concentration Overestimates
  Oxygen Carrying Capacity
  During Favic Crises 1075
  P. M. Taylor, L. G. Morphis, and
  K. Mandalenaki

Discussion of Subsession: Placental
  Oxygen Transfer 1083

Subsession: Oxygen Monitoring

Measurement of Oxygen in the Newborn 1089
  Jose Strauss, Anthony V. Beran,
  and Rex Baker

Oxygen Monitoring of Newborns by Skin
  Electrodes. Correlation
  between Arterial and Cutaneously
  Determined pO_2 1097
  Patrick Eberhard, Wolfgang Mindt,
  Franz Jann, and Konrad Hammacher

A Unique Electrode Catheter for Continuous
        Monitoring of Arterial Blood
        Oxygen Tension in Newborn Infants 1103
    Edwin G. Brown, Chung C. Liu,
    Francis E. McDonnell, Michael R. Neuman,
    and Avron Y. Sweet

Laboratory and Clinical Evaluation of a New
        Indwelling Oxygen Electrode for
        Continuous Monitoring of PaO_2 in
        Neonates 1109
    Thomas R. Harris and Michael Nugent

Continuous Intravascular PO_2 Measurements
        with Catheter and Cannula
        Electrodes in Newborn Infants,
        Adults and Animals 1113
    Albert Huch, Dietrich W. Lübbers, and
    Renate Huch

Routine Monitoring of the Arterial PO_2 of
        Newborn Infants by Continuous
        Registration of Transcutaneous
        PO_2 and Simultaneous Control of
        Relative Local Perfusion 1121
    Renate Huch, Dietrich W. Lübbers, and
    Albert Huch

Clinical Experiences with Clamp Electrodes
        in Fetal Scalp for Simultaneous
        pO_2 and ECG - Registration 1129
    W. Erdmann, S. Kunke, J. Heidenreich,
    W. Dempsey, H. Günther, and H. Schäfer

Discussion of Subsession: Oxygen Monitoring 1135

General Discussion of Session V 1137

Index 1145

WELCOME!

DR. MELVIN H. KNISELY

Ladies and Gentlemen:

It is a privilege to welcome you here in Charleston at the
beginning of this International Symposium on Oxygen Transport to
Tissue. It is a privilege to welcome you in the names of two great
cooperating universities, located more than 200 miles apart, Clemson
University and the Medical University of South Carolina. Permit
me to welcome you in the names of President Edwards of Clemson and
President McCord of the Medical University. The continuing strong
friendship of these two men for each other and the support of both
for studies of the limitations of the rates of oxygen supply to
tissues has been a major factor in making this symposium both
intellectually and economically possible.

Each of us comes to a conference with certain hopes, plans and
aspirations; to learn and to teach, and to gain new insights and
viewpoints on his own work and to perceive new directions for
investigation as they are opening up. It has been my privilege to
attend symposia and conferences in the general fields of anatomy,
physiology, pathologic physiology and clinical studies since 1935.
And, in addition to the purposes of conferences which are immediately obvious, I should like to point out that one of the tremendous
opportunities of every conference is the chance to make new, per —
sonal, lifelong friends. A young girl once defined a stranger as,
"A person I have not had time to become friends with yet." Sometimes persons see individuals with whom they come in scientific
conflict as potential enemies, but, as Professor R. R. Bensley once
said to Professor Mathews, the biochemist, "The fact that currently
we disagree over the details of this specific problem need not, of
course, in any way interfere with our lifelong friendship." Following Bensley's wisdom, we must see that most disagreements are
temporary. In looking over this audience, I am enjoying seeing the

faces of a great many persons from several countries, with whom I
have enjoyed very long-lasting friendships. Participants in this
symposium have come from many countries, clearly illustrating the
old, wise statement that: "Wherever mankind is loved, medicine will
always be studied." In welcoming you here, I now strongly hope and
urge that each and every one of you becomes as good friends with
each other as so many of those here have become with me. It is
particularly important that we enjoy our friendships and upon them
now, build strengthening bonds of mutual trust. This is essential
in a world in which so many different individuals and groups seem
devoted to developing paranoid fears and animosities. And so, in
welcoming you, I bid you not to forget that probably one of the
major accomplishments of this conference can be and should be the
cementing of all old friendships and the development of many new,
strong, lifelong friendships.

Let us pause a moment to remember and honor some of our
intellectual ancestors: William Harvey; Leeuwenhoek, who first
saw blood cells; Malpighi, who first saw living capillaries con-
ducting blood from arterioles to venules; Claude Bernard; Paul Bert;
Christian Bohr, of the "Bohr effect" and his great student, August
Krogh; Sir Joseph Barcroft; Nisimaru of Japan, a student of Barcroft;
J. B. S. Haldane; Cecil Drinker, for his studies of the lung and of
carbon monoxide poisoning; the neuropathologist, Cyril Courville (for
his classic book Cerebral Anoxia, 1953); and, of course, Opitz and
Schneider. Each of you will think of important men I have left out.
As we all know, the classic 1950 study by Opitz and Schneider set
the necessary stage for the further analysis of many processes of
normal and pathologic physiology. Less known, but I am told true,
is the fact that Gerhard Thews, at that time a young man, partici-
pated in and carried out the calculations for the Opitz and Schneider
1950 publication, and he did it "by hand," that is, without computers, a truly monumental undertaking. On this basis, if no other,
Thews must be considered one of our intellectual ancestors as well
as one of our contemporaries.

The studies leading toward understanding the limitations on
the oxygen supply to tissues, pioneered by our ancestors, have
blossomed, indeed, exploded in many directions, and as you can see,
contemporary leaders in the fields of study thereby opened up, are
now here all around us. A few, listed alphabetically, are: Duane
Bruley, Britton Chance, Leland Clark, Lars-Erik Gelin, Wolfgang
Grunewald, Carl Honig, Dietrich Lübbers, Masaji Mochizuke, Ian
Silver, Bill Whalen, and, as you well know, there are many others.
Further, undoubtedly, many new leaders in old and new directions
of study will identify themselves by their work in this symposium
as the conference progresses.

I should like to say a word in honor of colleagues who, because of pressing duties, cannot be here: Gerhard Thews, Chernukh of Russia, Harold Wayland of Cal. Tech., and my old friend Harald Harders, one of the best educated, most thoughtful and wisest of physicians, who is a product of, and who lives in Germany.

Why do we have this conference? What does it mean for the citizens of our respective countries, the people who pay their taxes and thereby support our separate studies and this combined meeting? This meeting aims in the long run at intensely practical results. Oxygen, which we breathe in through our noses, is absolutely necessary for many different, specific, chemical reactions which must take place inside of individual cells in different tissues and organs all over the body. Oxygen is necessary in order that many specific enzymatic reactions can take place. For example, Bauer and Lazarow, in 1961, found that oxygen is necessary during and for the synthesis of insulin by the beta cells of the pancreas. Oxygen is necessary for nerve cells to keep them firing and to keep them alive. Oxygen must come to mitochondria, which are inside tissue cells, if these mitochondria are to provide energy for cellular physiologic processes.

Many problems of medicine have been solved, and as a consequence, practicing physicians know how to treat many diseases successfully. However, we must recognize that many untreatable conditions remain. Among those not successfully treatable today are many cases of mental retardation, neurologic deficits, some of the endocrine deficiencies, many types of mental disease, and the inactivation or disintegration of parts of the nervous system, which are sometimes listed as "processes of aging," but which must clearly be described as inactivations and destructions of bits and pieces of the nervous system often by way of unknown causes during the passage of time. (The passage of time itself certainly is not a causative agent.) Incalculable amounts of money are now being spent supporting hospitals and other institutions in which patients in the above categories are receiving custodial care with but very little and often no successful treatment. According to Gorman, 1956, one half of all the hospital beds in the United States are permanently occupied by mental patients. As soon as one mental patient leaves, another takes his place. The total cash costs of all these items can hardly be estimated. Every country is burdened by continuing cash costs because of the above untreatable conditions.

Because oxygen is so necessary and must be delivered to specific points in the anatomy of the body at adequate rates, it now appears highly probable that studies of the factors which, cooper-

ating, guarantee, during health, adequate rates of oxygen delivery,
together with corresponding or correlative studies of factors of
disease and of toxic states which can and do interfere with, or
block, oxygen delivery to specific anatomic points, such studies
will open new understandings of what goes wrong and how to prevent
major classes of interferences with body functions, and damages to
the human body.

Keep in mind the problems related to the factors which initiate:
mental retardation, neurological deficits, endocrine deficiencies,
mental disease, the psychoses (among these, the post-partum
psychoses, the post-operative psychoses and the post-alcohol
psychoses) and senile dementia, in which latter condition cortical
nerve cell bodies in great numbers have been lost. These are some
of the clinical targets toward which our basic science studies are
aimed. Note that many clinicians participate in these basic science
studies. Clinical successes are like the tops of icebergs which
stick up above the surface of the water while enormous masses of
inconspicuous basic science studies under them support them and
keep their clinically-successful heads above water.

We have come together to share our wisdom, assumptions, both
recognized and unrecognized knowledge, mathematical and experimental
methods; and batches of data relating to basic science factors which
together determine the limitations on the rates of supply of oxygen
to tissue cells located in specific anatomic positions under three
specific conditions : during the physiology of maximal good health,
during reversible pathologic physiology and during non-reversible
pathology.

In summation, welcome to Charleston and Clemson. Welcome to
good science, good friendship, and the confident hope and expecta-
tion that the work we are doing is and will be of fundamental
importance to the health of human beings all over the world.

Session I

INSTRUMENTATION AND METHODS

Chairmen: Dr. Dietrich W. Lübbers, Dr. Leland C. Clark, Jr. and

Dr. William J. Whalen

THE OXYGEN MICRO-ELECTRODE

I.A. Silver

Department of Pathology

University of Bristol, England

The reduction of oxygen in a watery solution at a noble metal surface by a low voltage was first observed by Danneel in Nernst's laboratory in 1897. The application of this technique for biological purposes was instigated by Blinks and Skow (1938) in suspensions of plant cells and was developed for use in mammalian tissues by Davies and Brink (1942). These latter authors made a variety of electrodes which included small electrodes of 25 μm platinum wire enclosed in glass insulation which protruded a short distance beyond the end of the platinum. They called these 'recessed' micro-electrodes and successfully used them for measuring oxygen gradients on the surface of the brain of the cat. This type of electrode corresponded in its behaviour to the law of classical linear diffusion during its initial polarisation and was able to take its oxygen from very small regions. The disadvantage of this system was that the recess of the electrode was relatively long and readings could only be made at intervals of many minutes. However the readings that were obtained had real meaning and indicated that contrary to established physiological thinking at that time there were steep gradients of oxygen tension in organs such as brain, and that there were points even on the brain surface where the PO_2 was as low as 2 mm Hg. For more than a decade after Davies and Brink's work, little progress was made in the development of micro-electrodes other than that of Davies and Rémond (1947) who produced an antimony in glass probe of 14 μm diameter. However work was done by pioneers in the clinical field such as Montgomery and Horwitz (1950) with large oxygen

electrodes. The major problems with these were (a) that
they caused obvious tissue damage and (b) they were almost
impossible to calibrate, although among others, Cater and
his colleagues (1957; 1959) attempted to calibrate large
electrodes but were unsatisfied with the results. In an
effort to improve the resolution of open electrodes and to
examine oxygen environments at the cellular level they
first made a 10 µm platinum-in-glass electrode (Cater et
al. 1959) and then they constructed a probe based on the
micro-electrodes then being used for recording from single
nerve cells. This electrode was a stainless steel needle
electro-polished to a tip of approximately 1 µm, which was
then electroplated with a noble metal, either platinum,
rhodium or gold. The insulation was of Araldite 985E, and
the performance was significantly better than had been expected. Cater and Silver (1961) were able to show that
microelectrodes of this type when covered with a nitrocellulose membrane could be calibrated and would maintain
their calibration in a variety of fluids and tissues, and
provided that they were small enough, they were almost unaffected by stirring artefacts. A problem that was still
encountered with these electrodes was that of protein deposition by electrophoresis and also poisoning of the surface by sulphydryl compounds which particularly affected
platinum. An unsatisfactory feature of the plated needle
electrode was the frequent presence of micro-pores in the
plating which produced small galvanic cells. In 1956
Clark showed that the application of an oxygen diffusion
barrier over large electrodes eliminated many of the problems which had bedevilled the early development of absolute reading oxygen cathodes. Silver (1965) combined the
features of the platinum-in-glass microelectrode with
those of the 'Clark' electrode and produced an absolute
reading micro-probe which could be inserted into soft tissue or could be used for surface measurements. The platinum-in-glass microelectrode was further developed by Kunze
(1966; 1969) as a double probe system and he also applied
pulsed polarizing voltages to microelectrodes, a method he
had introduced previously (Kunze, 1965) for larger probes.
A slightly more robust form of the platinum-iridium-in-
glass electrode emerged from Lübbers' laboratory (Lübbers
and Baumgärtl, 1967).

     Another type of microelectrode is that described by
Whalen, Riley and Nair (1967) which is in direct line of
descent from the recessed electrode of Davies and Brink
(1942) and the metal-filled glass microelectrode of Davies
and Rémond (1947). This electrode consists of a metal-
filled micropipette in which the glass envelope protrudes

slightly beyond the end of the metal. The depth of the
recess can be adjusted by plating more or less gold onto the metal filling.   The external diameter of this
probe can be as small as 2 μm which allows it to be inserted into large cells (Whalen and Nair, 1967;   1970).
This electrode has the advantage over the open needle
that the recess can be filled with some kind of diffusion
barrier which prevents the deposition of protein and which
greatly reduces the accessibility of the catalytic surface
to sulphydryl compounds.   The disadvantage is that, at
least theoretically, its response time should be considerably longer than that of an open electrode.

      The wide availability of apparatus for evaporation
or 'sputtering' of metallic films onto glass surfaces has
led to the manufacture of glass micropipettes with platinum 'shielding' to reduce 'pick up' during bioelectrical
recording. When adequate external insulation is added to
such pipettes while the tip is left bare another type of
O_2 microelectrode is obtained which has the advantage of
an "internal" reference and is therefore particularly
suitable for intracellular work (Bicher and Knisely,
1970).   Electrodes of this design can be made with an
extremely small catalytic area and can be ground to an
oblique point on a diamond dust wheel by the same technique as that developed by Whalen and Nair (1967) for
putting points on their probes.   The major disadvantage
of the 'platinum-on-glass' electrode is the uncertain
insulating quality of the resins which are available to
form the outer coat of the probe.   One other problem,
common to all intracellular reference systems, is the
very high impedance of the column of electrolyte between
the reference Ag/Ag Cl wire and the platinised area, which
is an important consideration when designing the recording
system for such a probe.

      Multiple arrays of microoxygen electrodes have been
developed notably by Erdmann, Kunke and Krell (1973).

                        Technical Problems

      The essential features of a microelectrode are
1) a very small and chemically stable area for active reduction of oxygen and 2) a shape which introduces minimal
distortion to the tissue into which it is inserted.   There
seems little correlation between the performance of an
electrode in tissue and the shape of its current-voltage
plateau.   A persistent problem with micro-electrodes is
the hydration of the insulating material near the tip.

The most effective insulation is glass although many of
the platinum compatible glasses are of rather poor insulating quality.   Application of silicone to the surface
of the glass insulator reduces the hydration effect considerably.   The most successful preparation that we have
found is dimethyldichlorosilane applied as a vapour.   This
substance is also useful for coating intra-cellular electrodes since it enables the lipoid membrane of a cell to
seal very effectively against glass.   Another useful feature of this process is that it produces a surface on the
platinum which does not prevent oxygen reduction but which
considerably reduces protein deposition and sulphydryl
poisoning.   However even with silicone treatment the very
thin glass at the tip of the electrode eventually hydrates
and the electrode becomes unstable.   The zero currents of
oxygen electrodes are still the subject of some controversy.   Very clean electrodes which have been carefully
made, give very low currents in pure nitrogen and it is an
indication of poor electrode technique if zero currents
are high.   The commonest causes of these currents are leak-
ages in or along the insulation and contamination of the
catalytic surface.   Protein and sulphydryl contamination
remain a problem but the development of more effective
membranes should overcome this.

                          Biological Problems

     Any probe, however small, will excite an inflammatory
reaction and a foreign body response in living tissue.
This reaction will inevitably alter the local environment
(Silver, 1973) and is a serious problem when long term
observations are to be made.   Construction of microelectrodes with non-irritant smooth surfaces minimises but
does not eliminate tissue response.   The problem is
greatest in moving and highly vascularised tissue such as
heart, where mechanical irritation is continuous if the
electrode tip moves in relation to the tissue and causes
microdamage to cells and capillaries.   Various ingenious
floating electrodes have been used to overcome this but
damage during insertion is still a difficulty.   Zeuthen
and Silver (unpublished) have used a 'dart' electrode
weighing less than 3 mg inserted with a blow pipe, but
even with this, there is still evidence of cell damage
near the electrode tip.   The mechanical conditions are
especially difficult for intracellular electrodes, although Whalen et al. (1973) appear to have overcome
them.

   Intracellular electrodes must be very small in
relation to the cell in which they lie; the cell membrane must seal to the electrode surface and the polarizing voltage on the electrode must not disturb the cell
membrane potential. It is usually considered that electrodes larger than 1 μm diameter are unsuitable for intracellular work and that an intracellular reference
electrode is necessary to avoid membrane damage. Because
of the rather poor current-voltage plateau on most microelectrodes, it should be remembered that small changes of
D.C. bioelectric potential may appear as false changes of
oxygen current on the recording. Measurement of D.C.
shifts is therefore necessary as a control and great care
must be exercised with irritable tissue such as brain or
muscle so that the electrode does not cause increased or
decreased bioelectric activity, and especially that it
does not interfere with the 'sodium pump' mechanism.
Pulsed polarising systems give rise to special problems
in relation to membrane irritability.

   The question of whether a simple needle electrode
can be used with a reasonable degree of assurance was investigated by Silver (1965) who constructed an ultramicro Clark-type electrode with a maximum tip diameter
including membrane of approximately 3 μm and he was able
to show that this electrode (a) gave absolute readings of
PO_2 in fluid and in tissue and (b) that recordings made
with it were not significantly different from those obtained with 1 μm membrane-covered platinum-iridium probes
which did not have the elaborate second coating required
for a Clark-type electrode. A more critical method for
evaluating oxygen tension by a totally independent method
and for comparison of this with microelectrode performance is in the use of surface fluorescence systems which
measure the redox state of flavoproteins and pyridine
nucleotides. These methods which were developed extensively by Chance (Chance, Legallais and Schoener, 1962)
have been combined with oxygen microelectrode measurements both by the Dortmund group and by Silver and Chance
in Philadelphia and Bristol. It is clear from these
measurements that the oxygen diffusion gradient from the
capillary into the mitochondria is a fairly continuous
one and corresponds to the readings which can be obtained
by an electrode passed from the side of the capillary to
a cell at a given distance from that capillary. Furthermore, measurements in beating heart show that in the
underperfused organ where there is a minimum of oxygen
reserve in the perfusion fluid, the pyridine nucleotide
changes which occur during systole are exactly paralleled

by the fall of oxygen tension which can be recorded with
an oxygen electrode floating in heart muscle (Chance,
Salama and Silver, unpublished).

Diffusion onto needle O_2 electrodes appears to
approximate to a 'spherical' model in contrast to that seen
on the recessed type of electrodes which corresponds to
the 'linear' diffusion model. The behaviour of microelectrodes is often better than classical diffusion
theory would predict. This appears to be due to the static boundary layers which occur at the surface of the
electrode partly due to frictional forces and partly due
to electrical poly-layers and which become significant
when the electrode is of less than 3 µm diameter. Fatt
(1964) and Silver (1965) both agreed that the zone from
which at least 95% of the oxygen was drawn in electrodes
of 1 µm or less, is a sphere with a diameter approximately
6 x the radius of the measuring surface. Experiments
since then in which microelectrodes have been moved into
the vicinity of each other, (Silver, 1973) have also
shown that rather small diffusion zones exist around
microelectrodes and these zones have been analysed for
different situations by Grunewald (1973).

Future Developments

The oxygen microelectrode is established as a useful tool for the investigation of tissue microenvironment but it possesses a number of inherent disadvantages
which have been mentioned. One aspect, which is both a
strength and a weakness, is the fine resolution of small
probes. Combination of electrode measurements with computer models and data analysis seems likely to lead to
the next phase in an understanding of normal and pathological conditions at the cellular level. Because of
the complex relationship of oxygen supply to other physical factors in tissue, multiparameter investigations involving arrays of O_2 electrodes associated with pH and
other ion-specific probes are being developed. The synthesis of fluorescent potentiometric dyes of the mero-
cyanin type may be a pointer towards the development of
a non-destructive method of measuring intracellular PO_2
at the surfaces of organs. Some such method associated
with extracellular microelectrode measurements would
give us a clearer idea of the relationship between extracellular and intracellular oxygen environment.

Two problems which have still to be solved are seen in the phenomena of 'ageing' and in the development of sensitivity to various ions.   'Ageing' occurs when a new electrode is hydrated and polarised;   there is usually a period of increasing sensitivity for 2-6 hours, followed by a plateau in oxygen sensitivity over a further 10-20 hours which is succeeded by a slow decline in sensitivity. The process has not been adequately explained although the development of catalytic 'hot-spots' and hydration of the cathode surface are contributory factors.

Ion selectivity may develop when the very thin glass near the tip of a microelectrode becomes hydrated, and can be very misleading if large changes of ionic concentration occur in the vicinity of a probe with a poor current-voltage plateau.   We need more information on this process.   At present it can be limited by siliconising the tip of an electrode but if we could control the process it might lead to the development of a new range of ion sensitive probes.

REFERENCES

Bicher, H.I. and Knisely, M.H. (1970). J. appl. Physiol. 28, 387.

Blinks, L.R. and Skow, R.K. (1938). Proc. Nat. Acad. Sci. U.S. 24, 420.

Cater, D.B., Phillips, A.F. and Silver, I.A. (1957). Proc. Roy. Soc. B146, 289.

Cater, D.B. and Silver, I.A. (1961). In 'Reference Electrodes'. (Eds. Ives, D.J.G. and Janz, J.G.). (Academic Press, London.) Chap. 11.

Cater, D.B., Silver, I.A. and Wilson, G.M. (1959). Proc. Roy. Soc. B.151, 256.

Chance, B., Legallais, V. and Schoener, B. (1962). Nature 195, 1073.

Clark, L.C. (1956).   Amer. Soc. Art. Int. Org. <u>2</u>, 41.

Danneel, H. (1897-8).   Z. Elektrochem. <u>4</u>, 227.

Davies, P.W. and Brink, F. (1942).   Rev. Sci. Instrum.
  <u>13</u>, 524.

Davies, P.W. and Rémond, A. (1947).   Res. Publ. Assoc.
  Res. Nerv. Ment. Dis. <u>26</u>, 205.

Erdmann, W., Kunke, St., Krell, W. (1973).   In 'Oxygen
Supply' (Eds. Kessler, M. et al.).   (Urban and Schwarzenberg, München.) p. 169.

Fatt, I. (1964).   J. appl. Physiol. <u>19</u>, 326.

Grunewald, W. (1973).   In 'Oxygen Supply' (Eds.
  Kessler, M. et al.).   (Urban and Schwarzenberg,München)
  p. 160.

Kunze, K. (1965).   Pflügers Arch. ges. Physiol. <u>283</u>, 4.

Kunze, K. (1966).   Pflügers Arch. ges. Physiol. <u>292</u>, 151.

Kunze, K. (1969).   In 'Schriftenreihe Neurologie Ser.
  Vol. 3.   (Springer, Berlin).

Lübbers, D.W. and Baumgärtl, H. (1967).   Pflügers Arch.
  ges. Physiol. <u>294</u>, R.39.

Montgomery, H. and Horwitz, O. (1950).   J. Clin. Invest.
  <u>29</u>, 1120.

Silver, I.A. (1965).   Med. Electron. Biol. Engn. <u>3</u>, 377.

Silver, I.A. (1973).   In 'Chemical Engineering and
  Medicine'. (Advances in Chemistry Series. In press).

Whalen, W.J. and Nair, P. (1967).   Circulat. Res. <u>21</u>,
  251.

Whalen, W.J. and Nair, P. (1970).   Amer. J. Physiol.
  <u>219</u>, 973.

Whalen, W.J., Nair, P. and Buerk, D. (1973). In 'Oxygen
    Supply' (Eds. Kessler, M. et al.).   Urban and
    Schwarzenberg, Munchen,   p. 199.

Whalen, W.J., Riley, J. and Nair, P. (1967). J. appl.
    Physiol. $\underline{23}$, 798.

INTRACELLULAR OXYGEN MICROELECTRODES

William J. Whalen, Ph.D.

Director of Research, St. Vincent Charity Hospital
Cleveland, Ohio 44115
Adjunct Professor, Case Western Reserve University

In this presentation the work of many associates of mine will be discussed, most notably Dr. Pankajam Nair. I will say little about the construction of the micro O_2 electrode since the method is essentially the same as has been published (7). Rather, I will first briefly discuss tests of its reliability and new calibration techniques; then some of our recent findings.

In our laboratory we have constructed, tested and used a micro O_2 electrode (7, 6) which is apparently capable of measuring the oxygen tension inside a cell as small as 10μ (5). A microphotograph of the tip is shown in Figure I.

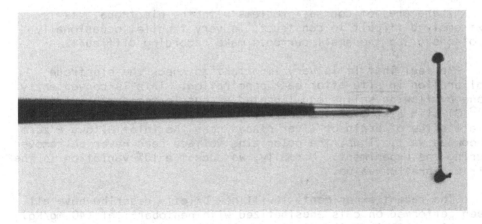

Figure I. Microphotograph of the tip of a relatively large tipped O_2 electrode. The bar represents 20μ.

The electrode is made by filling a glass-capillary with metal, drawing it out with a long shank and bevelling the tip which measures 1 - 3μ at the beginning of the bevel. A recess of 10 - 40μ is created at the tip and gold (the cathode in the polarographic system) is plated on the metal in the recess. Collodion in the recess acts as a filter. A separate Ag-AgCl anode is used. The current drawn is small (approx. 3×10^{-14} A/mm Hg) and probably for this reason the electrode is not sensitive to stirring, and has a rapid response time. There is little residual current (in fact, it is sometimes negative) and usually a nearly flat plateau in the current-voltage curve which is essential for accurate measurements of intracellular PO_2. The deflection on the oxygen current trace due to the action potential or the resting cell membrane potential can usually be used as an indicator of cell penetration (5). However, the creation of the proper recording conditions is difficult, and thus, in studies on skeletal muscle we often do not bother, since we have found that the electrode tip is in a cell about 70% of the time.

Our confidence in the electrode was greatly enhanced when we found that the PO_2 inside a surface cell of an isolated, superfused frog sartorius muscle was close to the PO_2 of the external solution (3). Still greater confidence came from the measurements of O_2 profiles in freshly-excised cat cerebral cortex (2). The calculated values for the coefficient of diffusion of O_2 and the oxygen consumption ($\dot{V}o_2$) obtained could not have been so reasonable if the electrode were not accurately recording the PO_2. A useful, simpler test of reliability using a yeast-agar mixture is described in the same paper (2).

There are, of course, problems with the electrode. It is extremely difficult to construct, is very fragile, occasionally "poisons", and the small currents make recording difficult.

We feel that it is very important to check the electrode calibration in situ after each penetration. This is conveniently done by flowing saline equilibrated at muscle temperature (34° - 36° C) with air, over the preparation between penetrations. A small slice of brain or liver placed near the inlet allows a zero check as well. Thus, the polarizing voltage need never be removed during the experiment. Normally, we accept a 10% variation in the air calibration value.

The recent experiments I will now briefly describe have all been performed on cats anesthetized with pentobarbital (40 mg/Kg) or pentobarbital-urethane. The animals are tracheotomized and kept warm.

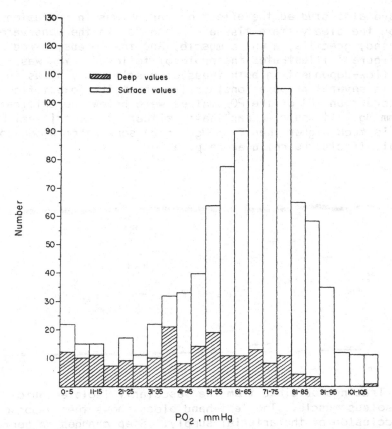

Figure 2. Frequency distribution of the PO_2 in 790 locations sampled in the surface (outer 200μ) and 190 locations deeper in the cat carotid body. Data from 27 cats.

Figure 2 shows a frequency distribution of the PO_2 values found in the carotid body while the cat breathed air spontaneously. Very few low values were found. When, in subsequent experiments, the cat was paralyzed with gallamine and ventilated with low O_2 gas mixtures, we obtained histograms skewed to the left, but still only about 5% of the values were below the "critical PO_2" of 5 mm Hg (4). We interpret these results to mean that classical hypoxic depolarization cannot be the mechanism of chemoceptor discharge. These results (and our conclusions) differ markedly from those of Acker <u>et al</u> (1) in Dr. Lübbers laboratory who reported finding a zone of very low PO_2 near the surface of the cat carotid body. This question needs to be resolved and both Dr. Lübbers and I hope that funds can be found for a collaborative effort.

We have also studied the effect of variations in perfusion pressure on the steady-state tissue PO_2 and $\dot{V}O_2$ in the denervated auto-perfused, gracilis, a white muscle, and the soleus, a red muscle. Figure 3 illustrates the protocol followed. $\dot{V}O_2$ was extremely flow-dependent in both types of muscle; varying as much as 6-fold in several preparations; yet, even at the lowest flow rates no more than 18% of the PO_2 values were below the critical PO_2 of 5 mm Hg. It would appear that: either 1) the critical PO_2 in muscle is much higher than 5 mm Hg; or 2) some other blood-borne constituent affects the cellular respiration.

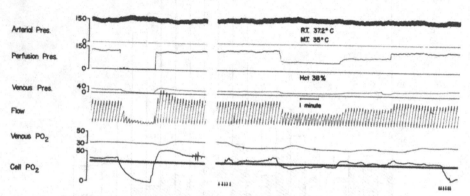

Figure 3. Tracings obtained from the vascularly isolated auto-perfused, soleus muscle. The left-hand block shows the response to complete occlusion of the arterial supply. Step changes in perfusion pressure are seen at right. Normally, the pressure steps were held for at least 8 minutes. Arrows at bottom indicate penetration steps into the muscle of 125μ each.

The values we found for tissue PO_2 in the soleus muscle in the above experiments were somewhat higher than we previously reported (5); those for the gracilis were markedly higher than in the previous studies (6). Experiments aimed at finding the reasons for the discrepancy are in progress. It appears that denervation yields higher values, but it alone cannot account for the different results on the gracilis. Repetition of the previous in situ experiments (6) has yielded even wider inter-individual variation than we previously reported (6). I am inclined now to the view that in this preparation tissue PO_2 is not usually the reference point in the blood flow control system. Rather, it may be that adjustments in blood flow are related more to the requirement for metabolic thermogenesis.

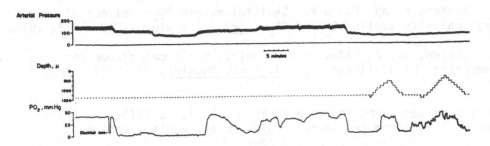

Figure 4. Response of the tissue PO_2 in the _in situ_ innervated gracilis muscle of the cat to step changes in arterial pressure induced by hemorrhage. Note also that the oxygen current zero is below electrical zero; an unexplained, occasional finding.

        As a part of the above search we are exploring the effect of variations in arterial pressure on tissue PO_2 in the gracilis muscle. After taking normal values the animal is bled to the desired level as illustrated in Figure 4. It is of special interest that in some locations, as seen here, tissue PO_2 falls to near zero for as long as 20 minutes when the arterial pressure is reduced only to what is considered a normal value of about 100 mm Hg. In denervated muscles this response has not been seen until arterial pressure was reduced to about 40 mm Hg. Overall, these results suggest that central control is important in the regulation of the tissue PO_2 in this preparation.

REFERENCES

1. Acker, H., D. Lübbers, and M. J. Purves. Local oxygen tension field in the glomus caroticum of the cat and its change at changing arterial PO_2. Pflugers Arch. 329: 136, 1971.

2. Ganfield, R., P. Nair, and W. Whalen. Mass transfer, storage, and utilization of O_2 in cat cerebral cortex. Am. J. Physiol. 219: 814, 1970.

3. Gore, R. and W. Whalen. Relations among tissue PO_2, Qo_2, and resting heat production of frog sartorius muscle. Am. J. Physiol. 214: 277, 1968.

4. Jobsis, F. Basic processes in cellular respiration. In: Handbook of Physiology. Respiration. Washington, D.C.: Am. Physiol. Soc., 1964, p. 111.

5. Whalen, W. Intracellular PO_2 in heart and skeletal muscle. The Physiologist, 14: 69, 1971.

6.   Whalen, W. and P. Nair.   Skeletal muscle PO$_2$:   effect of inhaled and topically applied O$_2$ and CO$_2$.   _Am. J. Physiol._   218:   973, 1970.

7.   Whalen, W., J. Riley, and P. Nair.   A microelectrode for measuring intracellular PO$_2$.   _J. Appl. Physiol._ 23:   798, 1967.

This work was supported in part by RR 05631, HL 13134, HL 12703, and HL 11906 from the United States Public Health Service.

The excellent work of Ms. Eloise Lerch and Mr. Frank Minnello in the preparation of the manuscript is gratefully acknowledged.

STANDARDIZATION OF PRODUCING NEEDLE ELECTRODES

E. Sinagowitz and M. Kessler
with the technical assistance of
K. Fehlau and B. Bölling
Max-Planck-Institut für Arbeitsphysiologie
Dortmund, West Germany

Platinum micro-electrodes insulated with glass for Po_2-measurements were first described by Cater and Silver (1961). Based on their work Lübbers and Baumgärtl (1967) developed a needle electrode with a tip diameter of 1 u for measurements of both oxygen and hydrogen tension in tissue.

In order to standardize the production we developed a new method for the manufacture of micro-electrodes.

According to the technique of Lübbers and Baumgärtl (1967, 1973), platinum wires of 200 u diameter are etched electrolytically by alternating current in a nearly saturated solution of KCN to a tip diameter of at least 1 u.

Prefabricated tubes of AR-glass, commercially available in a very accurate size, are used for insulating the Pt-wires. AR-glass has a coefficient of thermal expansion which is nearly the same as that of platinum so that tensions between glass and metal cannot develop.

For fusing the glass with the platinum an electromagnetic puller is used, which principally consists of a heating element and an electromagnet (Fig. 1). The heating element is a helix of 3 windings of Kanthal-A-1 wire, which has the advantage of very little emission of vapor during glowing, so that a very stable temperature can be maintained. During development of this method we found that a precise adjustment of the fusing temperature of $710^{\circ}C$ is extremely important. We check it frequently by means of a thermoelement. Even small movements of air cause changes of temperature in the center of the heating spiral within a range of

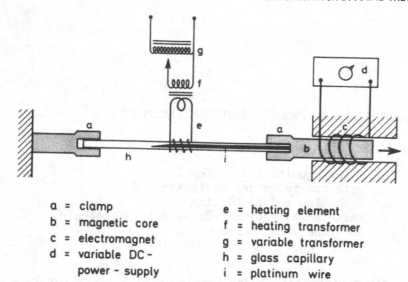

a = clamp   e = heating element
b = magnetic core   f = heating transformer
c = electromagnet   g = variable transformer
d = variable DC -   h = glass capillary
    power - supply   i = platinum wire

Fig. 1: Diagram of the electromagnetic puller

20 to 30°C. This is now avoided by covering the puller with a tube
of lucite. Good fusing can only be attained when the electromagnet
pulls continuously. In order to prevent pulling by forces other
than the magnetic one the puller is placed in a horizontal position.
The strength for pulling is 4p.

When the capillary tube containing the platinum wire is
brought into its exact position, the voltages for the heating
element and the electromagnet are adjusted. After switching on the
puller, the fusing process continues automatically. The helix is
heated, the glass melts, and by the constant pulling force of the
magnet the melting glass is drawn over the platinum tip in a very
thin layer. This procedure takes about 90 sec.

In order to prevent the developing of tensions in the glass
during cooling, which would lead to fissures during grinding, the
electrodes are tempered in an oven after fusing.

As suggested by Kessler (1973) the electrodes are ground in
order to sharpen the tip. A more acute tip makes inserting the
electrode into the tissue easier and less damaging. For grinding we
use a grinding machine based on the design developed by Ullrich
et al. (1969). The rotating disc (tin- lead -alloy) turns at a
rate of 1000 rpm, and the mechanical instability is less than 1 u.
The diamond paste used has a particle diameter of 0.25 u.

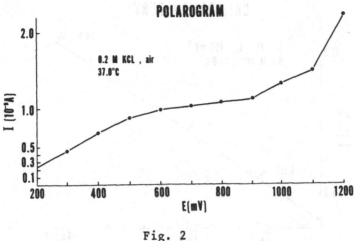

Fig. 2

The grinding process is observed under microscopic visualiza-
tion and controlled by measuring the d.c. resistance between
electrode and grinding machine. When the glass is removed an
acustic signal is heard. This indicates that sufficient grinding
has been accomplished.

The electrode is coated with a membrane by dipping it into a
solution of polystyrol in carbon tetrachloride.

RESULTS

The insulation resistance is in the range of 10^{11} Ohms. If
the electrode is stored in dist. water the resistance will decrease
to 10^{10} or 10^{9} Ohms after four weeks.

The polarographic plateau lies in a range of 500 to 900 mV
(Fig. 2), other electrodes may have a higher plateau. In order to
get the most accurate values, the polarogram of each electrode
should be determined before measuring.

The calibration curve (Fig. 3) is linear and shows a very
small zero current. The response time (T_{95}) is about 1 sec. The
electrodes show a drift of the signal up to 10 %/hr.

An example for tissue measurement is shown in Fig. 4 which
presents an ischemic reaction in the medulla of the rabbit kidney.
(Recently performed together with Strauss and Baker).

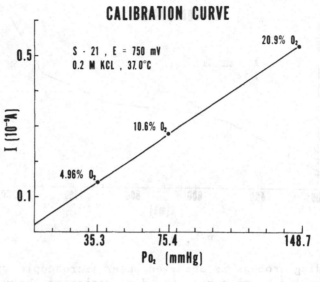

Fig. 3

After occlusion of the renal artery and vein the Po_2 decreases
continuously. After release a sharp increase occurs followed by a
decrease again, and finally the Po_2 returns to the control level.

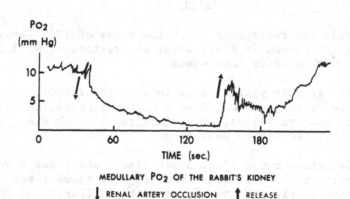

Fig. 4

REFERENCES

1. Baumgärtl, H., D.W. Lübbers: Platinum needle electrodes for
   polarographic measurement of oxygen and hydrogen.
   In: Oxygen supply, theoretical and practical aspects of oxygen
   supply and microcirculation of tissue, ed. by M. Kessler,
   D.F. Bruley, L.C. Clark Jr., D.W. Lübbers, I.A. Silver,
   J. Strauss, pp. 130-136. Urban & Schwarzenberg, München-
   Berlin-Wien 1973.

2. Cater, D.B., I.A. Silver: Electrodes and microelectrodes used
   in biology. In: References Electrodes, ed. by D.J.G. Ives
   and I.G. Janz, Chap. 11, p. 464, Academic Press, New York-
   London 1961.

3. Kessler, M.: Problems with the use of platinum cathodes for the
   polarographic measurement of oxygen. In: Oxygen supply,
   theoretical and practical aspects of oxygen supply and microcirculation of tissue, ed. by M. Kessler, D.F. Bruley,
   L.C. Clark Jr., D.W. Lübbers, I.A. Silver, J. Strauss,
   pp. 81-85. Urban & Schwarzenberg, München-Berlin-Wien 1973.

4. Lübbers, D.W., H. Baumgärtl: Herstellungstechnik von palladi-
   nierten Pt-Stichelektroden (1-5 µ Außendurchmesser) zur
   polarographischen Messung des Wasserstoffdruckes für die
   Bestimmung der Mikrozirkulation. Pflügers Arch. ges. Physiol.
   294, R39 (1967).

5. Ullrich, K.J., E. Frömter, K. Baumann: Micropuncture and micro-
   analysis in kidney physiology. In: Laboratory techniques in
   membrane biophysics ed. by H. Passow, R. Stämpfli, pp. 106-129
   Springer Verlag, Berlin-Heidelberg-New York 1969.

HIGH SPEED PULSATILE OPERATION OF MINIATURE OXYGEN ELECTRODES

Stanley H. Saulson

Univ. of Michigan, Ann Arbor, Mich., U. S. A.

This investigation has been an *in vitro* study of pulsatile amperometric techniques suitable for application in blood and tissue. Parameters of the study were selected to enhance spatial resolution, to obtain a faster time response to reveal changes in pO_2 within the cardiac cycle, and for low electrode O_2 consumption. Faster time response may provide new physiological information for possible future application in a research or clinical setting.

Pulsatile operation of electrodes is not a novel concept, having first been used by Davies and Brink in 1942. Most recently, Kunze (1969) used a pair of matched Clark-type electrodes feeding into a differential amplifier. Major pulsed electrode investigations are listed in a table which shows that the trend has been toward narrower pulse widths and higher repetition rates. This investigation included pulse widths down to 200 μ sec and repetition rates up to 120 Hz.

For ultimate application, electrodes must be simple and low cost. They must be readily fabricated, easily calibrated, and cheap enough to be considered disposable after a single use. Electrode miniaturization was considered very important so that a number of electrodes could be mounted on a needle or a standard size catheter, while, at the same time, leaving room for pressure sensors and an open lumen for indicator injection. To this end, electrode construction by embedment and by thin film techniques was explored.

METHODS

Any pulsatile electrode study requires a minimum system consisting of a cathode, anode, electrolyte, and the electronics which

PULSED ELECTRODE INVESTIGATIONS

INVESTIGATOR	YEAR	TIME ON	TIME OFF	RATIO OFF:ON	REPETITION RATE
Davies & Brink	1942	20 sec	20 min	60:1	3/hr
Olson, Brackett & Crickard	1949	3 sec *	6 sec	2:1	5/min
Carlson, Brink & Bronk	1950	12 sec	48 sec	4:1	60/hr
Kunze, Lubbers, & Windisch	1963	1.3 sec	4 min	200:1	15/hr
Evans & Naylor	1966	0.5 sec	10-20 sec	30:1	3-6/min
Fales & Penneys	1967	15-200 msec	—	--	—
Kunze	1969	0.6-1.8 msec	0.3-1 sec	550:1	3/sec

*3 sec negative polarity, followed by 3 sec off, 3 sec positive polarity, 3 sec off.

provides the pulse and amplifies the resulting current. Despite
the desire to change only one variable at a time, all elements of
the system are totally interrelated, and several also vary with
time. Due to these interactions, it was necessary to spiral into
an effective range of parameter values which would be suitable for
future research and clinical applications.

Gold cathodes were made by one of two methods. In the first,
gold wire was embedded in polycarbonate plastic and the assembly
polished to provide a flush electrode. Acid was used to remove
some of the gold thereby providing an open chamber to convert a
flush electrode into a recessed electrode. In the second method,
photofabrication techniques used in electronic circuit fabrication
were adapted to provide thin film electrodes. Glass or photopoly-
mers were used to insulate a gold conductor pattern formed on a
ceramic substrate. Holes etched into the insulator provided an open
chamber with the diameter of the etched hole determining the electrode diameter, while the recess depth was controlled by the insulator thickness. Cathodes were made by both methods with diameters
ranging from 12 μm to 500 μm and chamber depths from 0.5 μm to 10 μm.

Silver-silver chloride reference anodes were made by partial
electrochemical conversion of metallic silver. Conventional fabrication methods (Ives and Janz, 1961) did not perform well in pulsatile operation. An optimization program showed that very thin silver
chloride layers, made with a current density of 10 mA/cm^2 flowing for
a period of 30 seconds, were highly superior to thicker conventional
layers. Anodes were generally 10^4 larger in area than the cathodes.

A flexible electronic system, shown in Figure 1, was built.

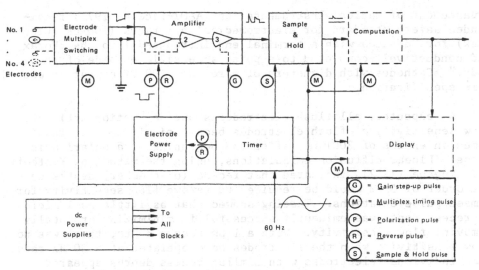

Figure 1. Electronic system block diagram.

It provided a train of polarization pulses with durations adjustable from 0.2 to 4.8 msec and a pulse rate from 3/sec to 120/sec. All pulses were synchronized to the 60 Hz power line to minimize noise pickup. A reverse polarity "cleaning pulse" with independent controls on pulse width and voltage was also available, but it was found to increase rather than reduce drift. Feedback capacitors in the first and second amplifier stages were optimized to permit fast charging of the electrode double layer and stray capacitances and to filter high frequency noise. During each pulse, after the initial charging current peaks had subsided, the gain of the third amplifier stage was increased 100-fold to provide further amplification of electrode current without the danger of amplifier saturation from spikes. Sample & Hold circuits converted the electrode current at a preselected time into a dc level. Multiplex switching provisions were made so that the system could handle up to four electrodes in succession.

Conventional test fixtures and instrumentation were used for flow sensitivity and step response studies. An automatic X-Y plotter was used to draw more than 500 polarograms.

RESULTS

The combination of electrodes and electronics described above achieved pO_2 sampling rates as fast as 120 Hz. Cathode diameters from 12 μm to 72 μm appeared similar in performance except for the expected difference in current. The increases in initial charging current time due to increased electrode diameter were not found to be significant after optimization of the electronics. Peak and average currents were well within the Association for the

Advancement of Medical Instrumentation (AAMI-Pacela, 1971) recommended safety standard for electromedical apparatus (100 µA pulse
peak) for "devices with a terminal end introduced into the thorax
and conductively connected to a point accessible outside of the
body." Cathodes with diameters of more than 100 µm appear to exceed
this specification.

As expected, all flush electrodes showed a "motion artifact."
Flow sensitivity of flush electrodes became significant at reading
times in excess of 200 µsec after the beginning of a polarization
pulse. Linear diffusion calculations, using the method of Kolthoff
and Lingane (1952), indicated that recess (or chamber) depths on
the order of 5 µm would be required to remove flow sensitivity for
2 msec pulse durations. Testing showed that as little as 1 micron
of recess depth was eminently successful in minimizing or totally
removing flow sensitivity. With a 1 µm recess depth, there was no
flow sensitivity when the electrodes were operated at a 30 Hz rate.
Some individual electrodes with similar recess depths appeared to
operate free of "motion artifact" at a 40 Hz rate. With a depth to
diameter ratio of 1:50, such shallow depressions hardly seem to
qualify for the term "recess"--yet they work!

Flow sensitivity can be further reduced by making the recess
in front of the electrode progressively deeper. Reduction in flow
sensitivity also implies an increase in response time to changes in
the external environment. Step response measurements are an effective way of determining how fast a system can respond to a large
change. For example, taking an electrode from air and plunging it
into saline will show how fast the electrode can respond to this
change. Electrodes, operating at a 120 Hz rate, came to their final
reading within the first pulse. Thus, they responded to this step
change within 8 msec. Moving from saline maintained at one level
of oxygen saturation to saline maintained at a different level of
oxygen saturation is a much more meaningful test. A series of step
response measurements were made going from a pO_2 of approximately
300 mmHg down to 150 mmHg. For these measurements, the electrode
was moved from a stationary beaker of saline at elevated pO_2 and
plunged, without wiping, into a second beaker of saline at room air
saturation. A magnetic stirrer was used to circulate the liquid in
the latter beaker. In this series of measurements, the electrodes
went from 0 to 90% of the correct new reading within 0.16 sec. Thus
the electrode responded to a step four times larger than the maximum expected in a physiological environment at a rate corresponding
to 6 Hz. If all elements of the electrode system were truly linear,
the size of the step would not be significant. Consideration of (a)
droplet carryover in the recess and on the electrode holder surface,
(b) consumption of oxygen in the recess, and (c) the practical
nature of the diffusion process suggests that the system is probably
not linear. If this is the case, response time for a physiological
pO_2 step of, say, 40 mmHg should be less than the value reported here.

Early measurements with pulsed electrodes produced results which were different from those predicted by extrapolation of previous work reported in the literature. As expected, the current produced by an oxygen saturated medium was substantially higher than the current measured from the same electrolyte exposed to room air. Nitrogen bubbled through the medium removed oxygen and reduced the current. The current did *not*, however, go to zero regardless of the length of time nitrogen was bubbled through. At first, this phenomenon was thought to be an artifact of the electronic circuits or an error in calibration procedure. Intensive investigation established conclusively that there was a "residual current" measurable in *all* electrodes operating in a short pulse mode. ("Residual current" discussed here appears to be the same phenomenon as the "background current" reported by Fales and Penneys (1967), but is an order of magnitude larger.) This was, perhaps, the most surprising outcome of this study!

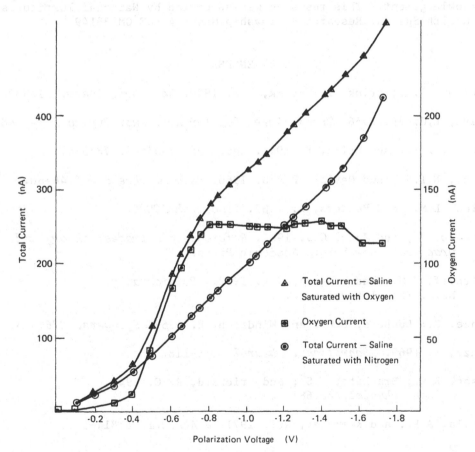

Figure 2. Typical polarograms hand plotted from DVM data (12 μm diameter recessed electrode).

Figure 2 shows the residual current on a typical polarogram. Within the range of pulse widths investigated in this study, the most favorable ratio of oxygen current to residual current generally occured at 2 msec. Large variations in residual current were seen between electrodes which were physically quite similar and which yielded similar levels of oxygen current. It is believed that ion movement during the establishment of the electrochemical double layer, and shielding within small surface cavities, may be responsible for the residual current phenomenon. Small differences in electrode geometry or surface texture could account for the large differences seen in residual current behavior.

A dynamic calibration technique, based upon "residual current", was identified which should permit continuous calibration while an electrode is in use.

Acknowledgement: This research was supported by National Institutes of Health Special Research Fellowship Grant 4 FO3 GM 39149.

REFERENCES

Carlson, F.D.; Brink, F.; Bronk, D.W. 1950. *Rev. Sci. Instr. 21*:932.

Clark, L.C.,Jr. 1956. *Trans. Amer. Soc. for Art. Int. Organs II*:41-48.

Davies, P.W., and Brink, F. 1942. *Rev. Sci. Instrum. 13*:524.

Evans, N.T.S., and Naylor, P.F.S. 1966. *Respir. Physiol. 2*:46-60.

Fales, E.M., and Penneys, R. 1967. *Proc. 7th ICMBE*.

Ives, D. J., and Janz, G.J. 1961. *Reference electrodes: theory and practice*. New York: Academic Press.

Kolthoff, I.M., and Lingane, J.L. 1952. *Polarography*. New York: Interscience.

Kunze, K.; Lübbers, D.W.; and Windisch, E. 1963. *Pflugers. 276*:415.

Kunze, K. 1969. *Schriftenr. Neurol. 3*:1-118.

Olson, R.A.; Brackett, F.S.; and Crickard, R. G. 1949. *J. Gen. Physiol. 32*:681

Pacela, A.F., and Kemmerer, W.T. 1971. *J.A.A.M.I. 5*:314-32.

ABSOLUTE PO$_2$-MEASUREMENTS WITH Pt – ELECTRODES APPLYING POLARIZING VOLTAGE PULSING

K. Kunze and D. W. Lübbers*
Department of Clinical Neurophysiology
Neurological Clinical University of Giessen
and
*Max-Planck-Institut für Arbeitsphysiologie
Dortmund, West Germany

The disadvantage of the normal polarographic measurement of oxygen pressure is that its reduction at the electrode surface consumes steadily oxygen. This results in an constant drain of oxygen out of the medium to be measured.
Using recessed electrodes DAVIES and BRINK have shown that this difficulty can be overcome by applying pulsing polarizing voltage. This has been applied too by other investigators so as OLSON and BRACKET; EVANS and NAYLOR; INCH, each of them using a different technique in pulsing the electrode.
In order to measure absolute PO$_2$-values the length of the pulse of the polarizing voltage should to be adapted to the depth of the recess and the diffusion characteristics of the solution. Furthermore one has to provide the formation of a steady polarizing layer at the electrode surface in order to gain reproducible results.
Our chamber electrodes had a depth of 400-200 u,using an electrode with a single Platinum-wire of 1mm diameter or a multi-wire electrode with 10 Pt-wires of 50 u. In order to obtain constant diffusion conditions, the chamber was completely filled with filter paper sucked with KCL-solution and fixed by a cuprophane membrane (fig.1).In order to get stable readings we had to apply the following measuring scheme : 4minutes measurement with a continuously polarizing voltage 5minutes resaturation of the chamber to the PO$_2$-value of the medium, and then the measuring impulse with a duration of 1,3sec. This provided sufficiently flat

polarograms and linear calibration curves (fig.2).

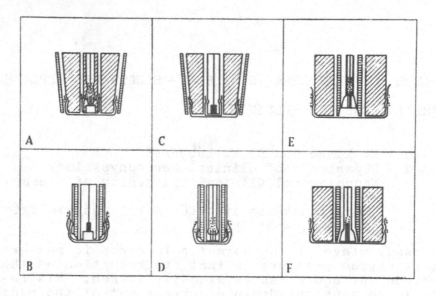

Fig.1:   Different PO$_2$-electrodes (schematically)
A multi-wire chamber electrode, B single-wire chamber
electrode, C single-wire continously measuring electrode, D multi-wire continuouly measuring electrode,
E chamber electrode in chamber position (E), F and
continously measuring position (F)

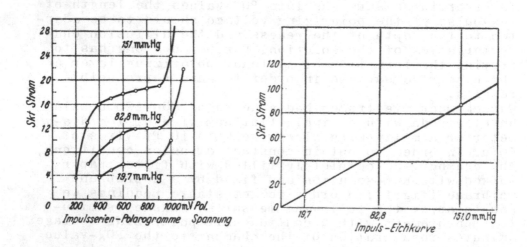

Fig.2:   Polarogram and calibration curve of the chamber electrode

An example for absolute PO_2 measurements in unstirred blood is shown in fig.3.

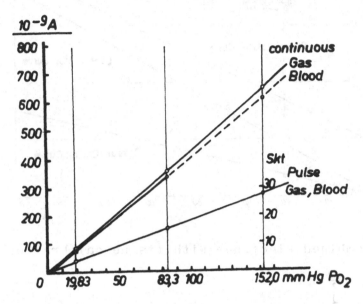

Fig.3:   Absolute PO_2 measurements with the chamber elec-trode in unstirred blood. In the upper part the con-tinuously measured PO_2 of the same electrode. In the lower part the absolute pulse measurements.

The absolute measuring chamber electrode can be com-bined with an ordinary Pt-electrode as it is demon-strated in fig.4. Applying the electrode to brain or heart surface, the continuously measuring electrode could be calibrated in situ by relating the PO_2 value obrained simultaneously by the absolute electrode. Thus the calibration curve for tissue measurements was established.
The reading of this chamber electrode may remain sta-ble for about 1day. Since the time constant of the electrode was very long, we tried to reduce the depth of the chamber. We succeeded in using the thin layers of cuprophane and teflon in front of the Platinum sur-face, together about 25 u, of our regular electrodes as a chamber. In this case we applied voltage pulses as short as 40-20msec using the following measuring scheme : 20 serial pulses at an interval of 1.2sec - 1 minute resaturation of the chamber- the measuring

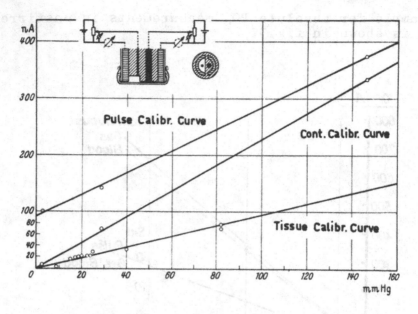

<u>Fig.4:</u> Combined electrode with tissue calibration curve

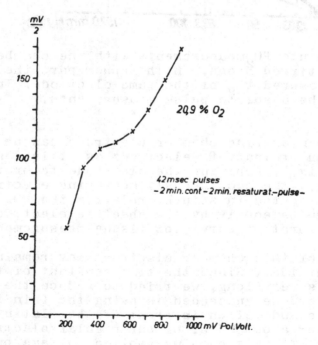

<u>Fig.5:</u> Polarogram of pulsing electrode with 42 msec
pulses.

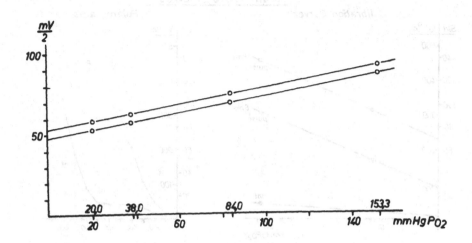

Fig.6: Calibration curves of the same electrode. The upper curve was found after the electrode had been switched off for 1 hour.

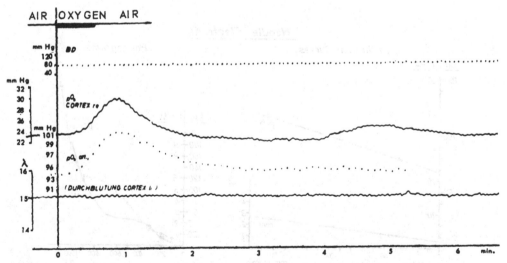

Fig.7: Pulsing electrode measuring absolute PO_2 in arterial blood in animal experiment. Response time (90%) 30 sec.(readings are indicated by dots).

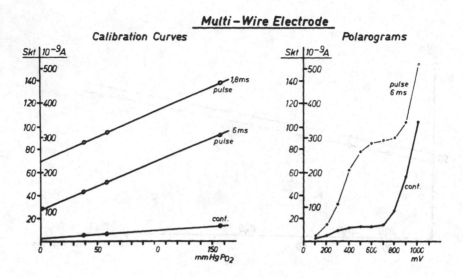

Fig.8: Calibration curves and polarograms with multi-wire electrodes using serial very short pulses.

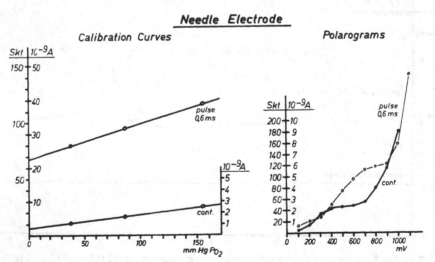

Fig.9: Calibration curves and polarograms with needle-electrodes using the same technique as in fig.8. Tip of the electrodes 2-5 µ.

Electrode Type	Cont.Measurement	Pulse Measurement		
	O_2- Sensitivity $10^{-9} Amps/100mm Hg$	Pulse Duration	O_2 Sensitivity $10^{-9} Amps/100mm Hg$
Recessed Electrode Pt ⌀ 1mm, Chamber ~400μ	55	1,3 sec Pulse Pattern	400
Recessed Multi-Wire Electrode 10 Pt-Wires ⌀~50μ Chamber ~400μ	40	1,3 sec Pulse Pattern	100
Multi-Wire Electrodes 9 Pt-Wires ⌀~30μ	25 - 40	0,6-80msec Pulse Series Depending on Pulse Duration up to 3/sec	27-37 Depending on Pulse Duration
Multi-Wire Electrodes 9-10 Pt-Wires ⌀~15μ	4 - 7	0,6-1,8 msec Pulse Series 1-3/sec	22 - 113
Needle Electrode Tip 2-5μ	0,38 - 3,8	0,6-1,8 msec Pulse Series 1-3/sec	2-87

Fig.10: O_2-sensitivity of different electrode-types in continuous and pulse measurement.

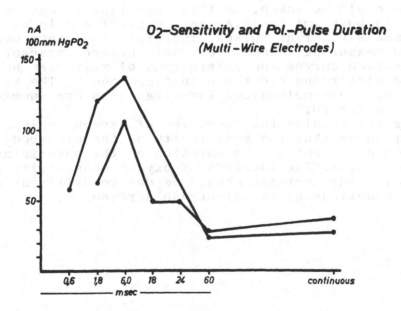

Fig.11: O_2-sensitivity of pulsing multi-wire electrode (serial pulses) with relation to pulse duration.

pulse, then the series of pulses again. The continuous
application of the forementioned measuring scheme was
necessary to obtain sufficient stability. An example
for a polarogram and a calibration curve is shown in
fig.5 and 6, the application in animals demonstrates
fig. 7.
These electrodes have a higher zero current than the
bigger ones. It could be proved that the shorter the
pulse the higher the zero current. This is due to
electrical loading of the double layer which is formed
in front of the Platinum surface.
For improving stability of the polarizing layer we
tried different buffers varying the pH between 6-9,
addition of catalase as well as reference electrodes
of different sizes. We applied also short circuiting
and changing of the polarity of the pulses. No reproducible influence of the stability was seen. We found
that only a better seperating of the reference electrode from the Platinum by agar or better by cuprophane
sucked in diluted KCL improved polarograms and stability.
By using two electrodes in an electrical bridge circuit
in which one electrode monitored a constant PO_2, but
the other one the PO_2 to be measured, even shorter
pulses could be taken. By this technique it was possible to buck out the high zero current and to apply
continuously serial pulses. Therefore the above mentioned measuring schemes were not anymore necessary.
Calibration curves and polarograms of multiwire and
needle electrodes are shown in fig.8 and 9. The results of these methodical investigations are summarized in fig.10.
During the loading the reduction of oxygen begins.
Fig.11 shows that the sensitivity of the electrode
changes dependent of the duration of the polarizing
voltage pulse. The increase of oxygen sensitivity and
the following decrease chould be due to different chemical reactions at the electrode surface.

Summary:

For absolute PO$_2$ measurements in blood and tissue
different types of Pt-electrodes using pulsing polarizing voltage are described and applications are demonstrated. Besides a chamber electrode with a long time
constant of 9 minutes, multiple wire electrodes employing short serial pulses of as short as 0.6msec
with a response time (90%) of 15sec have been employed.

References:

Davies, P.W.,and Brink,F., Microelectrodes for measuring local oxygen tension in animal tissues,Rev.
Scient.Instr.,13(1942)524.

Inch, W.R., Problems associated with the use of the
exposed platinum electrode for measuring oxygen tension in vivo.
Can. J. Biochem. Physiol. 36(1958)1009.

Kunze, K., D.W. Lübbers und E. Windisch
Die Messung des absoluten Sauerstoffdruckes mit der
Kammer-Pt-Elektrode in beliebigen Medien, insbesondere
im Blut und Gewebe.
Pflügers Arch.ges.Physiol. 276(1963)415.

Kunze, K., Das Sauerstoffdruckfeld im normalen und
pathologisch veränderten Muskel.
Schriftenreihe Neurologie, Neurology Series Vol.3,
Springer-Verlag Berlin-Heidelberg-New York 1969.

Naylor, P.F.D. and N.T.S. Evans
The Measurement of oxygen tension by rapid voltage
sweep polarography and bare platinum electrodes.
J. Polarographic Society, 2(1960)9.

Olson, R.A., F.S. Brackett and R.G. Crickard
Oxygen tension measurement by method of time selection
using the static platinum electrode with alternating
potential.
J. General Physiol. 32(1949)681.

SPECTROPHOTOMETRIC EXAMINATION OF TISSUE OXYGENATION

D. W. Lübbers
Max-Planck-Institut für Systemphysiologie
Dortmund, West Germany

Methods of absorption photometry are sensitive enough to measure natural pigments participating in oxygen supply, as hemoglobin, myoglobin and cytochromes in vivo. The influence of the light on the pigment can be mostly made so small that it can be neglected. Therefore, the history of in vivo measurements is rather long. We might recall the direct measurements performed by G.A. MacMunn (1880), D. Keilin and O. Warburg in the twenties. The results they obtained were very important, but they were mostly qualitative ones and the absolute evaluation remained a difficult problem. Later on, in the thirties, K. Kramer, K. Matthes and G.A. Millikan tried to overcome these difficulties by using the two-wavelengths method measuring on isolated vessels or on earlobe or partially isolated muscle, but all these methods required after each change of the preparation a new calibration with an absolute method. In the fifties, the two-wavelengths method was very much improved by B. Chance.

In order to explain the basic problems of the quantitative analysis of reflexion spectra, I will analyse the reflexion spectrum of the human skin which is mostly determined by hemoglobin present in the capillaries. The following photometric research was carried out together with Reinhard Wodick. The idea of our modus procedendi was to bring the hemoglobin within the skin in a state the spectrum of which is known. By analysing the changes of the spectrum we tried to find the laws behind these changes and to work out an appropriate evaluation method. In the best way, this known state was brought about by producing a hyperemic skin and fully O_2-saturated blood, for example, by heating up the skin and respiring pure oxygen.

Figure 1 shows the HbO_2 spectrum within the skin $G(\lambda)$ and the extinction spectrum of the corresponding HbO_2 solution $M(\lambda)$.

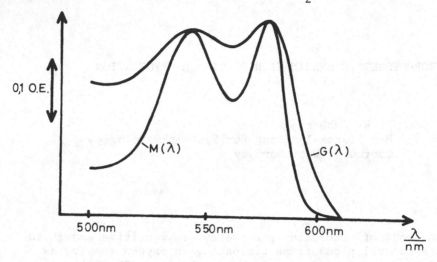

Fig. 1: Extinction spectrum of an oxygenated hemoglobin solution $M(\lambda)$ and oxygenated human skin in vivo $G(\lambda)$

The spectra were registered by the rapid spectroscope of Kieler Howaldtswerke which we developed together with Koehler and Niesel several years ago especially in order to measure reflexion spectra of moving organs (2). The scanning time for a single spectrum is only 1/100 of a second.

The difference between both spectra is obvious: The peaks of the HbO_2 solution are flattened in the skin spectrum (upper trace), similarly as it was observed in turbid solutions (1).

In order to quantify these changes we drew the function shown in Figure 2, relating wavelength by wavelength the extinction of the HbO_2 solution (abscissa: $M(\lambda)$) to the extinction of the HbO_2 within the skin (ordinate: $G(\lambda)$). This function represents the transformation $H(M)$ of the spectrum of the HbO_2 solution into the spectrum of the HbO_2 within the skin. One observes a monotonously increasing curve which has several branches in its upper part.

The construction showed the reason for this: for the same extinction of the solution one obtained different extinctions of the skin at different wavelengths. To understand the other changes we have to analyse,
1) the influence of the distributional factor: since hemoglobin is situated only in the capillaries, it is inhomogeneously distributed in the field to be measured, and,
2) the influence of the reflexion: since the light is reflected in

different depths of the skin, also the light path is inhomogeneous.

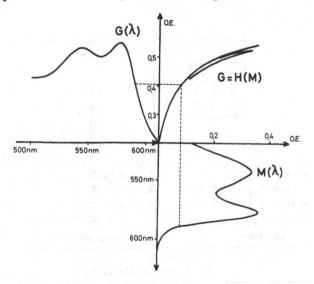

Fig. 2: Transformation of the extinction spectrum of an oxygenated
        hemoglobin solution M(λ) into a reflexion spectrum of the
        oxygenated human skin in vivo G(λ): G = H(M)

     To explain the influence of the distribution the next figure
specifies the basic photometric laws we are dealing with: On the
right side, three cells are placed one after the other. The incident
light L_o is attenuated in the first cell to L_1, being the product
of the incident light L_o times the transmission T_1. In the second
cell L_1 is attenuated to L_2, and, finally, in the third cell to L_3.
The total attenuation of the light equals the product $T_1 \cdot T_2 \cdot T_3$.
Therefore, in a photometric system this kind of mixing is called
multiplicative mixing and the system "multiplicative mixed" system
(abbreviated M-system). In a M-system each incident light beam has
the same way and meets the same amount and the same kind of dye-
stuff molecules. On the left side the three cells are put side by
side. In this case, only the fractions Ψ_1, Ψ_2 and Ψ_3 of the incident
light L_o are passing through the respective cells. The total transmission is given by the sum of the three fractional transmissions.
Therefore, this kind of mixing in a photometric system is called
<u>additive mixing</u>, and the system "additive mixed" system (abbreviat-
ed A-system).

     After the Bouguer-Lambert-Beer law the concentration of the
substance can be found from the extinction E. With multiplicative
mixing we obtain a sum of the different exponents which can be
solved by taking the logarithm. With additive mixing, however, we
obtain a sum of exponential functions the exponents of which can-

not be calculated without knowing all the coefficients involved.

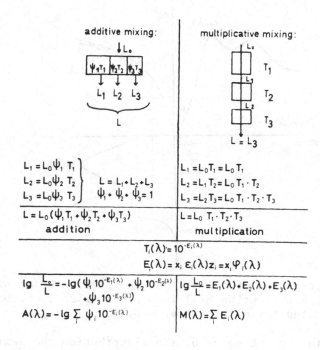

Fig. 3: Scheme of an additively and multiplicatively mixed system
(A- and M-system)

In order to find an evaluation method a combined additively-multiplicatively mixed system - abbreviated, A-M-system - was produced from a pure M-system by confining all hemoglobin molecules into a part of the cell (Fig. 4).

Fig. 4 shows also that the extinction spectrum $M(\lambda)$ has changed its form to $A(\lambda)$. Looking for the transformation of this A-system, we see that the straight line which holds for the M-systems is changed into a monotonously increasing curve having only one single branch. The important result is that the spectral changes caused by the distributional factor depend only on the magnitude of the extinction: equal extinctions in the M-system result in changed, but equally changed extinctions in the A-system. Therefore, the wavelength distances $\Delta\lambda$ (see Fig. 4) between equal extinctions remain the same in all M- and A-systems independent of the concentration and independent of the distribution.

If the spectrum of the M-system is composed of different components, the same holds for the transformation of the multi-component M-system into a multicomponent A-system. The wavelength

distances remain invariant against the distributional changes and
are influenced only by the relative concentration of the components
within the mixture.

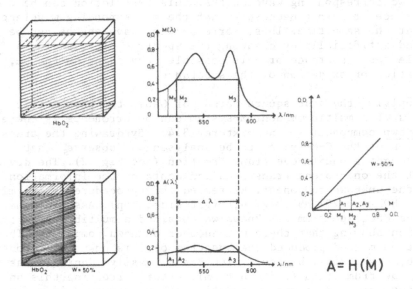

Fig. 4: Basic laws of Q-analysis

This finding is the basis for a new evaluation method, which
we called "Queranalyse" or, abbreviated Q-analysis (see for
literature 3,4). This means that we measure the interval between
two wavelengths having the same extinction. Such wavelengths are
called "corresponding wavelengths", abbreviated, C-wavelengths.
The next figure shows the Q-analysis of desoxygenated hemoglobin.

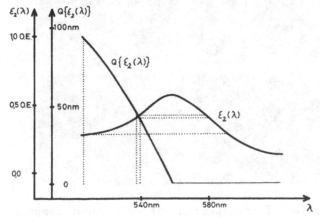

Fig. 5: Q-analysis and Q-curve Q $\{\varepsilon_2(\lambda)\}$ of desoxygenated
hemoglobin $\varepsilon_2(\lambda)$

Taking the shorter wavelength as x-coordinate, the distance
to the longer C-wavelength is the y-coordinate. Thus, we obtain
the Q-analysis curve, abbreviated, Q-curve. The Q-analysis in this
form is restricted to substances or mixtures which must have at
least two corresponding wavelengths. This restriction can be overcome, since it is not necessary that the corresponding wavelengths
exist at the same time. Thus, corresponding wavelengths can be
produced artificially by changing the spectrum after adding a
suitable test substance or - if possible - by changing the pH,
oxygenation or oxidation of the substance.

Applying the last square method of Gauss the photometric
analysis of a multicomponent M-system can be erroneous if there is
an unknown component in the mixture (3,4). By drawing the transformation of the G-M-system to be analysed one observes that there
is no longer a one-to-one transformation (see Fig. 2). The deviation of the one-to-one transformation contains the information
about the unknown component. We tested this procedure with a mixture
of 80% HbO_2 and 20% Hb (Fig. 6, right side, top). Assuming that
only the HbO_2 spectrum was known we obtained a multibranched transformation showing that there was another unknown component. The
evaluation method produced the spectrum of this unknown component
(Fig. 6, right side, bottom) which can be easily identified as to
be the spectrum of Hb (left, bottom). After correcting this unknown
component the transformation function of the M-system is a straight
linge (left side, top), the steepness of which corresponds in the
zero point of the coordinate system to the relative concentration
of the unknown component.

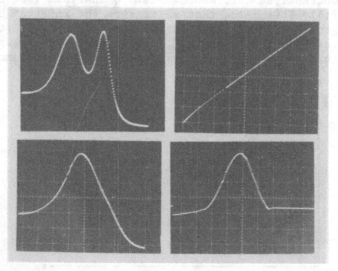

Fig. 6: Calculation of the spectrum of an unknown component by
        means of the Q-analysis

The latter method now can be applied to the HbO_2 spectrum of the skin $G(\lambda)$: the different branches show that there must be an unknown component. The spectrum of this component (Fig. 7) can be obtained similarly as the Hb-spectrum out of the 80% HbO_2 + 20% Hb spectrum.

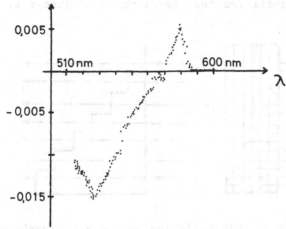

Fig. 7: Wavelength-dependent disturbance function of the human
        skin in vivo

We think that this spectrum represents the wavelength-dependent light scattering within the skin and the weak basic color of the skin.

After eliminating this component as a disturbance function we obtained the corrected spectrum $A(\lambda)$ which gives a one-to-one transformation (Fig. 8) and, thus, can be used as the basis for the quantitative analysis.

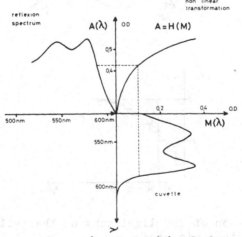

Fig. 8: Corrected transformation A = H(M) of the oxygenated human
        skin in vivo

    The second point was the inhomogeneous lightway. This can be
simulated by a staircase-shaped cell, partly filled with HbO_2
solution as shown in Fig. 9. The figure shows that the lightpaths
in reflexion are similar to those in the staircase cell. To quantify the distribution of the lightway within the probe, we can give
the different probabilities for the different lightpaths.

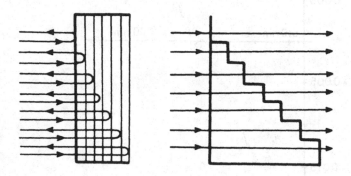

Fig. 9: Simulation of the reflexion by a staircase-shaped cell

In fig. 9 the probability for the seven different lightways is
equal and amounts to 1/7. Fig. 10 shows how the staircase cell
looks which simulated the lightpath distribution of the hemoglobin-
free perfused Guinea pig brain.

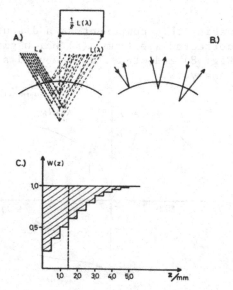

Fig. 10: Distribution of the lightpaths of the reflected light
       in the Guinea pig brain

In this case we have also to take into account that only the part $1/\gamma$ of the incident light reaches the photomultiplier (Fig. 10/A). Fig. 10/B demonstrates the different reflexion conditions. As it was shown, the staircase cell gave a one-to-one transformation, thus, the Q-analysis can be applied to these systems, too. The actual form of the transformation depends on the distribution of the probability of the different lightways. The transformation allows for calculating the lightway within the probe as well as the average lightway (6).

As an example of the new evaluation method, I would like to show the reflexion spectrum of a Hb-free perfused and reduced Guinea pig brain (Figure 11). You can see the cytochrome $a+a_3$ peak (605 nm) the cytochrome c (551 nm) peak and the cytochrome b shoulder. The other spectrum is calculated by just using the librarian spectra of cytochrome $a+a_3$, c, and b, and the transformation. The only deviation concerns the peak of cytochrome c, probably since we did not take into account cytochrome c_1.

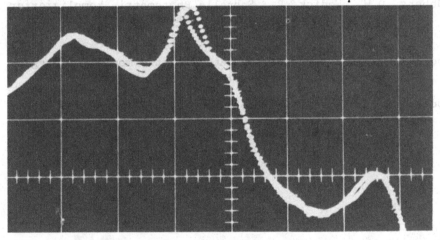

Fig. 11: Measured and calculated reflexion spectrum of a hemoglobin-free perfused, desoxygenated guinea pig brain

Summarizing we have shown that there are invariants against distributional and lightpath inhomogeneities which are independent of the total concentration changes, but dependent on the relative concentrations. Thus, they can be used as Q-analysis for quantitative reflexion spectrofotometry.

At the end, I would like to mention the limit of the just explained method. We have dealt only with systems where we have several different compartments but filled with the same colored substance. In reality, different substances may coexist in the different compartments. In his paper R. Wodick (5) will show how we think we can also deal with such more complicated systems.

REFERENCES

1. Duysens, L.N.M.: The flattening of the absorption spectrum of suspensions as compared to that of solutions. Biochem. Biophys. Acta 19, 1-11 (1956).

2. Lübbers, D.W., Niesel, W.: Der Kurzzeit-Spektralanalysator, ein schnell arbeitendes Spektralphotometer zur laufenden Messung von Absorptions- bzw. Extinktionsspektren. Pflügers Arch. 268, 286-295 (1959).

3. Lübbers, D.W., Wodick, R.: The examination of multicomponent system in biological materials by means of a rapid scanning photometer. Appl. Optics 8, 1055-1062 (1969).

4. Lübbers, D.W., Wodick, R.: Schnelle Photometrie komplizierter biochemischer Mehrkomponentensysteme. Z. Anal. Chem. 261, 271-280 (1972).

5. Wodick, R.: Stochastic versus deterministic models of oxygen transport in the microcirculation. This book

6. Wodick, R., Lübbers, D.W.: Methoden zur Bestimmung des Lichtweges bei der Photometrie trüber Lösungen oder Gewebe mit durchfallendem oder reflektiertem Licht. Pflügers Arch., in press.

A NEW HISTOCHEMICAL STAIN FOR INTRACELLULAR OXYGEN

I. S. Longmuir and J. A. Knopp

Department of Biochemistry, North Carolina State Univer-

sity, Raleigh, N. C. 27607 U. S. A.

The observation of Vaughan and Weber[1] that oxygen concentrations in the physiological range would quench the fluorescence of pyrenebutyric acid in solution suggested to us that this principle might be used to measure intracellular P_{O_2}. Such a technique could eliminate the disadvantages encountered with techniques using electrodes, namely tissue damage and alteration of oxygen tensions by consumption of oxygen, providing that the following criteria could be fulfilled: (a) Penetration of the fluorescent probe into the cell. (b) Absence of metabolic damage as determined by respiration rate. (c) The quenching of the fluorescence of the intracellular probe by oxygen should occur according to a known relationship, preferably Stern-Volmer[2].

To obtain absolute values directly, the following criteria are also necessary: (d) The probe be uniformly distributed within the cell. (c) The probe have a known quenching constant for oxygen, preferably the same in the sample as outside.

We have tested these criteria by studying the applications of solutions containing pyrenebutyric acid on isolated rat liver cells, prepared as described previously[3]. A preliminary report of this work has been presented earlier[4,6].

The first criterion was tested by exposing rat liver cells to various concentrations of pyrenebutyric acid in 0.1 M potassium phosphate buffer, pH 7.4. After varying periods of time, the cells were spun down and disrupted, and the concentrations of the probe were measured spectrophotometrically, using ε at 342 nm of $4.04 \cdot 10^4$ (ref. 5). We found that the cells took up the maximum concentration

of the probe more rapidly than they could be separated by centrifugation from the pyrenebutyric acid solution. The concentrations
found within the cells were approximately 200 times that in the ambient solutions. The range of concentrations found within the cells
was 0.04 to 4.0 mM.

The second criterion was tested by measuring the effect of various intracellular concentrations, measured after disrupting the
cells, on the respiration rate. These rates were determined by following the P_{O_2} *versus* time in a closed system[3]. We found that in
the presence of intracellular concentrations up to 0.8 mM pyrenebutyric acid, there was no diminution in respiration rate. Since this
concentration would be adequate for fluorescence measurements, we
studied none higher.

We tested the third criterion by measuring with an Aminco-Bowmen
spectrofluorimeter the fluorescence intensities of a suspension of
cells in a pyrenebutyric acid solution at different oxygen concentrations as measured by a Clark electrode. As expected from the distribution constant between free and intracellular pyrenebutyric acid,
essentially all of the fluorescence intensity is due to intracellular pyrenebutyric acid. Because rat liver cells respire linearly to
below 2 Torr[3], we do not expect differences of P_{O_2} between inside
and outside the cells greater than 2 Torr. Therefore, these experiments give us the intracellular oxygen quenching relationship. Specifically, we found a linear relationship between the reciprocal of
the fluorescence intensity and the oxygen concentration from 0 to
700 Torr in P_{O_2}, *i. e*. Stern-Volmer quenching. Furthermore, the
quenching constants as derived from these plots showed little difference between intracellular pyrenebutyric acid and pyrenebutyric
acid solutions containing no liver cells.

The question of homogeneity of probe distribution was examined
with a Leitz fluorescence microscope using top illumination. It was
found that the distribution was far from uniform. The nuclei apparently took up little dye, no more than fourteen times the concentration of that in the suspending fluid. Other structures took up a
great deal, as much as eight hundred times the ambient concentration.
Studies on isolated cell organelles, nuclei, mitochondria, micro-
somes, showed that those structures which take up the probe avidly
showed some diminution in quenching constant; a reduction in the
slope of the Stern-Volmer plot. This seemed at first to complicate
the problem of calibration since it now appears it will be necessary
either to calibrate the method at each point to be examined or to
make measurements of lifetime of fluorescence rather than simple
intensity. However, it does offer the possibility of a three-
dimensional approach to the problem, at least for those points showing high intensity.

In all methods of oxygen measurement, the question arises as to which parameter of oxygen is being measured, concentration or partial pressure. In the case of polarographic electrodes, Longmuir and Allen[7] have shown that the parameter is partial pressure; and we speculated that it might be this same parameter measured with this new method. We, therefore, applied the method of Longmuir and Allen[7] to this question and found that the quenching of the fluorescence of pyrenebutyric acid is a function of oxygen concentration in aqueous solutions. We also found that under certain circumstances, in non-aqueous solutions quenching was a function of partial pressure.

SUMMARY

We have examined pyrenebutyric acid as a possible fluorescent probe to determine intracellular concentrations of oxygen. Isolated rat liver cells rapidly take up pyrenebutyric acid, and the fluorescence of the cells is quenched by oxygen to a similar extent as is free pyrenebutyric acid. Therefore, this technique appears to be applicable to the physiological range of oxygen concentrations.

This work was supported in part by the following funds: Grant No. GM 19358-01 from the National Institutes of Health, Grant No. HE 10328-04 from the National Institutes of Health, and Projects No. 3319 and 3320 from the Agricultural Experiment Station of North Carolina State University.

REFERENCES

1. W. M. Vaughan and G. Weber, *Biochemistry*, 9 (1970) 464.
2. O. Stern and M. Volmer, *Z. Phys.*, 20 (1919) 183.
3. I. S. Longmuir, *Biochem. J.*, 64 (1957) 378.
4. I. S. Longmuir and J. A. Knopp, *Fed. Proc.*, 31 (1972) 365.
5. J. Knopp and G. Weber, *J. Biol. Chem.*, 242 (1967) 1353.
6. J. Knopp and I. S. Longmuir, *Biochim. Biophys. Acta*, 279 (1972) 393.
7. I. S. Longmuir and F. Allen, *J. Polarograph. Soc.*, VIII (1961) 63.

ANALYSIS OF GAS TRANSPORT IN LUNGLESS AND GILL-LESS

SALAMANDERS USING INERT GAS WASHOUT TECHNIQUES

Randall Neal Gatz and Johannes Piiper

Department of Physiology, Max-Planck-Institute

of Experimental Medicine, Goettingen, W. Germany

Most respiratory studies on intact vertebrate animals are concerned with the functional properties of the special respiratory organs-lungs or gills. We have become interested in the respiratory problems of a vertebrate animal which has neither lungs nor gills. Consequently all gas exchange occurs across the skin in the absence of a specialized ventilatory mechanism. This situation is found in the members of the amphibian family Plethodontidae (Wilder, 1894). We chose the species Desmognathus fuscus to characterize the relative roles of diffusion and circulatory convection in gas transport to tissues.

MATERIALS AND METHODS

Adult specimens of Desmognathus fuscus ranging in weight from 4. 1 to 7. 0 g (average weight 5. 8 g) were purchased from an animal dealer and shipped to the laboratory. The animals were housed in two large glass tanks partially submerged in a circulating water bath thermostated at 13°C. The animals were fed live mealworms and allowed a minimum of two weeks for acclimatization.

In order to characterize the roles of diffusion and circulatory convective transport, the washout kinetics of an inert gas (Freon 22 or acetylene) was measured from both alive and

dead animals. Specimens of <u>Desmognathus</u> <u>fuscus</u> were equilibrated in a filter-beaker with either 20% Freon 22 and 80%
oxygen or 30% acetylene and 70% oxygen (Figure 1).

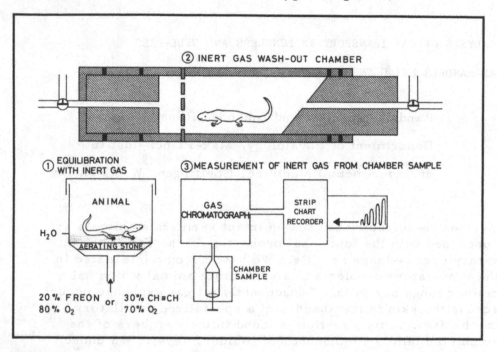

Figure 1. Experimental procedure for measurement of inert
gas washout from <u>Desmognathus</u> <u>fuscus</u>. The animals were
equilibrated with the inert gas mixture in a filter-beaker.
Thereafter, they were quickly transferred to a chamber designed for gas sampling. The gas samples were analyzed for
amount of inert gas in a gas chromatograph and the results
recorded on a strip-chart recorder.

Therefore, they were quickly transferred to a chamber designed
for the withdrawal of gas samples. Samples of the chamber gas
were withdrawn every ten minutes and the chamber was flushed
with air after each sample. The gas samples were analyzed for
inert gas concentration in a gas chromatograph and introduced
into the gas chromatograph via a modification of the Van-Slyke
manometric gas analysis apparatus according to Farhi <u>et</u> <u>al.</u>
(1966).

RESULTS

A semi-logarithmic plot of amount of inert gas remaining in
the alive or dead animal is plotted versus time in Figure 2. The
washout curve from the dead animal is a compound exponential
having a dominant slow component accounting for about 70% of
the total amount of gas contained in the dead animal. The rate
constant of the slow component from the dead animal is 0.0175/
min. It was assumed that this transfer rate was due solely to
diffusion from the body of the dead animal. The washout from
the alive animal is also a compound exponential having a dominant slow component with a rate constant of 0.046/min. It was
assumed that the transfer of inert gas out of the alive animal was
due to diffusion from the body and circulatory convection acting

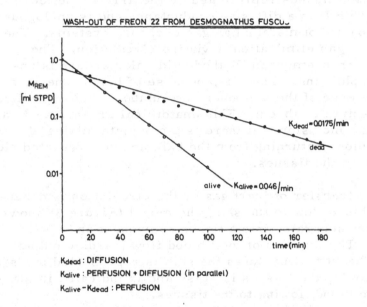

Figure 2. A semilogarithmic plot of the amount of inert gas
remaining in the animal plotted versus time in minutes. The
rate constant of the washout from the dead animal is assumed
to be due to diffusion alone. The rate constant from the alive
animal is assumed to be due to diffusion and circulatory convection in parallel.

in parallel. In order to evaluate the role of circulation the diffusive component (k_{dead} = diffusive transfer rate) is subtracted from the rate constant from the alive animal (k_{alive} = $k_{diffusion}$ + $k_{circulation}$).

MODEL AND DISCUSSION

A model of the tissues and the circulation in <u>Desmognathus fuscus</u> is shown in Figure 3. The tissues are represented by a volume V, where the amount of inert gas contained in the tissues is dependent on the solubility of the inert gas, α , the partial pressure of the gas, P, and the volume of the tissues, V. There are two parallel routes shown for the elimination of the inert gas contained in the tissues. The first is direct diffusion from the tissues represented by the arrow labelled D in Figure 3. This D is a diffusive conductance and is analogous to diffusion capacity of mammalian gas exchange systems. The other route of gas elimination is via the circulation. The circulatory arrangement in Plethodontid salamanders is unusual for amphibians. There is, because of lunglessness, a complete absence of the pulmonary circulation. Subsequently, the atrial septum is absent. This anatomical arrangement has led us to the conclusion that there is a complete mixing of oxygenated blood returning from the skin and deoxygenated blood returning from the tissues.

Since the transfer of inert gas by the circulation is dependent on the blood flow to the skin, the model (Figure 3) shows the blood flow separated into a tissue component and a skin component. The fraction of total blood flow (cardiac output) through the heart that perfuses the skin is represented by "s". The blood flow to the tissues is "1-s" and is indicated in the model as the blood flowing to the tissues.

It can be shown that the rate constants for both the circulatory and diffusive transfer of inert gas are conductance to capacitance ratios and are shown in the equations at the bottom of Figure 3. Utilizing the experimentally determined rate constants from the inert gas washout a diffusive conductance (diffusion capacity) for Freon 22 can be calculated as $24 \cdot 10^{-6}$ ml/(min$\cdot$torr$\cdot$g).

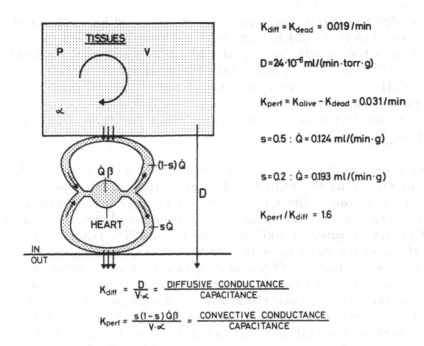

$K_{diff} = K_{dead} = 0.019\,/min$

$D = 24 \cdot 10^{-6}\,ml\,/(min \cdot torr \cdot g)$

$K_{perf} = K_{alive} - K_{dead} = 0.031\,/min$

$s = 0.5 : \dot{Q} = 0.124\,ml\,/(min \cdot g)$

$s = 0.2 : \dot{Q} = 0.193\,ml\,/(min \cdot g)$

$K_{perf} / K_{diff} = 1.6$

$$K_{diff} = \frac{D}{V \cdot \alpha} = \frac{\text{DIFFUSIVE CONDUCTANCE}}{\text{CAPACITANCE}}$$

$$K_{perf} = \frac{s(1-s)\dot{Q}\beta}{V \cdot \alpha} = \frac{\text{CONVECTIVE CONDUCTANCE}}{\text{CAPACITANCE}}$$

Figure 3. A model of the gas transport system of Desmognathus fuscus. The box represents the tissues of the animal containing a quantity of substance M, dependent on the partial pressure P, the solubility of the substance within the tissue compartment α, and the volume of the tissue V. The elimination of the substance may follow two paths: 1) M may diffuse directly out of the tissue in accordance with the diffusion parameter D, here termed the diffusive conductance or 2) it may be transported out of the animal via circulatory convection - here represented by the convective conductance. The circulatory arrangement is unusualy in lungless salamanders. Since there is no pulmonary circulation the blood flow may be divided simply into that fraction of the cardiac output perfusing the tissues and that fraction perfusing the skin. The fraction of blood flow perfusing the skin is here represented by the variable "s". Where $s \cdot Q$ is the blood flow to the skin and $(1-s)Q$ is the blood flow to the tissues. The diffusive rate constant (k_{diff}) is interpreted as a diffusive conductance to capacitance ratio and the transport due to circulatory convection is interpreted as a convective conductance to capacitance ratio. Assuming a fractional distribution of blood flow to the skin of 50% of the cardiac output, the blood flow through the heart or cardiac output needed to explain the washout curves could be calculated and was found to be 0.124 ml/(min·g). Assuming a skin blood flow of 20% of the cardiac output the blood flow through the heart must be 0.193 ml/(min·g) to explain the washout of inert gas. The convective to diffusive conductance ratio (k_{perf}/k_{diff}) = 1.6 indicating an approximately equal role of diffusion and circulatory convection in the elimination of an inert gas from <u>Desmognathus fuscus</u>.

Since these animals lack a pulmocutaneous artery, which is the vessel supplying the skin in other amphibians, the measurement of the fraction of the cardiac output perfusing the skin is difficult. Based on measurements of cutaneous blood flow measured directly in other amphibians (Shelton, 1970) fractional distributions of the cardiac output to the skin were assumed at upper and lower limits of 50% and 20% respectively. When the cardiac output required to explain the washout rate constants based on these assumed distributions is calculated the values are 0.124 ml/(min·g) for a distribution of 50% of the cardiac output to perfuse the skin and 0.193 ml/(min·g) for a distribution of 20% of the cardiac output to perfuse the skin. Both of these are in agreement with estimates of the cardiac output made by observing the volume of blood ejected with each cardiac contraction into a horizontal pipette inserted into the conus arteriosus (0.176 ml/(min·g).

The relative roles of diffusion and convection in the elimination of Freon 22 are assessed by the ratio of the rate constants for perfusion and diffusion. The ratio of the rate constants are a convective to diffusive conductance ratio and for Freon 22 is 1.6. This indicates an approximately equal role of diffusion and circulatory convection in the elimination of Freon 22 from <u>Desmognathus fuscus</u>.

In Figure 4 the analysis of oxygen transfer in the model proposed for the analysis of inert gas washout is shown. The circulatory arrangement is the same as the inert gas model but the symbols here indicate the oxygen content of the blood returning from the skin (C_a^-), and returning from the tissues (C_v^-). Because of the small size of the animal the direct measurement of these oxygen contents is difficult. However, because of the anatomical arrangement of the vessels, the blood in the heart was considered

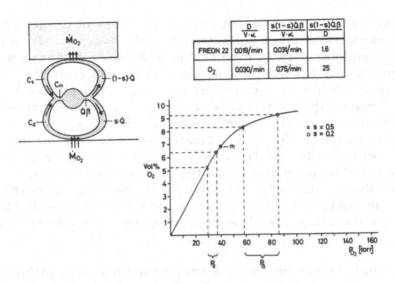

Figure 4. The analysis of oxygen transport in <u>Desmognathus</u> <u>fuscus</u> from inert gas washout. The model of the circulation is the same as the model proposed for the washout of Freon 22 except the concentrations of oxygen in blood are noted. The circulatory and gas exchange arrangement divides the blood into three categories according to the oxygen content. $C_{\bar{v}}$ is the oxygen content in the blood returning from the tissues. $C_{\bar{a}}$ is the oxygen content in the blood returning from the skin. C_m is the blood that results from the mixing of blood returning from the tissues and blood returning from the skin. From the direct measurement of partial pressure of oxygen in mixed blood (denoted by the solid black point on the oxygen-hemoglobin dissociation curve) and from assuming a skin-tissue blood flow distribution of 50% and 20% of the cardiac output to perfuse the skin the oxygen contents of blood returning from the skin and blood returning from the tissues can be estimated. Depending on the distribution chosen the partial pressure of oxygen in blood returning from the tissues ranges from 30 to 38 torr and from the skin ranges from 59 to 87 torr. From the experimentally determined washout curves for Freon 22 it is shown that the convective to diffusive conductance ratio for Freon 22 is 1.6. By substituting the correct physical constants for oxygen into this ratio the convective to diffusive conductance ratio for oxygen can be calculated as 25. This value indicates a major role of circulatory convection in the transport of oxygen to tissues in <u>Desmognathus</u> <u>fuscus</u>.

to be mixed sample. From the partial pressure of oxygen measured in samples of blood collected from the heart and from the oxygen hemoglobin dissociation curve, the values for oxygen partial pressures and contents of blood returning from the tissues and from the skin can be estimated. The estimated ranges shown on the partial pressure axis of the dissociation curve (Figure 4) are estimated assuming a 50% distribution of the cardiac output to the skin (indicated by "x" on the dissociation curve) and a 20% distribution of the cardiac output to the skin (indicated by open circles on the dissociation curve). Assuming these ranges for skin blood flow the range of partial pressure for oxygen in blood returning from the tissues is 30 to 38 torr and the range for blood returning from the skin is 59 to 87 torr.

The tabular inset in Figure 4 shows the measured diffusive conductance to capacitance ratio for Freon 22 in column 1. The convective conductance to capacitance ratio for Freon 22 is shown in column 2. The convective to diffusive conductance ratio for Freon 22 is shown in column 3. From the tissue solubility of oxygen and the diffusion coefficient for oxygen in tissue, the diffusive conductance to capacitance and the convective conductance to capacitance ratio can be estimated. From these ratios the convective to diffusive conductance ratios for oxygen in Desmognathus fuscus is estimated to be 25. This implies that about 96% of the oxygen is transported to the tissues by circulatory convection where about 4% is delivered to the tissues by direct diffusion to the tissues.

Wilder, H. H. (1894). Anat. Anz. 9: 216-220.

Farhi, L. E., A. W. T. Edwards and T. Homma (1963). J. Appl. Physiol. 18 (1): 97-106.

Shelton, G. (1970). Respir. Physiol. 9: 183-196.

MEASUREMENT OF TISSUE GAS LEVELS WITH A MASS SPECTRO-METER

William E. Donovan and Bert Myers

Department of Surg., LSU Med. School and the Surg.

Res. Lab. Vet. Admin. Hosp., New Orleans, LA.

The measurement of oxygen levels in tissue is a difficult task. Polarographic electrodes are not suited for determining the mean tissue gas partial pressures of tissue masses larger than a few cubic mm. The delicacy of electrodes also interferes with their use in clinical situations. A new instrument, the medical mass spectro-meter, offers opportunities for a more reliable, consistent measure-ment of tissue gas levels in vivo. This machine is specifically de-signed to quantitate gases with molecular weights ranging from 10 to 60 amu (atomic mass units) and to display these gas levels in terms of partial pressures.

In our studies gas levels of oxygen, carbon dioxide, and nitrogen were measured in the subcutaneous tissue of rabbits, swine, and humans.

MATERIALS AND METHODS

The principle of operation of the mass spectrometer is not compli-cated. Figure 1 shows a diagram of the essential structures of the mass spectrometer. Gas is drawn into the machine by a vacuum and ionized by a 2000v electron beam. The ionized gas sample is accel-erated past a magnetic field which changes the direction of the gas according to the mass of the individual gas molecules. Thus the gases of different molecular weights strike different targets and are elec-tronically counted.

The actual sampling part of the mass spectrometer consists of

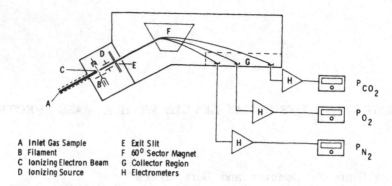

A Inlet Gas Sample   E Exit Slit
B Filament   F 60° Sector Magnet
C Ionizing Electron Beam   G Collector Region
D Ionizing Source   H Electrometers

Figure 1. Magnetic mass spectrometer.

a 6-foot cannula of Teflon coated stainless steel tubing leading from
the inlet of the ionization chamber of the machine to the connector to
which the sampling catheter is attached.   A catheter, one for each
of the two sampling parts of the machine, consists of a 22 gauge
stainless steel tube with the distal 1.5 cm perforated and the entire
tube covered with either Teflon or Silastic.   The proximal end of the
catheter is open and attaches to the cannula through airtight O-ring
fittings.   The plastic coating of the catheter adheres to the surface
of the catheter except at the distal tip where it forms a bubble
around the perforations.   Gas samples are drawn through the plastic
by the 10^{-6}mm Hg vacuum produced by the machine.

Two types of catheters are available.   Those with Silastic coat-
ings are used for blood gas determinations, but not for tissue as the
extreme permeability of Silastic would cause a rapid depletion of
gases in tissue.   Teflon-coated catheters have a much lower permeability and hence require lower flow rates for calibration or measurement of tissue gas tensions.   Since the Teflon catheter extracts a
smaller sample in a given time the response time of the Teflon catheter is much slower, 2-3 minutes for a 90% step change as compared
to 40 sec. in Silastic catheters.

The mass spectrometer is zeroed electronically before the calibration process.   The catheters are zeroed before calibrations by
placing them in two gases which do not contain respectively oxygen
and carbon dioxide or nitrogen.   That is, oxygen and carbon dioxide

controls are zeroed in nitrogen gas and the nitrogen readout zeroed
in oxygen gas.

Calibrations of both types of catheters is the same. Analyzed
gas mixtures identical to those used in commercial blood gas determination instruments are bubbled through a tonometer at 37°C. The
catheter reading tips are placed in the tonometer for 30 minutes,
the time required for equilibrium to occur. The partial pressures
of the calibration gases at the ambient barometric pressure and
water vapor pressure are calculated and the machine set to display
the partial pressures of the calibration gas mixture. The emission
control regulates the degree of ionization of the gas sample and the
gain controls determine the amplification of the signal from the mass
spectrometer collector area. To calibrate the oxygen the gain is fixed
at a value of 250 and the emission controls used to display the proper
partial pressure of oxygen. The carbon dioxide and nitrogen gain controls are then adjusted to give the proper readings. Separate emission
controls for each inlet of the machine allow correction of any slight
permeability differences between the two catheters. The two inlets can
be operated one at a time or at an automatic cycling rate of 90 sec.

Experiments with humans require that the catheters be sterilized.
Before sterilization the catheters were calibrated as has been described and then placed in air and the oxygen and nitrogen values for the
catheters in air and their emission and gain calibration settings recorded. The catheters were then gas sterilized. At the time of use
the previously determined settings of the emission and gain controls
were reset on the machine and the values in air checked. The presence of sterilization gas had an adverse effect on the accuracy of
the catheters and it was necessary to allow the catheters to remain
unused for at least 72 hours to eliminate any traces of the gas. During the procedures with animals sterilization was not done; the catheters were merely wiped with an alcohol sponge.

Insertion of the mass spectrometer catheters was performed
under general anesthesia in animals and local in humans. The local,
1% lidocaine, was saturated with sterile nitrogen gas to prevent oxygen contamination of the tissue. A 16-gauge venipuncture needle clad
with a 14-gauge Teflon catheter was inserted into the tissue to be
measured. The central needle was removed and the sampling catheter inserted through the catheter. The exterior catheter was removed
and the mass spectrometer catheter sutured or taped in place. Tissue
gas partial pressure readings were taken while the subject breathed

either room air or 99% oxygen by mask.   Rabbits were measured
while awake in a restrainer cage as well as under anesthesia.

RESULTS

With Teflon catheters the values did not show a depletion of
tissue gases over a period of three days.   Stabile readings could be
obtained in rabbits and pigs after an initial period of evacuation of
the catheter lines and equilibration with the tissue.   The average
time for this equilibration was 30 minutes.   In humans the equilibration period was usually between 30 and 60 minutes.

In rabbits readings were taken while the animals were awake or
under general anesthesia.   It was found that the tissue gas tensions
under general anesthesia were less variable with a smaller frequency
and magnitude of change in one sample area and a closer correlation
between two simultaneously measured areas.

The depth of anesthesia, especially in rabbits could be judged by
the tissue gas levels.   Deepening the level tended to lower PO_2 and
raise PCO_2, generally without any change in blood gases.

The values obtained for subcutaneous tissue gas levels in rabbits,
swine, and humans breathing either room air or 99% oxygen by mask
are in Figure 2.

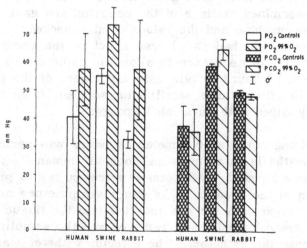

Figure 2. Effect of 99% oxygen breathing on subcutaneous tissue
         gas levels.

DISCUSSION

Although the area of tissue being measured cannot be called normal because of the wound required to insert the catheter, the trauma
to the area was minimal.   There was very little wound dead space
since the catheter filled the entire volume of the defect caused by the
14 ga. intercath.   Readings did not show any drop in PO_2 values after
three days to below 10 mm Hg as had been reported by Hunt.   This
indicates that the values obtained were true tissue readings rather than
those of wounds.   Breathing oxygen consistently led to a rise in PO_2,
whereas wounds show little or no change under similar circumstances.

Sudden loud noises resulted in a sharp drop in PO_2 and rise in
PCO_2 in unanesthetized rabbits, a transient effect previously reported
by Silver.   The changes under anesthesia indicate that tissue gas tensions may be useful clinically in determining depth of anesthesia in
patients under halothane or other agents which mask the usual signs.

The medical mass spectrometer possesses unique advantages for
measuring tissue gas partial pressures of a relatively large block of
tissue.   Polarographic electrodes for in vivo tissue gas level determinations limit the sample area to as little as 1-5 microns.   Large
variations, up to 60 mm Hg can be caused by microscopic movements
of the sampling device.   For this reason the fact has been stressed that
individual readings of the micro-electrodes are extremely variable and
that an oxygen tension field and oxygen tension gradient must be measured to obtain a true picture of the activities and state of the tissue.
The resultant oxygen tension distribution curves indicate the condition
of the tissue (Lubbers).   On the other hand the catheter tip of the mass
spectrometer has as a sampling area a cylinder 2 cm long and 1-2 mm
in diameter and thus indicates the average tissue gas partial pressure
of an area much larger than that which can be measured even with
numerous micro-electrode readings.

The stability of the mass spectrometer system is such that catheters used for extended experiments of 2 to 5 days have shown only a 2%
error upon recalibration.   The capability of measuring two separate
areas almost simultaneously with essentially identical sampling devices
provides the researcher with a close to ideal control measurement during experimental studies.   The catheters may be calibrated, sterilized,
and the calibration settings recorded for later use.   This plus their
sturdiness make them more suitable than polarigraphic electrodes for
animal use.   For example, intramyocardial PO_2 and PCO_2 have been

measured during coronary artery bypass operations in humans. Continuous readings for several days in experimental animals are possible since the animals need only be moderately restrained, not anesthetized.

Aside from the initial high purchase price of the system, the medical mass spectrometer has only a few minor disadvantages. Although the machine is simple to operate, trouble shooting any problem which occurs and performing some of the routine maintenance requires an elementary background in electronics. The electronics of the machine requires a stabile source of power within strict limits which electrical wiring in some older buildings may not meet. The machine must also operate constantly to maintain the necessary vacuum. It is never totally shut off except to move it to a different location or for repairs. While in operation the machine can develop small leaks in one of the two channels or both. If the leak is in both channels the vacuum gauge of the machine is usually adequate for diagnosing the problem. When only one channel has a slight leak the nitrogen readout shows a rise with the change in vacuum. Unexpected PO_2 and PCO_2 readings may be shown to be due to leakage when PN_2 values indicate a PN_2 of greater than 500 mm Hg.

SUMMARY

The medical mass spectrometer has proven to be a useful tool for the measurement of gas partial pressures in vivo at a tissue level. It is a quick, accurate method which will no doubt become more widely used in the future as more investigators become aware of its capabilities and possible applications.

References
1.   Davies, P.W. The oxygen cathode. In Ed. W.L. Nastuk. Physical Techniques in Biol. Res. Vol 4, pp. 137-179. Academic Press, NY, '62.
2.   Hunt, T.K., Zederfeld, B., Goldstick, T.K. Oxygen and Healing. Amer. J. Surg. Vol 118, Oct. '69; 521-525.
3.   Silver, I.A. The measurement of oxygen tension in healing tissue. Int. Sym. on Oxygen Pressure Recording Progr. Resp. Res. Vol 3, '69; 125-135.
4.   Lubbers, D.W. The meaning of the tissue oxygen distribution curve and its measurement by means of Pt electrodes. Int. Sym. on Oxygen Pressure Recording Prog. Resp. Res. Vol 3, pp 112-123, 1969.

ANALYSIS OF DIFFUSION LIMITATIONS ON A CATHETER

IMBEDDED IN BODY TISSUES

Robert D. Walker, Jr. and Yasar Tanrikut

Department of Chemical Engineering, University of

Florida, Gainesville, Florida, U.S.A.

INTRODUCTION

Accurate in vivo measurement of dissolved gases in body fluids and tissues has been a goal of biomedical research for many years. Until recently this search had been attended with relatively little success. Recently, however, Folkman and co-workers (1967) demonstrated that a catheter made of Medical Silastic could measure dissolved blood gases in vivo. Unfortunately, the size of the catheter required surgical insertion. Ernst and O'Steen (1970) developed a catheter of the same material which could be inserted through a 14 gauge hypodermic needle, and they showed that it could be used for in vivo monitoring of blood gases. These investigators also reported measurements taken after insertion into the peritoneal cavity of a dog and one of their observations of particular interest was that the partial pressure of oxygen in the peritoneal cavity declined from 110 mm Hg to 7 mm in 5 minutes when the dog was changed from breathing air to breathing pure nitrogen. It is of interest to inquire as to how much of the time lag they observed was due to equilibration in the tissues and how much was due to the mass transfer resistance of the catheter wall.

It is possible to consider two cases which may represent extremes likely to be encountered in in vivo gas measurements with such a catheter, namely, a catheter inserted in the lumen of a vein, and a catheter imbedded in tissue. We have considered the latter case in this paper.

Krogh (1918, 1959) showed that the capillaries in muscle tissue were fairly uniformly distributed throughout the tissue and that

73

they were generally parallel to the muscle fibers. Thus, he concluded that muscle tissue could be represented by a coaxial cylinder
of muscle fibers surrounding a capillary. He further estimated the
average diameter of the muscle fiber cylinder by dividing the transverse area of a section by the number of capillaries contained there-
in. The capillaries themselves were found to be 8-10 microns in
diameter and about one mm in length (Krogh, 1918; Wright, 1934).

MATHEMATICAL MODEL

We shall accept Krogh's basic view of muscle tissue and consider
an imbedded catheter as shown in Figure 1, where a ring of muscle
fiber bundles--each bundle containing a centrally-located capillary--
surrounds the catheter. However, to simplify the model further, we
shall consider that a solid ring of tissue divided into trapezoidal
sections, surrounds the catheter, and we shall approximate the fiber
bundles by calculating the dimensions of an equivalent square.

The radius of the fiber bundle can be calculated from the blood
perfusion rate and transit time by

$$R_b = R_{cap} \left[\frac{1 + xt}{xt} \right]^{1/2} \tag{1}$$

where R_b = radius of fiber bundle served by capillary, cm

R_{cap} = radius of capillary, cm

x = blood perfusion rate, cm^3 blood/cm^3 tissue - sec.

t = blood transit time, sec.

Muscle tissue perfusion rates are reported to be 2-5 ml blood per
100 ml tissue per min. and blood transit times are reported to be
about one second (Papper and Kitz, 1963). Substitution of these
values into Equation 1 leads to a fiber bundle radius of 180 microns.
(For R_{cap} = 4 microns, and x = 3 ml/100 ml - min.), and the side
of the equivalent square is 320 microns. ($\pi R^2_b = D^2$).

In order to model the process we make the following assumptions:

(1) The properties of the tissue are not changed by insertion of a
     catheter.

(2) Fiber bundles--each with a centrally-located capillary--are
     uniformly arranged around the catheter.

(3) Owing to their thinness, the diffusional resistance of the cell
     and capillary walls is negligible.

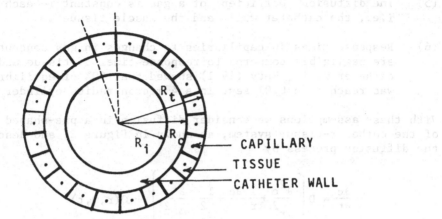

Figure 1:   Schematic Diagram of Catheter Surrounded
             by Muscle Fiber Bundles.

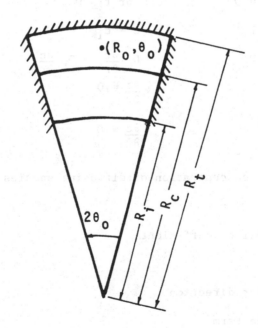

Figure 2:   Section of Catheter-Tissue System Used for Model

(4)   No axial concentration gradient in the capillaries.

(5)   The diffusion coefficient of a gas is constant in each phase, i.e., the catheter wall, and the muscle tissue.

(6)   Response times in capillaries to changes in gas concentration are negligible compared to response times of tissue and the catheter wall. Kety (1951) showed that 90% of equilibrium was reached in 0.01 sec. in a 4 micron radius cylinder of blood.

With these assumptions we consider diffusion in a pie-shaped section of the catheter-tissue system, as shown in Figure 2, and describe the diffusion process by

$$\frac{\partial c}{\partial t} = D\left[\frac{\partial^2 c}{\partial r^2} + \frac{1}{r}\frac{\partial c}{\partial r} + \frac{1}{r^2}\frac{\partial^2 c}{\partial \Theta^2}\right] + Q(r,\Theta,t) \qquad (2)$$

with the following initial and boundary conditions:

I.C.: $c = c_i = 0$ for $t \leq 0$ all r,Θ

B.C.1:   at $r = R_i$ $c = c_i$ $t > 0$

B.C.2:   at $r = R_c$ $D_c\frac{\partial c}{\partial r} = D_t\frac{\partial c}{\partial r}$ all t

B.C.3:   at $r = R_t$ $\frac{\partial c}{\partial r} = 0$ all t

B.C.4:   at $\Theta = 0$

          $\Theta = 2\Theta_o$ $\frac{\partial c}{\partial \Theta} = 0$ all t

where c = local concentration of diffusing species

       t = time

       D = diffusion coefficient

       r = radius

       Θ = angular direction

       Q = source term

       Subscripts i,c, and t refer to catheter lumen, catheter wall, and tissue ring, respectively.

We assume that the source term can be represented by a point source located at $r = R_o$, $\Theta = \Theta_o$ which is given a constant value, Q_o, at t = 0 so that Equation 2 becomes

$$\frac{\partial c}{\partial t} = D\left[\frac{\partial^2 c}{\partial r^2} + \frac{1}{r}\frac{\partial c}{\partial r} + \frac{1}{r^2}\frac{\partial^2 c}{\partial \Theta^2}\right] + Q_o q(r - R_o)q(\Theta - \Theta_o) \qquad (3)$$

where $q(r - R_o)$ and $q(\Theta - \Theta_o)$ are impulse functions of r and Θ, respectively, with the properties

$$q(x) = \begin{array}{l} 0 \text{ for } x \neq 0 \\ 1 \text{ for } x = 0 \end{array}$$

We let $c(r,\Theta, t) = \bar{c}(r,\Theta, t) + Q(r,\Theta)$. Then, if a series solution for $\bar{c}$ and $Q(r,\Theta)$ is assumed,

$$\bar{c} = \sum_n \sum_m B_{n,m}(t)\phi_{n,m}(r,\Theta) \qquad (4)$$

$$Q = \sum_n \sum_m E_{n,m} \phi_{n,m}(r,\Theta) \qquad (5)$$

where B(t) is a function of time, $E_{n,m}$ is a constant, and $\phi(r,\Theta)$ is a function of r and Θ and is the solution of the Hemholtz equation with the boundary conditions on c

$$D\nabla^2\phi(r,\Theta) + \beta^2\phi(r,\Theta) = 0 \qquad (6)$$

where β is a constant (eigenvalues of the Helmholtz equation). We assume that $\phi(r,\Theta)$ can be represented by the product of functions of r and Θ, respectively, such that

$$\phi(r,\Theta) = \tau(r)\psi(\Theta) \qquad (7)$$

where τ is a function of r only, and ψ a function of Θ only. Then Equation 6 yields

$$r^2\tau'' + r\tau' + \left[\frac{\beta^2 r^2}{D} - \alpha^2\right]\tau = 0 \qquad (8)$$

with the boundary conditions

at $r = R_t$ $\qquad \frac{d\tau_t}{dr} = 0$

at $r = R_c$ $\qquad D_c\frac{d\tau_c}{dr} = D_t\frac{d\tau_t}{dr}$

$\tau_c\Big|_{r=R_c} = \tau_t\Big|_{r=R_c}$

$\tau_c\Big|_{r=R_i} = 0$

and $\qquad\qquad\qquad\qquad\qquad \psi'' + \alpha^2\psi = 0 \qquad (9)$

with the boundary conditions

at $\Theta = 0$

$$\frac{1}{r}\frac{d\psi}{d\Theta} = 0$$

$\Theta = 2\Theta_o$

The solutions to these equations are

$$c_t(r,\Theta,t) = \sum_{n}^{\infty} \sum_{m}^{\infty} (E_{n,m})_t \{1 + \frac{1}{\beta_m^2}[1 - \exp(-\beta_m^2 t)]\}\phi_{n,m}(r,\Theta)_t \cos\alpha_n$$

$$\text{for } R_c \le r \le R_t \qquad (10)$$

and

$$c_c(r,\Theta,t) = \sum_{n}^{\infty} \sum_{m}^{\infty} (E_{n,m})_c \{1 + \frac{1}{\beta_m^2}[1 - \exp(-\beta_m^2 t)]\}\phi_{n,m}(r,\Theta)_c \cos\alpha_n$$

$$\text{for } R_L \le r \le R_c \qquad (11)$$

Equations 10 and 11 are the equations for the transient concentration profiles in the tissue and catheter wall, respectively. The steady-state concentration profiles follow directly when we note that as

$t \to \infty \exp(-\beta_m^2 t) \to 0$ so that Equations 10 and 11 become

$$c_t(r,\Theta) = \sum_{n}^{\infty} \sum_{m}^{\infty} (E_{n,m})_t \left[1 + \frac{1}{\beta_m^2}\right]\phi_{n,m}(r,\Theta)_t \cos\alpha_n\Theta \qquad (12)$$

and

$$c_c(r,\Theta) = \sum_{n}^{\infty} \sum_{m}^{\infty} (E_{n,m})_c \left[1 + \frac{1}{\beta_m^2}\right]\phi_{n,m}(r,\Theta)_c \cos\alpha_n\Theta \qquad (13)$$

RESPONSE OF CATHETER IMBEDDED IN TISSUE

The response of a catheter can be determined from the transient concentration profiles. From Equations 11 and 12 it can be shown that

$$c_m = \frac{-4D_{ic}L}{G_{He}} \sum_{n=0}^{\infty} \sum_{m=1}^{\infty} B_m(t)\frac{\sin\alpha_n\Theta_0}{\alpha_n J_o(\beta_m R_i)} \qquad (14)$$

where c_m = gas concentration in helium stream from catheter lumen

D_{ic} = diffusivity of species i in catheter wall

L = catheter length available for diffusion

G_{He} = volumetric helium flow rate, the carrier gas in chromatographic analysis.

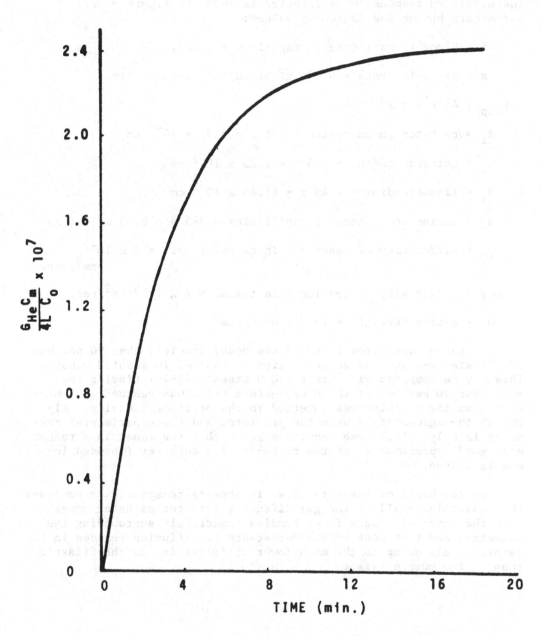

Figure 3. Plot of $\dfrac{G_{He}C_m}{4L\,C_o}$ versus time.

The predicted response of a catheter is shown in Figure 3 for parameters having the following values:

t = blood transit time in capillary = 1 sec.

x = perfusion rate = 0.03 cm^3 blood/cm^3 tissue - min.

R_{cap} = 4μ = 4×10^{-4} cm

R_i = catheter lumen radius = 571μ = 5.71×10^{-2} cm

R_c = catheter radius = 825μ = 8.25×10^{-2} cm

R_t = tissue radius = 1145μ = 11.45×10^{-2} cm

R_o = radius of centers of capillaries = 985μ = 9.85×10^{-2} cm

D_{ic} = diffusivity of species i in catheter wall = 2×10^{-7} cm^2/sec.

D_{it} = diffusivity of species i in tissue = 2×10^{-5} cm^2/sec.

Q_o = source strength = 10^{-3} g moles/cm^3

It can be seen from Figure 3 the model predicts that 90 percent of the steady-state gas concentration is reached in about 8 minutes. This may be compared with Ernst and O'Steen's (1970) finding that more than 90 percent of the steady-state value was reached in 5 minutes when the catheter was inserted in the peritoneal cavity. Although the agreement between the predicted and the experimental response is only fair, these results suggest that the model is a reasonably good approximation of the response of a catheter imbedded in muscle tissue.

On the basis of these results, it appears reasonable to conclude that essentially all of the gas diffusing into the catheter comes from the layer of muscle fiber bundles immediately surrounding the catheter, and that most of the resistance to diffusion resides in the catheter wall owing to the much lower diffusivities in the Silastic than in the muscle tissue.

BIBLIOGRAPHY

Ernest, E. A. and L. O'Steen. "Preliminary Evaluation of
In Vivo Peritoneal Gas Analysis Using Silastic Catheter
and Chromatography," Proc. Fed. of Am. Soc. Expt'l. Biol.,
29:1299 (1967).

Folkman, J., H. S. Winsey and B. Cohen. "Diffusion of Blood
Gases into an Intravascular Silicone Rubber Catheter: Rapid
Measurement of Anesthetic Level, PO_2 and P_{CO_2} Without Blood
Sample," Transactions of American Society for Artificial
Internal Organs, XIII:350-355 (1967).

Kety, Seymour S., "The Theory and Applications of the Exchange
of Inert Gas at the Lungs and Tissues," Pharmacological Reviews,
3:1-40 (1951).

Krogh, August, "The Number and Distribution of Capillaries in
Muscles with Calculations of the Oxygen Pressure Head Necessary
for Supplying the Tissue," J. of Physiology, 52:409-415
(1918-19).

Krogh, August, The Anatomy and Physiology of Capillaries, New
York: Hafner Publication Co. (1959).

Papper, E. M. and Richard J. Kitz, Uptake and Distribution of
Anesthetic Agents, New York, Toronto, London: McGraw-Hill Book
Co., Inc. (1963).

Wright, C. I., "The diffusion of Carbon Dioxide in Tissues,"
J. Gen. Physiol., 17:657-676 (1934).

DUAL WAVELENGTH MICRO-OXIMETER OF HAMSTER WHOLE BLOOD IN VITRO*

Herbert J. Berman, Stuart J. Segall, and Robert L. Fuhro

Department of Biology, Boston University, Boston,

Massachusetts, U.S.A.

INTRODUCTION

Difficulties of measuring oxygen saturation of circulating whole blood in microvessels have greatly limited past efforts to obtain such data. These difficulties are related to the small diameters of the vessels, the small, continuously changing volume of blood flowing in them, variations in the state of red cell orientation and suspension during flow, and numerous optical problems. In order to define some of the problems, establish specific relationships that may exist among the variables, and determine the sensitivity and reliability of our equipment and approach, we first studied certain important variables governing the measurement of oxygen saturation by transmitted light in small samples of whole blood in vitro, where conditions can be more readily and completely controlled than in vivo. The studies were first done with static blood in thin layer cuvettes and then with blood in flow in small diameter polyethylene tubes.

Dual wavelength oximetry was chosen as a feasible method to measure oxygen saturation (% sat) since it is a relatively simple approach and has been proven to be reliable and accurate (7,8). The method is based on the existence of isosbestic wavelengths -- spectral regions where the species of hemoglobin concerned (in this case oxyhemoglobin and reduced hemoglobin) have the same coefficient of extinction. If light transmittance is measured at an isosbestic wavelength and at a wavelength where there is a difference in absorption between the two species, the ratio of transmittance of the two wavelengths is proportional to the relative concentrations of the two species. A micro-oximeter was therefore

constructed to measure % sat in a non-invasive manner in whole
blood in cuvettes, tubes, and in blood vessels of thin membrane
preparations. The wavelengths chosen were 810nm, which is isosbestic for reduced hemoglobin and oxyhemoglobin, and 650nm, where
there is a ninefold difference in extinction coefficients between
the two species. These relatively long wavelengths have become
well established for use in oximetry, since their penetration of
tissue is appreciably greater and protein interference is less
than shorter wavelengths.

The first spectrophotometric measurements of hemoglobin oxygen saturation were made in the late 1800's by Vierordt (9,10).
Kramer made the first continuous oximetric measurements in large
blood vessels in 1934, using a single red wavelength band (3).
Dual wavelength oximetry was pioneered by Matthes (5,6) who first
used green light and then 800nm as an isosbestic wavelength. Since
then work has been done in vivo on large vessels and in vitro by
many investigators (7,8,11,12).

METHODS AND MATERIALS

A microscope stage with three replaceable holders in parallel
-- one for a short pathlength flat cuvette, a second for a neutral
density filter and a third for a small diameter tube -- was designed and built for a Leitz Ortholux microscope. The blood sample in
a cuvette or tube was transilluminated by a tungsten light source
(Osram 70239) regulated at 4.5 amperes. The light was then divided
by a beam splitter at the ocular and directed through one of two
narrow bandpass filters (I.L. Optikel type 20, 650nm and 810nm) to
two photomultiplier tubes (Hammamatsu Trialkali tubes with S-20
response). The electric signals at the two wavelengths were first
evenly balanced electronically with the light path unobstructed and
then equally amplified by two Kiethly 414 amplifiers. The neutral
density filter was used to check the system.

The amplified signals were processed on-line by a Wang 720B
programmable calculator. For most experiments, 650nm/810nm ratios
were averaged in groups of 100. When six consecutive groups showed
that a stable reading had been reached, these groups (600 ratios)
were averaged to give one data point. The ratio was then paired
with the reading of oxygen saturation obtained from an I.L. 182 co-
oximeter for the sample of the same blood. Hemoglobin concentration (Hb;gm%) was also determined with the co-oximeter.

Blood samples were taken from golden hamsters (Mesocricetus
auratus) by cardiac puncture and heparinized. The hemoglobin concentration (Hb) was adjusted, when necessary, by centrifugation and
drawing off of plasma or packed cells and remixing the remainder

of the sample. % sat was varied by tonometering with either nitrogen or room air.

Ratios were obtained from blood in flat cuvettes with a pathlength of 200μ (Hellma cells, 136-05) and in polyethylene tubes
279 and 584μ in i.d. (P.E. 10 and 50). Experiments in cuvettes
were done with static blood; those in tubes were done at various
flow rates with flow controlled by a variable speed Harvard
Apparatus syringe pump, model 902. Tubes were centered in the
light path and masked so that only light that passed through the
P.E. tubes could reach the photomultiplier tubes.

RESULTS

A. Cuvettes

Experiments with cuvettes showed that the system measured
% sat with good reliability. At a constant Hb, the plot of 650nm/
810nm ratios vs. % sat's measured by the co-oximeter was a slightly curved line which could be closely approximated by two straight
lines (derived by linear regression analysis, least-squaresmethod)
intersecting at 60% sat. The slopes of these lines varied directly, and the Y intercepts inversely, with Hb.

B. Tubes

Plots of ratio vs. % sat measured by the co-oximeter were
separated by Hb into groups of 1 gm% (Table I). An
example of the data for one group is given in Fig. 1. At a given
shear rate, the slopes and Y intercepts varied with Hb in the same
manner as in cuvettes. The ratios of the slopes of the regression
lines above 60% sat to those below 60% sat were constant. In the
smaller tube the slopes were smaller and Y intercepts greater than
in the larger tube, showing that the total content of hemoglobin
in the light path rather than the hemoglobin concentration, was the
determining variable. The regression lines calculated for the
several Hb groups converged toward some broad 'point' above 70%
sat. This is in accord with the observations of Kramer (4).
However, the convergence 'point' varied with each set of experiments, with experimental error possibly precluding the finding of
a perfect fan-shaped distribution of lines for each set of Hb's.

The wall shear rate (γ_w) was varied next. The range chosen
was that found for blood flowing in the small blood vessels of the
cheek pouch of the anesthetized hamster (2). No significant effect
on shear rate with respect to the ratio was found when γ_w was above

TABLE I

Calculated Regression Lines:

Relationship to Hemoglobin Concentration

Hb (gm %)	Below 60% Sat.		Above 60% Sat.	
	slope	Y intercept	slope	Y intercept
584μ tube γ_w=130 sec^{-1}				
9.40	.207	.400	.329	.327
10.43	.216	.383	.308	.332
11.45	.261	.348	.383	.280
12.42	.295	.328	.503	.188
13.32	.305	.320	.495	.196
279μ tube γ_w=1204 sec^{-1}				
9.66	.176	.509	.217	.479
10.54	.182	.486	.243	.444
11.55	.212	.458	.251	.428
12.62	.214	.466	.275	.427
13.23	.235	.436	.264	.420

N $\geq$ 20 for each Hb group

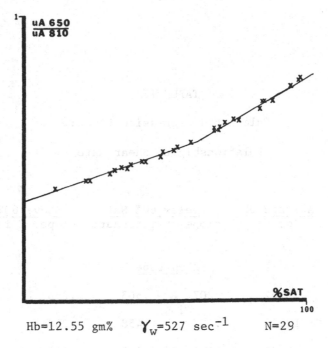

Figure 1: Relationship of measured ratio to oxygen
           saturation measured with the co-oximeter.

$200 \ sec^{-1}$ (Table II). However, when γ_w was below $200 \ sec^{-1}$, the
measured ratio fell appreciably over a period of several minutes
until a plateau was reached. We attribute this effect to settling
of erythrocytes in the tube. When a single blood sample was test-
ed at 2 γ_w's above $200 \ sec^{-1}$ (4817 and $241 \ sec^{-1}$ in the 279μ tube;
1304 and $263 \ sec^{-1}$ in the 584μ tube), only a slight effect was
noted -- an increase of 0.2 to 2.0% sat at the lower shear rate
(N=8). By comparison, transmittance at the individual wavelengths
varied linearly with the $\log_{10}$ of γ_w from 53 to $1304 \ sec^{-1}$ for
single blood samples, with transmittance increases of up to 25%
observed at the higher shear rates.

                C. Accuracy and Sensitivity of System

     By this procedure a series of standard graphs for the differ-
ent variables of interest were constructed. These relationships
were then used to determine the accuracy and reliability of the
approach. The ratios were measured with the micro-oximeter and %
sat's were calculated from the established relationships and then
measured for the sample of blood in the co-oximeter. Deviations
were then calculated by substracting the calculated % sat's from

TABLE II

Calculated Regression Lines:

Relationship to Shear Rate

γ_{w-1} (sec^{-1})	Average Hb (gm %)	Below 60% Sat.		Above 60% Sat.	
		slope	Y intercept	slope	Y intercept
		279μ tube			
4817	12.42	.207	.463	.265	.426
2409	12.28	.207	.458	.262	.422
1204	12.62	.214	.466	.275	.427
482	12.33	.216	.456	.266	.421
241	12.41	.202	.465	.281	.421
		584μ tube			
1304	12.47	.331	.355	.582	.193
527	12.55	.341	.350	.580	.201
263	12.53	.336	.350	.549	.218

$N \geq 20$ for each γ_w group

the measured % sat's. The accuracy of the system was found to be
reasonable for a prototype setup. 63.4% of the values calculated
from the ratios were within 2.5% sat of the values measured in the
co-oximeter and 94.4% were within 5% sat. Distribution was
Gaussian (Fig. 2), with a standard deviation of ± 2.63% sat. The
mean absolute deviation was 2.05% sat (N=395). A plot of calculated % sat vs. measured % sat shows that deviations from linearity
occur only at values above 95% sat and below 20% sat (Fig. 3). The
instrument could detect a change of 0.5% sat.

D. Aggregation

Heparinized blood was moderately aggregated by the addition
of a small amount of a concentrated solution of dextran (Mw=500,000)
and the sample flowed at γ_w's of 527 and 263 sec^{-1} in PE 50 tubes.
No change was found in the 650nm/810nm ratio between paired samples
of dextran treated and untreated bloods. In the aggregated samples
transmittance at both wavelengths was increased.

DISCUSSION

The ratio approach has been shown to compensate adequately
for many variables and has permitted the establishment of definite
relationships under in vitro conditions using cuvettes and tubes.
The results further show that the present instrument and approach
have potentially sufficient accuracy and sensitivity to determine
blood oxygen saturation in circulating whole blood in individual
vessels in membrane preparations. However, certain basic problems
must be solved before such measurements will be possible under
in vivo conditions. Because the 650nm/810nm ratio for a given %
sat varies with the hemoglobin content in the light path, development of a means of measuring this variable in individual vessels
is probably the most important problem to be solved. Densitometric
measurement at a single isosbestic wavelength (e.g. 810nm) would
not seem to be practicable for determining hemoglobin content,
since transmittance has been shown to vary both with shear rate and
with the state of erythrocyte aggregation, as well as with other
factors.

Another problem is the difficulty of characterizing the various parameters under conditions of creeping flow in vivo. Due to
the relatively large size and long length of tube needed for in
vitro studies, settling of erythrocytes occurs at low shear rates.
The tendency for settling and aggregation in vivo is minimal in the
normal hamster. However, it is present in accentuated form in
certain pathological states in man (2).

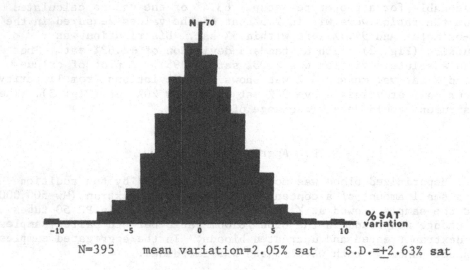

N=395   mean variation=2.05% sat   S.D.=±2.63% sat

Figure 2: Distribution of variation of calculated oxygen
           saturations from measured oxygen saturations.

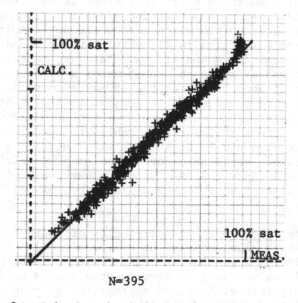

N=395

Figure 3: Calculated vs Measured Oxygen Saturation

SUMMARY

An oximeter for use in conjunction with a microscope was
built and various parameters affecting the measurement of the oxygen saturation in whole blood were studied in flat cuvettes and in
small diameter tubes. Definite relationships among the most important variables were found. The 650nm/810nm ratio was found to be
dependent upon hemoglobin concentration and light pathlength.
Variations in speed of blood flow and in red cell aggregation were
found to have minimal effect upon the determination of oxygen saturation by the ratio technique, although transmittance at the individual wavelengths could change appreciably. When experimentally
derived oxygen saturations were compared to those that were measured directly, the mean absolute variation was 2.05% sat. These
findings with the instrumentation and approach provide a basis for
measurement of oxygen saturation in individual blood vessels in
membrane preparations. The data suggest that, once a method for
measuring the hemoglobin content in the light path is developed,
the present system and approach has sufficient sensitivity and
reliability to make acceptable % sat measurements in vivo.

BIBLIOGRAPHY

1. Berman, H.J. and R.L. Fuhro. Velocity Profiles in Small Blood
    Vessels. Fed. Proc. 26: 496 (1967).

2. Knisely, M.H. Intravascular Erythrocyte Aggregation. Handbook
    of Physiology (W.F. Hamilton, P. Dow, ed.) Sect. 2, Circ.
    III: 2249-2292 (1965).

3. Kramer, K. Fortlaufende Registrietung der Sauerstoffsatigung
    im Blute am uneroffneten Blutgefassen. Klin. Wchnschr. 13:
    379-380 (1934).

4. Kramer, K. Ein Verfahren zur fortlaufenden Messung des Sauer-
    stoffgehalten in stromenden Blute an uneroffneten Gefassen.
    Ztschr. Biol. 96: 61-75 (1935).

5. Matthes, K. Uber den Einfluss der Atmung auf die Sauerstoff-
    satigung des Arterienblutes. Arch. Exper. Path. u. Pharmakol.
    179: 698-711 (1935).

6. Matthes, K. and F. Gross. Untersuchungen uber die Absorption
    von rotem und ultrarotem Licht durch kohlenoxygegesattigtes,
    sauerstoffgesatigtes, und reduziertes Blute. Arch. Exper.
    Path. u. Pharmakol. 191: 369-380 (1939).

7. Nilsson, N.J. Oximetry. Physiol. Rev. 40: 1-26 (1960).

8. Ofstad, J. The Measurement of Oxygen Saturation and Hemo-
    globin Concentration by Photometry of Whole Blood. Chr.
    Michelsens Institute # XXVIII, 3. 1-175 (1965).

9. Vierordt, K. Physiologische Spektralanalysin, VIII. Das
    Hamoglobinspektrum am lebendem Menschem. Ztschr. Biol. 11:
    195-197 (1875).

10. Vierordt, K. Physiologische Spektralanalysin, IX. Die Sauer-
    stoffzchrung den lebenden Gewebe. Ztschr. Biol. 14: 422-
    448 (1878).

11. Wood, E.H. Oximetry. In Medical Physics, ed. O. Glasser.
    The Yearbook Publishers, Inc., Chicago. Vol. 2: 664-680
    (1950).

12. Wood, E.H. Oximetry. In Medical Physics, ed. O. Glasser.
    The Yearbook Publishers, Inc., Chicago. Vol. 3: 416-445
    (1960).

*Supported by grant HL-902 and HL-09447 from the National
Heart and Lung Institute, National Institutes of Health, PHS, and
Grant NGR 22-004-018 from the National Aeronautics and Space
Administration.

P50 DETERMINATIONS: TECHNIQUES AND CLINICAL IMPORTANCE

K. D. Fallon, A. L. Malenfant, R. D. Weisel, and

H. B. Hechtman, Instrumentation Laboratory, Lexington,

Mass., Boston University Medical Center, Boston, Mass.

The oxyhemoglobin dissociation curve demonstrates the relationship between the partial pressure of oxygen and the percent hemoglobin carrying oxygen. The decrease in this percentage as blood passes from the arterial to venous side of tissue is indicative of the amount of oxygen delivered to that tissue. The four controlling factors governing oxygen delivery to tissue are: oxyhemoglobin concentration, blood flow, tissue PO_2 and hemoglobin affinity for oxygen.[1] If the affinity of hemoglobin increases, then compensation must occur or there will be a corresponding decrease in oxygen delivery to the tissue. The forms of compensation are increased blood flow (cardiac output), increased oxyhemoglobin concentration or decreased tissue PO_2.[1] P50 is the PO_2 at which hemoglobin is 50% saturated with oxygen. It's value defines relative changes in oxygen-hemoglobin affinity. To test the hypothesis that decreases in P50 are potentially harmful to an acutely ill individual, we developed procedures for rapidly and easily determining P50.

Materials and Methods

The definition of P50 requires establishing the percentage oxyhemoglobin at any given PO_2. When this has been determined at two or more PO_2.values, the points can be graphed and joined. The P50 can then be determined where the line crosses the 50% saturation point.

Blood is tonometered against a gas with an oxygen concentration which has been set by means of mixing system. The mixture is of two gases, one 20% O_2, the other 0% O_2. The actual percentage of

93

oxygen is read directly on the oxygen monitor. Carbon dioxide is
constant at 40 mm since both tanks have 5.6% CO_2. The number of
points that can be determined by this means is virtually unlimited.

The design of the tonometer allows for rapid equilibration of
blood and gas with minimal hemolysis. The removable sample cup can
hold up to 8 cc but normally only 3-4 cc of blood is used in order
to accelerate equilibration. The sample cup is cycled through one
second rapid rotation then one second stop. This provides for a
continuously changing thin layer of blood against the wall of the
cup exposed to the flowing gas stream.

Blood PO2 measurements are made with a Clark electrode, the
accuracy of which is determined by reading blood tonometered to
equilibration with analyzed gases. Deviations from pH 7.4 are
corrected using the standard Severhinghaus nomogram for pH.

Oxygen saturations are determined on a dedicated photometer
which measures absorbance of the automatically hemolyzed sample at
3 wavelengths. The wavelengths of choice are 548 which is isobestic
for reduced hemoglobin, oxyhemoglobin and carboxyhemoglobin, 568
which is isobestic for reduced hemoglobin and oxyhemoglobin but not
for carboxyhemoglobin, and 578 which is isobestic for reduced carboxyhemoglobin but not for oxyhemoglobin. Thus, the absorbance at
548 is indicative of the total hemoglobin, the absorbance at 568 is
indicative of the carboxyhemoglobin and the absorbance at 578 is
indicative of the oxyhemoglobin. A calibrated analogue matrix
solves the necessary equations and generates the signals which allow
the instrument to read out total hemoglobin, % carboxyhemoglobin
and % oxyhemoglobin directly. The accuracy of the system has been
and is continuously checked against Van Slyke determinations.

Since the PO2 is read simultaneously with the % HbO2, there is
no need to equilibrate completely the blood with the gas in the
tonometer. Three or more samples are obtained sequentially and
anaerobically directly from the tonometer into the measuring
systems. The PO2 is corrected and the points plotted on a work
sheet. P_{50} is determined.

Observations and Results

Using this system, extensive studies were done on patients
admitted to the Trauma Unit at University Hospital, Boston University Medical School, Boston, Massachusetts. Theoretically, an
acute decrease in P_{50} would cause:

1. Increase in mixed venous oxygen saturation.

2. Decrease in arterial-venous oxygen content difference.

3.   Decrease in oxygen consumption.

4.   (Probably) Hypoxia to heart and brain.

To maintain oxygen consumption normal compensation would involve:

1.   An increase in cardiac index and/or

2.   Decrease in venous oxygen tension.

Fifty-eight acutely ill patients in four categories are included in this study. Of 25 patients undergoing cardiac surgery, 24 had significant decreases in P50 (to less than 24 mm Hg). Patients demonstrating post-traumatic respiratory insufficiency showed decreased P50 six times in seven cases. Four patients in five undergoing major abdominal surgery developed low P50 values. Significant shifts were seen in sixteen of twenty-one septic patients.(Fig. 1.)

Incidence of Acute Decrease in P50 (24 mmHg)		
Total Patients	86%	(50/58)
Cardiac Surg	96%	(24/25)
Sepsis	71%	(15/21)
Past Traumatic		
Respirator Insufficiency	86%	(6/7)
Major Abdominal Surgery	80%	(4/5)

Figure 1.

Mortality was 100% in those patients with decreases in P50 who also demonstrated both a decrease in $P\bar{v}O2$ and oxygen consumption. This occurred in eight patients. A much smaller mortality was seen in patients who had either a drop in PvO2 (3 of 26) or a decrease in O2 consumption (3 of 10).(Fig. 2 - 6.)

Cardiac Surgery - Intra - Operatively			
No significant change in flow during pump perfusion 11/12 had fall in P50 during perfusion			
No. Patients	Physiological	Response	Mortality
n = 11	$P\bar{v}O2$	$\dot{V}O2$	
6	+	0	0
4	0	+	1
1	+	+	1

Figure 2.

Cardiac Surgery: Post-Operative (13)

13/13 had decreased P50 from control values

No. Patients	Physiological	Response	Mortality
n = 13	$P\bar{v}O2$	$\dot{V}O2$	
5	0	0	0
6	+	0	1
2	+	+	2

Figure 3.

Acute Respiratory Insufficiency (7)

No. Patients	Physiological	Response	Mortality
n = 6	$P\bar{v}O2$	$\dot{V}O2$	
4	+	0	0
1	0	+	0
1	+	+	1

Figure 4.

Major Abdominal Surgery (5)

4/5 had decreased P50

No. Patients	Physiological	Response	Mortality
n = 4	$P\bar{v}O2$	$\dot{V}O2$	
4	+	0	0

Figure 5.

Sepsis (21)

16/21 had decrease P50
15/16 had high fixed C.I.

No. Patients	Physiological	Response	Mortality
n = 15	$P\bar{v}O2$	$\dot{V}O2$	
6	+	0	2
5	0	+	2
4	+	+	4

Figure 6.

Conclusion

Significant decreases in P50 are common in acutely ill patients. When the patient's ability to compensate for the decreased oxygen delivery to tissues is reached, oxygen consumption will decrease and mortality can be predicted.

Bibliography

1. Finch, C. A. & C. Lenfant, Oxygen Transport in Man, N. E. J. Med., 286; 407-415, 1972.

CATHETERIZABLE ABSOLUTE PHOTOMETER

B.Rybak

Zoophysiologie , Université de Caen , 14032
Caen , France

The direct and continuous measurement _in situ_ of
the oxygen saturation of haemoglobin has to be considered
in clinical explorations and controls as well as in
foundamental physiology of respiratory gases ,chiefly
the oxygen acting as an electrons detoxicant (1) .

Since the time I initiated the left thoracotomized
rabbit preparation (2) (3) permitting to accede directly
to a mammal heart irrigated by the own blood of the
animal – blood being then oxygenated by the residual
right lung – it was possible to catheterize an incan-
descent microlamp inside the right auricle and, by-
passing the auricle ,to locate such light source into
the quasi-laminar flow of the inferior vena cava blood
(4) . Then it is possible to follow the change in oxygen
content of haemoglobin with the highly sensitive
Lallemand's photomultiplier (5) , the evaluations being
however restricted to a venous blood ,the transparent
vessel of which being the "cuvette" of the system (6) .
But because there is _one_ arterial blood which belongs
to haematosis (reference blood) and as many venous
bloods as there are organs – following the different specific metabolism of each – , it was necessary to develop
a new technique concerned with miniaturization of a
photometric device .

The first generation of catheterizable microcolori-
meters (and micro-opacimeters) (7) (8) was therefore

built - with a photodiode as photocell - and calibrated,
with some difficulties , in vitro with a running sample
of blood , the difficulties being in the rather large
time consumed and in the fact that the cell morphology,
the velocity in the pump-circuit and the P_{O_2} / P_{CO_2} of
the sample have to be very carefully checked . This kind
of photo-device is not very sensitive but , even so , it
gives a better light transmittance than the optic fibers
catheter - mainly for intravascular use - I developed
at that time (9) .

It is to notice that the reflex induced by intravenous injection of adrenaline or by a transient nasal
inhalation of CO_2 in the rabbit detected thanks to
the original micro-P_{O_2}-probes (2) (10)(11) (12) is also
well observed : 1º) with the intravenous microlamp-
photomultiplier device , 2º) with the single microcolo-
rimeter . This reflex was also revealed by hemes reflectance and even , simultaneously , at the reduced
coenzyme I intracellular level (13) by induced fluorescence monitored by the combined fluorometer and
double-beam spectrophotometer of Chance , Legallais
and Schoener (14) .

To improve the sensibility and to make metrologi-
cal the catheterizable photometer , I developed a new
generation of micro-photometers giving absolute values
and operating with photoresistive cells . Figure I shows
the shape of the active head . There are two photoresistive cells with cadmium sulphide , one located at the
distal part of the opened cuvette , the other one located at the proximal part of the second opened cuvette ;
in between two identical micro-lamps (DC : 1.5 V ,20 mA)
are positioned in direction of the photocells . The
photoresistive elements are catathermized by a convenient
filter and , as for the double monochromatism we are
dealing with , it is to notice that , the maximum spectral
region of the used photoresistive element being at 580
nm , one cell is not optically filtered whereas the other
photocell catches the light through a Wratten filter at
645 nm. These two photocells are plugged in differential to an appropriate recorder . This device is not
only 1000 times more sensitive than the previous photodiode colorimeter , it represents now an absolute photometer which - after easy calibration in vivo (intravenously) with rabbits or dogs - gives : (a) rectilinear

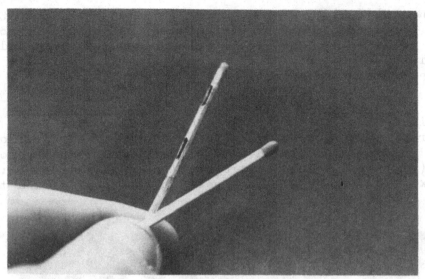

Figure I. Original catheterizable photometer. Size comparison with an ordinary match.

proportionality in function of the oxygen content of
haemoglobin [the device of 1968 demonstrated already
that there is a linear relationship between extinction
and oxygen saturation of haemoglobin of the erythrocytes,
and this has been confirmed by Huckauf , Hutten and
Waldeck with isolated red blood cells (15)] ; (b) the
kinetics or the rates of oxygenation and deoxygenation
and (c) the coefficient of utilization .The calibration
is done : 1º) by increasing the percentage of oxygen
inhalated by the anaesthetized and heparinized animal ;
2º) by decreasing the percentage of oxygen inhalated
by the anaesthetized and heparinized animal giving it
hypoxic mixture of gases to breath,nitrogen being the
diluent (in this case it is convenient to catheterize
the photometer inside the descending aorta). In vivo
simultaneous controls by P_{O_2} catheters are managed .

     The actual external diameter of the instrument va-
ries between 2.2 mm - 1.8 mm.The response time corresponding to the lighting resistance is 350 ms from the
obscurity resistance (for 1 lux). The thermic coefficient is lying between 0.01 %/C and 1 %/C.

OTHER APPLICATIONS OF THE DIRECT INTRAVASCULAR PHOTOMETRY
    Blood volume may be evaluated by one single injec-
tion of an index substance (Evans blue or a so-called
"radiopaque" material for angiography) at a definite
concentration and after in vitro calibration .

    Blood velocity - in addition to circulation time
obtained "top" to "top" of the oxygenation wave from
arterial to venous haemoglobins - can be measured . For
this purpose a double cuvette catheter has been developed (figure II) and "cardiogreen" used as indicator :
if x figures the distance between the proximal and the

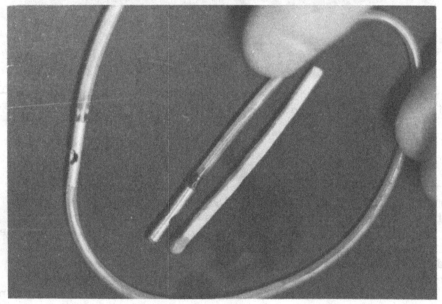

Figure II . Original catheterizable photospeedometer
Two circulating cuvette-lamps-photocells are located
on the same catheter at a definite distance :"cardiogreen" gives a top on the recorder when penetrating
inside the first cuvette and another top when penetrating inside the second cuvette .

distal cuvettes , one gets dx / dt , result which can
not be obtained with catheterizable optic fibers. The
diameter of the photometer (actually 1.8 mm) does
not sensibly interfere with the blood flow when catheterization occurs inside relatively large vessels .

In addition , using an <u>ad hoc</u> photosensitive cell
(CdSe) at 805 nm - which corresponds to the intersection
of the two curves of oxygenated and deoxygenated bloods
plotting light absorption <u>versus</u> wave length -,"cardiogreen", the actual best pigment for dye-dilution measurements in this case , as well as "contrast" material
["radiopaque" particles; cf. also (16)] with a CdS
photocell , is useful with intravascular photometer -
eventually working as a nephelometer - for accurate
evaluation of <u>cardiac output</u> without sampling .

RÉSUMÉ

Les événements colorimétriques et néphélométriques
qui se déroulent dans le sang peuvent être mesurés en
continu et en zone profonde grâce à des photomètres ab-
solus originaux ayant actuellement∿2 mm de diamètre.Ces
photomètres sont constitués par deux cellules photo-
électriques convenablement filtrées pour les longueurs
d'ondes caractéristiques d'emploi ainsi que pour parer
aux éventuels développements de chaleur,faibles d'ailleurs
et constamment éliminables par le flux sanguin , du dis-
positif d'éclairage.Celui-ci est placé en position cen-
trale par rapport à deux systèmes de fenêtres pratiquées
dans la génératrice du cylindre et formant cuvettes à
circulation ;les éléments photo-électriques miniatures
sont disposés de part et d'autre de ces fenêtres en regard
de la source lumineuse et les signaux sont enregistrés en
différentiel. Ces photomètres cathétérisables permettent
ainsi des mesures en continu du rapport $[HHb] / [HbO_2]$;
la calibration se fait aisément par étalonnage <u>in vivo</u>
dans le sang veineux de la veine cave inférieure, dont
on connaît la P_{O_2} , avec des mélanges gazeux renfermant
des taux connus d'oxygène et en procédant par inhalations
nasales chez le Lapin ou le Chien anesthésiés. Mais de
plus - et en conséquence ces photomètres miniatures
sont d'un emploi plus étendu que les fibres optiques -
ils permettent aussi , en disposant convenablement sur
un même cathéter à distance connue deux dispositifs du
type décrit , la mesure de la vitesse du sang . En plus,
par l'usage d'index colorés ou opacifiants appropriés
et par injection sans soutirage d'échantillon de sang,
ces micro-photomètres autorisent la mesure du débit
cardiaque , de la masse sanguine et du temps de circulation .

BIBLIOGRAPHY

(1) B.Rybak,Principles of Zoophysiology,Vol.I;Pergamon Press,Oxford (1968).

(2) B.Rybak,Mesures simultanées en continu de la P_{O_2} encéphalique et de la P_{O_2} cardiaque d'un Mammifère en ventilation autonome.Life Sc.(1964)3,725.

(3) B.Rybak,Tactique opératoire pour la thoracotomie gauche du Lapin.Proc.Can.Fed.Biol.Soc.(1967)10,28.

(4) B.Rybak,Sonde-lampe pour cathétérisme intravasculaire profond.Possibilités offertes.Proc.Can.Fed.Biol.Soc.(1966) 9,96 .

(5) A.Lallemand, Photomultipliers. In:Astronomical Technique,W.A.Hiltner Ed.;Univ.Chicago Press (1962) II,6,426.

(6) B.Rybak,Premières estimations directes et continues de l'état d'oxygénation du sang veineux profond in situ par spectrophotométrie à large bande. C.R.Acad.Sc.(Paris)(1967)264,398.

(7) B.Rybak,Contrôle direct,simultané et in situ du taux d' oxyhémoglobine en milieux artériel et veineux profonds.Experientia (1968)24,204.

(8) B.Rybak, Instrumental Methods for Minimum Interference Physiology, Trans.New York Acad.Sc.(1971) 33,nº4,371.

(9) B.Rybak,Cathéter à fibres de verre pour photométrie intravasculaire.J.Physiol.(Paris)(1968)60,298.

(10) B.Rybak & L.Le Camus,Sonde pour la détermination continue de la pression partielle d'oxygène ainsi que pour la mesure d'autres paramètres physiques au sein d'un milieu. Brevet C.N.R.S.(1966).

(11) B.Rybak,Mise en évidence d'un réflexe végétatif complexe (pulmo-cardio-vasculaire)par polarographie d'oxygène.Abstr.23rd Int.Cong.Physiol.Sc.Tokyo, (1965) 240.

(12) B.Rybak,Evolutions polyphasiques des P_{O_2} artérielle et veineuse à l'application nasale où sous-laryngée de gaz carbonique chez le Lapin. J.Physiol. (Paris)(1967) 59,495 .

(13) B.Rybak,B.Chance,B.Paddle & A.Kaplan, A Molecular Respiratory Reflex and a Fluorescent Signal of Severe Hypoxia.Life Sc. (1970) 9,557 .

(14) B.Chance,V.Legallais & B.Schoener,Combined Fluorometer and Double-beam Spectrophotometer for Reflectance Measurements.Rev.Sc.Instrum.(1963)34, 1307.

(15) H.Huckauf,H.Hutten & F.Waldeck,Beitrag zur mikropho-
      tometrischen O_2-Sättigungsbestimmung an einzelnen
      Erythrocyten. Pflüger's Archiv(1969) 305,fasc.2,
      190.
(16) A.Jarløv, T.Mygind & E.D.Christiansen, Left Ventricu-
      lar Volume and Cardiac Output of the Canine Heart.
      Application of a Mathematical two Compartment Mo-
      del and a New Dye Dilution Technique.Med.& biol.
      Engng.(1970) 8,221.

CLINICAL USE OF A NEW INTRA-ARTERIAL CATHETER ELECTRODE SYSTEM[*]

Haim I. Bicher, Joseph W. Rubin and Robert J. Adams

Departments of Anatomy and Surgery, Medical University

of South Carolina, Charleston, South Carolina, U.S.A.

INTRODUCTION

Until the recent development of continuously recording oxygen electrodes, the clinical monitoring of blood oxygen tensions depended on the findings from isolated blood specimens. The acquisition of such data was limited, expensive and often unreliable because of the unavoidable delay between sampling and reading.

Since Clark introduced a gas permeable membrane-covered oxygen electrode (1), numerous reports have appeared on different attempts to use miniaturized versions for continuous monitoring (3, 4, 5, 6, 7, 8, 9, 10). The main problems encountered were those of drift, calibration, miniaturization and mass production.

A new oxygen catheter electrode system in which these problems are minimized has been developed. The special characteristics of this system include a new type of semi-pervious membrane, dried electrolyte and a unique geometrical configuration. The description and clinical application of this new system constitutes the basis of this report.

MATERIAL AND METHODS

Figure 1 is a schematic drawing of the polarographic electrode system employed. The electrode consists of an Ag-AgCl-plated Cu anode and an Ag-plated Cu cathode exposed to an electrolyte chamber enclosed by a membrane which is pervious to O_2 but only semipervi-

[*]Work performed under a grant from Mediscience Technology Corporation, Collingswood, New Jersey, USA

ous to water. As shown in Figure 1, the system is completed by
the polarizing cell and a current amplifier with a digital ammeter
which may be calibrated to read pO_2. The sensor tip of the electrode

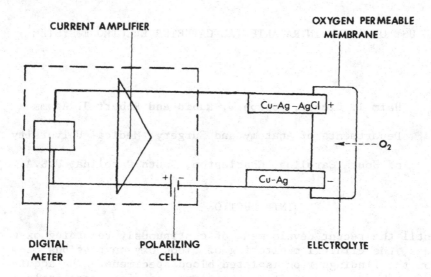

Fig. 1

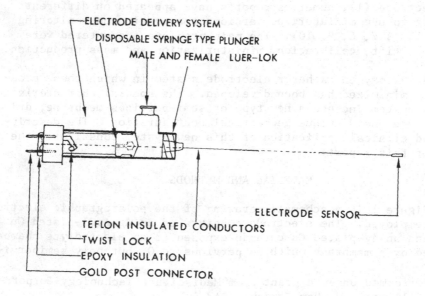

Fig. 2

is made using an epoxy cast as the base for depositing KCl electrolyte gel which is allowed to dry. A semipervious membrane is
layered on over the electrolyte by dipping the sensor tip in Form-
var®, a polyvinyl formal resin. The final membrane is applied by
dipping the tip into a specifically formulated solution of Silastic®,
a medical adhesive Silicone Type A. As shown only the ends of the
electrode wires are exposed at the tip within the sensor membrane
and the entire electrode surface is covered, either by the teflon,
in which the wires are embedded, or by the Silastic exterior of
the sensor tip.

This catheter electrode, with an outer diameter of 0.5 mm,
fits easily through a 20 gauge cannula. Figure 2 depicts the delivery head complementing the catheter. This head not only permits completion of the electrode circuit, but also allows access
to the cannula for blood sampling and recording of arterial pressure. The entire electrode unit is disposable and not intended
for reuse.

The electrode is test calibrated in vitro and its stability
checked. Figure 3 is an in vitro calibration curve showing the
output response after transferring the electrode from N_2 at 36 mm Hg
to O_2 at 320 mm Hg. The two-thirds response time is 60 seconds
and in vitro drift over 24 hours is approximately 10%. Electrodes
have been kept active for three days with little change in sensitivity.

The polarogram of this electrode configuration (Figure 3b)
shows a plateau in current output between .55 and .75 volts. The
response (Figure 3a) is linear from 15 to 350 mm Hg pO_2.

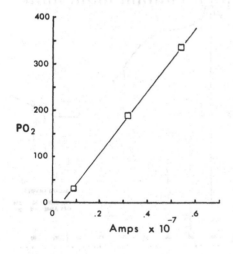

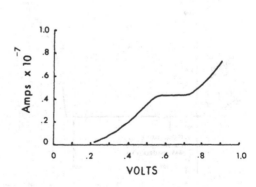

Fig. 3a   Fig. 3b

Once tested and calibrated _in vitro_ the catheter electrode may be dried, packaged and gas sterilized for subsequent clinical use. In clinical PaO_2 monitoring, electrodes have been placed within a radial artery of adults through a previously inserted cannula. In neonates, the sensor was advanced into the descending aorta via an umbilical artery catheter.

Prior to intra-arterial placement, the electrodes are reactivated in saline. After insertion into the blood stream, the electrode output is allowed to stabilize. A two-point calibration is then made _in situ_ which permits allowance for flow, temperature and positioning artifacts. Calibration is performed using PaO_2 values, measured by conventional methods in the hospital laboratory, while varying the patient's respiratory O_2 concentration. Because of the very low drift, calibration is then checked only once every 8 hours.

RESULTS

Electrodes have been tested in 20 dogs for periods of up to 10 hours. The electrode pO_2 measurements correlated to within 12% with pO_2 values of blood samples measured in a conventional gas analyzer during this study.

Figure 4 shows a penrecorder tracing of the output of a calibrated electrode in clinical use. The electrode had been placed in the radial artery for monitoring PaO_2 in a patient on a respirator following open heart surgery.

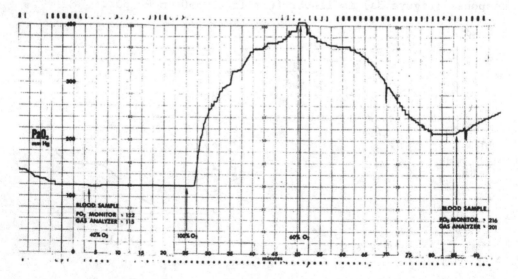

Fig. 4

Clinical trials of the electrode were performed in 18 patients, during and after major cardiovascular and pulmonary operations, and in 3 neonates in acute respiratory distress. In the post-operative patients, trial periods varied from 2 to more than 30 hours. Three electrodes malfunctioned and no data could be obtained. Table I summarizes the results from 18 patients and data received from 195 hours PaO_2 monitoring by the electrodes. PO_2 values from individual patient trials were averaged and weighted. The weighted mean PaO_2 values from each trial were then averaged to give an electrode pO_2 mean of 149.8 mm Hg. The mean pO_2 from conventional gas analysis was 151.3 mm Hg. This represented a 0.99 $\pm$ 7.11% (S.D.) difference between the means.

	MEAN MMHG	STD. DEV. MMHG
PO_2 MONITOR	149.8	
GAS ANALYZER	151.3	
DIFFERENCE	-1.5	10.76
% DIFFERENCE	.99%	7.11%

TOTAL HOURS: 195

NO. OF PATIENTS: 18

Table I

Three complications occurred during the clinical trials. When one of the electrodes was withdrawn a thrombus was adherent to the shaft. This thrombus may have originated in the cannula because of its dimensional resemblance to the cannula. Two patients complained of pain around the arterial puncture site and had significant tenderness and induration of the region. No late sequelae were noted.

COMMENT

The new intra-arterial oxygen catheter electrode has several advantages over previously described electrodes (1 to 10). The device is of simple construction and relatively inexpensive to produce. It may be calibrated in vitro, then sterilized and stored for unlimited time. For practical clinical purposes, it may be considered drift-free.

SUMMARY

An indwelling arterial electrode for monitoring PaO_2 useful for controlling oxygen content in respired air of infants in incubators and adults on respirators has been developed by using a new semi-pervious membrane and a special geometrical configuration. The problems of drift and miniaturization inherent to these systems have been minimized.

REFERENCES

1. Clark, L.C., Jr. Monitor and control of blood and tissue oxygen tensions, Trans. Amer. Soc. Art. Int. Organs, 2:41 (1956).

2. Severinghaus, J.W. Recent developments in blood O_2 and CO_2 electrodes, A Symposium on pH and Blood Gas Measurements. London: J.E.A. Churchill, Lts., pp. 126-149 (1959).

3. Purves, M.J. Information of physiological value derived from continuous measurement of oxygen tension of blood in vivo, in Oxygen Pressure Recording in Gases, Fluids, and Tissues, F. Kreuzer, ed. Basel/New York: Karger, pp. 79-88 (1969).

4. Schuler, R. and F. Kreuzer. Rapid polarographic in vivo oxygen catheter electrodes, Resp. Physiol., 3:90 (1967).

5. Parker, A.K. and R. Davies. A disposable catheter tip transducer for continuous measurement of blood oxygen tensions in vivo, Bio. Med. Eng., 6:313 (1971).

6. Smith, L.L., D.M. Walton, D.R. Wilson, C.C. Jackson and D.B. Hinshaw. Continuous gas and pH monitoring during cardiovascular surgery, Am. J. Surg., 120:249 (1970).

7. Huch, A., D.W. Lubbers and R. Huch. A catheter electrode for the continuous measurement of oxygen pressure in the aorta of the newborn infant, in Oxygen Pressure Recording in Gases, Fluids, and Tissues, F. Kreuzer, ed. Basel/New York: Karger, pp. 110-112 (1969).

8. Neville, J.R. A simple, rapid, polarographic method for blood oxygen content determination, Rev. Soc. Instr., 33:51 (1962).

9. Koeff, S.T., M.V. Tsoao, A. Vadnay, T.O. Wilson, and J.L.
    Wilson. Continuous measurement of intravascular oxygen ten-
    sion in normal adults, J. Clin. Invest., 41:1125 (1962).

10. Harris, T.R. and M. Nugent. Laboratory and clinical evalua-
    tion of a new indwelling oxygen electrode for continuous mon-
    itoring of PaO_2 in neonates, in Oxygen Transport to Tissue,
    H.I. Bicher and D.F. Bruley, eds. New York: Plenum Press
    (in press).

PROBLEMS OF TRANSCUTANEOUS MEASUREMENT OF ARTERIAL BLOOD GASES

D. W. Lübbers, R. Huch, and A. Huch*
Max-Planck-Institut für Systemphysiologie
Dortmund, West Germany
and
*Frauenklinik der Universität Marburg

Applying the dropping mercury electrode is has been previously tried to measure the arterial Po_2 by measuring the Po_2 of heated water which was brought in close contact with the skin (1,11) Using solid electrodes, Po_2 measurements on the skin surface turned out to be extremely difficult to perform, since even a rather light electrode had the tendency to compress some of the skin capillaries. Therefore, Evans and Naylor (3) mounted the electrode on a spring balance. We succeeded in reducing the pressure by increasing the contact area of the electrode using plastic material (Xantopren). Similar to Evans and Naylor (4) we found that the blood of the normal skin is regulated in such a way that the oxygen pressure on the skin surface covered by an oxygen-impermeable layer is only a few Torr (4,6). The highest value measured so far was 7 Torr, more frequently the values ranged between 0 and 2.5 Torr. During O_2 respiration skin Po_2 did not rise. Interruption of blood flow decreased the skin Po_2 to zero; after releasing the cuff, the skin Po_2 rose up to 10 Torr, and then fell to the starting point again. Thus, under normal physiological conditions, skin blood flow is so regulated that it supplies just the amount of oxygen needed for the O_2 consumption of the skin. Since all these experiments had shown that O_2 diffuses through the skin, the question arose to which degree it would be possible to measure arterial Po_2 through the intact skin. Fig. 1 shows schematically which way the oxygen must diffuse in order to reach the Po_2 electrode. It leaves the capillary and permeates through the respiring skin (shown by the mitochondrium) and then through the upper part of the epidermis together with the membranes of the electrode. It can be easily predicted that vasodilatation without changing skin respiration must increase the skin surface Po_2. But how close this value will reach the arterial Po_2 depends on the composition of blood, on the blood flow, and on the O_2 consumption of the skin.

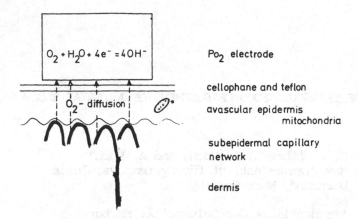

Fig.1 Scheme of the skin surface Po$_2$ measurement

The influence of blood flow and respiration can be minimized by reducing respiration and by increasing blood flow. Evans and Naylor
(10)reduced skin respiration by administration of barbiturates, but
these drugs did not affect the intact skin. We tried therefore to
produce hyperemia by local application of a derivate of nicotinamide (Finalgon, Anasco, Wiesbaden) hoping that the Po$_2$ gradient
through the skin (5) becomes also smaller. Under the influence of
these drugs the skin surface Po$_2$ rose to 38.1 ± 8.1 Torr (n=77) in
adults. These values were absolute Po$_2$ values, since a new technique
enabled us to calibrate the Po$_2$ electrode in situ (6). The relative
stability of these values showed that both tissue respiration and
local blood flow remained sufficiently constant to reflect all Po$_2$
changes in the arterial blood correctly, but in order to obtain values closer to the absolute arterial Po$_2$ chemically induced hyperemia was not satisfying. The conclusion of these experiments was
1) we had to look for a stronger hyperemic agent, 2) we should control the local blood flow to distinguish between flow changes and
arterial Po$_2$ changes. Hyperemia due to locally warming up the skin
to a constant temperature of ca. 42-43°C produced promising results
(7). This was later on confirmed by Eberhard, Hammacher and Mindt
(2). In order to control simultaneously local perfusion we used
the reverse Gibbs principle: we heated our electrode setup, for example, to 40°C, and measured the electrical current which is necessary to maintain this temperature against the cooling effect of the
local blood perfusion. Since this measurement is a temperature measurement, it is influenced by all possible temperature changes, but
under our measuring conditions it proved to be mainly influenced by
the local blood perfusion. Thus, with this device we could control
the relationship between local blood perfusion and skin surface Po$_2$.

If blood perfusion changes without changing skin surface Po_2, then
- assuming an unchanged skin respiration and an unchanged ambient
temperature - the arterial Po_2 (minus the local gradient caused by
the respiring part of the skin below the electrode) should be correctly measured at the skin surface. In other words, with our measuring device we are able to control the perfusion efficiency in respect to the arterial Po_2. Sufficient perfusion efficiency is the
main condition for a correct transcutaneous measurement of arterial
blood gases.

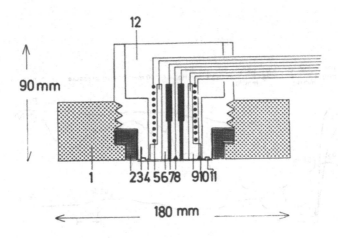

Fig. 2. Device for the non-invasive measurement of arterial Po_2 at
        the skin surface (1,2, O-rings; 3, lucite; 4, membranes;
        5, heating coil; 6, glass; 7, Pt wire 15 μ in diameter;
        8, NTC in central position; 9, silver anode; 10, NTC with-
        in the silver tube; 11, space for electrolyte).

Fig.2 shows the electrode device which enabled us to measure the
perfusion efficiency with respect to the skin surface Po_2 and thus,
as we think, the arterial Po_2. The whole Po_2 electrode is heated
from outside using an electrical wire coil [5] being in heat contact with the silver anode [9] of the Po_2 electrode. The temperature is monitored by thermistors or NTC resistors [8, 10] . Three
15 μm Pt wires [7] were fused in glass ; [1,2,3] and [12] formed
the housing of the electrode, [11], the grove for the electrolyte.
With increasing temperature blood perfusion increased. When we locally reached 43°C, then an optimal vasodilatation seemed to be established. We have controlled this by reducing stepwise the flow,
inflating a cuff wrapped round the upper arm. Fig. 3 shows that
blood flow can be reduced stepwise (marked by arrows) to 70 to 80%
without changing the skin surface Po_2 and Pco_2. As expected, higher
flow reduction decreases the tissue Po_2 and correspondingly increases the Pco_2. Unfortunately, the warming up of the skin alters the

arterial Po_2 corresponding to the temperature coefficient of blood
and tissue. Therefore, the transcutaneously measured Po_2 of the skin
arterialized by local heating, is a complicated function of the
true arterial Po_2 at body temperature. This function may be measured by simultaneous blood analyses, but this would be a considerable draw-back of our goal to find a non-invasive method for blood
gas analyses.

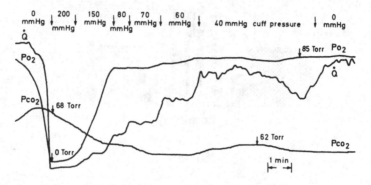

Fig. 3. Control of the perfusion efficiency with regard to Po_2
and Pco_2 at the skin surface.

Fortuneately, our experiments showed that hyperemia outlasted heating for several minutes. Thus, after interrupting heating, the perfusion efficiency remained high enough to measure the arterial Po_2
at body temperature. This was controlled by simultaneously performed measurements of arterial Po_2 and arterialzed skin surface
Po_2. Together with A.and R.Huch we could show that with this electrode the arterial Po_2 could be monitored under clinical conditions
sufficiently well (8,9). Thus, the Po_2 gradient in the skin caused
by tissue respiration is probably smaller than Evans and Naylor assumed (5).

    The other important blood gas is the Pco_2. Since it can be
measured by membrane-covered pH electrodes, we tried a similar device for measuring Pco_2 (Fig.4). Fig.3 shows that such measurements
are possible. The transcutaneous Pco_2 measuring device requires
further refining, but the simultaneous and continuous measurement
of arterial Po_2 and Pco_2 will allow a non-invasive control of the
patients' acid-base state, since knowing Po_2 and Pco_2 at body temperature allows the use of nomographs to determine the acid-base
state. This just discussed principle is not restricted to the Po_2

or Pco_2 electrodes, but it can be applied to other methods of gas analyses.

In summary our experiments have shown that with the aid of our specially developed electrodes it is possible to measure transcutaneously arterial Po_2 and Pco_2, if the perfusion efficiency is maintained at the necessary high level. The perfusion efficiency is controlled by the simultaneous measurement of blood gas tension and relative local blood perfusion. The efficiency is sufficient, if changes in blood perfusion do not change the measured skin surface Po_2 or Pco_2. The necessary perfusion efficiency is brought about by local hyperthermia of ca. $43°C$, and remains at a sufficiently high level after stopping heating to measure at body temperature. This enables us to obtain data on the acid-base state nomographically without puncturing a blood vessel.

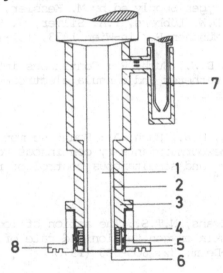

Fig.4. Device for non-invasive measurement of arterial Pco_2 at the skin surface (1, pH electrode; 2, space for the electrolyte; 3, housing; 4, silver tube with heating coil; 5, O-ring; 6, membranes; 7, reference electrode; 8, lucite ring for fixing the electrode by suction).

REFERENCES

1) Baumberger, J.P., Goodfriend, R.B.: Determination of arterial oxygen tension in man by equilibration through intact skin. Fed. Proc. 10, 10 (1951)

2) Eberhard, P., Hammacher, K., Mindt, W.: Deutsches Patentamt (Bundesrepublik Deutschland) Deutsche Klasse: 30a, 4/01, Offenlegungsschrift 2145400 (Hoffmann - La Roche)

3) Evans, N.T.S., Naylor, P.F.D.: The systemic oxygen supply to the human skin. Respir. Physiol. 3, 21-37 (1967).

4) Evans, N.T.S., Naylor, P.F.D.: Steady states of oxygen tension in human dermis. Respir. Physiol. 2, 46-60 (1966/67).

5) Evans, N.T.S., Naylor, P.F.D.: The oxygen tension gradient across human epidermis Respir. Physiol. 3, 38-42 (1967).

6) Huch, R., Lübbers, D.W., Huch, A.: Quantitative continuous measurement of partial oxygen pressure on the skin of adults and new-born babies. Pflügers Arch. 337, 185-198 (1972).

7) Huch, R., Lübbers, D.W., Huch, A.: An electrode for prolonged bloodless Po_2 measurements on the skin and a method for in situ calibration in: Oxygen Supply ed.by M. Kessler, D.F. Bruley, L.C. Clark, Jr., D.W. Lübbers, I.A. Silver, J. Strauss. Urban & Schwarzenberg, München-Berlin-Wien 1973, 101-103.

8) Huch, A., Lübbers, D.W., Huch, R.: Continuous intravascular Po_2 measurement with catheter and cannula electrodes in new-born, adults and in animals.
this book

9) Huch, R., Lübbers., D.W., Huch, A.: Rountine monitoring of the arterial Po_2 of newborn infants by continuous registration of transcutaneous Po_2 and simultaneous control of relative local blood perfusion.
this book

10) Naylor, P.F.D., Evans, N.T.S.: The action of locally applied barbiturates on skin oxygen tension and rate of oxygen utilization Br.J-Derm. 82, 600-605 (1970).

11) Rooth, G., Sjöstedt, S., Caligara, F.: Bloodless determination of arterial oxygen tension by polarography. Science Tolls. The LKW Instrument J. 4, 37-45 (1957).

FLOW LIMITED PROPERTIES OF TEFLON AND SILICONE DIFFUSION MEMBRANES

D. Nelson, L. Ostrander, E. Ernst, W. Baetz

Departments of Biomedical Engineering and Anesthesiology

Case Western Reserve University, Cleveland, Ohio 44106

INTRODUCTION

The mass spectrometer equipped with a diffusion catheter can detect partial pressures of gases in tissues and blood vessels. The catheter consists of a small gauge stainless steel conduit with small openings at one end covered by a thin teflon or silicone membrane. The entire catheter can be inserted through the lumen of a sixteen gauge needle.

Gas pressures inside the catheter are maintained on the order of 10^{-6} torr. Gases in the medium surrounding the catheter diffuse through the membrane and are transported by molecular flow to the mass spectrometer detector. Under steady state conditions the mass spectrometer reading is directly proportional to the gas tension at the membrane surface. An important point in our study is that this system removes gas molecules from the medium in which it is placed and depletes gases in the vicinity of the membrane surface. In the steady state gases removed at the surface of the catheter membrane may be replaced by convective flow in the medium and diffusion from parts of the medium further removed from the catheter's influence.

The purpose of the study is to use the concept of depletion at the membrane surface to accurately measure gas concentrations and/or fluid flow in the catheter vicinity.

METHODS

A sketch of the experimental setup is presented in Figure 1. Citrated blood, heparinized blood, or water in a 500 ml modified Florence flask was equilibrated with air or calibrated gas mixtures

by bubbling the gas through it for at least four hours. Catheters
to be tested were centered in the outlet ports and secured in
place. Harvard withdrawal pumps provided adjustable fluid flow
rates and allowed simultaneous study of two catheters. During the
studies, the internal diameter of the tubes through which the
fluid was drawn ranged from four to twenty mm. The entire assembly was immersed in a water bath for temperature control.

    Calibration of the mass spectrometer before each experiment
was accomplished by stirring the fluid with a submersible magnetic stirrer placed in an Erlenmeyer flask. Care was taken to keep
the calibrated gas bubbles from the diffusion membrane surface.
The rate of stirring was increased until maximal readings were
obtained and this was called the 100% reading. Increasing the

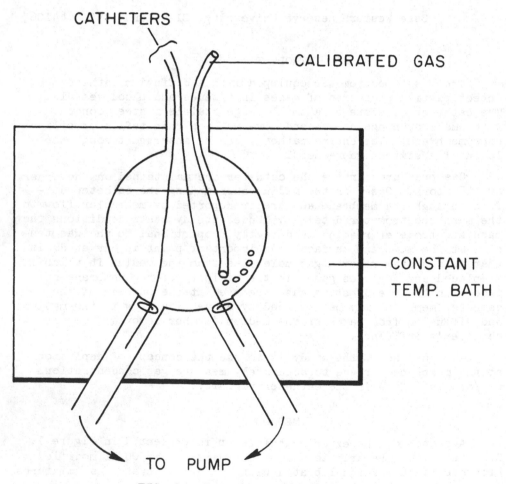

FIG. 1. Experimental Set Up

rate of stirring beyond this point did not increase the readings.
The readings of the mass spectrometer at any given flow rate was
measured as a percentage of the 100% reading.

RESULTS

Plotting the percent readings from the mass spectrometer
against the flow rate yields the typical graph displayed in Figure
2. Teflon (upper curve) harvests less gas and so is less flow dependent than silicone. Three regions of flow dependency are exhibited. In the region of high flow rates, convection replenishes
gas at the membrane surface and the concentration there is very
close to the actual gas concentration in the medium. In the middle
region there is a log-linear relationship between flow rate and
mass spectrometer readings with a curving off at both ends of the
region. In the third region at low or no flow rate, convection
contributes little or no gas to the outer surface of the membrane
and the molecules are delivered by diffusion through the medium.

The standard deviation at any given flow rate in the middle
region is 1.5%. From day to day the standard deviation was 3%.
One cause for variation is the position of the catheter in the
tube. As the catheter is moved from the center of the tube to the
wall there is a 3-5% decrease of the readings in the middle region.
This is presumably due to a change in the flow profiles near the
membrane which results in a net decrease in replenishment of gases.
Figure 3 compares data obtained from 10 mm tubing (solid lines)
with 18 mm tubing (dashed line) and Figure 4 displays data from
smaller tubing. As tubing size was changed, the slope of the curve
in region 2 did not change appreciably.

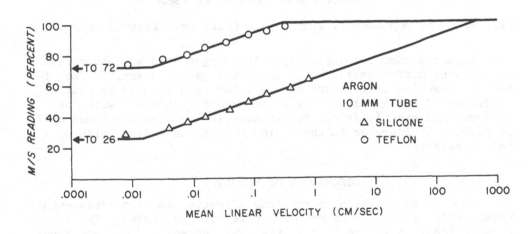

FIG. 2. Flow Dependency, 10 mm tube - fluid equilibrated with air

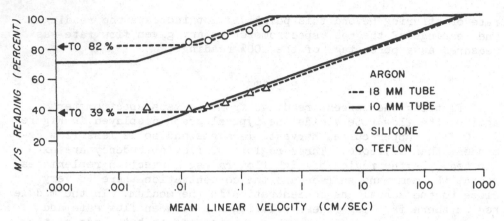

FIG. 3. Flow Dependency, 18 mm tube - fluid equilibrated with air

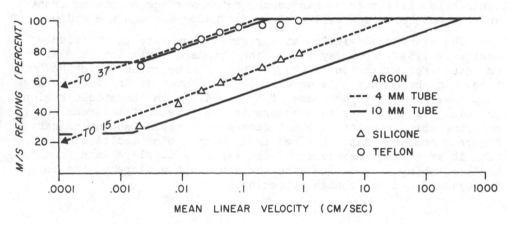

FIG. 4. Flow Dependency, 4 mm tube - fluid equilibrated with air

Figure 5 compares argon data with oxygen data and shows that measurement differences between these two gases is small. The effect of lowering temperature of the water bath from 37 degrees to 23 degrees C had little effect on the results obtained with the silicone membrane (a fairly temperature insensitive membrane) and produced a 5% increase in the region of flow dependency with a teflon catheter.

DISCUSSION OF RESULTS

Some of the physical conditions affecting in vivo measurements using teflon and silicone membrane have been presented. There is no question that the membranes have some degree of flow dependency for flow rates encountered in the vasculature. On the other hand

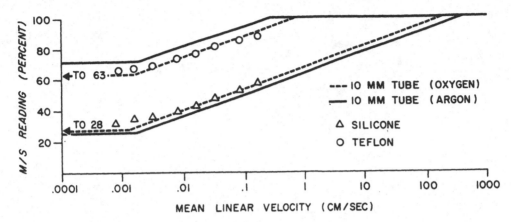

FIG. 5. Oxygen and Argon compared - fluid equilibrated with air

during air breathing the actual partial pressure of argon, a non-
metabolite, should be the same in the blood vessels as in the inspired air. The per cent reading from the mass spectrometer for
argon will indicate flow rates in the vicinity of the membrane.
This can provide a correction factor to determine the actual partial pressure of another gas, or estimate the flow rate within a
vessel. As can be seen in Figure 5, the percent reading for oxygen equals the percent reading for argon plus 3%. Division of
mass spectrometer gas tension readings by the percent readings expressed as a fraction yields the corrected gas tension reading.
Preliminary in vivo studies comparing corrected readings with simultaneous Radiometer PO_2 determinations support this approach.

When the diffusion catheters are placed in tissue, depletion
effects at the membrane surface are also encountered. The measurement conditions have similarity to the no or low flow conditions of the present study. Assessing depletion affects and true
gas tensions requires an appropriate modeling approach coupled
with knowledge of the physical performance of the catheters as
provided by the present study.

ACKNOWLEDGEMENTS

    This work was supported by National Institutes of Health
GM-19599, GM-47364, and GM-01090.

DIFFERENTIAL ANODIC ENZYME POLAROGRAPHY FOR THE MEASUREMENT OF GLUCOSE

Leland C. Clark, Jr. and Eleanor W. Clark

Children's Hospital Research Foundation - University of

Cincinnati College of Medicine

The coupling of enzymes to polarographic and other electro-chemical sensors has been a happy one (1-7). The first such union occurred in 1962 (8). The electrochemistry involved lends sim-plicity to the detecting equipment while in the sensor itself the enzyme provides the specificity, often a degree of specificity which cannot be obtained by any other means. In addition, and very importantly this type of sensor lends itself to miniaturiza-tion to the point where it may be used intracellularly.

From the by now rather extensive list of substances which can be measured by enzyme-electrode combinations we have selected the measurement of glucose as typifying those problems which will be encountered when polarographic enzyme sensors are placed in or on living tissue.

In order to illustrate the polarographic principles involved, the direct measurement of glucose in whole blood will be describ-ed. Preliminary continuous measurement of glucose concentration on the surface of the brain will also be reported. First, by means of a commercially available instrument (9) based upon the Clark anodic glucose electrode, which uses a 20 μL blood sample and gives a glucose reading in less than one minute and is based upon injection of this sample into a thermostated 250 μL cuvet. Because this method is based upon dilution several problems in-herent in direct measurement in blood or tissue are circumvented, but a number of factors can be studied which are relevant to tis-sue or undiluted whole blood. The role of the compensation elec-trode, or the role of differential anode polarography, will be an-alyzed since it may or may not become important in the accurate measurement of glucose in whole blood and living tissue.

127

We will make no attempt to review the thousands of papers on glucose analysis, a testimony perhaps to the problems that have plagued this measurement of glucose for half a century or perhaps testimony to the fact that next to hemoglobin it is the substance most frequently analyzed. A critical review of glucose analytical methods is to be found in an excellent monograph (10).

The analysis of glucose by the anode polarographic, or voltammetric if you prefer, electrode is based upon the fact that hydrogen peroxide allows a current to flow in proportion to its concentration. This discovery was first reported by Britton Chance (15). Secondly, that glucose oxidase (from either <u>Penicillin notatum</u> or <u>Aspergillus</u> <u>niger</u>) generates H_2O_2 from glucose. By trapping an excess of glucose oxidase between the platinum surface and a membrane, glucose is converted to H_2O_2. One then obtains a glucose <u>diffusion controlled</u> anode which very rapidly reaches an equilibrium state where the concentration of glucose in the sample produces a proportionate peroxide concentration on the platinum surface and hence a current proportional to the glucose concentration in the substance in contact with it.

Since H_2O_2 diffuses back into the sample catalase must be added to the buffer or standard. Addition of catalase is not necessary for measurement of glucose in blood (except for the dog, duck, and certain strains of mice) due to its high catalase content. There appears to be an excess of catalase activity in all tissue studied to date.

The membrane also serves to keep the glucose oxidase physically and/or chemically immobilized and to prevent large molecular weight H_2O_2 decomposing catalysts such as catalase from traversing the membrane.

The stoichometric chemical reaction upon which this glucose sensor is based is:

$$\text{GLUCOSE} + O_2 \xrightarrow[\text{OXIDASE}]{\overset{\overset{H_2O}{\text{GLUCOSE}}}{}} \text{GLUCONIC ACID} + H_2O_2$$

Since many small (<1000MW) molecules can diffuse through the membranes on the anode, a way is found to subtract these currents from the enzyme currents. This is readily accomplished by having an electrode identical in all respects to the sensor except that no enzyme is present. Hence the anodic current, however small, from ascorbate or other substances oxidized by the anode can be electrically substracted from the enzyme anodic current. For many practical purposes the compensation current is not required.

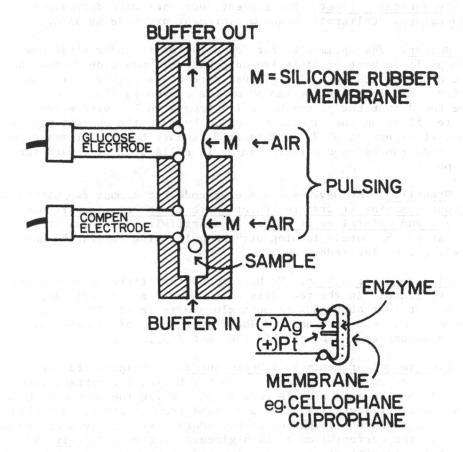

BUFFER OUT

M = SILICONE RUBBER MEMBRANE

GLUCOSE ELECTRODE

← M ← AIR

COMPEN ELECTRODE

← M ← AIR

}PULSING

SAMPLE

ENZYME

BUFFER IN (−)Ag

(+)Pt

MEMBRANE eg. CELLOPHANE CUPROPHANE

Effect of oxygen. The oxygen required for the enzyme's action comes from the buffers and also from the Silastic rubber stirring diaphram. The pO_2 in the cuvet remains at about 150 torr. Because the electrode is glucose diffusion controlled there is very little if any effect from increasing or decreasing the pO_2. Of course if there were no oxygen present the reaction would stop. When the pO_2 of the cuvet's contents is recorded as increasing amounts of glucose are added no change in pO_2 is found. If, however, the pO_2 of the enzyme electrode is measured as glucose is added, it is found to decrease. This effect has been used to measure glucose in solution (11,12). When the electrode is used on the brain, enough oxygen is provided by the tissues.

Stirring effect. The stirring effect is much less with a large anode glucose sensor than a large oxygen cathode. It can be reduced or eliminated by reducing the exposed Pt area and by selecting proper membranes.

   Temperature effect. The current decreases with decreasing
temperature. Calibrations and measurement are made at 38°C.

   Buffer. The optimum buffer for dilution is under study now.
Perhaps it is best if it is isotonic but this may depend upon the
type of blood studied. The glucose current is higher in isotonic
buffer. Although the optimum pH of the enzyme is about 5.6 we
have found that the pH can be varied from 4 to 7.5 with very
little effect on the glucose current. In fact the current may be
somewhat higher at pH 7.5. This is fortunate because it means the
electrode can be used directly on or in cells without regard for
the pH.

   Stability. We have used one electrode for almost two months
without removing it from the cuvet where it was continually polarized and maintained at 38°C. If sensitivity decreases it can
be restored by merely turning off the polarizing current by unplugging the electrode.

   Glucose distribution. We have found that there is very little,
if any, glucose in the red cells of the goat, sheep, cat, and
mouse, but that about 80% as much glucose is in the RBC as in the
plasma in man and the monkey. The distribution of glucose has
been a controversial subject in the past (13).

   Glucose measurements on a brain surface. Compared to the current from an oxygen cathode in or on the brain, the current from
an anode of the same size is very small. While the oxygen cathode
shows distinct waves (14) none are found from an anode. But when
a glucose electrode is placed on the brain distinct waves are seen.
   That the current from a brain glucose electrode largely reflects the concentration of glucose, and not some other polarographically active substance can be seen from the effect of insulin (figure 2).

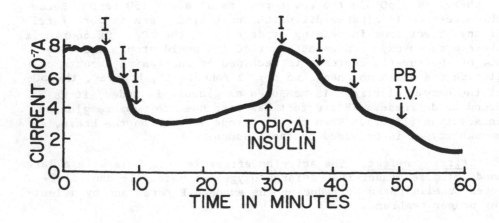

The current from a glucose electrode on the brain of a pento-
barbitalized mouse falls within 10 seconds after the intravenous
injection of 4 units of insulin. Repeated injections induce convulsions at the low levels shown in the curve. There is no effect
of oxygen breathing. When the animal was sacrificed with intravenous pentobarbital the current fell to about 1/8th of normal.
This residual current may be partly due to other polarographically
active substances and to the residual current in the electrode itself. Regardless of its nature it can be subtracted by the use of
a non-enzyme electrode which is calibrated with ascorbic acid.

Ascorbic acid. The most common anodic polarographically active substance encountered in biology is ascorbic acid. The current obtained from ascorbate (at pH 5.6) is much less than from
glucose as shown in figure 3.

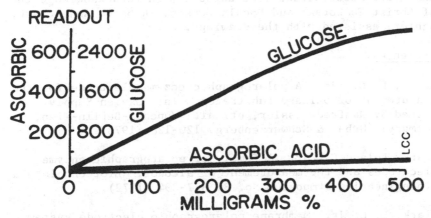

In order to use differential polarography to subtract the
effect of ascorbate (or other such substances) one adjusts the
"sensitivity knob" of the non-enzyme electrode so as to give the
same reading as the glucose electrode to a given concentration of
ascorbate. It can be shown that after this calibration procedure
the effect of ascorbate is eliminated. The small effect of ascorbate can be appreciated from figure 3 and from the fact that there
is about 1/20 as much ascorbate in blood as glucose.

Other enzymes. There is a long and growing list of oxygen
oxidoreductases, enzymes which use oxygen and produce H_2O_2. We
have already used alcohol oxidase, uricase, and the amino acid
oxidases.

Summary. The polarographic glucose oxidase anode is an accurate and rapid means to measure blood glucose. Readings may be
obtained in one minute using a 20μL sample which is diluted automatically in a 250μL cuvet. The response is linear up to about

200 mg% in the sample. The enzyme membrane, soaked in tetra-
cycline, has a life of perhaps 2 months. The glucose electrode
can be adapted to measure glucose on living brain but because of
the high glucose concentration there the response of the present
electrode is non-linear. Nonetheless it gives rapid and meaningful responses. It is concluded that it is entirely possible from
an electrochemical, electronic, and physiological standpoint to
make an intracellular glucose electrode. Because of the growing
list of oxygen oxidoreductases it is anticipated that there will
be a large number of intracellular electrodes based on this principle.

    Acknowledgements. The Yellow Springs Instrument Co., partic-
ularly Alan Brunsman, designed the instrument used. They have
been most helpful in this research. This research is supported
in part by HL12419 NIH grant and the Southwestern Chapter of the
American Heart Association. The authors wish to acknowledge the
help of Christ Tamborski and Donald Denson. Rebecca Anne Clark,
my daughter, assisted with the drawings.

    References.

1. Clark, L. C., Jr. A polarographic enzyme electrode for the
    measurement of oxidase substrates. In: Oxygen Supply,
    edited by Manfred Kessler, et. al. Munchen-Berlin-Wien,
    Germany: Urban & Schwarzenberg, 120-128 (1973).

2. Clark, Leland C., Jr. A family of polarographic enzyme
    electrodes and the measurement of alcohol. Biotechnology &
    Bioengineering Symposium No. 3, 377-394 (1972).

3. Clark, L. C. Jr. Membrane polarographic electrode system
    and method with electrochemical compensation. U.S. Patent
    No. 3,539,455, issued November 10, 1970.

4. Clark, L. C., Jr. Method of an apparatus for polarographic
    analysis. British Patent No. 1,167,317, issued October 15,
    1969. Improvements in or relating to apparatus for electro-
    chemical analysis. British Patent No. 1,169,140, issued
    October 15, 1969.

5. Clark, L. C., Jr. Method and apparatus for polarographic
    analysis. Japanese Letters Patent No. 610,201, issued
    November 11, 1970.

6. Clark, L. C., Jr. Future horizons of analytical electro-
    chemistry in the neurophysiology of mental retardation.
    American Journal of Mental Deficiency 77(5), 633-634 (1973).

7. Guilbault, C. G. (Ed.) Enzymatic Methods of Analysis.
    Oxford, England: Pergamon Press (1970).

8. Clark, L. C., Jr. and Champ Lyons. Electrode systems for
    continuous monitoring in cardiovascular surgery. Annals of
    the New York Academy of Sciences 102, 29-45 (1962).

9. The enzyme electrode analytical instrument used in this re-
    search is a prototype. It is about to go into production as
    Model 23 and is available from the Yellow Springs Instrument
    Co., Yellow Springs, Ohio 45387, U.S.A.

10. Cooper, G. R. and V. McDaniel. Methods for the determination
    of glucose. Public Health Service, Atlanta, Georgia (1966).

11. Clark, L. C., Jr. and George Sachs. Bioelectrodes for
    tissue metabolism. Conference on Bioelectrodes. Annals of
    the New York Academy of Sciences 148, 133-153 (1968).

12. Hicks, G. P. and S. J. Updike. Enzyme electrode. U.S.
    Patent No. 3,542,622, issued November 24, 1970.

13. Hedin, G. G., J. E. Johansson and T. Thunberg, editors.
    Hammarsten, O: Lehrbuch der Physiologischen Chemie,
    Chapter 5 entitled Das Blut, "Glucose in erythrocytes and
    plasma", p. 264. Munchen und Wiesbaden: J. F. Bergmann
    (1922).

14. Clark, L. C., Jr., George Misrahy and R. Phyllis Fox.
    Chronically implanted polarographic electrodes. Journal
    of Applied Physiology 13, 85-91 (1958).

15. Chance, B. The properties of the enzyme-substrate compounds
    of horseradish peroxidase and peroxides. IV. The effect
    of pH upon the rate of reaction complex II with several
    acceptors and its relation to their oxidation-reduction
    potential. Archives of Biochemistry 24, 410-421 (1949).

PROBLEMS INVOLVED IN THE MEASUREMENT OF MICROCIRCULATION BY MEANS OF MICROELECTRODES

HUTTEN, H., Physiologisches Institut, Universität Mainz
KESSLER, M.,Max Planck-Institut für Arbeitsphysiologie, Dortmund
THERMANN,M.,Chirurgische Klinik, Universität Marburg

Until now, the interpretation of local wash-out curves, measured by means of microelectrodes and using hydrogen as diffusible indicator, is an unsettled problem. It has been shown, that even the simultaneous measurement by means of a surface-multiwire-Pt-microelectrode at the isolated and hemoglobin-free perfused rat liver yields different wash-out curves (4). These differences occur with regard to the height of the curves as well as to the moment, when the maximum of the indicator's concentration is seen by the microelectrode. Fig.1 represents four simultaneously recorded curves. The difference in sensitivity of each microelectrode has been compensated by a computer. The fast curve corresponds the real input function to the liver and is directly measured in the inflow by means of a non-compensated electrode. Usually the evaluation of local hydrogen wash-out curves is performed in the same way as the evaluation of those clearance curves, which are measured by a large-scale detector, using 85-Krypton or 133-Xenon as indicator. The most commonly used methods are the slope-method (2) and the height-over-area-method (5). Application of these methods to local hydrogen wash-out curves yields different values for the local perfusion rate. Fig.2 shows the comparison between the mean perfusion rates, determined by means of the total inflow, and the local perfusion rates. In fig.2A the local perfusion rates were calculated using the height-over-area-method, whereas in fig.2B the slope-method was applied to the same curves.

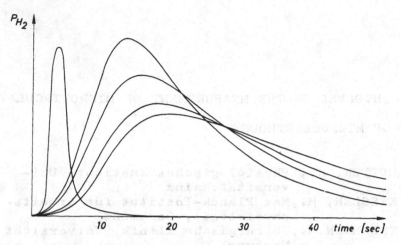

Fig.1: **Four simultaneously recorded local wash-
out curves measured by means of microelectrodes and compensated for different sensitivity by a computer. The fast curve
gives the input function to the liver.**

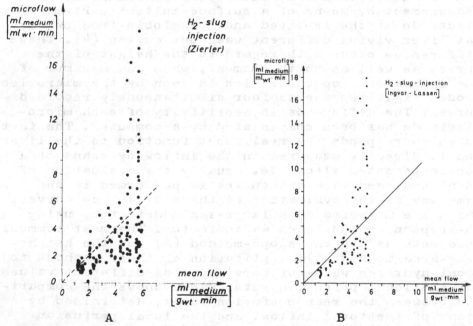

Fig.2: **Comparison between the experimentally determined values. Abscissa: mean flow. Ordinate: local flow.
A: Evaluation by the height-over-area-method
B: Evaluation by the slope-method**

The correlation between these values is not quite obvious. In the most cases, the local perfusion rates
are considerable higher than the mean perfusion rates.

METHOD

During the wash-out of the indicator, the nonsteady transcapillary exchange corresponds to a coupled
convection-diffusion-system. The mathematical description of such a system leads to partial differential
equations (1). The solution of these equations requires
the introduction of boundary conditions. The most
simple boundary conditions are those of the KROGH's
cylinder (3). Although the geometry of the KROGH's
cylinder is different from the real capillary archi-
tecture in the liver, it has been shown that the
diffusion of the indicator in radial direction is
sufficiently fast and, therefore, in this case the
limitation to the cylindric form does not mean any
restriction of the validity of the results (1). For
the mathematical procedure the assumption is made that
the size and the oxydation rate of the microelectrodes
are infinitely small. The following values are used
for all numerical calculations:
a) diffusion coefficient $D_{H_2(37^oC)} = 4,8 \cdot 10^{-5}$ cm^2/sec

b) tissue-perfusate partition coefficient $\lambda_{H_2} = 1$

c) radius of the capillary $r_o = 8 \cdot 10^{-4}$ cm

d) radius of KROGH's cylinder $r_z = 24 \cdot 10^{-4}$ cm

RESULTS

After the slug injection the indicator enters the
capillary from the arterial side. Nearly immediately
the indicator leaves the capillary by diffusion and
distributes in the surrounding tissue. Therefore, only
a very small quantity of the indicator reaches the
venous side of the capillary and the tissue around it
during the first passage of the perfusate. This means,
that in the first few moments after the injection the
indicator concentration is extremely high at the arterial side, whereas at the venous side it is nearly zero.
The indicator-free perfusate, which now is entering the
capillary, washes out some of the indicator's substance
and carries it closer towards the venous side of the
capillary. During the passage, however, the indicator

again diffuses into the tissue. This means with regard
to the microelectrode, that the maximum of the indicator's concentration is gradually passing along the
capillary, while at the same time it is decreasing more
and more. Finally, after reaching the venous side, the
indicator leaves the system together with the perfusate.
Therefore, microelectrodes located at the arterial
side, at the middle and at the venous side must see
different wash-out curves. Tab.1 is calculated for a
capillary with the length 360 /um and a passage-time of
the perfusate from 1 sec (corresponding a perfusion
rate of 6,67 ml/g/min). The location of the maximum of
the indicator concentration, expressed as the distance
from the arterial side, and the relative height of the
maximum are compared for distinct moments after the
injection.

Tab.1: The location, expressed as the distance
from the arterial side, and the relative height
of the maximum of the indicator concentration for
distinct moments after the injection.

Time after injection	location	relative height
1,1 sec	50 /um	100
2,8 sec	144 /um	58
5,0 sec	360 /um	40

A microelectrode, located at the venous side, sees
only 40% of the original maximum after a delay time
of 5,0 sec.

Although calculated wash-out curves show different
shapes, which mainly depend upon the location of the
test point, they can always be approximated over a wide
range by a monoexponential function. The time constant
during this phase of the wash-out process is independent upon the location of the test point. However, decreasing the real perfusion rate by 8:1 lowers the
slope and hence the calculated local perfusion rate by
more than 8:1.

The decrease in height from the arterial to the
venous side is more distinct, when the capillary becomes longer. In addition, the longer the capillary,
the shorter is the time constant of the wash-out curves,
even when the real perfusion rate remains unchanged.

DISCUSSION

If evaluation of local hydrogen wash-out curves is performed, using the height-over-area-method, the real perfusion rate is overestimated for all wash-out curves, which are obtained when the microelectrode is located between the arterial side and the middle of the capillary. Overestimation is enlarged if the perfusion rate is increased. Furthermore, it depends also upon the length of the capillary and may amount to 5:1. On the other hand, evaluation of wash-out curves, which are measured with microelectrodes located at the venous side, leads to a slight underestimation of the real perfusion rate. Fig.3A shows the comparison between the real perfusion rates and those perfusion rates which are calculated using the height-over-area-method. Most of the local perfusion rates are considerable higher

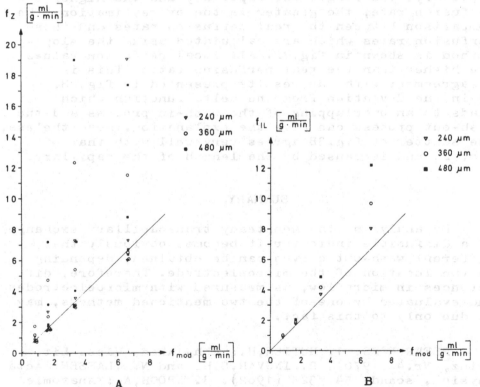

Fig.3: Comparison between the calculated flow
values. Abscissa: mean flow. Ordinate:
local flow.
A: Evaluation by the height-over-area-method
B: Evaluation by the slope-method

than the real perfusion rates. The scatter agrees very
well with that of fig.2A and is caused by a) the location of the microelectrode, and b) the length of the
capillary. The main difference is, that in the case of
the experimentally obtained results the local flow
values which are lower than the mean flow are more
numerous. This can be explained, however, by the fact
that the input function of the model was always assumed
to be an ideal delta function, whereas the real input
function shows a distinct deviation (fig.1). If the
same local wash-out curves are evaluated, applying
this time the slope-method, the real perfusion rate is
overestimated for all wash-out curves independent on
the microelectrode's position. The influence of the position is eliminated by using the best monoexponential
part of the curve. However, overestimation depends on
the real perfusion rate as well as on the length of the
capillary. The longer the capillary and the higher the
perfusion rate, the greater is the overestimation. The
comparison between the real perfusion rates and those
perfusion rates which are calculated using the slope-
method is shown in fig.3B. All local perfusion values
are higher than the real perfusion rates. This is in
disagreement with the results presented in fig.2B.
Again the deviation from the delta function which
leads to an overlapping of the wash-in process and the
wash-out process can give the explanation. Nevertheless,
the scatter of fig.3B agrees very well with that of
fig. 2B and is caused by the length of the capillary.

SUMMARY

By analyzing the nonsteady transcapillary exchange
of a diffusible indicator it becomes obviously that
different wash-out curves can be obtained, depending
on the location of the microelectrode. Therefore, differences in microflow, as measured with microelectrodes
and evaluated by one of the two mentioned methods, may
be due only to this fact.

REFERENCES: 1. HUTTEN,H.: Abh. Akad. Wiss. Lit.
Mainz, Nr.4 (1970). 2. INGVAR,D.H. and N.A.LASSEN: Acta
physiol. scand. 54, 325 (1962). 3. KROGH,A.: Anatomie
und Physiologie der Kapillaren. Springer-Verlag, Berlin
(1924). 4. THERMANN,M. and M.KESSLER: In: Oxygen supply.
Urban und Schwarzenberg, München und Berlin, University Park Press, Baltimore, 117 (1972). 5. ZIERLER,K.:
Circulat. Res. XVI, 309 (1965).

DISCUSSION OF SESSION I

Chairmen: Dr. D. W. Lübbers, Dr. L. C. Clark and Dr. W. J. Whalen

DISCUSSION OF PAPER BY I.A. SILVER

Lübbers: To avoid the tissue damage we are using Clark type multi-wire platinum surface electrode with Pt wires of a diameter of 5-15 microns. After our experience, the surface pO_2 histogram resembles the tissue O_2 histogram in most organs.

Strauss: Regarding your statement and that of Dr. Knisely on tissue damage induced immediately after implantation of electrodes. Following Dr. Clark's and collaborator's work, we have implanted electrodes chronically and found little or no damage after months of maintaining the electrodes in and recording from tissues. In the kidney, by light microscopy, at the most one cell layer can be seen affected. Would you care to speculate on how long the initial tissue damage lasts? Finally, we implant electrodes in ear lobes of neonates and record with good blood tissue correlations about 60 mins. later. Do you think that there are tissue differences in their response to the electrode?

Silver: We find that in brain there is relatively little inflammatory response and this disappears after about 24-36 hours. In other tissues, the electrode provokes a typical mild foreign body reaction with coating of the probe with macrophages. Subsequently, the macrophage response is converted to fibroblast proliferation with some fiber deposition. The fibrous layer is very thin and incomplete, but we always see something. Epithelial tissue, such as liver and kidney, give less reaction than connective tissue. I think that the distortion of the oxygen diffusion field by microfibrosis is probably of no significance to the oxygen but may lower the supply of O_2 to the implanted electrode by a small amount.

Panigel: Could you give us any information about the electron microscopic aspect of cells in tissues chronically implanted with microelectrodes?

Silver: We have looked at ultrastructural changes after chronic electrode implantation only in healing tissue. The electrode becomes surrounded by macrophages which are very resistent to alterations of microenvironment and show no changes of structure. However, if fibroblasts come to lie close to the electrode, they show changes in mitochondial structure after polarization of the electrode for more than 1-2 hours. The most sensitive cells are the fibroblasts

which are dividing or synthesizing collagen. Very small electrodes
with a cathode size of less than 1.0 μm do not produce ultrastructural damage provided that they are kept quite still.

Duling: Dr. Silver, would you elaborate on the problem of electrode
hydration and ion selectivity?

Silver: Ion selectivity develops in some electrodes as a result of
hydration of the insulating glass near the tip. Selectivity for
different ions varies with the glass used. It can be reduced by
siliconization of the glass near the electrode tip but cannot be
eliminated. It is important to recognize the development of ion
selectivity as a source of artifact. Hydration does not necessarily
lead to ion selectivity; it is most commonly associated with drift
in calibration or zero current.

Kessler: How can we determine that the in vitro calibration value
does not change under in situ conditions?

Silver: We calibrate our electrodes before and after use in tissue
and reject anything which has changed its calibration by more than
5-10%. This is not a real answer to the question, and we have tried
to check that tissue calibration is the same as in vitro calibration
by using the probe first as a surface electrode on thin layers of
tissue with wide capillary spacing and then inserting the electrode
into the tissue in sites whose surface pO_2 has already been measured.
We found that the reading in the tissue was virtually the same as
the surface reading in tissue layers 12-15 microns thick.

Schuchhardt: What was the mechanical sensitivity of the tissue-
pO_2-electrode for inserting into or moving within tissue?

Silver: We see movement artifacts on bare microelectrodes if the
tip is larger than about 1 micron. Routinely we cover our electrodes with polytyrene or Rhoplex or dichlorodimethyl silane, but
if electrodes have a tip of less than 0.5 microns they are usually
insensitive to mechanical movements even if they have no membrane.
The current reading is the critical measurement, if probe gives a
current of 10^{-13} to 10^{-14} amp/mmHg pO_2 it is unlikely to show
involvement sensitivity.
    In beating heart we have made measurements with a 'dart' elec-
trode which is inserted with a 'blowpipe' to avoid the shearing
force which develops if an electrode is inserted with a micromanipulator. Although a floating electrode of this type does not show
movement artifacts, it does cause microdamage to tissue near its tip.
    Advancing an electrode through tissue may give rise to capil-
lary compression artifacts which are real changes of pO_2.

Chance: My comment is to both Drs. Whalen and Silver. Calibration of "zero oxygen" by perfusion with N_2 may give a false zero point. We find that CO perfusion may be essential to secure intracellular anoxia in an exposed tissue that is at or near its resting state. Perfusion with CO-saturated solutions is simply and strongly recommended.

Silver: While CO may produce functional tissue anoxia, it may paradoxically increase the pO_2 by blocking O_2 uptake. If CO is played onto the surface of brain the pO_2 increases which the pyridoxine nucleotide fluorescence indicates mitochondrial hypoxia.

DISCUSSION OF PAPER BY W. J. WHALEN

Chance: My comment is to both Drs. Whalen and Silver. Calibration of "zero oxygen" by perfusion with N_2 may give a false zero point. We find that CO perfusion may be essential to secure intracellular anoxia in an exposed tissue that is at or near its resting state. Perfusion with CO-saturated solutions is simply and strongly recommended.

Whalen: I agree that there are problems with using N_2. We used the zero obtained in a brain or liver slice placed in the well over the exposed surface to be explored.

Lübbers: How did you protect the muscle against outside diffusion of oxygen and disturbance of microcirculation? The muscle seems to be especially sensitive in our laboratory. Follert made similar measurement about the oxygen consumption of the resting, flow-free, perfused heart. We found that you may find an increased oxygen consumption by increasing the flow if there is not correct protection against O_2 losses by diffusion.

Whalen: The muscle (at least the graciles) is placed on a warmed glass plate and covered with Saran, which is essentially impermeable to O_2. The solus was left in situ since it is damaged, according to Hudliska, by removing it. Saran was placed on the exposed parts, and even the hole in the Saran for electrode penetration was covered with pluronics F 127, a clear gel.

Honig: The flow dependence of $\dot{V}O_2$ of muscle may reflect species differences in $\dot{V}O_2$ of whole animal. In rat graciles, the phenomenon is easily demonstrated in our laboratory. It cannot be shown for dog graciles.
 (1) Have you observed animals smaller or larger than cat?
 (2) To what extent can the frequency histograms of tissue pO_2 account for flow dependence?

Whalen: (1) In 3 dog graciles muscles we found $\dot{V}O_2$ was flow-dependent, but the slope was much less than in the cat.

(2) We do not think that they can account for the blood flow-dependency in terms of the classical value for critical pO_2, namely about 5 mm Hg.

Kunze: Your experiments with the denervated muscle have been performed in acute or chronic denervation. In chronic denervated muscle of man I found higher oxygen pressures in the distribution and a little higher resting blood flow but especially an overshoot of repayment after ischemia.

Whalen: We have used only acutely denervated preparations, studied 15 minutes or more after applying procaine and cutting. We seldom see muscle activity upon cutting. Your observations on over-payment after ischemia are interesting. We saw little overshoot in blood flow after a period of 8-15 minutes at low perfusion pressure (e.g. 40 mm Hg). Only when flow was stopped did we see an overshoot ("reactive hyperemia") which was very marked. Overall we saw little "auto regulation" of blood flow.

Schuchhardt: We observed, with these pO_2 electrodes, a mechanical sensitivity of these electrodes when inserted into tissue or other media, and my question is, to the others who have made the same findings, if they observed dependence of this mechanical influence compared with the solidity of the tissue when the electrode moved with it.

Whalen: Really, not. An induction artifact is something that is a little hard to separate out when you have these small currents. You do, sometimes, get a little induction, and you see the induction when one moves one's hand and so on, but in the case of the heart I think we have ruled those out because if we weren't seeing an action potential with the electrode, then it was fairly quiet. It was only when we were inside a cell that we saw something that went up and down with the beating of the heart and I am sure that that was a combination of utilization of oxygen and the influx of oxygen into the tissues and, of course, the action potential, which is an artifact in that sense.

Silver: If the electrodes were larger than about .8 micron and you don't have a membrane over them, you certainly see a movement arti- fact. But if they are very small, around about .5 micron or less, and even without a membrane they seem to be fairly stable, but we normally put either a polystyrene or Rhoplex or some other membrane on the electrodes and that would seem to reduce the movement arti- fact. In beating heart we have tried using a dart electrode, which weighs about 3 milligrams, and we put it in with a blowpipe. That avoids the shearing damage that you get if you try to put it into the beating heart with a micromanipulator. Even so, we still find we get slight tissue damage. We also find that we can record the action potentials, but we have never been able to hold the intra-cellular position with our electrodes. I think that there is a difference in movement artifact according to the type of tissue that you are in. But, if you have an adequate diffusion membrane, then I think you can very much reduce it. Whalen's electrodes are better than mine because they have got a recess.

Whalen: It really is the current, not exactly the tip size.

Kessler: We did studies, together with Dr. Messmer of Munich, in hemodilution and also in our laboratory during hemorrhage. We measured oxygen supply in different organs and we always found that microcirculation and oxygen supply to the skeletal muscle is extreme-ly sensitive. For instance, when already the trauma of laporatomy can cause decrease in blood flow and in microcirculations so that we have severe hypoxia, but the interesting fact is that, when hemo-dilution is used, then we always get an almost normal flow pattern and we think this is the reason why microcirculation is re-estab-lished. Another point is that in the anesthetised animal, we have to be extremely careful in replacing enough water volume, especially if no infusion is made during the experiment of saline or something like that, then we also observe a very early decrease and we find a lot of hypoxic values in skeletal muscle.

DISCUSSION OF PAPER BY E. SINAGOWITZ AND M. KESSLER

Bicher: Your electrode showed a residual current when calibrating at low pO_2 value. Will that influence the exact calibration in this region?

Sinagowitz: As far as I know, all micro pO_2 electrodes show a more or less pronounced zero current. In thousands of measurements, we had the experience that the really good electrodes show a very low zero current which remains constant over a period of several hours. There are many factors which can influence the zero current in a negative way. One very important factor is the disturbance which is caused by electrical pulses or noise.

Kessler: I would like to point out that we did simultaneous measurements with the needle electrodes and with our surface Clark-type electrodes. The results show that both readings are corre-sponding well to each other. It is very important, however, that the animal is well grounded, but without producing grounding loops.

Lübbers: In continuation of Dr. Bicher's question, I think this electrode is linear until the very low values and there is a difference I have seen with the other calibration curve. The question probably arises, is this zero point stable over a certain period of calibration time, or is it instable?

Sinagowitz: It is stable and it is reproducible at your own calibration. One of the main points is that the animal is grounded very well, that we do not have any potential in the animal.

Chance: The increase and decrease of pO_2 following recovery from anoxia in the ischemic kidney is a phenomenon readily observed with surface fluorescence as well and may involve a component of excess mitochondrial respiration as well as circulatory alterations.

Sinagowitz: Our studies do not allow us yet to determine which component is the major one. In one experiment we found the slope of pO_2 independent of general kidney flow, in another one a parallel behavior of pO_2 and flow was observed. Further studies are needed.

DISCUSSION OF PAPER BY S. H. SAULSON

Wodick: How do you measure the response time?

Saulson: Response to a step change in pO_2 measured from 0 to 90% response level.

Holness: Were temperature effects taken into consideration during calibration of the electrode system?

Saulson: No. Temperature effects should, however be lower because a diffusion gradient is not established with short pulses.

Kunze: As far as I have seen from your slides, you have only a small distance between cathode and anode. Do you get interference from that during the peak currents of pulses?

Saulson: I worked with reference electrodes shown as close as on that one micrograph up to reference electrodes some 40 inches away and looked for differences in performance as a function of spacing. This I was not able to find. The geometry was arranged to try to minimize the pick-up of stray currents that may exist between the anode and cathode. Therefore, I tried to stay with a very symmetrical geometry.

DISCUSSION OF PAPER BY K. KUNZE AND D. W. LÜBBERS

Barr: What causes the high residual current when using pulsing techniques? Is this current subtracted from oxygen recordings in the same way that it is for continuous recording electrodes?

Kunze: This high residual current, depending on the pulse deviation, goes up the shorter the measuring pulses are. It has nothing to do with oxygen itself, because you find this high residual current in pulse measurements in nitrogen atmosphere too.

For pO_2 measurements, this residual current is subtracted and especially this is performed by using two different electrodes, one measuring at a constant pO_2 and the other at a pO_2 to be measured. In this case both electrodes must have the same characteristics.

Flower: Several years ago, Richard Albanese, et al., published a technique for obtaining absolute tissue pO_2 measurements by observing the current decay immediately following application of the polarizing potential. I would like to know if either you or Dr. Saulson have any comment about this particular technique.

Kunze: Yes, we have tried this. Of course current decrease is very steep driving the first phases of the pulse. We did not find the small differences we measured as different pO_2 sensitive enough for sufficient calibration curves. Perhaps this was due to the amplified systems we employed at that time.

Lübbers: If you look on an oscilloscope, the current decay does change the pulse; you can see that it is influenced (1) by a factor which does not depend on the pO_2 of the medium (2) by the pO_2 of the medium. So far as I remember, both factors are not independent, so it will be rather difficult to get a correct answer out of one decay curve. We saw that repeated pulses change their slope. Therefore, we measured series of pulses.

Chance: It is possible to employ a pulsed sample and hold curcuit for measuring the electrode current at any time after the polarizing pulse. We used this inflow stream up to 10M/sec with sintered glass and base electrodes with surprisingly good results.

Hutten: If the assumption is correct, which Dr. Lübbers made, that the residual current is only determined by the current which is needed for charging the double layer, then the O_2-tension must be equal to the difference between the time integral over the "on" pulse and the "off" pulse, provided that "off" means switching the voltage exactly to zero. Have you ever tried to measure the O_2-tension in this way?

Kunze: No, we did not do such measurements up to now.

Saulson: Yes, we tried this method. Even with nitrogen equilibrated saline, the integrated area of the "on" pulse was much
larger than the area of the "off" pulse.

DISCUSSION OF PAPER BY D. W. LÜBBERS

Chance: What is the theoretical basis for the Q analysis--how is
it related to theories of multipath scattering and self-absorption
screening according to Doysons?

Lübbers: The Q-analysis includes all effects predicted on grounds
of distributional factors and inhomogeneous light ray. It does not
need any theoretical assumption or a special model. By using the
transformation of the system, one is able to detect unknown components or wavelengths depending on scattering or reflection. Since
these values can be directly measured, no special assumptions are
necessary. The transformation allows, furthermore, calculations of
the average light path within the probe.

DISCUSSION OF PAPER BY I. S. LONGMUIR AND J. A. KNOPP

Chance: What is the minimum O_2 concentration at which the pyrene
fluorescence can be observed to be quenched in cells and tissues?

Longmuir: We have certainly measured accurately down to 5 mm Hg
(but this is only limited by the sensitivity of the fluorescence
measurement), with quenching constant of .0018. That means that
one atmosphere of oxygen in saline will quench about 60% of the
fluorescence.

Chance: This is too high for identifying cell anoxia which occurs
at about $10^{-7}M$. However, I am really excited about the use of pyrene
for regional two-dimensional O_2 concentrations as in the liver.
Also, the determination of the O_2 diffusion constant in the cell or
more important, in the membranes, is also of great importance.
     However, we put forward evidence against diffusion of O_2 with-
in the cell limiting the mitochondrial activity by comparing the
speed of reaction of cytochrome A_3 with O_2 in ascites cells and the
speed of the reaction of O_2 with mitochondria isolated from the same
cells. The speeds were the same, speaking against O_2 diffusion
within the cell limiting cytochrome oxidase activity.

Longmuir: I am glad to hear oxygen diffusion is not limiting.

Kessler: Is it necessary to make a correction for the inhomogeneous concentration of your stain which is caused by the heterogeneous form of the cells and which might mean that the length of the light ray differs?

Longmuir: Inhomogenenous distributions and varying quenching constants are corrected by calibration at each point.

Panigel: The scans shown were obtained on suspension of cells in saline. Did you obtain similar pictures using monolayered cell cultures developing in differently oxygenated culture media?

Longmuir: We have not looked at cultured cells.

DISCUSSION OF PAPER BY R. N. GATZ AND J. PIIPER

Song: Have you tried, in different environmental temperatures, to alter the perfusion component?

Gatz: No, we have not tried different temperatures. All of these measurements were made at 23°C. We plan, in the near future, to alter the convective component of gas transport by varying temperature.

DISCUSSION OF PAPER BY W. E. DONOVAN AND B. MYERS

Clark: Do you calibrate it in a quiet solution or a stirred solution?

Donovan: It is bubbled through. The calibration gas bubbles through an aerator in saline.

Lübbers: How can you be sure that you are measuring the average tissue oxygenation? Did you compare your values with a pO_2 histogram obtained under the same condition? In my opinion, the insertion of such a big catheter must disturb microcirculation considerably, thus the so-measured pO_2 values could be influenced by many factors which are not controlled.

Donovan: Results in subcutaneous tissue compare favorably with readings obtained by Dr. T. K. Hunt with tonometry of implanted coils. Values were compared with blood gas determinations, multiple readings under many conditions. Agreed, the catheter would do a great deal of damage to microcirculation. We have, so far, measured coils only in subcutaneous tissue.

Whalen: To follow up on Dr. Clark's question, was there a difference in the calibration reading if the solution was not stirred?

Donovan: No, as long as the concentration of calibration gases in the tonometer remained constant, stirring or not stirring had no effect.

Barnikol: Did you cover, when calibrating, the range of measurement with several points or did you calibrate with only one gas, assuming that the relation between gas content, e.g., O_2 or CO_2 is linear?

Donovan: Since the mass spectrometer is inherently linear, only one gas mixture and a zero point is necessary for calibration. The depletion of O_2, CO_2, N_2 with teflon catheters is slight, about 2×10^{-6} cc/sec.

DISCUSSION OF PAPER BY R. D. WALKER AND Y. TANRIKUT

Wodick: You say $\delta(x) = 0$ for $x \neq 0$ and $\delta(x) = 1$ for $x = 0$
I think that is not right.
    For Dirac δ function is valid:
        $\delta(x) = 0$ for $x \neq 0$
        $\delta(x) = \infty$ for $x = 0$
    and $\int_{-\infty}^{\infty} \delta(x) \, dx = 1$

Walker: Dr. Wodick's concern is a valid one and we thank him for raising the question. The problem appears to have arisen, at least partly, out of our choice of notation in which we used the delta function notation to represent a unit source function rather than a unit impulse function. What is required in the development of our model is the introduction of a step change in the source concentration (capillary at R_0, θ_0) at zero time. To avoid any possible misunderstanding arising from the use of delta notation, we have, in the revised manuscript, used the notation $q(r - R_0)$ and $q(\theta - \theta_0)$.

Hutten: If I understood your assumptions correctly, then the assumption was made that the diffusion resistance in the tissue and the capillary is negligible. Therefore, it seems to me that, the result that the diffusion resistance is mainly represented in the catheter wall is already included in your assumptions. Furthermore, the secondary condition for the exchange between the inner side and the outer side of the catheter is valid only if the solubility coefficients are the same.

Walker: We did not assume that the diffusion resistance in tissue was negligible. We did assume that the diffusional resistance of capillary and cell walls was negligible, primarily because they are so thin as compared to the total thickness of tissue considered. In assuming that the capillary could be represented by a point source,

we have also assumed no radial concentration gradients in the capillaries but this is substantiated by Kety's finding that a 4 micron
radius column of blood (on capillary radius) reached 90% of equilibrium in about 0.01 sec.

In respect to your second point concerning our boundary condition at the interface between the catheter wall and the tissue, we
have assumed continuity of mass flux at this interface. That
assumption does not require equal solubilities in the two phases.

DISCUSSION OF PAPER BY H. J. BERMAN, S. J. SEGALL AND R. L. FUHRO

Chance: (1) What is the linear polarization of the light as
incident upon the sample of blood?
(2) Could this polarization plus flow birefringence account
for the observed effects?

Berman: (1) Linear polarization was not measured.
(2) Such a possibility exists. Birefringence and polarization
certainly affect the intensity of transmitted light. Scatter, reflection, refraction and diffraction should also be considered. With
increasing rate of flow, the red cells are increasingly oriented and
more light is transmitted. However, the effect on the ratio seems
to be minimal, with the measured % sat increasing only by 0.2 to 2.0%
sat when the γ_w is decreased from 1304 to 263 sec^{-1} in 584 μ tubes.

Clark, J.:   Do you recalibrate the oximeter for each animal?

Berman: The calibration is checked before each experiment and at the
end of each experiment. The work reported here was done in vitro.
An 'experiment' comprised all work done on the blood taken from one
hamster. The lamp voltage and alignment of the light, sample, and
optics are critical in obtaining reproducible results.

Lübbers: (1) Can you use the calibration curve once established
for later measurements in different animals?
(2) Have you a theoretical explanation for the systematic
deviation at the lower and upper part of your curve?

Berman: (1) Yes, as long as experimental conditions--the spectral
quality of the light and the path of the light through the sample--
are the same.
(2) At least part of the deviation can be accounted for by
inaccuracy in the 2-regression line approach. Approximation of the
curve by two lines would result in such a variation at the ends of
the curve. Approximation by more lines would reduce the deviation
but would render data analysis more cumbersome. Above 95% sat,
however, there seems to be more deviation than can be accounted for

in this manner. It is possible that the greatly decreased O.D. at
high % sat's with a 650 nm filter may result in inaccuracies and
greater deviations in the ratio approach.

DISCUSSION OF PAPER BY K. D. FALLON, A. L. MALENFANT, R. D. WEISEL
       AND H. B. HECHTMAN

Chance: I was concerned about two omissions in your otherwise
excellent talk: (1) The "n" values may contain even more important
findings than the P_{50} values.
       (2) Many of us are deeply concerned about sickle cell disease.
What are the correlations there?

Fallon: (1) Preliminary data indicate that the "n" value does, in
fact, change. Since our methodology does develop a portion of the
curve, significant deviations in "n" values are either seen with the
naked eye or can be determined mathematically. We do see changes in
"n" values and are investigating this.
       (2) Sickle cell hemoglobin has a decreased P_{50}. Dr. Peter
Gillette of New York is using this same system to study P_{50} in
sickle cell disease. We have done nothing on this.

Messmer: Would you please comment a little more on the time
relation of the P_{50} values observed in your different groups of
patients, especially as far as blood transfusions are concerned?

Fallon: Decreases in P_{50} are associated with transfusion with
blood more than three days old. However, many changes in P_{50}
cannot be directly associated with transfusions. We have seen
changes of 15 mm Hg in P_{50} in open heart cases which received no
more blood (transfusion) than others who shifted only 4-6 mm Hg.

DISCUSSION OF PAPER BY H. I. BICHER, J. W. RUBIN AND R. J. ADAMS

Huch: I have just seen that your intravascular electrode protrudes
far beyond the disposable needle. How can you avoid the coagulation
risk by infusing heparin solution or NaCl solution against the blood
stream? You do not reach the tip of your electrode.

Rubin: The heparin-saline infusion is meant to help maintain the
patency of the arterial cannula for blood sampling and pressure
measurement. The sensor tip is advanced proximially to insure free
flow of blood around it with least disturbances. No buildup of
proteinaceous material or other debris has been noted on any of the

sensor tips. When we used shorter electrodes, there were more
artifacts due to the presence of the cannula.

DISCUSSION OF PAPER BY D. W. LÜBBERS, R. HUCH AND A. HUCH

Bicher: Will the usefulness of the electrode be limited in extreme
clinical conditions, like shock, major chest surgery, and hyaline
membrane disease in the newborn, by the fact that skin is one of
the first organs to be shut down and appear cyanotic?

Lübbers: Our device allows control, if the perfusion efficiency is
sufficient, thus you can control, if the measurements are correct.
Even if the perfusion efficiency is lower than needed, you can
measure all changes of pO_2 relatively, which can be checked by a
blood gas analysis. The test is a rather effective vasodilating
agent. There is certainly a limit of application during heavy
circulation disturbances but we do not know at the moment where
the limit is.

Strauss: Regarding the earlier discussion on catheter electrodes
vs. skin (transcutaneous or intracutaneous) electrodes, a possible
way of using each one at their best time may exist if, indeed,
there are limitations. Although this subject will be discussed in
Session V, would you think that the intravascular electrode should
be used in the acute phase of a patient's problem (shock, birth
asphyxia, etc.) and a less invasive technique in the more chronic
situation when even hyperoxia can be a problem?

Lübbers: The electrode monitors perfusion efficiency in regard to
pO_2. If the perfusion efficiency is high enough, the electrode
can be applied.

Strauss: Regarding the comment on dissemination of oxygen, either
intravascularly or in the skin, and the problem that is created
when that measurement is done in patients with shock or complications of various types, I think we can say that probably in the
acute moment when there are serious problems, an intravascular
measurement may be prefereble, but the problems do not stop then.
The problems of hyperoxia also exist at various times and probably
at those times the non-invasive techniques, either the surface of
the skin or maybe earlobe, may be useful.

Lübbers: I forgot to mention that the electrode measures relatively
correct values, even if the perfusion efficiency is not 100%. It
mirrors perfectly all the changes of the arterial pO_2 but then it
needs an inverse calibration by taking blood and analyzing. Then
you have calibrated your skin electrode in the same way as you

calibrate your catheter electrode. But the advantage of this
electrode is that you can steadily control your pO_2 value. If you
need to under certain conditions, then you can make a blood gas
analysis to be sure. In severe shock, you probably do not get even
the correct blood without putting a catheter inside the arterial
blood vessel system; so it is not true that the electrode does not
monitor something related to the arterial pO_2 if the blood pressure
is high or low.

DISCUSSION OF PAPER BY L. C. CLARK, JR., AND E. W. CLARK

Silver: We have made some micro-glucose electrodes of the type that
you suggested except that they were pointed. We found that they did
vary in tissue with position, and I suspected that possibly they
were sensitive to the oxygen gradients because we found in some
tissue that we got fairly consistent results and in other tissues,
where subsequently there were steep oxygen gradients, we did not get
good results. I wondered if possibly this was because there was not
enough oxygen. You mentioned a cut-off at about 5 mm of oxygen. I
just wondered whether this was a reasonable explanation for some of
the results that we were getting because we were a wee bit disap-
pointed.

Clark, L. C.: Keep at it! It may be that you did not have enough
enzyme there.

Silver: We coated the surface of the electrode and we dipped a
nitrocellulose membrane on. I think we should have had an excess
but electrodes did seem to be position-sensitive, and it did not
seem to be necessarily the excess of glucose. But I suspected it
seemed to go with the oxygen gradient, and your mention of 5 mm is
the answer.

Clark, L. C.: There is, of course, a point where there is insufficient oxygen to run the enzymatic reaction. This point depends
upon a number of things such as the type of membrane. But, generally speaking, it is quite low, maybe below 8 or 10 mm or oxygen.
And there may be steep gradients in glucose as well. We have been
astonished to find that the glucose on the surface of the brain
varies so widely from minute to minute and so rapidly. There seems
to be about 2 cycles per minute, while with oxygen, there are about
6 or 8 per minute. Anodic currents per se do not exhibit waves
from brain.

Bicher: I just want to report another failure! We also tried. We
got it to be quite linear in vitro up to 100, and in vivo, they
behaved very much like an oxygen electrode, that is, with the

cathode. I am quite sure that with the anode, everybody will be luckier. It looks very nice.

Clark, L. C.: You used the enzyme-coated cathode?

Bicher: I did with a cathode what Silver did with an anode, but using my design putting a coating on the outside with Rhoplex, but basically also platinum.

Clark, L. C.: Yes, the glucose oxidase coated oxygen cathode or the differential glucose oxidase cathode are influenced too much by the changing pO_2 of the blood. The anode which I have described is completely independent of the pO_2 except at extremely low tensions. Mrs. Clark and I have done thousands of glucose analyses with the new system and are quite satisfied with the results. Of course, there are special problems with in vivo calibration of any catheter sensor but they can usually be overcome.

Chance: I am struggling to remember whether or not we got a better differentiation between oxygen and H_2O_2 in post-operation. It is something to think about.

Lübbers: Have these electrodes a striking temperature coefficient? Are they very sensitive against temperature or not?

Clark, L. C.: No, they are not, because I think that when you measure the temperature coefficient, it seems lower than it should be. They are not very sensitive to temperature, and I think that may be again because there is so much enzyme there that although you may lose maybe half of its activity by lowering its temperature, it has no effect on it. The main thing is the temperature dependence of the diffusion through the membrane.

Between 15° and 50° C the glucose current given by the electrode in a 40 mg% glucose solution increases from 135 to 650 meter units. The average increase for a 10° C increase is about 155%. This is about 4% per degree C. Incidentally, the enzyme is stable for days at 50°C.

Kessler: I have a question concerning the sensitivity of the peroxide anode. Down to a peroxide concentration of 10^{-7}M/L one obtains very accurate linear calibration curves. We have found that hydrogen peroxide can be detected at a concentration of 10^{-12}M/L but at this low concentration, reproducible calibration curves cannot be obtained. Do you know of any way in which these electrodes can be improved?

Clark, L. C.: No, but, partly because of the new interest in peroxide-generating enzymes, several investigators are working on stabilizing polarographic anodes for this purpose. Dr. G. G.

Guilbault, in New Orleans, has referred to a new type of Pt anode which he has reported to be more stable.

Messmer: May I ask if you have placed your electrode on tissues, the pH of which is far from the pH optimum from the enzyme used?

Clark, L. C.: Yes, surprisingly, we have found that the electrode is quite insensitive to pH changes. For example, in changing the cuvette buffer from pH 5.6, the optimum pH, to 7.4, there was, in fact, a slight increase in glucose anode current. This is, of course, good news for those who will be measuring tissue glucose.

We have been very satisfied with the reproducibility. We have used one electrode for six weeks and have done literally thousands of measurements with it. The one question that remains, as far as the instruments are concerned and as far as we might be concerned in biology, is whether or not a compensating electrode is required. One gets about 1/400 reading on a gram per gram basis, glucose to ascorbate, so it is only 1/400 and whether that is worth compensating for or not, we are not yet sure.

Berman: What are the permeability characteristics of the cellophane membrane you use? Do you need to be concerned with the reconditioning of the membrane? What is the relationship of the enzyme to the membrane?

Clark, L. C.: The subject of membrane permeability and enzyme geometry with respect to the membrane is complex. We have worked with cuprophane, cellophane, collagen millipora and other glucose-permeable membranes with enzymes bound to the membrane or merely placed on the Pt surface. We have used one electrode as long as six weeks with no sign of deterioration. Incidentally, washing the membrane in situ often reactivates an electrode. Pluronic F68 is a good detergent for this. Merely unpolarizing (unplugging) the electrode activates it.

Chance: How are you going to improve the linearity at high glucose concentrations?

Clark, L. C.: We expect that linearity for high concentrations of glucose can be improved by some engineering of the membrane, such as changing its porosity towards glucose and the exact geometry of the enzyme-membrane interface. Dr. Lübbers has just suggested that linearity may be improved by increasing the temperature. But, of course, otherwise it will be necessary to use calibration curves for use in or on tissue.

DISCUSSION OF PAPER BY H. HUTTEN, M. KESSLER, AND M. THERMANN

Wodick: I question your first slide. Our theoretical conclu-
sions showed $\int_{-\infty}^{\infty} P\,(\vec{V},t)dt = k(\text{constant})$ for all values of $\vec{V}$ if
you have the same calibration and no loss of H_2 over the surface.

Hutten: For the local wash-out curves calculated with the computer for the model presented here the area is always constant
and independent of the position of the microelectrodes. With
regard to the experimentally measured wash-out curves it must be
taken into account that the electrodes are corrected by computer
for the same sensitivity.

Grunewald: For your calculation you assume concurrent perfused
capillaries (Krogh cylinder). How does the assumption of
countercurrent perfused capillaries influence your results.   I
believe in this case the diffusion shunt of indicator from
arterial to venous parts of capillaries can lead to other results.

Hutten: As long as the perfusion is homogenous the Krogh cylinder is an excellent model for these calculations. Only when the
perfusion becomes inhomogeneous, it may be important whether
there is a concurrent or a countercurrent system. However, there
are some hints that the rat liver is perfused homogeneously over
a wide range of perfusion rates.

Song: Did you get consistent results in terms of area of clearance curve and monoexponential components independently of the
amount of slug indicator $[H_2]$ injected?

Hutten: For the calculated wash-out curves where the input-
function always was identical to the delta-function, the results
were independent of the amount of injected indicator. For the
experimentally determined wash-out curves the input-function
never did correspond to the delta-function even by using a slug
injection. Therefore application of the simple height-over-area
formula yields erroneous results and deconvolution should be performed. However, for doing this the real input-function must be
known. Another dependence upon the amount of the indicator does
not exist as long as it is in the range of physical solubility.

Session II

PHYSIOLOGY OF OXYGEN TRANSPORT TO TISSUE

Subsessions: DPG

                BRAIN

                ABDOMINAL ORGANS

                MUSCLE

                SHOCK

                HEART

                VASCULAR CHEMORECEPTORS AND
                OXYGEN BARRIER

Subsession: DPG

Chairmen: Dr. Jørn Ditzel and Dr. Ian S. Longmuir

EFFECT OF PLASMA INORGANIC PHOSPHATE ON TISSUE OXYGENATION DURING RECOVERY FROM DIABETIC KETOACIDOSIS

Jørn Ditzel

Department of Medicine

Aalborg Regional Hospital, Denmark

INTRODUCTION

As early as in 1939 Guest and Rapoport emphasized that a striking decrease occurs in the content of 2,3-diphosphoglycerate (2,3-DPG) of the red blood cells of diabetics in ketoacidosis (1). The physiological implication of this finding has only recently emerged based on an appreciation of the allosteric behaviour of hemoglobin during oxygenation and of the unique effect of 2,3-DPG on the affinity of hemoglobin for oxygen (2,3). An increase in the concentration of 2,3-DPG in the red blood cells will produce a shift to the right in the oxyhemoglobin dissociation curve (ODC), thus facilitating oxygen release at the tissue level. A decrease in the 2,3-DPG content will increase the affinity of hemoglobin to oxygen, cause a shift of the ODC to the left, thus making less oxygen available. 2,3-DPG is formed as an intermediary product of glycolysis in the red cells and this fraction is decreased in acidosis due to the inhibitory effect of increased hydrogen ion and dehydration on glycolysis. In diabetic ketoacidosis there is also a significant depletion of the phosphorus stores in the body as shown by the immediate response of plasma and urinary phosphorus to insulin. With insulin treatment there occurs a precipitous fall in both plasma and urinary phosphorus level, and the plasma phosphate level may remain subnormal for as long as a week. Since inorganic phosphate (Pi) is known to act as a cofactor in the glycolysis of the red cells by stimulating both the phospho-fructo-kinase and the glyceraldehyde-3-phosphate-dehydrogenase

163

(4,5,6) and thereby the formation of 2,3-DPG, the concentration of Pi may be a determining factor for the rate of resynthesis of red cell 2,3-DPG and the normalization of the affinity of hemoglobin for oxygen. In evaluating this possibility we have studied the interrelationship between the concentration of plasma inorganic phosphate, red cell 2,3-DPG, and the position of the oxyhemoglobin dissociation curve in patients in and during recovery from severe diabetic ketoacidosis.

PATIENTS AND METHODS

Ten patients admitted to the hospital because of severe diabetic ketoacidosis constituted our material. The ages of the patients varied from 16 to 72 years; 8 were females and 2 were males. None of them had severe anemia or renal insufficiency. The duration of their diabetes varied from 0 to 19 years, one being diagnosed just before admission.

The blood sampling was carried out immediately on admission and thereafter each morning prior to breakfast and insulin administration. Arterial blood samples were drawn for pH and blood gas measurements. Venous blood was drawn into heparinized syringes and was analyzed for plasma phosphate and for 2,3-DPG according to the method by Ericsson and de Verdier (7). The parameters of the reaction of hemoglobin with oxygen were measured by the dissociation curve analyzer (type DCA-1, Radiometer,Copenhagen) providing a continuous print out of the ODC of whole blood (8). From the recorded curves P50 at pH of 7.40 and the in vivo pH were calculated from the formula: log P50 = log T + 0.38 (pH - 7.40), where T is the pO_2 corresponding to 50 % saturation (9,10). The student's t-test was used for statistical analyses.

RESULTS

Figure 1 shows the typical pattern of changes occurring in plasma phosphate, red cell 2,3-DPG content, and the P50(7.40) of the ODC on admission and following treatment with insulin and neutral fluid replacement in diabetic ketoacidosis. Pi on admission was normal or slightly increased, but immediately following insulin administration there occurred a pronounced drop in the plasma Pi to values not infrequently below 1 mg/100 ml. The plasma phosphate may remain at such low levels for

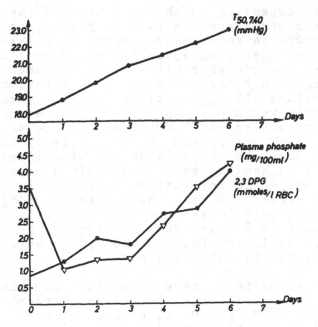

Fig.1: Changes in Pi, red cell 2,3-DPG and P50(7.40)
of ODC during treatment of diabetic ketoacidosis.

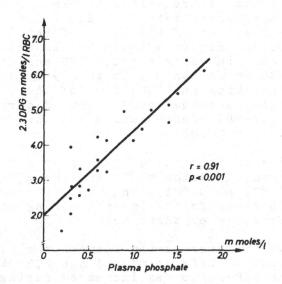

Fig.2: Correlation of Pi and red cell 2,3-DPG after
insulin administration during recovery from
diabetic ketoacidosis.
Regression line: y = 2.02 + 2.36x

several days, depending on the condition of the patient, and thereafter the plasma level slowly increased. The red cell 2,3-DPG content was decreased in all ketoacidotic patients, averaging approximately 2 mmol/l RBC on admission. The concentration slowly increased during the following 6 to 8 days to reach concentrations above the normal values. P50($\underline{in\ vivo}$) was usually normal on admission. This was due to the low concentration of 2,3-DPG counteracting the Bohr effect on the position of the ODC. P50(7.40) of the ODC was markedly below normal, approximately 18 to 19 mm Hg. With insulin treatment the pH usually became normalized approximately 24 hours after the initiation of treatment, and the P50($\underline{in\ vivo}$) became lowered. The values of P50($\underline{in\ vivo}$) and P50(7.40) slowly increased towards normal during the following 6 to 8 days. This pattern of changes between Pi, red cell 2,3-DPG, and the ODC do suggest that these changes may be interrelated.

Figure 2 shows that there is a close correlation between the concentration of Pi and the concentration of red cell 2,3-DPG (r = 0.91, p < 0.001). The high coefficient of correlation suggests that Pi may control the resynthesis of red cell 2,3-DPG.

Figure 3 shows that there exists a very close relationship between the concentration of 2,3-DPG of the red cells and the position of P50(7.40) of the ODC (r = 0.94, p < 0.001). Figure 4 indicates an individual case of diabetic coma in which the 2,3-DPG concentration was 0.93 mmol/l RBC on admission. It took 9 days before the 2,3-DPG concentration and P50(7.40) of the ODC became normal. In this case the coefficient of correlation between the 2,3-DPG concentration and the P50(7.40) of the ODC was 0.97, p < 0.001.

Figure 5 indicates that there is a close correlation between the concentration of Pi and the P50(7.40) of the ODC (r = 0.80, p < 0.001). Thus the Pi concentration may be an important factor in determining the release of oxygen from the erythrocytes.

Figure 6 shows the correlation between the blood lactate/pyruvate ratio (L/P-ratio) and the 2,3-DPG concentration. The L/P-ratio was increased during and shortly following diabetic ketoacidosis indicating a state of absolute tissue hypoxia in this condition. The correlation between the L/P-ratio and the 2,3-DPG concentration is significant(r = -0.56, p < 0.01).

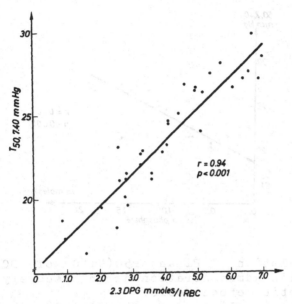

Fig.3: Correlation of red cell 2,3-DPG content and
        P50(7.40) of ODC during recovery from diabetic
        ketoacidosis. Regression line: y = 15.74+1.94x

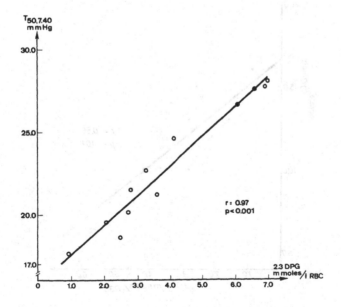

Fig.4: Correlation of red cell 2,3-DPG content and
        P50(7.40) of ODC during recovery in an individual
        case with diabetic ketoacidosis.
        Regression line: y = 14.70 + 2.35x

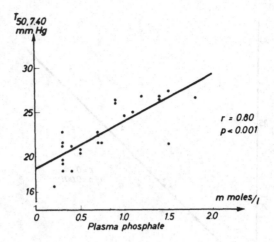

Fig.5: Correlation of Pi and P50(7.40) of ODC after
       insulin administration during recovery from
       diabetic ketoacidosis.
       Regression line: y = 18.65 + 5.28x

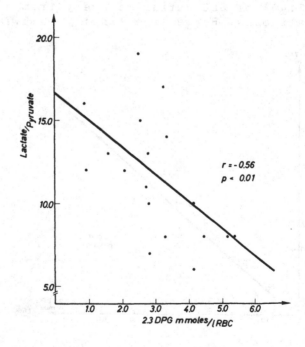

Fig.6: Correlation of red cell 2,3-DPG content and
       L/P-ratio during diabetic ketoacidosis.
       Regression line: y = 16.65 - 1.63x

More direct evidence that the concentration of Pi
is an important determining factor for the resynthesis
of the 2,3-DPG concentration and thereby for the tissue
oxygenation would be to demonstrate an immediate effect
of intravenous administration of phosphate to cases
showing hypophosphatemia. Figure 7 illustrates such an
effect in a 72-year-old woman who was admitted to Aalborg Regional Hospital in a prolonged severe ketoacidosis. On admission she was unconscious, her blood sugar
was 520 mg%, the arterial pH was 7.12, the standard bicarbonate 8.0 mmol/l. She was treated with large doses
of crystalline insulin and fluid, and despite the fact
that she had an almost normal blood sugar level, normal
blood pH, and normal concentration of serum sodium and
potassium she remained stuporous. On the third day of
her admission it was noted that she had a low Pi of
1.2 mg/100 ml. The P50(7.40) and P50(in vivo) of her
ODC was 20.5 mm Hg, i.e. the oxygen release capacity
from blood was below normal. To exclude edema of the
brain as a reason for her unconsciousness, lumbar puncture was performed showing a normal cerebrospinal fluid
pressure. She was then given 1 liter of sodium potassium
phosphate intravenously and to our surprise regained
consciousness during the latter part of the infusion
and became completely alert. On the following day the
Pi was normal and the P50(7.40) was normal. We have observed one more case in which phosphate infusion was
followed similarly by a rapid clearing of the mental
state.

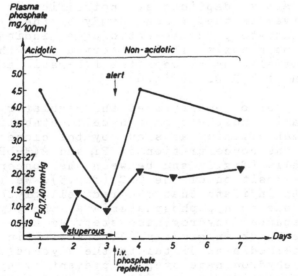

Fig.7: Changes in Pi and P50(7.40) of ODC before and
       after i.v.phosphate repletion.

DISCUSSION

In normal man, factors involved in oxygen transport include pulmonary function, cardiac output, hemoglobin
concentration, and hemoglobin oxygen affinity. These
factors are in equilibrium to maintain normal tissue
oxygen tension under varying oxygen requirements. When
a single component within this system is altered, compensatory changes occur. Factors within the red cell
environment such as 2,3-DPG concentration may change
in a manner to decrease oxygen release. Cardiac output
may then increase and those circumstances in which
oxygen loading of the blood is incomplete may be improved by increased ventilation.

This and other studies (1, 11, 12, 13, 14, 15)have
shown that diabetic ketoacidosis is associated with a
marked decrease in the content of red cell 2,3-DPG and
that during treatment the concentration of this organic phosphate compound may only rise slowly. The present study indicates that this decrease in 2,3-DPG is
strongly correlated to an increase in the red cell
affinity for oxygen (fig.3). Normally this decrease in
oxygen release capacity would easily be compensated for
by an increase in the cardiac output leading to an improved tissue perfusion and a normalization of tissue
oxygenation. These compensatory changes do take place
during diabetic coma, but due to dehydration, acidosis,
and changes in the microcirculation of many tissues
these compensatory adaptions are not efficient enough.
This is observed in the present study by the transient
rise in the lactate/pyruvate-ratio as an indication of
absolute tissue hypoxia. It is observed that there is
an inverse correlation between the L/P-ratio and the
concentration of 2,3-DPG (fig.6).

This study also demonstrates the regulatory role of
plasma inorganic phosphate on red cell metabolism and
red cell oxygen affinity as shown by the close relationship between the concentration of Pi and 2,3-DPG content
of the red cells (fig.2) and between the concentration
of Pi and the position of the ODC (fig.5). We interpret
our results to indicate that the red cell glycolysis
is inhibited due to hypophosphatemia at the glyceral-
dehyde-3-phosphate dehydrogenase step. As a result of
this relative block in glycolysis, the rise in 2,3-DPG
and other intermediates distal to the glyceraldehyde-
3-phosphate dehydrogenase step is prevented. Apparently
the 2,3-DPG repletion is markedly favoured by giving
intravenous phosphate infusion thus normalizing the Pi
(fig.7).

Other investigators have reported an influence of plasma inorganic phosphate on red cell organic phosphate compounds, 2,3-DPG and ATP (20,16,17). Travis and co-workers (18) demonstrated a relation between red cell organic compounds and red cell affinity for oxygen as a consequence of hypophosphatemia in patients, receiving intravenous hyperalimentation.

The striking clinical effect in clearing the mental state in two patients following phosphate infusions with subsequent normalization of 2,3-DPG concentration and oxygen release capacity of the blood is of considerable clinical significance. It is difficult to attribute this effect of the phosphate administration alone to its effect on the red cell and its oxygen release capacity. However, when an increased supply of phosphate is made available to the central nervous system, an increased efficiency of phosphorylations and hence of carbohydrate utilization may result. The presented metabolic improvement might be reflected in the clearing of consciousness. The present observation of the important effect of inorganic phosphate on the function and metabolism of the erythrocytes may only exemplify the importance of the organic phosphate compounds and their role in the intermediary metabolism of all cells. The result of this study emphasizes the suggestion originally brought forward by Franks et al.(19) and others that the therapeutic regimen in severe diabetic coma should include the parenteral administration of sodium phosphate 4 to 8 hours after the first dose of insulin.

SUMMARY

In order to study the determining factors for the rate of resynthesis of 2,3-DPG in diabetic ketoacidosis we have daily determined acid-base status,Pi, erythrocytic 2,3-DPG and the ODC during treatment of diabetic coma.

A significant interrelationship was found between Pi, 2,3-DPG and the position of ODC. The resynthesis of 2,3-DPG and thereby a shift of the ODC to the normal position facilitating oxygen release, was significantly correlated to Pi ($r = 0.91$, $p < 0.001$). Intravenous phosphate administration was able to normalize the 2,3-DPG content and the ODC within 24 hours and to accelerate mental recovery. For this reason phosphate infusions are recommended as an additional treatment in cases of severe diabetic ketoacidosis.

ACKNOWLEDGEMENTS

This study was partly supported by the Danish Heart Association, P.Carl Petersen's Fund and the Northern Jutland County Research Fund.

REFERENCES

1.   Guest,G.M., Rapoport,S. Amer.J.Dis.Child.58:1072, 1939.
2.   Benesch,R., Benesch,R.E. Biochem.biophys.Res. Commun.26:162,1967.
3.   Benesch,R., Benesch,R.E. Nature 221:618,1969.
4.   Rose,I.A., Warms,J.V.B., O'Connell,E.L. Biochem. biophys.Res.Commun. 15:33,1964.
5.   Tsuboi,K.K., Fukunaga,K. J.biol.Chem.240:2806,1967
6.   Schrier,S.L. Biochim.biophys.Acta 135:591,1967.
7.   Ericsson,Å., de Verdier,C.-H. Scand.J.clin.Lab. Invest. 29:85,1972.
8.   Duvelleroy,M.A., Buckles,R.G., Rosenkaimer,S., Tung,C., Laver,M.B. J.appl.Physiol. 28:227,1970
9.   Garby,L., Robert,M., Zaar,B. Acta physiol.scand. 84:482,1972.
10.   Siggaard-Andersen,O., Salling,N. Scand.J.clin.Lab. Invest. 27:361,1971.
11.   Guest,G.M., Rapoport,S. Proc.Amer.Diabetes Ass. 7:97,1948.
12.   Bellingham,A.J., Detter,J.C., Lenfant,C. Trans.Ass. Amer.Phycns. 83:113,1970.
13.   Ditzel,J. in Microcirculatory Approaches to Current Therapeutic Problems(edited J.Ditzel & D.Lewis), p.123, Basel 1971.
14.   Ditzel,J. Lancet, II:925, 1971.
15.   Alberti,K.G.M.M., Darley,J.H., Emerson,P.M., Hockaday,T.D.R. Lancet II:391, 1972.
16.   Lichtman,M.A., Miller,D.R., Freeman,R.B. New Engl. J.Med. 280:240,1969.
17.   Lichtman,M.A., Miller,D.R., Cohen,J., Waterhouse,C. Ann.intern.Med. 74:562,1971.
18.   Travis,S.F., Sugarman,H.J., Ruberg,R.L., Dudrick,S.J. Delivoria-Papadopoulos,M., Miller,L.D., Oski,F.A. New Engl.J.Med. 285:763, 1971.
19.   Franks,M., Berris,R.F., Myers,G.B. Arch.intern.Med. 81:42, 1948.
20.   Astrup,P. Advanc.in Exp.Med.& Biol. 6:67,1970.

EFFECTS OF REDUCED 2,3 DIPHOSPHOGLYCERATE ON OXYGEN RELEASE FROM BLOOD OF ALLOXAN DIABETIC RATS: MYOCARDIAL CELLULAR HYPOXIA

T.B. Allison, S.P. Bruttig, J.C. Shipp, R.S. Eliot and M.F. Crass III. Departments of Biochemistry and Medicine, Univ. of Nebraska College of Medicine, Omaha, Nebraska 68105

INTRODUCTION

The extent of tissue oxygenation in patients with diabetes mellitus has been the subject of several recent reports in the literature (Alberti, et al., 1972; Ditzel, 1972; Bellingham, et al., 1970). The criterion of tissue oxygenation used in these studies was the P_{50}, the oxygen tension at 50% hemoglobin saturation. Interpretation of these results is difficult in that both increased and decreased P_{50}'s were reported. The conditions varied from acute ketoacidosis to non-acidotic, ambulatory patients receiving insulin. An increased P_{50} was associated with the acute ketoacidotic stage of diabetes while a decreased P_{50} was associated with insulin treatment.

Two factors in diabetic ketoacidosis affect the oxygen equilibrium curve. Acidosis shifts the curve to the right, indicative of increased tissue oxygenation. Low 2,3 diphosphoglycerate (2,3 DPG) shifts the curve to the left, indicative of decreased tissue oxygenation. Tissue oxygenation depends on which of these factors has the greatest influence on oxygen-hemoglobin affinity.

The aim of this study was to examine the effects of diabetic ketoacidosis on the rate of oxygen release from blood. Previously we observed that myocardial high energy phosphates, ATP and creatine phosphate, CP, were reduced to critically low levels in acute alloxan diabetic rats (Allison, et al., 1972). We felt that tissue hypoxia may be a major contributing factor in reduction of the high energy phosphates in the heart.

173

MATERIALS AND METHODS

Fed, male albino Sprague-Dawley rats (Holtzman Co., Madison, Wisconsin) were injected intravenously with alloxan (60 mg/kg). Acute ketoacidotic diabetes was established within 48 hours following injection. Chronic, non-acidotic diabetes was produced by insulin injection (4u/day x 10 days; Lente, E.I. Lilly) 24 hours after alloxan. Blood gas analysis and tissue high energy phosphates (Bergmeyer, 1965) were determined using conventional methods. 2,3 DPG was determined enzymatically (Keitt, 1971). Kinetics of oxygen release from blood was determined in a Durrum-Gibson stopped-flow apparatus (Salhany, et al., 1971).

RESULTS

The rate of oxygen release was decreased in ketoacidotic diabetes. In addition, arterial and venous oxygen content was increased and the arteriovenous oxygen content difference was reduced to a level approaching zero. Further, myocardial high energy phosphates were decreased by 45 to 60 percent.

Table 1 compares changes in arterial pH, 2,3 DPG and k_d, the rate constant of oxygen release from hemoglobin, between control, acute diabetic and chronic diabetic rats. In the diabetic, pH, 2,3 DPG and k_d were reduced.

Blood oxygen data is shown in Table 2. Both arterial and venous values are shown. Blood oxygen tension and content were increased in the diabetic group. The blood oxygen levels were normalized after insulin administration.

	pH	2,3 DPG (mm/L RBC)	k_d (sec^{-1})
CONTROL	7.38 ±0.01	7.0 ±0.4	5.8 ±0.2
DIABETIC	7.10 ±0.03	4.0 ±0.4	4.5 ±0.2
CHRONIC DIABETIC	7.39 ±0.01	7.2 ±0.2	-

TABLE 1: Effects of ketoacidotic diabetes on arterial blood pH, 2,3 DPG and k_d. Average of ten animals. $p < 0.01$ for control vs. diabetic and for chronic diabetic vs. diabetic. No significant difference between control and chronic diabetic.

	pO_2 (mm Hg)		% SAT.		O_2 CONTENT (ml/100 ml)	
	A	V	A	V	A	V
CONTROL	76.9 ±2.3	51.8 ±1.8	94.9 ±0.4	79.5 ±4.9	15.4 ±0.8	11.8 ±0.8
DIABETIC	108.1 ±7.1	79.0 ±7.6	95.1 ±0.8	91.5 ±1.3	19.9 ±0.9	19.4 ±0.5
CHRONIC DIABETIC	80.4 ±1.9	53.8 ±1.3	95.4 ±0.8	81.0 ±2.1	18.5 ±0.6	15.8 ±0.6

TABLE 2: Effects of ketoacidotic diabetes on arterial and venous oxygen levels. Average of ten animals. Diabetic differed from both control and chronic diabetic, $p < 0.01$, for all values. A = arterial. V = venous.

Table 3 shows the effects of diabetes on the levels of myocardial ATP and CP. ATP was reduced by 45 and CP by 60 percent in the acute diabetic rats. Insulin restored high energy phosphates to control values.

	ATP	CP
	μmoles/g dry wt.	
CONTROL	20.4 ±0.4	13.7 ±0.2
DIABETIC	11.1 ±0.6	5.8 ±0.3
CHRONIC DIABETIC	20.4 ±0.4	13.4 ±0.3

TABLE 3: Effects of ketoacidotic diabetes on myocardial ATP and CP levels. Average of ten animals. Diabetic differed from control and chronic diabetic, $p < 0.01$. No significant difference between control and chronic diabetic.

DISCUSSION

P_{50} has become the accepted reference for tissue oxygenation. Increased P_{50} signifies increased tissue oxygenation or decreased oxygen-hemoglobin affinity. Decreased P_{50} signifies the opposite; decreased tissue oxygenation or increased oxygen-hemoglobin affinity. Factors which influence the hemoglobin-oxygen affinity include pH, 2,3 DPG, CO_2, CO, other ligands and alterations in the subunits of hemoglobin. P_{50} describes an equilibrium condition which can be described mathmatically as follows:

$$K_{eq} = \alpha P_{50}$$

The equilibrium constant can be written as the ratio of the overall kinetic dissociation constant, k_d, to the overall kinetic association constant, k_a, as shown in the following equation:

$$K_{eq} = k_d/k_a$$

These two equations may be combined to yield a relationship between equilibrium, in terms of P_{50}, and kinetics of association and dissociation:

$$P_{50} = \beta(k_d/k_a)$$

where $\beta = 1/\alpha$. From this equation, it can be seen that significant changes can be made in both k_d and k_a which would leave P_{50} unchanged.

We have used the alloxan diabetic rat as a model to study the effects of acidosis versus low 2,3 DPG on the rate of release of oxygen from blood. It has been established that acidosis causes a depletion of 2,3 DPG in red cells. The relationship between acidosis and 2,3 DPG is such that a prediction equation may be written relating pH to 2,3 DPG concentration (Alberti, et al., 1972; Bellingham, et al., 1970). We observed the same correlation in our studies, $r = 0.83$. The rate of oxygen release was reduced in ketoacidotic diabetes despite the observed decrease in arterial pH (Table 1). This observation implied that low 2,3 DPG exerted a tighter control on hemoglobin-oxygen affinity than did pH. Salhany, et al. (1971) showed that the effect of decreased extracellular pH on the kinetics of oxygen release in 2,3 DPG-poor red cells was about 20% of that in red cells with normal 2,3 DPG. We have observed the same phenomenon in blood. Changing the extracellular pH from 7.4 to 7.0 had no significant effect on the k_d of the diabetic blood (pH 7.10; low 2,3 DPG) whereas the same extracellular pH change in normal blood (pH 7.38; normal 2,3 DPG) increased the k_d significantly.

The decreased rate of release of oxygen from blood (Table 1) was reflected in the increase in oxygen tension and content of both arterial and venous blood (Table 2). The arteriovenous oxygen content difference of 3.6 ml/100 ml of blood in the control group is comparable to human arteriovenous O_2 content differences. In the ketoacidotic group, the arteriovenous O_2 content difference was reduced to 0.5 ml/100 ml of blood. Furthermore, venous O_2 content was increased by 65% while the arterial O_2 content was increased by only 30%. The increase in venous oxygen content was evident in the increased calculated oxygen saturation (80% → 91.5%). The observed changes in the oxygen content of arterial and venous blood and arteriovenous differences might have been sufficient to cause a general tissue hypoxia. The reduction of high energy phosphates in the heart (Table 3) are of the same magnitude as found under anoxic conditions in perfused hearts in vitro (Opie, et al., 1971).

Other factors in diabetic ketoacidosis may be responsible for, or contribute to the decrease in myocardial high energy phosphates which were observed. An increase in long chain fatty acyl CoA has been shown to inhibit oxidative phosphorylation in the heart (Shug and Shrago, 1973). However, these authors indicated that anaerobiosis or cyanosis was required to initiate the inhibitory effects of fatty acyl CoA esters.

Insulin administration to alloxan diabetic rats completely restored arterial pH and 2,3 DPG to control values (Table 1) and preliminary studies have indicated that oxygen release rates were similar to controls. The latter is supported by the insulin-induced normalization of myocardial ATP and CP.

We are currently examining the relationship between the kinetics of oxygen release and equilibrium, in terms of P_{50}, in a variety of experimental conditions.

SUMMARY

Diabetic ketoacidosis produced a decreased rate of release of oxygen from blood as a result of low 2,3 DPG in the red cell. This result tends to oppose the concept of increased tissue oxygenation based on P_{50} values in diabetic patients. Since many factors influence the equilibrium of hemoglobin with oxygen we propose that the use of P_{50} as the criterion of tissue oxygenation be reconsidered. We have observed 1) a decreased rate of oxygen release from blood, 2) a decrease in arteriovenous oxygen content difference and 3) decreased myocardial high energy phosphates in ketoacidotic diabetic rats. These observations individually and collectively suggested tissue hypoxia, not increased tissue oxygenation.

REFERENCES

Alberti, K.G.M.M, Emerson, P.M., Darley, J.H. and Hockaday,
    T.D.R. (1972). The Lancet. No. 7774:391.

Allison, T.B., Shipp, J.C. and Crass, M.F. III. (1972). Circulation
    46: Suppl. II:II-255.

Bellingham, A.J., Detter, J.C. and Lenfant, C. (1970). Trans.
    Assoc. Am. Physns. 83:113.

Bergmeyer, H.U.(ed.) (1965). Methods of Enzymatic Analysis. Aca-
    demic Press, New York.

Ditzel, J. (1972). The Lancet. No. 7753:721.

Keitt, A.S. (1971). J. Lab. Clin. Med. 77:470.

Opie, L.H., Owen, P. and Mansford, K.R.L. (1971). Cardiovasc.
    Res. Suppl. I:87.

Salhany, J.M., Keitt, A.S. and Eliot, R.S. (1971). FEBS Letters
    16:257.

Shug, A.L. and Shrago, E. (1973). J. Lab. Clin. Med. 81:214.

2,3-DPG-INDUCED DISPLACEMENTS OF THE OXYHEMOGLOBIN DISSOCIATION CURVE OF BLOOD: MECHANISMS AND CONSEQUENCES

Jochen Duhm

Department of Physiology, Medical Faculty

Technical University, Aachen (Germany)

In this paper an attempt will be made to analyze the effect of 2,3-diphosphoglycerate (DPG) on the oxygen affinity of intact human erythrocytes. Furthermore, the DPG-induced changes of oxygen release and P_{O_2} in the tissues will be estimated quantitatively in a theoretical approach. Finally, an experimental procedure is proposed which might be suitable to elucidate experimentally the physiological importance of the DPG mechanism.

TRIPLE EFFECT OF DPG ON THE OXYGEN AFFINITY OF HUMAN ERYTHROCYTES

DPG influences not only the oxygen affinity (5,8) but also the Bohr effect of hemoglobin (2,3,6,7,17,21, 25). This is shown in Figure 1 which demonstrates the changes in the P_{50} of hemoglobin solutions caused by DPG as well as by alterations of the pH. Note that the hemoglobin concentration in these experiments was close to that in intact human erythrocytes. As can be seen, the P_{50} increases a) with rising DPG concentration at all pH values studied, and b) with lowering of the pH due to the Bohr effect of hemoglobin at all concentrations of DPG. However, the increase in the absolute value of the P_{50} with rising DPG concentrations is associated with an increase in the slope of the lines which relate log P_{50} and pH, indicating changes in the Bohr coefficient.

These DPG-induced changes in the Bohr coefficient Δ log P_{50}/Δ pH are quantitated in Figure 2. Obviously, the Bohr coefficient rises from -0.22 in the absence of DPG to about -0.47 at 8 mM DPG. With further increase of

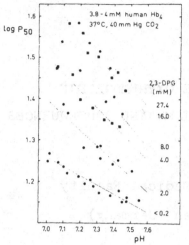

Figure 1: Effect of DPG on the P_{50} of solutions of human hemoglobin at different pH values.- Washed erythrocytes were hemolyzed by freezing in liquid nitrogen and thawing. Membranes were removed using toluene. The hemolysates were dialyzed for three days (4°C) against solutions containing 130mM KCl and 18mM $NaHCO_3$ (final molar ratio DPG/Hb_4 < 0.1). The P_{50} values were calculated from Hill plots computed from 3-5 measurements of O_2 saturation in the range of 20-80% HbO_2. The pH was varied by adding 0.3M $NaHCO_3$ or 0.3n HCl.

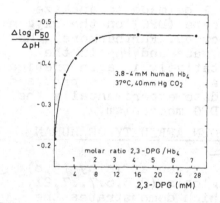

Figure 2: Effect of DPG on the Bohr coefficient of human hemoglobin.- The values were obtained from the regression lines given in Figure 1.

DPG concentration the Bohr factor remains constant indicating that the maximal effect is reached at a molar ratio DPG/hemoglobin tetramer of two, whereas the oxygen affinity of hemoglobin becomes still further reduced at higher molar ratios (Figure 1). The effect of DPG on the Bohr coefficient of human hemoglobin may be explained by an influence of DPG on the O_2-linked carbamate formation (3,21,25) and by an effect on the pK values of the residues of hemoglobin involved in the preferential binding of DPG to deoxyhemoglobin (2,7).

In intact erythrocytes, the oxygen affinity of hemoglobin is altered by DPG not only due to the direct interaction with the hemoglobin molecule but also, indirectly, through changes of the red cell pH which in turn influence the oxygen affinity because of the Bohr effect of hemoglobin (13,16). It has been demonstrated that the red cell pH decreases linearly with rising DPG levels by about 0.017 pH units per μmole DPG (plasma pH 7.4). This

decrease of the red cell pH can be explained in the following way: The DPG molecule which carries about four negative charges cannot penetrate across the red cell membrane. Consequently, with rising concentrations of DPG the
Donnan equilibrium of penetrating anions and hydrogen ions
is displaced. As a result the intracellular pH must decrease with rising DPG levels. As could be shown the pH
values calculated from the concentrations, net charges and
osmolarities of the non-penetrating cell constituents by
use of a modified equation of van Slyke closely corresponded to the measured values even under conditions differing considerably from the normal (10,11,13,16).

From all these findings it is evident that the DPG-
induced changes of the oxygen affinity of intact erythrocytes must be caused by three different mechanisms, namely 1) by the direct effect of DPG on the oxygen affinity
of hemoglobin, 2) by the influence of DPG on the Bohr
effect of hemoglobin, and 3) by the DPG-induced decrease
of the red cell pH. The contribution of each of the three
mechanisms is demonstrated in Figure 3. Curve A gives the
relationship between the P_{50} and the concentration of red
cell DPG in human blood determined at a plasma pH of 7.4.
As can be seen the P_{50} value of blood increases from 15
to 45 mmHg when DPG levels were elevated from 0 to 25
µmoles/g erythrocytes. Curve B is calculated from curve A
by correcting the P_{50} to a constant intracellular pH of
7.27 (the red cell pH in the absence of 2,3-DPG at a
plasma pH of 7.4) using the Bohr coefficients given in
Figure 2. Thus, the distance between the abscissa and
curve B is a measure of the direct allosteric effect of
DPG on the oxygen affinity of hemoglobin. The distance
between the curves A and B reflects the changes in the
P_{50} values which are brought about by the two other
effects of DPG.

Curve C is computed by correcting curve B to the

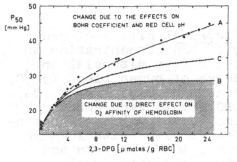

Figure 3: Triple effect of
DPG on the P_{50} of human blood.
Curve A: Measured values
(37°C, 40 mmHg O_2, plasma
pH=7.4).
Curves B and C: see text.

actual intracellular pH using the Bohr coefficient of
-0.22 determined in the absence of DPG. In this way the
alterations of the P_{50} which are due to the DPG-induced
changes of the Bohr coefficient can be eliminated from
curve A. Therefore, the distance between curve B and
curve C can be regarded to reflect the changes in the
P_{50} values resulting from the DPG-induced alterations of
the red cell pH at a constant Bohr coefficient of -0.22.
The distance between the curves A and C indicates the
changes in the P_{50} caused by the influence of DPG on the
Bohr effect of hemoglobin which become only visible, however, due to the fact that the red cell pH decreases with
rising 2,3-DPG levels.

When comparing the curves given in Figure 4 it is
obvious that the direct allosteric effect of DPG on the
oxygen affinity of hemoglobin (curve B) predominates by
far at DPG concentrations between 0 and 6 μmoles/g. However, with rising concentrations of DPG the influence of
DPG on the red cell pH and the Bohr effect becomes increasingly more important. At DPG concentrations above
10mM these two mechanisms are almost exclusively responsible for the further increase of the P_{50} values.

CONSIDERATIONS CONCERNING THE PHYSIOLOGICAL CONSEQUENCES
OF A SHIFT OF THE OXYHEMOGLOBIN DISSOCIATION CURVE

It is generally assumed that in the human adult a
right hand shift of the oxygen dissociation curve which
is caused by an elevation of red cell DPG levels leads
to an improvement of oxygen supply of tissues (cf.17,23).
Conclusive evidence proving this assumption, however, is
rather difficult to obtain in vivo. Therefore it seemed
of interest to estimate the magnitude of the changes in
oxygen release and in capillary P_{O_2} which can be expected
to result in vivo from an isolated DPG-induced shift of
the oxyhemoglobin dissociation curve.

The experimental data (13,16) allowing a theoretical

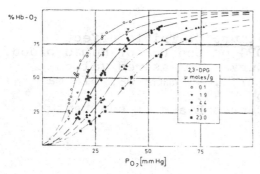

Figure 4: Effect of red
cell DPG concentration on
the oxygen dissociation
curve of human blood (37°C,
plasma pH 7.4, 40mmHg CO_2).
DPG levels were changed by
incubation without substrates (o ▽) or with 10mM inosine, 10mM pyruvate and
50mM phosphate (▲ ■).

calculation are shown in Figure 4. It is apparent that a
displacement of the curve to the right can affect
1) the amount of O_2 released at a given O_2 tension, and
2) the O_2 tension at a given O_2 release, or both parameters. Since the magnitude of the effects depends considerably on the P_{O_2} at which the cells had been oxygenated,
the results for two different P_{O_2} values used for oxygenation are given in Figures 5 and 6 as examples. It has
to be pointed out, however, that the curves shown in these Figures demonstrate the changes of O_2 release and P_{O_2}
resulting from an increase or decrease of red cell DPG
concentration in vitro from its normal value of 4.4 μmo-
les/g erythrocytes at constant pH, P_{CO_2} and temperature.
Since the latter three factors are different in the lungs
and in the capillaries in vivo, the results of these calculations cannot be applied to the conditions in vivo
without reservations.

Figure 5 demonstrates the DPG-induced changes in the
amount of oxygen released at a given P_{O_2} (oxygen releasing capacity). As can be seen the oxygen releasing capacity increases with rising DPG levels and decreases at
subnormal DPG concentrations. A reduction of the P_{O_2} used
for oxygenation from 100 to 60 mmHg is associated with a
decrease in the magnitude of the effects. Interestingly,
the DPG-induced changes of oxygen releasing capacity exhibit a maximum at P_{O_2} values between 20 and 40 mmHg under both conditions. At lower P_{O_2} values the effects of
DPG tend to disappear or even become reversed.

The highest and lowest DPG concentrations found as
yet in man in vivo are about 12 and 2 μmoles/g erythrocytes, respectively (1,9,12,18). The alterations in oxygen releasing capacity which can result from such changes
of DPG levels under the in vitro conditions of our experiments amount, maximally, to about + and - 15 % of the
total O_2 capacity (see Figure 5). If this change in oxygen releasing capacity would also occur in vivo it should
be of sufficient magnitude to cause measurable changes of

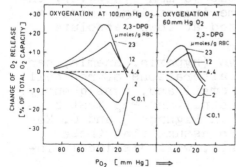

Figure 5: Changes in oxygen
release due to increase or
decrease of red cell DPG
concentration from its normal
value of 4.4 μmoles/g RBC.-
The curves were computed from
the data given in Figure 5.

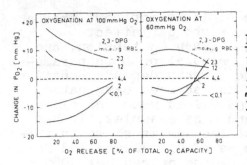

Figure 6: Change in P_{O_2} due to increase or decrease of red cell DPG concentration from its normal value.-
The curves were computed from the data given in Figure 5.

capillary oxygen release and P_{O_2} (at constant blood flow) or of the capillary blood flow required to provide a certain amount of oxygen at a given oxygen tension.

Figure 6 shows the changes of P_{O_2} at a given oxygen release which can result from alterations of DPG levels in vitro. The DPG-induced alterations of P_{O_2}, like those of oxygen release, depend on the P_{O_2} during oxygenation. Firstly the effects calculated for erythrocytes oxygenated at 100 mmHg O_2 shall be considered. Obviously, elevation of red cell DPG levels leads to an increase of P_{O_2} whereas a decrease of DPG concentration exerts the opposite effect. The magnitude of the changes becomes smaller the more oxygen is released from hemoglobin. In cells oxygenated at 60 mmHg O_2 the effects are less pronounced. It is interesting to note that under these conditions both, an increase and a decrease of DPG levels lead to an elevation of P_{O_2} when more than 50 to 60 % of the total O_2 capacity are released. If it is assumed that the actual changes occurring in vivo are quantitatively comparable to the calculated values, an elevation of DPG levels to 12 µmoles/g should lead to an increase in the capillary P_{O_2} of about 5 mmHg when 30 - 80 % of total O_2 capacity are released from hemoglobin. This change should only slightly influence tissue oxygenation in organs with a capillary oxygen release of 20 - 30 % of total O_2 capacity and a corresponding P_{O_2} of about 40 mmHg. However, the increase of 5 mmHg O_2 might become increasingly more important the more oxygen is released at lower absolute oxygen tensions.

Under most conditions in vivo (hypoxia, anemia, cardiopulmonary diseases, etc.) the alterations of red cell DPG concentration are relatively small and, consequently, the changes in oxygen release or capillary P_{O_2} must be less pronounced than those shown in Figures 5 and 6. Nevertheless, it may be justified to assume that these changes, although numerically small, will distinctly in-

fluence tissue oxygenation. On the other hand, the inspection of the curves given in Figures 5 and 6, which
demonstrate only the maximal changes to be expected, reveals that the effects of displacements of the oxyhemoglobin dissociation curve on tissue oxygenation should
not be overestimated.

The question whether a DPG-induced right hand displacement of the oxyhemoglobin curve of blood can, in
fact, induce an improvement of tissue oxygenation and a
reduction of cardiac work in vivo has not yet been elucidated. One promising approach to the problem might be
studies on tissue function in animals after exchange
transfusion with blood containing very high DPG levels.
A necessary prerequisite to such studies is a method for
elevating red cell levels. Since incubation of erythrocytes in the presence of inosine, pyruvate and inorganic
phosphate had been reported to be a suitable tool for the
rapid elevation of DPG concentration to very high values
in human red blood cells (10,11,15), the effect of such
an incubation procedure on DPG levels in erythrocytes
from various species was investigated.

As can be seen from Figure 7, erythrocytes of mouse,
rabbit and pig accumulate DPG like human erythrocytes during incubation with inosine, pyruvate and phosphate. In
contrast, DPG levels do not increase under these conditions in erythrocytes of rat, guinea pig, dog, cat, beef
or sheep (17). These species differences can be explained
by differences in the membrane permeability for the substrate inosine (17) and by different activities of the
red cell enzyme purine nucleoside phosphorylase (17,19,
22,24) which catalyzes the first step involved in the
metabolic pathway converting the ribose moiety of inosine to DPG. According to these results mouse, rabbit, pig
and also the monkey (19,24) can be used as test animals
in experimental studies designed to investigate the effect
of DPG-induced displacements of the oxyhemoglobin dissociation curve of blood on tissue oxygenation and on tissue function.

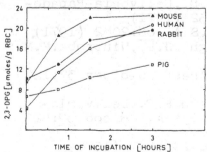

Figure 7: Increase of DPG levels in erythrocytes from various species during incubation
of the cells with 10mM inosine,
10mM pyruvate and 50mM inorganic
phosphate (hct.10%, pH 7.35,
37°C).

1) Alberti,K.G.M.M.,Darley,J.H.,Emerson,P.M.,Hockaday,
   T.D.R.: Lancet:391 (1972).
2) Bailey,J.E.,Beetlestone,J.G.,Irvine,D.H.: J.Chem.
   Soc. (A) 756 (1970).
3) Bauer,Ch.: Life Sci. 8:1041 (1969).
4) Bellingham,A.J.,Detter,J.C.,Lenfant,C.: Trans.Assoc.
   Am.Physicians 83:113 (1970).
5) Benesch,R.,Benesch,R.E.: Biochem.Biophys.Res.Commun.
   26:162 (1967).
6) Benesch,R.E.,Benesch,R.,Yu,C.I.: Biochemistry 8:2567
   (1969).
7) DeBruin, S.H.,Janssen,L.H.M.,VanOs,G.A.J.: Biochem.
   Biophys.Res.Commun. 45:544 (1971).
8) Chanutin,A.,Curnish,R.R.: Arch.Biochem.Biophys. 121:
   96 (1967).
9) Delivoria-Papadopoulos,M.,Oski,F.A.,Gottlieb,F.A.:
   Science 165:601 (1969).
10) Deuticke,B.,Duhm,J.,Dierkesmann,R.: Pflügers Arch.
    326:15 (1971).
11) Deuticke,B.,Duhm,J.: In:Oxygen Affinity of Hemoglobin
    and Red Cell Acid Base Status. M.Rørth,P.Astrup,eds.,
    p. 576, Munksgaard: Copenhagen and Academic Press:
    New York, 1972.
12) Ditzel,J.: Lancet: 721 (1972).
13) Duhm,J.: Pflügers Arch. 326:341 (1971).
14) Duhm,J.,Gerlach,E.: Pflügers Arch. 326:254 (1971).
15) Duhm,J.,Deuticke,B.,Gerlach,E.: Transfusion 11:147
    (1971).
16) Duhm,J.: In: Oxygen Affinity of Hemoglobin and Red
    Cell Acid Base Status. M.Rørth,P.Astrup,eds., p.583,
    Munksgaard: Copenhagen and Academic Press: New York.
17) Duhm,J.:In: Erythrocytes, Thrombocytes, Leukocytes;
    Recent Advances in Membrane and Metabolic Research.
    E.Gerlach,K.Moser,E.Deutsch,W.Wilmanns,eds. G.Thieme:
    Stuttgart, p. 149, 1973.
18) Oski,F.A,Marshall,B.E.,Cohen,P.J.,Sugerman,H.J.,
    Miller,L.P.: Annals Int.Med. 74:44 (1971).
19) Oski,F.A.,Sugerman,H.J.,Miller,L.D.: Blood 39:522
    (1972).
20) Oski,F.A.,Travis,S.F.,Miller,L.D.,Delivoria-Papado-
    poulos,M.,Cannon,E.: Blood 37:52 (1971).
21) Riggs,A.: Proc.Nat.Acad.Sci.,U.S.A. 68:2062 (1971).
22) Sandberg,A.A.,Lee,G.R.,Cartwright,G.E.,Wintrobe,M.M.:
    J.Clin.Invest. 34:1823 (1955).
23) Shappell,S.D.,Lenfant,C.J.M.: Anesthesiology 37:127
    (1972).
24) Sugerman,J.J.,Pollock,T.W.,Rosato,E.F.,Delivoria-
    Papadopoulos,M.,Miller,L.D.,Oski,F.A.: Blood 39:525
    (1972).
25) Tomita,S.,Riggs,A.:J.Biol.Chem. 246:547 (1971).

EVIDENCE FOR A RELATIONSHIP BETWEEN 2,3-DIPHOSPHOGLYCERATE-DEPLETED

RED BLOOD CELLS, SLOW OXYGEN RELEASE AND MYOCARDIAL ISCHEMIA

J.W. Holsinger, Jr., J.M. Salhany, and R.S. Eliot

Division of Cardiology, University of Nebraska Medical

Center and Department of Biophysics, Univ. of Chicago

Following the reports of Chanutin and Curnish (1) and Benesch and Benesch (2) in 1967, numerous reports have emerged extending our knowledge of the molecular physiologic and clinical aspects of 2,3-diphosphoglycerate (DPG). Some of these molecular findings may now be tested physiologically using an animal model. The first part of this paper will consider the molecular basis for oxygen release from the red cell while the second will deal with a physiologic model and the question of whether a decrease in the rate of release of oxygen from the red cell can induce myocardial ischemia in the dog.

KINETIC BASIS FOR OXYGEN RELEASE FROM THE RED BLOOD CELL

It is now well established that DPG reduces the oxygen affinity of stripped, dilute hemoglobin solutions (1,2). The site of binding to hemoglobin appears to be established as the central cavity between the beta chains of deoxyhemoglobin (3,4,5). Indeed, in non-cooperative hemoglobins such as carboxypeptidase digested hemoglobin and hemoglobin reacted with bis (N-maleimidomethyl) ether, DPG shows no effect on the hemoglobin-oxygen equilibrium curve (6,7). These hemoglobins are "locked" in the liganded protein conformation independent of the state of heme ligation. Thus the above results indicate that a necessary condition for DPG to affect the oxygen affinity is a change in the conformation of the protein from the liganded to the unliganded, or perhaps an intermediate (8) protein conformation.

Such large changes in the oxygen affinity, clearly must have a kinetic basis. The first demonstration that DPG increases the rate of deoxygenation of human hemoglobin solutions was reported

187

in 1970. As in hemoglobin solution, DPG significantly reduces the oxygen affinity of hemoglobin within the red blood cell. The whole blood equilibrium studies of Duhm (10), measured P_{50} as a function of intracellular DPG from near zero to 24 μmoles per gram RBC. Simultaneously Salhany, Keitt and Eliot (11) measured the rate of deoxygenation of red blood cells as a function of intracellular DPG and pH.   The shape of the curve of P_{50} vs DPG concentration (10, Fig.2) is almost identical to the plot of k_c (the cellular pseudo first order deoxygenation rate constant in sec^{-1}) vs DPG concentration (11, Fig.2). It is now clear that intracellular variation in DPG produces changes in intracellular pH via shifts in the Donnan equilibrium (10,11,12). Salhany et al (11) measuring ΔpH (13) vs intracellular DPG (14) found the following linear equation to fit the data:

$$\Delta pH = 0.007 \text{ (DPG μmoles/gm Hb)} + 0.129$$

This equation agrees closely with that obtained by Duhm (15).

The question thus arises concerning how much of the change in P_{50} and k_c is due to a direct effect of DPG on intracellular hemoglobin and how much is due to the indirect effect of DPG; i.e., the change in intracellular pH and the consequent increase in P_{50} and k_c via the Bohr Effect. Duhm (10) and Bellingham, Detter, and Lenfant (12) calculated, based on the known changes in P_{50}, DPG and intracellular pH, that the direct effect of DPG was present only up to about 19 μm/gm Hb. Salhany et al (11), using the rapid kinetic technique, were not only able to separate the direct effect of DPG from the indirect effect, but were also able to determine the effect of DPG on the "kinetic Bohr Effect" of red cells. They too observed that the direct effect of DPG on k_c occurs up to about normal red cell levels at any constant intracellular pH below a pH of about 7.7. DPG greatly increased the "kinetic Bohr Effect" of intracellular hemoglobin in a manner quite analogous to solution kinetic studies (9). Thus from these three studies we can suggest that the function of DPG within the normal red cell is to maintain an adequate Bohr effect for intracellular hemoglobin by direct stoichiometric binding to the protein. Thus at physiologic pH a sufficient P_{50} and rate of deoxygenation will be present to meet tissue needs. When DPG is present at levels well above normal, the Bohr effect will be maintained, but the P_{50} will drop and the rate of cellular deoxygenation (k_c) will increase solely due to the additional protons present consequent to the shift in the Donnan equilibrium. With these points in mind, we shall now describe the physiologic model used in this study.

PHYSIOLOGIC MODEL

The animal is prepared such that an anterior myocardial infarction is produced. Later, the same animal is studied by partially constricting the circumflex coronary artery, thereby

producing a near failing left ventricle. Finally, DPG depleted
blood, with a measured slow rate of oxygen release is perfused
through the left coronary arterial system. The effect of the DPG
depleted blood on the myocardium is then determined.

This preparation is carried out by sterilely placing an ameroid
constrictor (16,17) near the origin of the left anterior descending
coronary artery of 20–25 Kg dogs. An acute anterior myocardial
infarct is thus produced. From 3 to 9 weeks later, the circumflex
artery is dissected free. Utilizing Hood's method (18), a coronary
artery occluder consisting of a 6.5 x 7.0 mm silastic balloon
attached to a 6.5 x 30 mm dacron-reinforced belt with the balloon
bonded to a 28 mm silastic tube is placed around the circumflex
artery. To monitor circumflex artery blood flow, a Biotronix 1.75 mm
blood flow transducer is placed distal to the balloon coronary
artery occluder. Left ventricular pressures are obtained by placing
a pigtail catheter in the left ventricle via direct puncture of the
ventricular wall. Baseline left ventricular pressures, circumflex
coronary arterial flow, and an electrocardiogram are obtained.

In step-wise increments, the balloon occluder is slowly inflated
with saline until a stable LVED pressure elevation is recorded. As
reported by Hood (19), a stable elevation of LVED pressure is
defined by maintenance of the elevated pressure for five minutes.
By this method, the amount of saline necessary to elevate the LVED
pressure is determined and the saline is then withdrawn from the
occluder. While the occluder is thus partially inflated, the
circumflex artery flow distal to the partial occlusion is measured.
This level of flow is then used throughout the experiment as the
baseline flow during partial circumflex artery occlusion.

Via the right carotid artery a medium right Judkins coronary
artery catheter is placed into the ascending aorta. Under fluoro-
scopic control and utilizing radiopaque contrast material, the
catheter is placed in the ostium of the left coronary artery. The
balloon occluder is then inflated with the previously determined
amount of saline. Immediately on placing the catheter in the left
coronary artery, previously prepared, fully saturated, blood with
depleted red cell DPG and a reduced rate of oxygen release is perfused into the left coronary arterial system by way of a Sarns pump.
Simultaneously LVED pressure, ECG and circumflex artery blood flow
are measured. By controlling the speed of the pump, the flow through
the circumflex artery is maintained equal to that determined as the
baseline flow with the occluder partially inflated. The LVED
pressure, circumflex artery flow and the ECG are recorded utilizing
Statham physiologic pressure transducers, Model P23Db and a
Biotronix Laboratory flowmeter.

The DPG depleted blood was prepared by drawing fresh dog blood
under sterile conditions into a 500 cc plastic bag containing 75 cc
of acid citrate-dextrose (Fenwall Laboratories). The blood is
stored at $4^{\circ}C$ for 7 to 10 days. The level of DPG in the red blood
cells was measured (14) and the rate of deoxygenation measured as

described previously using the modified Durrum-Gibson stopped flow
apparatus (11). Blood was not utilized unless the level of DPG and
the rate of deoxygenation were reduced compared with dog norms.
Not only will such rapidly perfused DPG depleted blood have a lower
rate of deoxygenation at the same extracellular pH compared with
normal but it will also have a reduced "kinetic Bohr Effect".

RESULTS AND DISCUSSION

The results of four experimental animals is presented here.
With each dog acting as its own control, DPG was reduced from a mean
($\pm$SD) normal value of 18.85 $\pm$ 1.99 μmoles/gm Hb to 0.20 $\pm$ 0.04 μmoles/
gm Hb prior to utilization in these experiments. The value of k_c
was reduced from a mean ($\pm$SD) control of 1.90 $\pm$ 0.16 sec^{-1} (measured
in vitro in isosmolar Tris-buffer, extracellular pH 7.5 and temperature 23°C) to a value of 1.03 $\pm$ 0.04 sec^{-1} (Fig.1).

In all animals in which a transmural myocardial infarction was
noted histologically a rise in LVED pressure was also noted when
the circumflex artery balloon occluder partially occluded the lumen
of this vessel (Fig.2, panel B). This compares with the results of
Hood (19) who found that partial occlusion of the circumflex artery
in the face of a previous anterior myocardial infarction resulted in
a stable state of left ventricular decompensation for at least 5
minutes. They noted tachycardia, increased LVED pressure and
hypotension, which was reversible on termination of the constriction.

With perfusion of the experimental blood in the studies
presented herein, the left ventricle of all animals with proven
transmural infarction failed (Fig. 2 panel C). As may be seen in
Fig. 2, the circumflex artery flow distal to the balloon occluder,
although not measured, was matched before and during the perfusion
of the experimental blood. In the animal shown in this figure, it
is most interesting to note that ischemia is present with partial
occlusion of the circumflex artery as well as when blood with a
decreased rate of oxygen release (and decreased kinetic Bohr Effect)
is perfused through the left coronary arterial system as indicated
by the inverted T-waves of the ECG. Of even more interest is the
evidence of an injury current with ST-segment elevation noted in the
ECG in Panel C (Fig. 2) occurring during perfusion of blood with the
altered functional properties described.

In summary, we can state that DPG-depleted blood greatly affects
the degree of myocardial oxygenation as determined by LVED pressure
and ECG. However, it would seem to go without saying that any
sweeping conclusions concerning a cause and effect relation between
oxygen release and myocardial ischemia, although extremely tempting,
must be guarded. In particular, we must be concerned about the
rheologic state of DPG-depleted cells (to our knowledge a yet
undetermined aspect) before it becomes possible to make conclusions
about the cause and effect relation between DPG, oxygen release from
the red cell, and the observed ischemic damage to the dog myocardium.

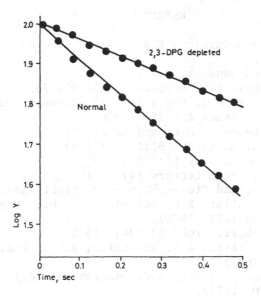

Figure 1. The rate of deoxygenation of dog fresh and DPG depleted blood in isotonic tris-HCl buffer pH 7.5 at 23°C. Plotted as the natural log of the percent saturation (Y) versus time in seconds.

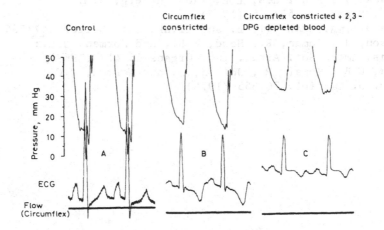

Figure 2. The effect of partial occlusion of the circumflex artery and DPG depleted blood on Left Ventricular end-diastolic pressure.
Panel A - Control: ECG and flow are normal, LVED 0 mm Hg.
Panel B - Partial constriction of circumflex artery: Moderately decreased arterial flow, ischemic t-waves, LVED 13 mm Hg.
Panel C - Partial constriction of circumflex artery plus infusion of DPG depleted blood. Flow matched with that of Panel B, ischemic t-waves and ST-segment elevation indicating injury, LVED 28 mm Hg.

REFERENCES

1. Chanutin, A. and Curnish, R.R.:   Arch. Biochem. Biophysics
    121:96 (1967).
2. Benesch, R. and Benesch, R.E.:
    Biochem. Biophys. Res. Commun. 26:162 (1967).
3. Bunn, H.F. and Briehl, R.W.: J. Clin. Invest. 49:1088 (1970).
4. Perutz, M.F.:   Nature 228:734 (1970).
5. Benesch, R., Benesch, R.E. and Enoki, Y.:
    Proc. U.S. Nat. Acad.Sci. 61:1102 (1968).
6. Imai, K.:   Biochemistry 12:798 (1973).
7. Salhany, J.M.:   FEBS Letters 14:11 (1971).
8. MacQuarrie, R., and Gibson, Q.H.:   J. Biol. Chem. 246:5832 (1971).
9. Salhany, J.M., Eliot, R.S. and Mizukami, H.:   Biochem. Biophys.
    Res. Commun. 39:1052 (1970).
10. Duhm, J.:   Pflügers Arch. 326:341 (1971).
11. Salhany, J.M., Keitt, A.S. and Eliot, R.S.:   Fed. Euro. Biochem.
    Soc. Letters 16:257 (1971).
12. Bellingham, A.J., Detter, J.C. and Lenfant, C.:   J. Clin.
    Invest. 50:700 (1971).
13. Hilpert, P., Fleischmann, R.G., Kempe, D. and Bartels, H.:
    Amer. J. Physiol. 205:337 (1963).
14. Keitt, A.S.:   J. Lab. Clin. Med. 77:470 (1971).
15. Duhm, J.:   Pflügers Arch. 319:2 (1970).
16. Litvak, J., Siderides, L.E. and Vineberg, A.M.:
    Amer. Heart J. 53:505 (1957).
17. Vineberg, A., Mahanti, B. and Livak, J.:   Surgery 47:765 (1960).
18. Joison, J., Kumar, R., Hood, W.B., and Norman, J.C.:
    Trans. Amer. Soc. Artif. Int. Organs 15:417 (1969).
19. Hood, W.B., Kumar, R., Joison, J. and Norman, J.C.:
    Amer. J. Cardiol. 26:355 (1970).

THE OXYGEN-AFFINITY OF HEMOGLOBIN: INFLUENCE OF BLOOD REPLACEMENT

AND HEMODILUTION AFTER CARDIAC SURGERY

F. Jesch, M.D., L.M. Webber, PhD, J.W. Dalton, M.D.,
J.S. Carey, M.D.
From the Thoracic Surgery & Chest Sections, Wadsworth
VA Hospital Center, and the UCLA School of Medicine,
Los Angeles, California. Supported in part by U.S.
Public Health Grant #14043-02.

Red cell 2,3-diphosphoglycerate (2,3-DPG) is an important factor
affecting the affinity between oxygen and hemoglobin (2). The
infusion of stored blood during and after operations employing
cardiopulmonary bypass produces a decrease in the 2,3-DPG concentration in erythrocytes (4,5). Low concentrations cause an
increase of the oxygen affinity for hemoglobin resulting in a left
shifted oxygen dissociation curve. From a high arterial oxygen
tension to a given tissue pO_2, less oxygen is unloaded from the
blood to the tissue. In addition, blood loss and fluid replacement during and after surgery cause an acute decrease of hemoglobin, lowering the arterial oxygen content. Oxygen transport to
the tissues may be compensated by an increase in cardiac output or
oxygen extraction. Reduced hemoglobin concentration has been
found to decrease affinity of oxygen for hemoglobin by adaptive
rise in red cell 2,3-DPG (6,9). The purpose of this study was to
examine the possible compensation of the progressing hemodilution
by a decreasing oxygen affinity to hemoglobin in order to maintain
a sufficient oxygen supply to the tissue.

METHODS

Measurements were performed on 10 males undergoing open heart
surgery for coronary artery bypass grafts, 6, or cardiac valve
replacement, 4. All patients, ranging in age from 43 to 61 years,
underwent general anesthesia, thoracotomy and cardiopulmonary
bypass. The pump was primed with one-to-three day old blood
stored in acid-citrate-dextrose (ACD), bicarbonate and various
crystalloid and colloid solutions.

Venous blood samples were obtained after the start of

193

anesthesia, after the finished operation, and on the morning 3, 6, and 13 days postoperatively. An additional sample was taken from the priming blood.

The oxygen affinity of hemoglobin was determined as the oxygen partial pressure (pO_2) at a hemoglobin saturation (HbO_2) of 50% (P_{50}). Increased affinity of hemoglobin for oxygen would lower the P_{50} value shifting the oxygen dissociation curve (O_2-DC) to the left, and a decreased affinity would shift the O_2-DC to the right indicating lower oxygen affinity of hemoglobin. Six ml of each blood sample were equilibrated in a tonometer* for 30 minutes at 37°C with two gas mixtures which produced an oxyhemoglobin saturation of approximately 65 and 35% and a CO_2 partial pressure (pCO_2) of 40mmHg. This saturation, the hemoglobin concentration (Hb) and the CO saturation of hemoglobin (HbCO) were measured spectrophotometrically*. The pH, pO_2, and pCO_2 for each equilibrated blood sample were measured using a digital pH/blood gas analyzer*. Each pO_2 value was corrected to a standard plasma pH of 7.4. The oxygen dissociation curve was linearized using Hills equation (1) and the P_{50} was calculated by computer. The values in 8 non-smoking young adult males ranged from 25.6 to 27.0mmHg (mean 26.2+0.1mmHg). Prior to equilibration, the concentration of red cell 2,3-DPG of each sample was determined by a spectrophotometric procedure (8). The values in the 8 normals ranged from 9.5 to 14.6µmoles/gHb (mean 11.8+0.7µmoles/gHb). The oxygen release to a normal mixed venous pO_2 of 40mmHg was calculated from actual arterial oxygen content by % deoxygenation and expressed as ml oxygen per 100 ml of blood. The data are mean values with standard error of the mean (SEM) and analyzed by means of students t-test with p=0.05 as the level of significance.

RESULTS

The blood volume (measured by I-131 albumin) preoperatively averaged 5560+293ml. The blood loss during the operation was replaced by 2680+532ml ACD blood including pump prime blood. By the third postoperative day additional 1750+133ml whole blood were infused. All the blood used for replacement ranged in age from 1-3 days.

The replaced blood during the operation was found to have a hemoglobin concentration of 14.4+0.3%, a P_{50} of 22.2+0.5mmHg, a 2,3-DPG concentration of 8.8+1.5µmoles/gHb, and a HbCO of 3.8+0.7%. Fig. 1 represents the alterations in P_{50}, 2,3-DPG, Hb and HbCO from preoperatively to second week after the operation. An additional sample was taken from the priming blood. The mean

*Instrumentation Laboratory Inc., Lexington, Mass.

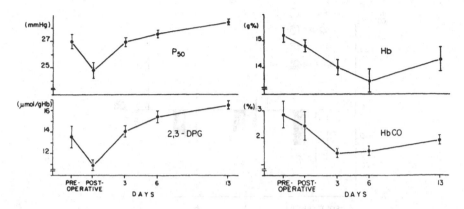

Fig. 1: Changes in hemoglobin affinity for oxygen (expressed by
P_{50}), red cell 2,3-diphosphoglycerate (2,3-DPG), hemoglobin concentration (Hb), and carbon monoxide saturation of hemoglobin
(HbCO) in 10 patients who had undergone open heart surgery (mean
values $\pm$ SEM).

control level for P_{50}, 27.0 ± 0.5mmHg, was elevated above the normal
mean in our laboratory. The affinity of hemoglobin for oxygen
immediately after the operation was increased as indicated by a
lower P_{50} (24.8 ± 0.6mmHg) shifting the O_2-DC at a 50% saturation to
the left by 2.2mmHg against the control level. On the third postoperative day the P_{50} reached the control level (26.9 ± 0.3mmHg)
progressively increasing until the second week (28.4 ± 0.2mmHg)
causing a right shift of the O_2-DC at the saturation of 50% from
the postoperative value by 3.6mmHg. Statistically significant was
the increased affinity after the operation and the decreased
affinity two weeks postoperatively ($p< 0.02$). The alterations in
red cell 2,3-DPG were closely related to the changes in P_{50}
(Fig. 1). From a control level elevated above normal (13.6μmoles/
gHb) the concentration decreased significantly ($p<0.05$) after the
operation ($10.9\pm0.4\mu$moles/gHb) and achieved the highest level two
weeks postoperatively ($16.5\pm0.3\mu$moles/gHb), significantly elevated
above the control level ($p<0.05$). During the operation forced
oxygen breathing slightly lowered the carbon monoxide saturation
from 2.9 ± 0.5% to 2.5 ± 0.5%. In the early postoperative period the
HbCO decreased to 1.4 ± 0.2, ($p<0.02$). By replacement of half the
blood volume the postoperative mean of P_{50} and 2,3-DPG is midway
between preoperative and replaced blood. The hemoglobin concentration decreased on the 6th postoperative day (15.3 ± 0.3 to
13.5 ± 0.4, $p<0.01$), probably as a result of fluid replacement and
elimination of pump damaged red cells. Two weeks after the
operation the Hb concentration had risen, but a slight hemodilution
remained (14.3 ± 0.5%Hb). Fig. 2 shows the changes in % of control

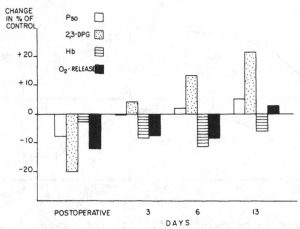

Fig. 2: Alterations in % of control for P_{50}, 2,3-DPG, hemoglobin
concentration (Hb) and oxygen release immediately and 3, 6, and
13 days after the operation.

for P_{50}, 2,3-DPG, Hb concentration and oxygen release at a normal
venous pO_2 of 40mmHg. In spite of the marked decrease in the
2,3-DPG concentration of the red cells immediately after the
operation (20%) the alteration of P_{50} did not achieve the expected
amount (8%). This behavior was observed during the whole postoperative period: the changes in P_{50} never reached the extent
expected by changes in 2,3-DPG. Immediately after the operation,
both the high oxygen affinity and the slight hemodilution caused a
deficit of 12% in oxygen release compared with the control level,
if the venous pO_2 or the cardiac output did not change for compensation. During the following week the oxygen affinity decreased,
but was not able to compensate for the progressing hemodilution.
After two weeks a slight increase in oxygen release resulted from
a 5% decrease in oxygen affinity in spite of a remaining small
hemodilution.

DISCUSSION

During an uncomplicated open heart operation the affinity of
oxygen for hemoglobin, indicated by a lowered P_{50}, is significantly
increased and may impair tissue oxygenation. The main determining
factor for alterations in oxygen affinity appears to be the concentration of red cell 2,3-DPG. After replacement of almost half the
blood volume with ACD preserved blood, the postoperative range of
P_{50} and 2,3-DPG is nearly midway between preoperative values and
replaced blood. The increased affinity could be in part attributed
to a direct influence of the pump oxygenator system on the 2,3-DPG
concentration (4). Hemolysis occurring during cardiopulmonary

bypass may also contribute to increased oxygen affinity after the
operation. However, the quantitative significance of those
factors was not determined in this study. The CO level, elevated
in the replaced blood, was significantly lowered by forced oxygen
breathing. Only in the immediate postoperative period could this
decrease counteract the increasing right shift of the oxygen dissociation curve, because after the third postoperative day the
oxygen affinity progressively decreased in spite of a slight
increase in carbon monoxide saturation.

The hemoglobin concentration decreased continuously until the
6th postoperative day resulting in a lower oxygen capacity of the
whole blood. Thus, the available oxygen for the tissues would be
reduced unless compensated by a higher flow rate. It has been
shown experimentally that until a hematocrit of 20%, tissue pO_2
remains unchanged indicating a sufficient tissue oxygenation (7).
Cardiac output, however, has to rise compensatorily. For cardiac
patients during the cirtical recovery phase this demand could be
a deleterious factor. In comparison to other possible mechanisms,
such as increased oxygen extraction, the most harmless compensatory
mechanism would be a decreased oxygen affinity of hemoglobin.
Reduced hemoglobin concentration results in a decreased affinity
of hemoglobin for oxygen (6,9), mediated by an increase in 2,3-DPG.
In addition, the 2,3-DPG after transfusion of stored blood rises
rapidly following its initial drop (10). It was, therefore,
expected that decreased oxygen affinity would undertake at least
partly the compensation for the progressing hemodilution. During
the first postoperative week the expected compensation was not
efficient enough, but after two weeks the remaining slight hemodilution was fully compensated by decreased oxygen affinity without
further need of other mechanisms.

SUMMARY

Alterations in the oxygen affinity of hemoglobin (P_{50}), red
cell 2,3-diphosphoglycerate (2,3-DPG), hemoglobin concentration
(Hb), and carbon monoxide saturation of hemoglobin (HbCO) were
studied in 10 patients undergoing open heart surgery. P_{50} and
2,3-DPG concentration decreased significantly immediately after the
operation, reached the control level on the third postoperative day,
and increased during the following two weeks. Immediately after
the operation increased oxygen affinity of hemoglobin and slight
hemodilution caused a potential deficit in oxygen release to the
tissue. After the 3rd postoperative day, decreased oxygen affinity
alone was not able to compensate for the progressing hemodilution.
Full compensation of a mild persisting hemodilution by decreased
oxygen affinity alone was reached two weeks after the operation.

REFERENCES

1. Bartels H, Harms H: Sauerstoffdissoziationskurven des Blutes
   von Säugetieren. Pflüg. Arch. ges. Physiol. 268:334-365 (1959).

2. Genesch R, Benesch RE: The effect of organic phosphates from
   the human erythrocyte on the allosteric properties of hemoglobin. Biochem. Biophy. Res. Commun. 26:162-167 (1967).

3. Bohr C, Hasselbalch K, Krogh A: Über einen in biologischer
   Beziehung wichtigen Einfluss, den die Kohlensaurespannung des
   Blutes auf dessen Sauerstoffbindung übt. Skand. Arch.
   Physiol. 16:402-412 (1904).

4. Bordiuk JM, McKenna PJ, Giannelli S, Ayres SM: Alterations in
   2,3-DPG and O_2 hemoglobin affinity in patients undergoing open-
   heart surgery. Circulation, Sup I, Vols. XLIII & XLIV:
   1-141 - 1-146 (1971).

5. Ecker RR, Rea WJ, Sugg WL, Miller WW: Changes in 2,3-DPG after
   cardiopulmonary bypass. Ann. Thor. Surg. 13:364-370 (1972).

6. Edwards MJ, Canon B: Oxygen transport during erythropoietic
   response to moderate blood loss. N.E.J.M. 287:115-119, (1972).

7. Messmer K, Sunder-Plassmann L, Jesch F, Gornandt L, Sinagowitz
   E, Kessler M: Oxygen supply to the tissues during limited
   normovolemic hemodilution. Res. exp. Med. 159:152-166 (1973).

8. Sigma Tech. Bul. 665 1/72.

9. Torrance J, Jacobs P, Restrepo A, Eschbach J, Lenfant C,
   Finch CA: Intraerythrocytic adaptation to anemia. N.E.J.M.
   283:165-169 (1970).

10. Valeri CR, Hirsch NM: Restoration in vivo of erythrocyte
    adenosine triphosphate, 2-3-diphosphoglycerate, potassium ion,
    and sodium ion concentrations following the transfusion of
    acid-citrate-dextrose-stored human red blood cells. J. Lab.
    Clin. Med. 73:722 (1969).

11. Woodson RD, Torrance JD, Shappell SD, Lenfant C: The effect
    of cardiac disease on hemoglobin-oxygen binding. J. Clin.
    Invest. 49:1349-1356 (1970).

ANALYSIS OF 2,3 DIPHOSPHOGLYCERATE-MEDIATED, HEMOGLOBIN-FACILITATED OXYGEN TRANSPORT IN TERMS OF THE ADAIR REACTION MECHANISM

Jerry H. Meldon, Kenneth A. Smith and Clark K. Colton

Department of Chemical Engineering, Massachusetts

Institute of Technology, Cambridge, Mass.   02139

Since the initial observations ($\underline{1},\underline{2}$) of the effect of 2,3 diphosphoglycerate (2,3 DPG) upon the oxygen affinity of hemoglobin, considerable interest has focussed on the importance in the gas exchange process ($\underline{3},\underline{4}$) of this species and other organic phosphates. This paper summarizes a theoretical analysis of the influence of 2,3 DPG on O_2 transport in hemoglobin solutions. The physical system analyzed is the same as that used in previous treatments of hemoglobin-facilitated oxygen transfer ($\underline{5}$). A thin film of solution separates two phases containing differing partial pressures of oxygen (p_{O_2}). Hemoglobin, although mobile, is constrained to remain within the liquid film. As a result of O_2-Hb interactions, the diffusion of O_2 from the high to the low p_{O_2} boundary induces a parallel diffusion of oxyhemoglobin. If 2,3 DPG is present, there are gradients in the concentrations of free and of hemoglobin-bound 2,3 DPG as a result of the gradients in oxy- and deoxyhemoglobin and preferential binding of 2,3 DPG to the latter ($\underline{6}$). In this study, the concentrations of free and bound 2,3 DPG were taken to be constant across the film.

MATHEMATICAL ANALYSIS

Mass conservation equations in the absence of electrical, convective, and coupled diffusive effects take the form:

$$D_i \frac{d^2 C_i}{dx^2} = r_i \quad (i = 1,2,3 \ldots ,n) \qquad (1)$$

199

where D_i is the diffusion coefficient of component i (n of which participate in the chemical reactions), C_i is its molar concentration, r_i is its local rate of depletion by chemical reaction, and x is the position in the film. Boundary conditions are:

$$\text{at } x = 0; \quad C_{O_2} = C_{O_2}^0, \quad \frac{dC_i}{dx} = 0 \quad (i \neq O_2)$$

$$\text{at } x = L; \quad C_{O_2} = C_{O_2}^L, \quad \frac{dC_i}{dx} = 0 \quad (i \neq O_2)$$

where 0 and L refer to the upstream and downstream boundaries.

In the limit of reaction rates sufficiently high relative to diffusion rates, a state of reaction equilibrium prevails throughout the film and it can be shown (7) that the solution is:

$$J_{O_2} = \left[\frac{D_{O_2}}{L} (C_{O_2}^0 - C_{O_2}^L) \right] \left[1 + \frac{4 \, D_{Hb} \, C_{Hb}^T}{D_{O_2}} \left(\frac{S^0 - S^L}{C_{O_2}^0 - C_{O_2}^L} \right) \right] \quad (2)$$

where J_{O_2} is the O_2 flux, D_{Hb} is the hemoglobin diffusivity (assumed equal for all forms), C_{Hb}^T is the total concentration of oxy and deoxy-hemoglobin in the film and S^0 and S^L are the up- and downstream fractions of oxygenated heme sites. Equation (2) can be derived independent of kinetic mechanism. The total flux is increased in proportion to the slope of a chord joining the two boundary conditions on a saturation curve.

Most analyses of hemoglobin-facilitated O_2 transport which account for the finite kinetics (e.g. 8,9) have approximated O_2-Hb interaction kinetics by $O_2 + Hm \rightleftarrows HmO_2$ where Hm represents the reactive heme site, four of which are present in undissociated hemoglobin. A one-step kinetic scheme implies a hyperbolic saturation curve expressed by:

$$S_{1-step} = \frac{K_{eq} \, C_{O_2}}{1 + K_{eq} \, C_{O_2}} \quad (3)$$

where K_{eq} is the association equilibrium constant. Since the physiological saturation curve is sigmoidal and cannot be fit over any appreciable range of p_{O_2} by a hyperbola (see Figure 1), the Adair (10) "intermediate compound" scheme has been used here:

$$O_2 + Hb(O_2)_{i-1} \; \underset{b_i}{\overset{k_i}{\rightleftarrows}} \; Hb(O_2)_i \quad (i = 1,2,3,4) \quad (4)$$

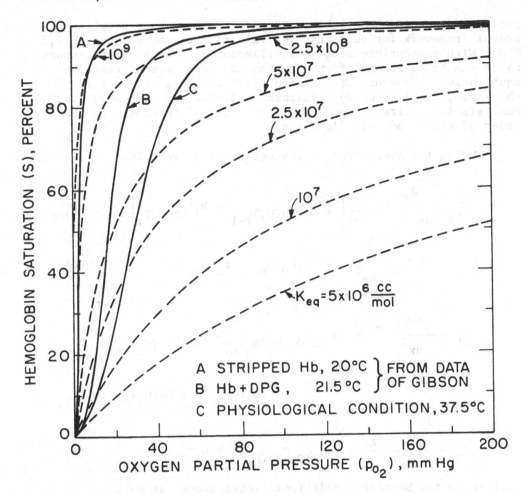

FIGURE I. COMPARISON OF VARIOUS SATURATION CURVES
AND ATTEMPTED FITS WITH HYPERBOLAE (BROKEN LINES)

where k_i and b_i are the respective forward and reverse rate constants
of the ith oxygenation reaction, and the corresponding equilibrium
constants are given by $K_i = k_i/b_i$ (i = 1 to 4). In the Adair scheme,
the hemoglobin saturation is a function of all four K_i and the oxygen concentration. A set of K_i values can be derived so as to give
a reasonably close fit to physiological saturation curves (11).

The function in O_2-Hb interaction of 2,3 DPG and other phosphates has been interpreted (11) in terms of their effect upon the
apparent equilibrium constants. In the presence of 2,3 DPG, there
was a marked decrease in K_1, K_2, and K_3, with K_4 remaining unchanged.
The kinetic studies of Gibson (12) showed that 2,3 DPG increased
the rates of dissociation of the last three oxygen molecules from

fully saturated oxyhemoglobin. The Adair scheme thus provides a useful framework for quantitative evaluation of the effects of 2,3 DPG. With appropriate sets of equilibrium constants, O_2 transport rates can be calculated from equation (2) for cases of reaction equilibrium. However, with finite reaction rates and/or film thickness, the rate of O_2 transport is decreased. A nonequilibrium analysis is required, especially with films of thickness on the order of red blood cell dimensions.

Using the Adair scheme, the equations to be solved are:

$$D_{O_2} \frac{d^2 C_{O_2}}{dx^2} = \sum_{i=1}^{4} \left[k_i C_{O_2} C_{Hb(O_2)_{i-1}} - b_i C_{Hb(O_2)_i} \right] \tag{5}$$

$$D_{Hb} \frac{d^2 C_{Hb}}{dx^2} = k_1 C_{O_2} C_{Hb} - b_1 C_{HbO_2} \tag{6}$$

$$D_{Hb} \frac{d^2 C_{Hb(O_2)_m}}{dx^2} = k_{m+1} C_{O_2} C_{Hb(O_2)_m} - b_{m+1} C_{Hb(O_2)_{m+1}}$$

$$\tag{7}$$

$$- k_m C_{O_2} C_{Hb(O_2)_{m-1}} + b_m C_{Hb(O_2)_m} \quad (m = 1,2,3)$$

$$D_{Hb} \frac{d^2 C_{Hb(O_2)_4}}{dx^2} = -k_4 C_{O_2} C_{Hb(O_2)_3} + b_4 C_{Hb(O_2)_4} \tag{8}$$

subject to the boundary conditions listed above, as well as

$$\int_0^L \left[\sum_{i=1}^{5} C_{Hb(O_2)_{i-1}} \right] dx = C_{Hb}^T L \tag{9}$$

An exact analytical solution to this non-linear problem is not possible. Therefore, two approximate solutions were derived. The first makes use of regular power series expansions in terms of a perturbation parameter proportional to L^2. Termed "thin film theory," it measures the effect of reaction on a process which is predominantly diffusive. The second, termed "thick film theory," makes use of a singular perturbation and the method of matched asymptotic expansions. It measures the effect of diffusion for a case in which reaction effects predominate. Results from the two theories, together with a minimum of interpolation between them, produce an excellent estimate of the O_2 flux at any film thickness. Details of these analyses, as well as a similar approach to CO_2

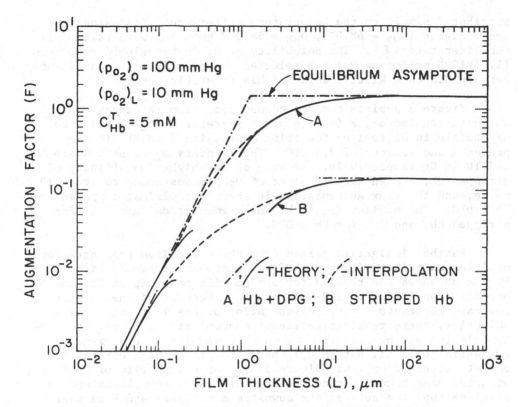

FIGURE 2. EFFECT OF 2,3 DPG ON DEPENDENCE OF
AUGMENTATION FACTOR ON FILM THICKNESS.

transport in buffered alkaline solutions, are available (13).
Application of these techniques to facilitated transport systems
characterized by single-step kinetics is discussed elsewhere (14).

RESULTS AND DISCUSSION

For the purpose of evaluating the effect of 2,3 DPG upon
oxygen transport rates, calculations were made using the kinetic
constants reported by Gibson (12). The values for stripped hemo-
globin (k_1 = 1.47, k_2 = 3.52, k_3 = 1.58, k_4 = 3.3 cc/mol-sec$\times 10^{10}$;
b_1 = 136, b_2 = 15.7, b_3 = 138, b_4 = 50 sec^{-1}) were from experiments
run at 20°C, while those undertaken in the presence of 2,3 DPG
(approximately equimolar with C_{Hb}^T; k_1 = 1.77, k_2 = 3.32, k_3 = 0.49,
k_4 = 3.30 cc/mol-sec$\times 10^{10}$; b_1 = 1900, b_2 = 158, b_3 = 539, b_4 = 50
sec^{-1}) were at 21.5°C. The 1.5°C temperature difference lessens the
comparability of the two sets of data. However, differences in
reaction rates due to 2,3 DPG are much greater than could be

attributed simply to the temperature difference. Diffusion
coefficients (D_{O_2} = 6×10^{-6}, D_{Hb} = 5×10^{-8} cm^2/sec) were taken from
the literature (**9**). The solubility of O_2 in hemoglobin solutions
(1.06×10^{-9} mol/cc-mm Hg) was selected so as to provide consistency
between Gibson's kinetic data and his saturation curves.

Figure 2 depicts the dependence upon film thickness of the
augmentation factor, F (the relative increase in O_2 flux due to
oxyhemoglobin diffusion) for films containing 5 mM Hb, in the
presence and absence of 2,3 DPG. The boundary O_2 pressures are 100
and 10 mm Hg respectively. Because of the higher O_2 affinity of
stripped Hb, a significant amount of O_2 remains bound to it at 10
mm Hg, and the flux augmentation is therefore minimal compared to
Hb + DPG. The maximum (equilibrium) augmentations are 0.13 for
stripped Hb, and 1.4 for Hb + DPG.

Further insight is gained from the normalized concentration
profiles calculated from thick film theory and shown in Figure 3.
Figure 3a shows the results for a 5 μm film of stripped Hb, and O_2
boundary conditions of 100 and 0 mm Hg. Because of the relatively
low rate constants for the dissociation of the last three oxygen
molecules, there remain significant concentrations of all the oxy-
hemoglobins at the downstream boundary, despite a zero oxygen
concentration. All but $Hb(O_2)_4$ have the predominant effect of
back-transfer of oxygen. Figure 3b is for a 5 μm film of Hb + DPG,
with the same boundary conditions. All the oxyhemoglobin concentrations approach zero at the downstream boundary and F is nearly
F_{eq} because of the higher dissociation rates.

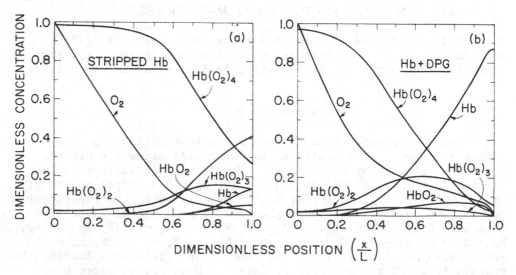

FIGURE 3. DIMENSIONLESS CONCENTRATION PROFILES FOR
L = 5 μm, C_{Hb}^T = 5 mM, $(p_{O_2})_0$ = 100 mm Hg, $(p_{O_2})_L$ = 0
($C_{O_2}/C_{O_2}^0$ AND $C_{Hb(O_2)_i}/C_T$ vs. x/L)

The results must be qualified by several limitations. First, the kinetic data employed in the calculations were for temperatures significantly below physiological levels. At a higher temperature the reaction rates are increased more than diffusion rates, and there is a closer approach to chemical reaction equilibrium for systems with and without 2,3 DPG. Secondly, the analysis was based on a neglect of the gradients in 2,3 DPG concentration. The extent of error introduced by such approximation is difficult to estimate without quantitative data giving the functionality of reaction rates with DPG concentration. Finally, the Adair scheme is itself a simplification to the kinetics of O_2-Hb interaction, and the recent work of Gibson (15) indicates the necessity for a re-evaluation of the mechanism in terms of the widely different reactivities of α and β chains. Despite these qualifications, it is believed that a semi-quantitative evaluation of the effect of 2,3 DPG on O_2 transport rates has been presented.

ACKNOWLEDGEMENTS

Supported by the National Science Foundation, E.I. DuPont de Nemours Company, and Camille and Henry Dreyfus Foundation.

REFERENCES

1. Benesch, R. and Benesch, R.E. (1967) Biochem. Biophys. Res. Commun. 26, 162.
2. Chanutin, A. and Curnish, R.R. (1967) Arch. Biochem. Biophys. 121, 96.
3. Forster, R.E. (1972) in Benzon Symp. IV, Rorth, M. and Astrup, P., eds., Munskgaard, Copenhagen, p. 518.
4. Rossi-Bernardi, L., et al. (1972) in Benzon Symp. IV, Rorth, M. and Astrup, P., eds., Munskgaard, Copenhagen, p. 224.
5. Kreuzer, F. (1970) Resp. Physiol. 9, 1.
6. Perutz, M.F. (1970) Nature, 226, 726.
7. Olander, D.R. (1960) AIChE J. 6, 233.
8. Kreuzer, F. and Hoofd, L.J.C. (1972) Resp. Physiol. 15, 104.
9. Kutchai, J., Jacquez, J.A., and Mather, F.J. (1970) Biophys. J. 10, 38.
10. Adair, G.S. (1925) J. Biol. Chem. 63, 529.
11. Tyuma, I., Imai, K., and Schimizu, K. (1972) in Benzon Symp. IV, Rorth, M. and Astrup, P., eds., Munskgaard, Copenhagen, p. 139.
12. Gibson, Q.H. (1970) J. Biol. Chem. 245, 3285.
13. Meldon, J.H. (1973) Sc.D. Thesis, MIT, Cambridge.
14. Smith, K.A., Meldon, J.H., and Colton, C.K. (1973) AIChE J. 19, 102.
15. Gibson, Q.H. (1973) Proc. Nat. Acad. Sci. 70, 1.

Chairmen: Dr. Jørn Ditzel and Dr. Ian S. Longmuir

DISCUSSION OF PAPER BY J. DITZEL

Longmuir: What happens to the plasma calcium?

Ditzel: Generally very little, Si calcium might decrease 0.2 - 0.3 m
moles and we have not seen any clinical signs of hypophosphatemia.
This might be because the infusion often is made in an acidotic
situation.

Salhany: Would you care to comment on the possibility that the
injection of inorganic phosphate you give to your patients may be
influencing DPG metabolism, not only as a substrate for DPG synthesis, but also as a buffer for the low blood pH? We do know that
increasing alkalinity will increase intracellular DPG.

Ditzel: There is no doubt that the effect of the phosphate infusion
is due to its effect on 2,3 DPG resynthesis and not just due to
increased alkalinity.

Holland: (1) Is lactate/pyruvate ratio reliable to estimate tissue
hypoxia in diabetic ketoacidosis when carbohydrate metabolism is
disturbed?
    (2) Can we be sure improvement in L/P ratio is due to DPG
resynthesis, when circulation is being improved at the same time
as DPG is resynthesized?
    (3) It is hard to accept a venous P_{50} of 80 Torr due to low
DPG. One would expect a left-shifted curve to give normal O_2
extraction at the low pO_2 or low O_2 extraction at normal pO_2.

Ditzel: As to your first question, one cannot be sure that the
lactate to pyruvate ratio in this situation gives a correct estimate
of tissue hypoxia. I am, however, inclined to theorize that the
figures presented for the L/P ratio underestimate rather than over-
estimate the actual hypoxic situation.
    As to your second question, you might be correct that this
relationship might be due to a simultaneous improvement of the
microcirculation rather than due to a decrease in the 2,3 DPG
content. However, these patients were not in shock and were regularly well-hydrated and out of their acidosis after 24 hours of
treatment, and despite this, the L/P ratio remained increased.
    As to your third question, a venous pO_2 of 80 Torr is high and
we were also astonished to see this. However, you have to realize

that this is not mixed venous blood, but blood taken from a deep
brachial vein. Total oxygen consumption is generally not decreased
in diabetic acidosis, but the oxygen consumption is rather deranged,
and the oxygen consumption of the liver is, in contrast to that of
muscle, very high.

Duhm: I would like to comment on some therapeutic consequences
which might be postulated from your findings: In severe acidosis,
the decreased levels of DPG compensate for the right-hand shift of
the oxyhemoglobin dissociation curve which is caused by the decrease
of the blood pH. Upon a sudden return of blood pH to the normal
range, the DPG induced shift becomes "unmarked" and can thus display
its possible disadvantageous effects on tissue oxygenation for
several days until the red cell DPG pool is restored. Therefore,
one might postulate from this very specialized point of view, that
a severe acidosis should be therapeutically compensated only slowly,
thus allowing a continuous regeneration of DPG which could be
accelerated by your phosphate infusion.

DISCUSSION OF PAPER BY T. B. ALLISON AND S. P. BRUTTIG

Murthy: (1) Did you measure cardiac output?
       (2) Without measuring cardiac output, just based on A-V O_2
difference it is difficult to decide regarding O_2 supply to tissue
because marked changes in cardiac output can compensate for decrease
in release of oxygen from blood.

Allison: (1) No.
       (2) In order to normalize oxygen delivery to the myocardium
with the decrease in A-V O_2 content we observed would require an
increase in cardiac output of approximately 7 fold. We do not feel
that this is likely in view of the fact that heart rate was not
increased.

Chance: A very simple test for your hypothesis on the role of DPG
in diabetes can readily be controlled by transfusing with normal
rat blood. Did you do this control?
       Without such a control, I am very doubtful that such a small
decrease of the "off" velocity constant could have such a large
effect on heart metabolism. Do you agree?

Allison: (1) No. I agree that this would be a desirable experiment to perform.
       (2) The small decrease in the rate of oxygen release from
ketoacidotic diabetic blood compared to control blood in in vitro
experiments using dithionite may possibly become large differences

in rates of release <u>in vivo</u> where the major stimulus to oxygen release is the O_2 gradient to the tissue.

<u>Holland</u>: I cannot accept that a decrease in the release velocity constant is of importance. The slide showed results at 23° C. I measured these rates with the Lawson and Forster some years ago over a range of temperatures and it is much faster at 37° C. There is good reserve in normals for all reasonable values of capillary transit times. I do not really think that the paper has shown that the "off" velocity constant is of importance in this disease.

<u>Allison</u>: I agree that increasing the temperature to 37° C will increase the rates of oxygen release. However, the relationship we observed between control and low 2,3 DPG blood should be maintained at 37° C. In the heart of normal individuals coronary sinus pO_2's of 20 mm Hg represent the lower limit of oxygen dissociation from blood. Our hypothesis is that a 20-30% decrease in the rate of oxygen release may be sufficient to compromise ventricular function. The observed decrease in ATP and CP does compromise ventricular function and may be due to hypoxia induced by a decreased rate of oxygen release from blood.

<u>Lübbers</u>: It is difficult to understand that such a small change in the P_{50} results in a tissue hypoxia. Normally microcirculation buffers small changes in the dissociation curve. Why did this mechanism not work in your cases?

<u>Allison</u>: If one examines the oxygen content data, one sees that the A-V O_2 difference is reduced by nearly 7 fold. An increase in capillary density may account for this, but hypovolemia should result and with a widening of the A-V O_2 difference. Several other authors, including Dr. Ditzel, have shown that this is not the case.

<u>Kessler</u>: I am skeptical about your interpretation of your results. Following our experience, I suggest that the severe disturbances of metabolism which you observed cause disturbances of microcirculation and consequently partial hypoxia in tissue.

In our own experiments, in which the influence of the shift of the dissociation curve on tissue oxygen supply was investigated, we found that the effect on the local oxygen distribution curve is relatively small. Did you make any investigations on local microcirculation on a local tissue oxygen supply in your experiments?

<u>Allison</u>: No, we have not. However, anoxia is a potent stimulus to vasodilatation. Our oxygen content data and pO_2 data shows that there is not a systemic hypoxemia. I am not aware of data indicating vasodilatation due to tissue hypoxia. Acidosis alone will produce vasodilitation. Therefore, in these studies, I would not consider decreased microcirculation to be a safe limiting factor.

DISCUSSION OF PAPER BY J. DUHM

Salhany: I would like to comment on Dr. Duhm's excellent paper.
When we make calculations of oxygen transport to tissue we must ask
the question as to whether the blood-oxygen system is at equilibrium
in vivo, in the relatively short times for oxygen release to such
high oxygen consuming tissue as brain and the myocardium. If the
blood-oxygen system is not at equilibrium, then measurement of
oxygenation and deoxygenation rates appear relevent. If, on the
other hand, the blood-oxygen system is at equilibrium, then red
cell deoxygenation rate measurements are purely academic.

Duhm: It was one aim of my paper to point out that the cases given
in Figures 5 and 6 show the 2,3-DPG-induced changes in oxygen release
and pO_2 calculated from oxyhemoglobin dissociation curves determined
in vitro at equilibrium. In case the "contact time" of the erythrocytes in the capillaries (time for effective gas exchange) exceeds
0.5 sec, one can certainly assume that the equilibrium is obtained
almost completely. Under these conditions, not the changes in the
velocity of the "off reaction" ($HbO_2 \rightarrow Hb+O_2$), but rather of the
ratio of the "off" and "on" reactions, which determines the O_2 saturation of hemoglobin at a given pO_2, should alter the amount of
oxygen released in the capillaries. However, as already mentioned,
it remains to be elucidated whether a 2,3-DPG-induced shift of the
curve can, in fact, alter tissue oxygenation in man and animals in
vivo.

Chance: Thank you for the suggestion of your extra slide since we
have done just the experiment you suggest, with low and high DPG
human blood, however, we used the working perfused heart, with work
and flow measurements, and, most important, measured the delivery
of oxygen to the tissue by surface fluorometry of mitochondrial NADH.
The latter was adjusted to incipient anoxia (10-50% extra NAD reduction) with high DPG blood and the switching to low DPG blood, both
equilibrated with the same pO_2 (more HbO_2 will be present in low
DPG blood). Under these conditions, the two blood samples gave
indistinguishable tissue oxygenation. The explanation is that at
very low tissue pO_2's, there is very little difference due to low
and high DPG cells, as indeed some of your data showed. At higher
pO_2's, DPG may raise tissue pO_2's but the perfused heart is adequately
oxygenated.

Duhm: This slide is included as Figure 7 in the paper. Your results
could be due to the fact that isolated hearts can increase their
coronary flow when perfusing them with erythrocytes depleted of 2,3
DPG. You can "trim" the experimental conditions in such a way that
isolated hearts respond to changes of red cell DPG levels. According to our own studies, performed more than one year ago, an isolated,
working rat heart which is perfused at a constant pressure with saline

solutions containing human erythrocytes with low (< 1 mg) or high
(> 1 mg) DPG levels (oxygenated at 100 mm Hg O_2) shows no changes
in flow rate or heart work when hematocrit was 30-40%. At hematocrit values between 5 and 10%, however, the coronary flow increased
by about 100% when high DPG cells were replaced by DPG-depleted
erythrocytes. These results do not bare evidence that the "DPG
mechanism" might be effective in vivo under normal conditions.
However, they may indicate that changes of the position of the
oxyhemoglobin dissociation curve can be important for the oxygenation of the heart at very low hematocrit values in vivo.

DISCUSSION OF PAPER BY J. W. HOLSINGER, R., J. M. SALHANY AND
R. S. ELIOT

Messmer: Unfortunately, I could not find out from your slide what
the coronary flow values have been in absolute values and if the
decrease in coronary flow after transfusion of stored blood was
significant. Therefore, I wonder if you could comment on the
hematocrit values of your animals as compared with the hematocrit
of the transfused blood.

Holsinger: Coronary blood flow was measured qualitatively and not
quantitatively. Thus, I have no absolute value of the blood flow.
There was no significant difference in hematocrit between the dog's
own blood and the infused stored blood.

Coburn: I think it is most difficult in this type of experiment to
match your low DPG blood with your control blood. Was pH and O_2 the
same? Is it possible vasoactive substances were liberated in your
low DPG blood and this could have influenced or explained your
results? Red blood cells probably were smaller and the infused low
DPG blood may have had different pressure-flow characteristics.

Holsinger: ATP in the infused blood was minimally reduced. pO_2 and
O_2 saturation are normal at the time of infusion due to O_2 being
bubbled through the boood prior to infusion. pH was titrated to
7.3 - 7.4 prior to infusion using Na bicarbonate. Vasoactive substances may be released and their effect on the model is unknown.

Subsession: BRAIN

Chairmen: Dr. Ian A. Silver, Dr. Goran M. Kolmodin

and Dr. Britton Chance

AUTOREGULATION OF OXYGEN SUPPLY TO BRAIN TISSUE

(INTRODUCTORY PAPER)

Haim I. Bicher

Departments of Anatomy and Medicine, Medical University

of South Carolina, Charleston, South Carolina, U.S.A.

INTRODUCTION

The availability of oxygen throughout the brain is far from homogeneous, oxygen tensions varying 30 or 40 mm Hg within a distance of a few microns (1-4). However, the pO_2 at a given micro-area of cerebral tissue is remarkably constant, and can be changed only through major alterations in blood supply or the composition of respiratory gases (1,4,10). We have defined the different processes arrived at maintaining the constant brain cell oxygen micro-environment as "oxygen autoregulatory mechanisms."

Prior experimental investigations in the brain cortex and spinal cord of cats with a new ultramicrooxygen electrode (1-2-4) have produced surprising results.

(1) Tissue pO_2 during a short period of anoxia was initially decreased, but then leveled out at a relatively constant plateau, even when arterial pO_2 values neared zero.

(2) As arterial tension increases from depressed levels near zero, tissue tension responds; but on returning to normal tissue concentrations, oxygen tension overshoots the pre-existing normal value and then slowly decreases to line out at the pre-existing normal level.

(3) Measurement of local electrical activity and tissue oxygen tension with the same microelectrode indicates a significant reduction in electrical activity when tissue tension is in the "plateau" region.

In previous theoretical investigations based on the above experimental data (9), we demonstrated that the overshoot phenomena could be explained as a time delay in the flow rate versus arterial blood curve (steady state), i.e., hyperemia for a short period of time after arterial blood had returned to normal conditions. Later, based on the assumption that decreased electrical activity during reduced tissue oxygen tension was an indication of reduced oxygen utilization, we inferred that the plateau region of tissue pO_2, in spite of decreasing arterial tension, could be explained as a reduction in cerebral oxygen consumption.

These experiments and theoretical reasoning led to the assumption that there is in brain tissue an oxygen "sensor," able to regulate flow and neuronal activity according to TpO_2 changes. Experiments hereby reported relate to properties of this hypothetical O_2 sensor under normal and hyperbaric oxygen conditions.

METHODS

The experiments were performed on 40 cats and 20 dogs, nembutalized (nembutal, I.P., 60 mg/Kg), curarized (flaxedil, 6 mg/Kg) and put under positive pressure breathing. Femoral artery, blood pressure, ECG and carotid artery blood flow were recorded on a Beckman S_{II} Dynograph using standard transducers. Blood and tissue pO_2, as well as the electrical activity of single cortical neurons, were determined using our ultramicroelectrodes as described before (4). The data was finally registered on a tape recorder as well as the Dynograph. The different respiratory mixtures tested were administered through the artificial respiration pump, or in our hyperbaric chamber at 70 p.s.i., and all solutions were injected into the cannulated Femoral vein. In the hyperbaric chamber experiments, only pO_2 action potentials and blood pressure were measure, these animals being anesthetized with chloralose, 50 mg/Kg, I.P.

In an additional experimental series, in 10 nembutalized, curarized cats, TpO_2 and neuronal activity were determined in the right prefrontal cortex, while TpO_2 was also measured in the left prefrontal cortex. TpO_2 was lowered locally in a small area of the left cortex by applying locally an N_2 jet, and the TpO_2-neuronal activity response determined in the contralateral side.

RESULTS

A. Anoxic-anoxia:

Cat studies (recording of pO_2 and electrical activity as well as other parameters).

Figure 1 represents studies of anoxic-anoxia in which arterial

pO_2, initially at normal conditions, decreases to very low values before returning to the pre-existing normal. In comparison to the arterial change, tissue pO_2 is seen to lag arterial pO_2 for a relatively long period of time, then decrease slightly, line out, increase with increasing arterial pO_2, overshoot normal values, and finally return to the pre-existing normal conditions. Flow increases in the carotid artery can be seen to initially lag arterial pO_2, increase at approximately the same time as tissue pO_2 begins to decrease, peak at the same time the lowest values of arterial and tissue pO_2 are attained, decrease sharply to values slightly above normal when arterial and tissue pO_2 begin increasing, and then slowly decrease to the preceding normal steady-state value. Note that tissue pO_2 is still slightly elevated after arterial pO_2 returns to normal values.

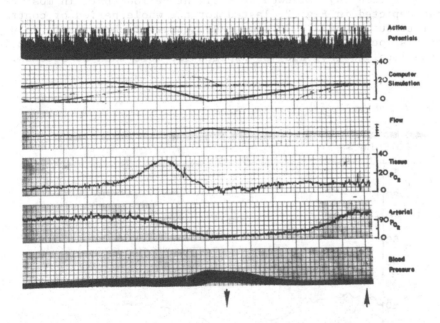

Fig. 1: Simultaneous recordings of biological and computer responses to anoxic-anoxia as a function of time. Read from right to left with respect to increasing time. From top to bottom neuronal action potentials, computer simulation of tissue pO_2, blood flow in the internal carotid artery, tissue pO_2, arterial pO_2.

B.   Hyperbaric Oxygen:

Cats breathing pure oxygen in the hyperbaric chamber showed, as
pressure was increased from one to 6.5 ATS, first a slight decrease
in cortical pO_2, then a prolonged increase to about ten times the
initial value when the highest pressure levels were reached. Shortly
before oxygen convulsion appeared, a more pronounced rise in tissue
pO_2 appeared with stabilization or were decreased in cortical pO_2
levels when the electrical activity of the cortex was increased
during the period of the oxygen fit.

C.   Effect of localized hypoxia on contralateral neuronal activity:

In the experiments in which pO_2 was lowered in one side of the
brain while TpO_2 and neuronal electrical activity recorded in the
contralateral motor cortex (Fig. 2) a diphasic response was observed.
TpO_2 was lowered in the side affected by the N_2 jet. No change in
TpO_2 occured in the contralateral side. The neuronal activity in
the contralateral side showed the bursts of "injury potentials" as
described before (4) followed by a silent period that, in most cases,
as that depicted in Fig. 2, lasted for the whole period of contralateral tissue hypoxia. In some cases, however, bursts of "injury
potentials" occured periodically during the silent period, especially
when the localized hypoxia was applied for more than 30 seconds.

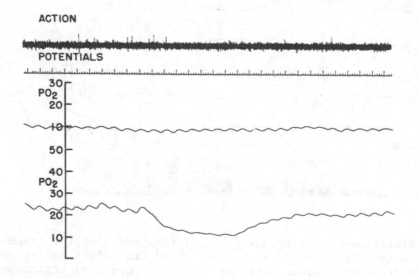

Fig. 2: Recording (from top to bottom) of action potentials, TpO_2
homolateral side of action potentials and pO_2 contralateral side
where TpO_2 has been lowered locally by an N_2 jet.

DISCUSSION

Among the different brain functions regulated by circulation changes, oxygen supply seems to be the most carefully guarded. Only a major departure from physiological conditions can alter it, and then for only very short periods of time. Hypoxic periods of 6 min or more are needed to alter the carefully guarded "autoregulation" mechanisms.

When analyzing the different "built in" compensation factors involved, we have to bear in mind the fact that pO_2 determinations made with our microelectrode represent an artificial equilibrium in one microarea of a nonhomogeneous organ, between the amount of O_2 supplied and the amounts utilized by the tissue.

If, at a certain moment in time, we change the equilibrium by diminishing the oxygen supply (anoxic anoxia experiments), different compensation mechanisms seem to be immediately activated. From the data reported here and in previous publications (1-2-3-4), the following factors seem to interact to maintain constant pO_2 levels:
(a) arterial pO_2 (representing the amounts of oxygen available);
(b) blood flow velocity, especially in the small arterioles and capillaries (representing the supply rate); and
(c) oxygen consumption by the tissue.

The fact that the arterial blood flow to the brain increases when arterial pO_2 is reduced has been reported by Opitz and Schneider (10). These authors found a twofold increase in cerebral blood flow under anoxic anoxia conditions in humans. We have confirmed their findings in our experiments, and also established that, in a normal animal, arterial blood flow increases only when pO_2 begins to fall in the brain tissue itself. When carefully observing the records in Fig. 1, we can see that when the animal is respired pure nitrogen, the drop in tissue pO_2 lags in time after the arterial pO_2 decreases. This delay can be as much as 60 sec in some experiments, but never less than 30 sec. Since both oxygen microelectrodes have the same frequency response (less than a second) (2), we consider that the delay in tissue pO_2 drop represents a true physiological mechanism to protect the brain ("delay mechanism") (6,12,14), different than the blood flow increase.

When interpreting our anoxic anoxia experiments, we have to assume then, that the decreased availability of oxygen in the arterial blood is only reflected in brain tissue after their "transport delay" is overcome. At this point, tissue pO_2 begins to fall and the next defense mechanism is started, namely the increase in arteblood flow. As this mechanism fails, because by that time arterial pO_2 is nearing zero, the electrical activity of the brain is stopped in a very sharp way. This "shut-off" point is very reproducible at a given microarea of brain tissue and usually occurs when the given pO_2 in that area is reduced by about 20% (4) (see Fig. 1).

The assumption is then made that brain electrical activity is related to tissue oxygen consumption, and electrical silence means a sharp decrease in oxygen utilization. Two facts in the results presented tend to support this assumption: (a) the pO_2 level in cortex stabilizes when neuronal firing stops, and (b) computer simulations match the actual pO_2 values almost exactly when the consumption term is made equal to zero (R = 0), instead of being kept at a constant.

If the electrical silence is a compensatory mechanism, then there are two possibilities for its function: (a) neurons are very sensitive to their O_2 atmosphere, and a slight drop is enough to silence them, or (b) this is an inhibitory reflex, in which case a tissue pO_2 receptor should be theorized.

Present experiments offer further proof to the existence of the tissue oxygen sensor and its ability to actively inhibit neuronal firing, even at distant brain regions. The fact that lowering pO_2 locally in the right cortex can produce a period of "silence" in neurons firing in the contralateral motor cortex, where TpO_2 was unchanged, could be interpreted as a process of active inhibition emanating from the anoxic area.

Opitz and Schneider (6) have assumed that such a receptor exists in tissue and predicted that it is possibly located at the venous end of the capillaries; if it exists, it should have the capability of both increasing blood flow and the reflex inhibition of synaptic or neuronal potentials.

Under hypoglycemic conditions, the regulatory mechanisms described hitherto are markedly altered. The electrical activity is only sporadic, and does not change much with a decrease in oxygen supply. Blood flow compensation occurs very early, paralleling in time the changes in arterial pO_2. The delay mechanism is absent (4). Our conclusions are that under those circumstances, the main compensation mechanism is blood flow.

Experiments performed under hyperbaric conditions showed the same regulatory mechanisms working in an opposite direction.

CONCLUDING REMARKS

This paper is one of a series aimed at establishing the mechanisms regulating oxygen supply to brain tissue. Under normal conditions, the regulatory mechanisms for a change in oxygen supply seem to be:

(1) delay mechanism

(2) change in arterial blood flow

(3) change in tissue oxygen consumption

(4) the O_2 receptor for the regulation of the above seems to be located in brain tissue

SUMMARY

The regulatory mechanisms involved in maintaining a constant brain oxygen supply were studied in anesthetized, curarized cats and dogs. Physiological parameters (tissue pO_2 and firing in the same microarea of cortex, arterial pO_2 in the carotid artery blood flow and blood pressure) were determined in some experiments; and in others the response to hyperbaric oxygen administration was determined.

Compensation for anoxic-anoxia in the brain was based on a delay mechanism, increased blood flow, and diminished cellular activity, and found to be quick and accurate. Animals placed under hyperbaric conditions showed the same regulatory responses working in an opposite direction. The basis for the autoregulatory mechanism seems to be a tissue oxygen sensor, able to regulate blood flow to microareas of brain tissue and actively inhibit neuronal firing.

REFERENCES

1. Bicher, H. I. and M. H. Knisely. Brain Tissue Reoxygenation, Demonstrated with a new Ultramicro Oxygen Electrode, J. App. Phys., 28:387-390, 1970.

2. Bicher, H. I., D. D. Reneau and M. H. Knisely. Brain Tissue Oxygenation as Determined with a new Ultramicro Oxygen Electrode, Blood Oxygenation. New York; Plenum Press, 201-217, 1970.

3. Bicher, H. I., D. F. Bruley, D. D. Reneau and M. H. Knisely. Effect of Microcirculation Changes on Brain Tissue Oxygenation, J. Physiol., 217:689-707, 1971.

4. Bicher, H. I., D. F. Bruley, D. D. Reneau and M. H. Knisely.
    Brain Oxygen Supply and Neuronal Activity under Normal
    and Hypoglycemic Conditions, Am. J. Physiol., 224:275-282,
    1973.

5. Bruley, D. F., H. I. Bicher, D. D. Reneau and M. H. Knisely.
    Auto-regulatory Phenomena Related to Cerebral Tissue
    Oxygenation, Biomed. Eng., Chemical Engineering Symposium
    Series, 67:195-201, 1971.

6. Opitz, E. and M. Schneider. Ueber Sauerstaffversorgung des
    Gehirns und den Mechanismus von Mangelworkingen. Ergeb.
    Physiol. Biol. Chem. Exptl. Pharmakol., 46:126-260, 1950.

7. Reneau, D. D., D. F. Bruley and M. H. Knisely. Chemical Eng-
    ineering in Medicine and Biology, New York: Plenum Press,
    135-148, 1967.

8. Reneau, D. D., D. F. Bruley and M. H. Knisely. A Digital
    Simulation of Transient Oxygen Transport Systems (Cerebral
    Gray Matter), A. I. Ch. E. J., 15:916-925, 1969.

9. Reneau, D. D., H. I. Bicher, D. F. Bruley and M. H. Knisely.
    A Mathematical Analysis Predicting Cerebral Tissue Reoxygen-
    ation as a Function of the Rate of Change of Effective
    Cerebral Blood Flow, Blood Oxygenation. New York: Plenum
    Press, 175-200, 1970.

10. Silver, I. Some Observations on the Cerebral Cortex with an
    Ultramicro, Membrane-Covered Oxygen Electrode, Med. Elec-
    tron. Biol. Eng., 3:377-387, 1965.

LOCAL PO$_2$ IN RELATION TO INTRACELLULAR pH, CELL MEMBRANE POTENTIAL AND POTASSIUM LEAKAGE IN HYPOXIA AND SHOCK

I. A. Silver
Department of Pathology
University of Bristol
Bristol, England

In many disease conditions it is ultimately hypoxia at cellular level which leads to reversible or irreversible damage. While searching for the factors which may be of primary importance in inducing this damage, we have examined a number of changes that occur during tissue hypoxia. We have used as our models (a) intact animals during respiratory hypoxia and hemorrhagic shock and, (b) tissue cultures in graded hypoxia. Hemorrhagic shock produces profound hypoxia in many tissues complicated by changes in blood flow, by leakage of fluid into the tissues and by build up of CO_2. The two tissues which we have studied in some detail are (a) the population of fibroblasts, endothelial cells and macrophages at the edge of healing wounds, and (b) the neurones and glial cells of the cerebral cortex of the rat.

The experiments were designed to measure the local PO$_2$ and to see if changes could be detected in cell membrane potential, in intra-cellular pH, in extra-cellular potassium levels and in spontaneous electrical activity during hypoxia, and if so could they be correlated with any changes in the ultrastructure of the tissue under examination. While it is easy to demonstrate that long term severe hypoxia causes changes in cells, not only in fine structure but also at the level of the light microscope it is much less easy to demonstrate alterations of intracellular structure during the initial stages of hypoxia and to discover whether these changes are a reflection of reversible or irreversible damage.

MATERIALS AND METHODS

Measurements were made in the cerebral cortex of rats anesthetised with urethane or with barbiturates and held in a modified Baltimore stereotaxic headholder. The skin over the skull was removed, holes were drilled through the frontal and parietal bones and the dura was removed under the holes. Platinum-iridium membrane-covered oxygen microelectrodes were inserted under stereotaxic control to a depth of approximately 1mm into the cortex until positive going action potentials were recorded from them which ensured that they were in close proximity to active neurones. Through the same hole and also through a hole symmetrically placed on the opposite side of the mid-line, were inserted (1) a standard potential-measuring glass micro-pipette filled with 3 M KCl, external diameter 0.3-0.5 μm, (2) a pH sensitive electrode with similar dimensions and (3) two potassium sensitive electrodes with an external diameter of approximately 0.5 μm. The electrocorticogram, electrocardiogram and respiration were also monitored by standard methods.

The healing wound model was the rabbit ear chamber. Plastic chambers, based on the design described by Wood et al. (1966), but made from polymethylpentene (TPX) were inserted into the ears of half-lop rabbits. When growth of new tissue could be seen on the transparent "table" of the chamber the cover slips were removed under heavy mineral oil and electrodes as described for the brain, were inserted along the growing edge of the tissue under direct microscopic observation.

The third model was composed of fibroblasts growing in tissue culture. Similar measurements to those which were carried out in the healing wound were made at the edge of a mono-layer culture of mouse fibroblasts.

Electrodes

The oxygen electrode was a platinum-iridium needle, external diameter approximately 0.5 μm which was covered by a Rhoplex AC 35 (Rhom Haas, Philadelphia, Pa.) membrane and insulated with glass to within 1 μm of the tip. It was polarized with -700 mV D.C.   The pH electrode was based on the design of Thomas (1970) in which a standard borosilicate glass (Corning 0120) pipette is drawn to a fine point and then a second glass pipette made of pH-sensitive glass (Corning 0150) is drawn with similar but

very slightly smaller dimensions. The tip of the pH glass
cone is sealed by heat, the end is cut off and is dropped
down inside the pyrex glass so that the tip of the pH-
sensitive glass stops just short of the end of the pyrex
glass. The two glasses are then fused together where they
touch and the electrode is filled with 3 M KCl electrolyte and allowed to hydrate for a few hours. The filling
is difficult by conventional means but is relatively
simple by the method of Zeuthen (1971). This consists of
distillation of water from the body of the electrode into
the cool tip by an external heating coil followed by
substitution of the distilled water by electrolyte.

The potassium electrodes were made either on the same
pattern as the pH electrodes but using a potassium-sensi-
tive glass (Corning NAS27-4) or by using the method described by Walker (1971) in which a pyrex pipette is drawn
to a point which is not less than 0.5 μm external diameter.
The tip is coated with a silicone preparation and initially we used Siliclad (Clay, Adams Inc., N.Y.) 1% in
1-chloronaphthalene, as described by Walker (1971) but
found that this tended to clog the electrode tip and not
to produce an even water-repellent surface. Recently we
have used dichlorodimethylsilane (B.D.H. Chemicals, Poole,
U.K.) which is evaporated onto the electrode surface and
produces a very highly water resistant finish in a few
seconds. The treated electrode is dipped into a liquid
potassium ion-exchanger (Corning 477317) of which a column
about 50 μm long is taken into the tip of the electrode by
capillarity. The shaft of the electrode is then filled by
the method of Zeuthen (1971). Connections from both the
pH and pK electrodes were made through a silver chlorided
wire inserted into the electrolyte through the back of the
electrode. Reference electrodes of silver chlorided silver
wire were placed in the subcutaneous tissue of the animal.
Alternatively double barelled electrodes were drawn by
twisting together two pyrex glass tubes and pulling them
to give a total tip diameter of approximately 0.6 μm. One
of these electrode barrels was coated on the inside with
dimethyldichlorosilane and the other was protected with
glycerol. The electrodes were dipped into potassium liquid
ion-exchanger and filled with electrolyte after removal of
the glycerol. This gave an intracellular electrode with
an intracellular reference. Double barrelled electrodes
containing a pH glass cone and an open barrel were also
produced but the fusion of the pH glass and pyrex was difficult and a compromise of fixing the pH to the outer glass
with wax was adopted although this has not yet proved very
satisfactory.

Recording

Records were obtained from the ion-selective and DC-potential channels via electrometer amplifers (Analog Devices 311K) with suitable bias adjustment. The impedence of these amplifiers is nominally $10^{14}\Omega$, but they gave a satisfactory performance even with the high impedence pH glass electrodes. The DC-potential measuring electrode was necessary because, in brain, during hypoxia there are shifts of DC potential which are not related to potassium leakage and these are detected by the potassium electrodes and have to be subtracted from the true potassium potential readings.

Potassium readings were made extracellularly because normally the extracellular potassium concentration is low and small changes are easy to observe. The pH electrodes were used both intracellularly and extracellularly.

Electron microscopy

Serial biopsies were taken from the surface of the cortex after periods of hypoxia and also from the edge of the healing tissue. They were processed by fixation in 4% glutaraldehyde and treated routinely. Sections were cut at approximately 6-800 Å and examined in a Phillips EM300.

Hypoxia

Respiratory hypoxia was produced by varying the gas flow to the animal via a tracheotomy cannula. Gas mixtures consisted either of air and 5% CO_2 or nitrogen and 5% CO_2. The animals were given the anoxic mixture until bradycardia was observed and spontaneous respiration ceased. The gas was then turned off and if necessary artificial respiration and oxygen was applied until spontaneous breathing was resumed.

Hemorrhagic shock was induced by cannulating the femoral artery and bleeding the animal into a siliconised reservoir to the point at which its blood pressure was 30-35 mm Hg for rats and 50-55 mm Hg for rabbits.

In tissue cultures hypoxia was produced by replacing the gas over the culture with a stream of 5% CO_2 in nitrogen.

RESULTS

(1) Brain

During hypoxic episodes there was a rapid fall in PO_2 to zero over the course of 25-30 sec. After approximately 15 sec of hypoxia there was a change in the DC potential of the brain and this was followed shortly afterwards by an increase in the extracellular potassium concentration. A slight change only (5-10 mV) occurred in the extracellular pH during this period although changes of as much as 0.5 pH units were seen with longer periods of milder hypoxia. It was very noticeable that in the first hypoxic episodes the change in extracellular potassium concentration was minimal, but that when hypoxia was repeated, even if long recovery periods were allowed between episodes, there was a progressive increase in potassium leakage and a progressive decrease in the return of the potassium into the cells during recovery. Electron micrographs of brain biopsies taken during these hypoxic episodes showed no obvious changes in the structure of intracellular organelles, although occasionally a swollen mitochondrium was found.

(2) Wound Tissue

In wound tissue virtually no change in extracellular potassium levels could be detected during short periods of hypoxia and there was little or no change in the intracellular pH of fibroblasts at the edge of wounds. The only rapid changes which occurred in this tissue were in the oxygen gradients. As has previously been reported (Silver, 1973a) systemic hypoxia especially affects wound tissue where there is almost immediate vasoconstriction during the stress of hypoxia. It was clear that in contrast to brain, fibroblasts even in the dangerous environment of a healing wound are very much more resistant to hypoxia in terms of membrane leakage than is brain. Membrane potential studies with intracellular pipettes on fibroblasts in situ showed virtually no changes during short periods (i.e. $\frac{1}{2}$-1 minute) of hypoxia. This was in direct contrast to what happened in the brain.

In hemorrhagic shock there was a long term change in the environment of the wound which included an early progressive fall in PO_2 during hemorrhage followed first by a change in the intracellular pH and finally by a change in membrane potential of the cells, which was accompanied by potassium leakage into the extracellular fluid. In

macrophages, the pH and PO_2 changes were not followed by
membrane potential failure or potassium leakage. Biopsies taken from the wound during the development of shock
showed that fibroblasts at the growing edge of the tissue
were particularly susceptible to the effect of deprivation of oxygen or to the subsequent changes in pH, in
that their mitochondria swelled and the cristae became
disrupted; the endoplasmic reticulum became hydrated;
the chromatin of the nucleus became marginated and the
nuclear membrane became crenated. These alterations were
correlated with a fall of intracellular pH below about
6.7. They did not appear to be directly correlated with
the oxygen tension since this had been near zero, usually
for several hours before the ultrastructural changes could
be detected. In contrast to the fibroblasts, pericytes
at the surface of capillaries and macrophages both in the
tissue and in the wound dead space, survived these conditions without ultrastructural change.

Dividing fibroblasts in tissue cultures appeared to
be much more resistant to hypoxia than did those in the
wound edge. Several hours of total hypoxia did not lead
to major changes in extracellular potassium concentration
although intracellular pH fell to about 6.7 from a resting value of 7.1, and neither were there obvious changes
in ultrastructure.

DISCUSSION

It is clear from these measurements that rather
different sequences of changes can occur in different
populations of cells in relation to hypoxia. In the
brain, hypoxia appears to lead directly and rapidly to
changes in membrane potential and to leakage of intracellular potassium without major changes in local pH.
In contrast to this, prolonged hypoxia in fibroblasts in
culture leads to little, if any change, either in the
membrane potential or in potassium leakage. It is of
course possible that cells which grow in tissue culture
are a selected population and tend to be clones which
have a natural tolerance of adverse conditions; perhaps
those cells that are more sensitive and delicate are
eliminated in the fight for survival in artificial media.
Actively synthesizing fibroblasts in wound tissue on the
other hand are well adapted to tolerate relatively short
term hypoxia which is obviously of survival value to the
organism. On the other hand growing fibroblasts suffer
extensive damage if hypoxia and particularly ischemic

hypoxia is prolonged. The most significant change during
hypoxia in wound healing appears to be the intracellular
pH change which develops slowly when oxygen is withdrawn
and is presumably the result of anerobic metabolism. The
fibroblast can maintain its membrane potential for some
hours during the development of hemorrhagic shock but it
slowly loses this capacity as the intracellular pH
becomes more acid. At a critical point of around pH
6.7-6.6, there is a failure of the sodium pump and potassium can be found leaking out into the medium. If this
process continues for more than an hour or two, ultrastructural damage can be observed which may be irreversible and most obviously affects mitochondria and endoplasmic reticulum.

The macrophages represent a population which can
survive extreme conditions of both the intracellular and
extracellular environment. They can live in wound dead
space where the PO_2 is zero for long periods and they
maintain their membrane potential even when the intracellular pH falls to below 6.0. Macrophages are capable
of maintaining phagocytic activity in total anoxia but
they become unable to digest or kill many of the bacteria
they ingest. Oxygen is presumably needed to maintain the
peroxidase systems which they normally employ to kill
microorganisms. The pericytes which may be considered as
pleuripotential primitive mesenchyme cells, provide an
interesting source for speculation. They survive prolonged hypoxia undamaged when the fibroblasts around them
show severe ultrastructural changes and possibly they may
serve as a source of new cells when the hypoxic period is
over.

Neuronal changes in the central nervous system during hypoxia must necessarily be considered in relation to
the changes occuring in the glial cells around them. It
is perhaps not always appreciated that approximately 98%
of the cells in the C.N.S. are glia and possibly the
changes in extracellular potassium that one detects
during hypoxic periods are due to leakage from these
cells since it would be difficult to account for the
quantity of potassium ion movement if it was all derived
from neurones. Perhaps the K^+ leakage secondarily
affects the ability of neural cells to maintain their membrane potential and hence their ability to transmit information. Extracellular rather than intracellular potassium
concentration was measured in this study because (a) the
intracellular potassium levels are high and small changes
are difficult to detect and (b) it was thought probable

that the extracellular changes were the ones that might
prove most significant in terms of cell damage. We are
currently examining the behaviour of cultured glial cells
separated from neural cells to see how they respond to
local hypoxia. We are also looking at the effects on
neural cells in culture which result from local hypoxia
induced by bringing micro-oxygen electrodes near to the
cell surface. The system permits a study of the effects
of local hypoxia induced and measured by microelectrodes
on intracellular organelles in different parts of cells
with extensive ramifications such as neurones and astro-
cytes, to see whether organelles in special regions, such
as synapses may be more susceptible to hypoxia than those
in other parts. It has been shown by Grossman et al.(1971)
Silver (1973b) and by Bicher, et al. (1973) that oxygen
deprivation acts in a specific sequence on the C.N.S.,
first inducing a transient increase in irritability shown
by increased firing of cells. This period corresponds to
an increase of membrane potential and a fall in extracellular potassium. Further hypoxia destroys spontaneous
electrical activity but cortical cells can still be induced to fire by a peripheral stimulus.   More prolonged
oxygen deprivation blocks transmission from the lower
parts of the brain to the cortex, although cortical cells
will still fire if the cell body is directly stimulated.
During this period potassium leakage into the extracellular environment can be detected.   Finally, as the
hypoxic period lengthens cortical cells lose altogether
their ability to respond to stimuli and at the same time
their membrane potentials fall drastically. We are examining the possible reasons for this progressive change
particularly in relation to the suggestion that the syn-
apse may be especially susceptible to hypoxia.

        Our morphological findings conflict with those of
Brown and Brierly (1971) who found microvacuolation
(mitochondrial disruption) in cells of the cortex after
a few minutes of hypoxia. It is possible that their
hypoxic model (a Levine preparation) was more severe than
ours, but the preliminary findings of Mela (Personal communication) on mitochondrial activity in brain after prolonged ischemia suggest many cortical mitochondria must
survive hypoxia intact.

ACKNOWLEDGMENT. This work was supported in part by U.S.P.H.S.
Grant 1 P01 NS 10,939-01.

REFERENCES

Bicher, H.I., Bruley, D., Reneau, D.D. and Knisely, M. (1973). Regulatory Mechanisms of Brain Oxygen Supply in 'Oxygen Supply' (Eds. Kessler, M. et al.), (Urban and Schwarzenberg, Munchen) p. 180.

Brown, A.W. and Brierly, J.B. (1971). The Nature and Time Course of Anoxic-Ischaemic Cell Change in the Rat Brain. An Optical and Electron Microscope Study, in 'Brain Hypoxia' (Eds. Brierly, J.B. and Meldrum, B.S.) (Spastics International Medical Publications) p. 49.

Grossman, R.G. and Williams, V.F. (1971). Electrical Activity and Ultrastructure of Cortical Neurones and Synapses in Ischaemia in 'Brain Hypoxia' (Eds. Brierly, J.B. and Meldrum, B.S.), (Spastics International Medical Publications) p. 61.

Silver, I.A. (1973a). Local and Systemic Factors Affecting Fibroblast Proliferation and Maturation, in 'The Biology of the Fibroblast' (Eds. Kulonen, E. and Pikkarainen, J.), (Academic Press, London and New York) in Press.

Silver, I.A. (1973b). Brain Oxygen Tension and Cellular Activity in 'Oxygen Supply' (Eds. Kessler, M. et al.) (Urban and Schwarzenberg, Munchen) p. 186.

Thomas, R.C. (1970). A New Design for a Sodium-Sensitive Glass Micro-electrode. J. Physiol. Lond. 210, 82P.

Walker, J.L. (1971). Ion Specific Liquid Ion Exchanger Microelectrodes. Analyt. Chem. 43, 89A.

Wood, S., Lewis, R., Mulholland, J.H. and Knack, J.(1966) Assembly, Insertion and Use of a Modified Rabbit Ear Chamber. Bull. Johns Hopkins Hosp. 119, 1.

Zeuthen, T. (1971). A Method to Fill Glass Micro-electrodes by Local Heating. Acta Physiol. Scand. 81, 141.

ENERGY-RICH METABOLITES AND EEG IN

HYPOXIA AND IN HYPERCAPNIA

Ursula Schindler, E.Gärtner and E.Betz

Institute of Physiology I, Univ.Tübingen

Tübingen, W.- Germany

In the present communication we report the effect of controlled hypoxia, of severe hypercapnia and its recovery upon the metabolic state and the electrical activity of the cerebral cortex in cats. We investigated also the influence of high carbon dioxide tensions in brain metabolites and EEG, maintaining a sufficient oxygen supply to the brain. In the hypoxia experiments the pCO_2 was low. The oxygen tension was decreased to such a degree that the EEG disappeared. Isoelectric EEG was also obtained by high CO_2 concentrations (2,6,8).

METHODS

The techniques of operation, freezing and sampling of cortical tissue and the analysis of the metabolites have been reported elsewhere in detail (7).

The experiments with hypoxia were conducted on spontaneously respiring, anaesthetized cats, whereas in the hypercapnia experiments the cats were ventilated artificially. The EEG was taken from symmetrical sites of both hemispheres. In the four groups of experiments the conditions prior to tissue sampling were as follows:
1) Hypoxic group: Exposure to 3% O_2, 3,5% CO_2 and 93,5% N_2 for 14 min.
2) Hypercapnic group: Exposure to increasing concentrations of CO_2 up to 50% CO_2 in pure oxygen (mean 40%

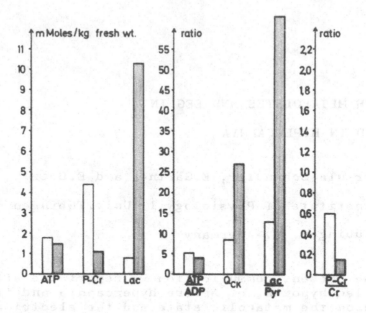

Fig.1: Metabolic state of the brain cortex in hypoxia.
The left column represents metabolite levels and ratios in controls (n = 10) and the right column those
in the hypoxic animal. P-Cr, phosphocreatine; Lac,lac-
tate; Q_{CK}, apparent equilibrium constant of the creatine kinase reaction.

    CO_2) til the EEG had been isoelectric for at least
    10 min.
3) Recovery group: Exposure to 40% CO_2 for 45 min followed by the administration of normal air for 45 min.
4) Control group.

                    RESULTS AND DISCUSSION

     Fig.1 represents a typical hypoxia experiment. The
pO_2 of the cortex in the measuring area had dropped to
1-6 mm Hg and the EEG was isoelectric for about
5-10 sec. The level of P-creatine and the ratio P-creatine to creatine were both reduced by about 75%. The
ATP concentration and the ratio ATP/ADP were lowered
too, but not to the same extent. It is likely, that
the glucose level is also diminished, since, in general,
the order of depletion of the compounds of the energy
reserve is P-creatine, glucose, ATP. The markedly increased lactate concentration and the high lactate

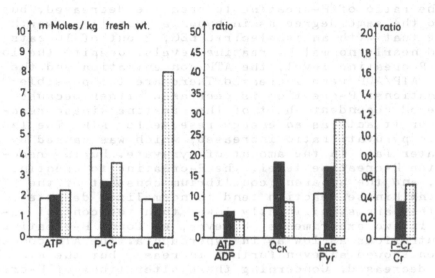

Fig.2: Metabolic state of the brain cortex in hypercapnia and in recovery. In the three columns the different experimental conditions are shown: left, controls (n = 20); middle, hypercapnia (n = 16); right,
recovery (n = 8). For abbreviations see fig.1.

to pyruvate ratio suggest a higher glycolytic rate compared with results obtained during ischemia (3).

In hypercapnia with mean pCO_2 exceeding 200 mm Hg,
the pH of the arterial blood fell from 7.31 to 6.51.
The mean arterial pO_2 was 280 mm Hg and in CSF we recorded 144 mm Hg. The cortical pO_2 measured at different spots was not lower than 30 mm Hg. Under these
conditions the EEG disappeared completely in most cases. Only with a few cats could very low and slow potentials be recorded under high amplification. In the
recovery phase the values of pO_2 and pCO_2 in arterial
blood and CSF were again nearly identical with those
of the control group, whereas the arterial pH reached
only 7.16 instead of 7.31 in the control group. The
electrical activity of the cortex had returned.

Fig.2 shows the mean metabolite levels and ratios
of the controls, the hypercapnic group and the group
after recovery. In hypercapnia the level of P-creatine

and the ratio of P-creatine to creatine decreased, but
not to the same degree as in hypoxia. But it is worth
noting that with an isoelectric EEG, 3 out of 16 cats
showed nearly normal P-creatine levels. Despite the lowered P-creatine level, the ATP concentration and the
ratio ATP/ADP were increased.There are two possible
explanations: P-creatine is decreased either because
of the pH dependent shift of the creatine kinase reaction, or it acts as an energy reserve for ATP. The lactate to pyruvate ratio increased, which was caused by
a greater fall in the amount of pyruvate. During recovery the P-creatine level, the P-creatine to creatine
ratio, and the apparent equilibrium constant of the
creatine kinase reaction tend to normalize, despite
that they are significantly lower than the control values. In two experiments, however, we found P-creatine
concentrations as low as in hypercapnia. The ATP concentration showed an even further increase, but the ATP/ADP
ratio decreased. Concerning these alterations of P-creatine and ATP levels and their corresponding ratios with
respect to the status of EEG, we conclude that P-creatine and ATP are a necessary but not a sufficient condition for maintaining EEG potentials in the cortex.
Because the low energy potential in hypoxia is an explanation for the disappearance of the EEG potentials, the
conditions during hypercapnia were of greater interest
concerning the relation of electrical and energetic cortical functions. The energy charge potential (1) remained unchanged during hypercapnia but it decreased
from 0.901 to 0.862 after recovery.

The concentrations of the intermediates of glycolysis and citric acid cycle are shown in fig.3. In hypercapnia both arterial glucose and cortical glucose
concentration rose; also glucose-6-phosphate and fruc-
tose-6-phosphate increased. With the exception of 3-P-
glycerate and P-enolpyruvate, the concentrations of all
other metabolites are lowered. These results indicate
that the intracellular acidosis, produced by hypercapnia,
inhibits a rate limiting step in the glycolysis between
glucose and pyruvate. Since the first metabolite concentration that is lowered, is fructose-1,6-diphosphate,
it seems that the phospho-fructokinase step is inhibited.
This enzyme has been shown to be influenced by pH in
vitro and in vivo (4,5). The decrease in aspartate and
glutamate levels may be related to the decreased concentrations of the citric acid cycle intermediates. In
the recovery group the glucose, glucose-6-phosphate and
fructose-6-phosphate levels were normal or nearly normal. Since the concentrations of all substrates beyond

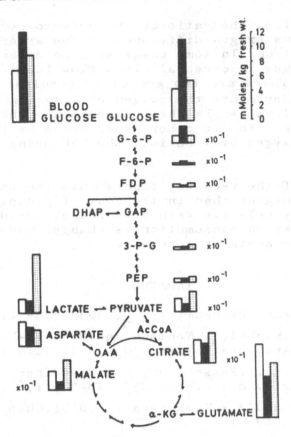

Fig.3: Levels of the glycolytic and citric acid cycle
intermediates in controls, in hypercapnia and in recovery from hypercapnia. Arrangement of the columns is
as in fig.2. Abbreviations are as follows: G-6-P, glu-
cose-6-phosphate; F-6-P, fructose-6-phosphate; FDP,
fructose-1.6-diphosphate; GAP, glyceraldehyde-3-phos-
phate; DHAP, dihydroxyacetone-phosphate; 3-P-G, 3-phos-
phoglycerate; PEP, phosphoenol-pyruvate; α-KG, α-keto-
glutarate (GLUCOSE indicates cortical tissue glucose).

fructose-6-phosphate increase, it is likely that under
these circumstances the inhibition or "deinhibition"
of the phospho-fructokinase reaction should lead to a
decreased or increased glycolytic rate, respectively.

     In order to receive a rough parameter of the oxy-
gen demand of the cortex we measured the oxygen

utilization, i.e. the ratio of the arterio-cerebral
cortical venous oxygen difference to the arterial oxygen concentration. In some cases we also determined the
relative changes in cerebral blood flow (CBF) during
hypercapnia. There are two groups of results: In about
50% of the experiments the oxygen utilization rose above the control value. In these experiments the CBF decreased; whereas in the other experiments we found a
decrease in oxygen utilization, the CBF being increased.

    In all of the recovery experiments the oxygen uti-
lization was higher than in the control group. Since
these are only relative values we cannot decide whether
the overall oxygen consumption is changed under conditions of hypercapnia or recovery.

LITERATURE

(1) D.E.Atkinson: Biochemistry 7, 4030-4034 (1967).

(2) E.Betz, U.Knebel, L.Neumann and H.Ngyen-Duong:
    Pflügers Arch.ges.Physiol 307, R 117-118 (1969).

(3) O.H.Lowry, J.V.Passonneau, F.X.Hasselberger and
    D.W.Schulz: J.Biol.Chem. 239, 18-30 (1964).

(4) O.H.Lowry and J.V.Passonneau: J.Biol.Chem. 241,
    2268-2279 (1966).

(5) J.Scheuer and M.N.Berry: Am.J.Physiol. 213,
    1143-1148 (1967).

(6) U.Schindler, E.Betz, H.Pfeiffer and M.Strohm:
    Europ.Neurol. 6, 83-87 (1971/1972).

(7) F.W.Schmahl, E.Betz, H.Talke and H.J.Hohorst:
    Biochem.Z. 342, 518-531 (1965).

(8) F.W.Schmahl, E.Betz, E.Dettinger and H.J.Hohorst:
    Pflügers Arch.ges.Physiol. 292, 46-59 (1966).

Supported by a grant of the 'Deutsche Forschungsgemeinschaft'.

A NEW LONG-TERM METHOD FOR THE MEASUREMENT OF NADH FLUORESCENCE

IN INTACT RAT BRAIN WITH CHRONICALLY IMPLANTED CANNULA

A. Mayevsky and B. Chance*
Johnson Research Foundation, School of Medicine
University of Pennsylvania, Philadelphia, Pennsylvania

The method developed by Chance et al. (1) which measures the oxidation-reduction state of NADH in vivo by surface fluorometry is in use in many laboratories. In all cases, acute preparations are used.

The purpose of the present study has been to develop a method by which the NADH fluorescence could be measured on the brain surface of chronically operated rats, and of unanesthetized rats as well. Using this method, one can measure the NADH fluorescence in the same animal over an interval of several days and compare the effect of various physiological and behavioral situations on the oxidation-reduction state of NADH in the brain (2).

METHOD

The air-turbine driven time-sharing fluorometer designed by Chance et al. (3) was employed here. This fluorometer permits the measurement of NADH fluorescence and light scattering changes at the excitation wavelength (366 nm) on the surface of the brain cortex. In this mode of operation the light is guided by a Y-shaped flexible (quartz fiber) light pipe with a total length of 20 cm and a common part of 5 cm. The outer quartz fiber diameter of the common part is 4 mm and the inner quartz fiber diameter is 2 mm for each limb. One limb carries the 366 nm excitation light to the cannula and the other carries the fluorescence emission (450 nm) and reflectance (366 nm) back to the air-driven disk where time-sharing wavelength resolution is accomplished by appropriate filters (4). The plexiglass cannula which fits the common part of the light pipe is shown in Figure 1. The thread in the bottom of the cannula enables the cannula to be screwed into the skull and to make a better connection with the acrylic cement. A 0.2 mm step holds the light pipe in at a constant distance from the brain.

*Support from NINDS 10939-01.

239

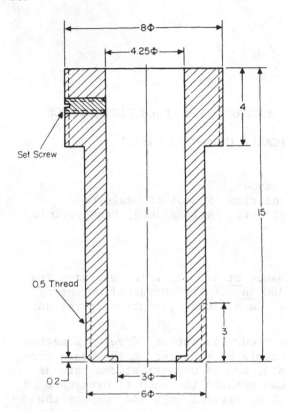

Figure 1. The construction of the implanted cannula. All dimensions in millimeters. The set-screw is used to fix the light pipe to the brain surface.

Male Wistar rats were used (200-250 g). The animal was anesthetized (Equi-thesin, 0.75 ml) and mounted to a head-holder. The skull was exposed and a hole of 6 mm diameter was drilled in the parietal bone on the right side of the brain. Only animals which showed a clear, hemoglobin-free brain surface were used. The cannula was screwed into the skull (1 mm deep) above the dura. Two metal screws were used for EEG recording from the contralateral as well as from the ipsilateral hemisphere. Acrylic dental cement fixed the cannula and the screws to the skull. A suitable plexiglass plug closed the exposed area until measurements were made. Blood pressure was measured by cannulation of the femoral artery. In the chronic preparation, blood pressure was not measured.

During measurements, the common part of the light pipe was plugged into the cannula in contact with the dura, to minimize brain movement or fluid accumulation which would interfere with the measurement. A nitrogen cycle was produced by exposing the animal to N_2 for 60 seconds. During the N_2 flushing, the animal stopped breathing, and 20-30 seconds later the animal started breathing spontaneously.

A spreading depression was obtained by flushing a solution of 0.2 to 0.4 M KCl through a small reservoir in the bottom of the cannula so that the solution was localized externally.

RESULTS AND DISCUSSION

Two distinctive conditions of the brain cortex were observed and interpreted to differ with respect to the microcirculatory response to anoxia. The first and simpler case occurs in the later phases of repetitive anoxia where, as shown in Figure 2, there are scarcely any systematic changes in the reflectance trace (top) as compared with the uncorrected fluorescence trace (second from top) during the cycle of anoxia, both traces being recorded on the same sensitivity (percent of maximum signal). Therefore the corrected fluorescence trace (third from top) appears nearly identical to the uncorrected trace, the reflectance being subtracted from the uncorrected fluorescence at a 1:1 ratio (5,6).

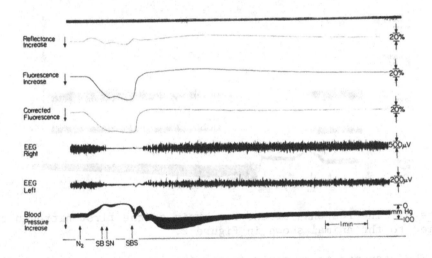

<u>Figure 2</u>. A typical response of the rat brain and the systemic blood pressure to a nitrogen cycle (#12). The corrected fluorescence trace is obtained by subtracting the reflectance change from the fluorescence change on a 1:1 basis. SB, stop breathing; SN, stop nitrogen; SBS, start breathing spontaneously.

The characteristic transition from normoxia to anoxia is slow and extends over an interval of about 30 seconds. The EEG maintains a constant level until the fluorescence increase reaches approximately 80% of maximum, and by the time 95% of maximal fluorescence is reached, no further EEG can be observed. The transition from normoxia to anoxia is slow because the oxygen tension is reduced from the normoxic value to a very low value by a combination of washout of the oxygen and tissue oxygen consumption. The return from anoxia to normoxia is very rapid, since the "front" of oxygen concentration in the freshly oxygenated hemoglobin is high, and the very small span of mitochondrial oxidation-reduction states (from 5×10^{-8} to 5×10^{-7} M oxygen) is bridged in a short time. As indicated in an accompanying paper (3), calibration of the NADH fluorescence increase in isolated mitochondria identifies the point of 50% reduction of NAD with an oxygen concentration of approximately 10^{-7} M (0.07 mm) and with virtual cessation of energy coupling. Thus, only about 10 seconds elapse between the cessation of energy coupling, the complete reduction of NADH, and the cessation of the EEG signal. The conditions of this experiment are very similar to those employed by Chance and Schoener (7,8) whose uncorrected fluorescence traces were also taken in later phases of the anoxic response where reflectance artifacts are negligible.

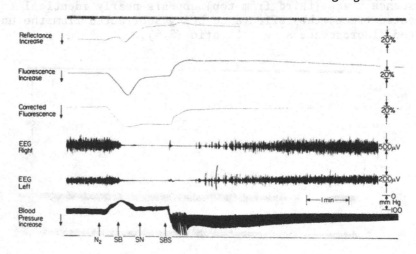

Figure 3. The response of the rat brain to the first nitrogen cycle applied to the animal shown in Figure 2.

The response to an early anoxia (#1 for this particular animal) is indicated in Figure 3. Here, the blood pressure pattern is generally similar but the microcirculatory response is such that shortly after the beginning of the pyridine nucleotide reduction, a large reflectance decrease causes a fluorescence decrease of comparable magnitude. These effects very nearly counter-balance each other on a 1:1 basis on the corrected trace, with similar changes of reflectance also appropriately cancelled out in the recovery from anoxia. Other features of the recovery from anoxia are the same as in Figure 2, except it should be noted that the recovery of the EEG is considerably delayed.

This change in the reflectance from cycle #1 to #12 may be caused by some damage to the autoregulatory mechanism controlling the blood flow to the brain. The arterial blood pressure of this

animal is not involved, since quite stable values are observed from
cycle #1 to cycle #12 during this interval, 110 - 80 mm Hg in the
first nitrogen cycle of Figure 3, as compared with 110-90 mm Hg in
the twelfth cycle shown in Figure 2. The amplitude of the EEG cycle
decreases with time.

     Preliminary experiments have been done in order to correlate
the redox state of NADH with the level of electrical activity of
the brain. In these experiments, we perfused a small area of the
dura (2 mm^2) with 0.4 KCl solution. The distance from the perfused
area to the NADH fluorescence measurement was 2 mm. A typical response to spreading depression is shown in Figure 4.

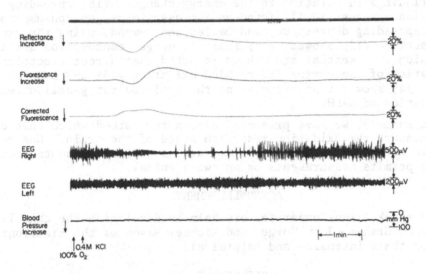

Figure 4. The response of the brain to the application of KCl
(0.4 M) on the dura surface.

     The animal was breathing pure oxygen or normal air during this
part of the experiment, so the oxygen supply was in the normoxic
range. The change in the reflectance and the NADH fluorescence
appears 30 to 40 seconds after the application of the KCl solution.
The changes in the right EEG (upper) begin even earlier since the recording was made from a point near the KCl application site. From
the changes in the reflected light, we assume that the response to
spreading depression is biphasic; in the beginning there is a short
increase in reflectance, followed by a longer decrease. The large
reflectance changes introduce an artifact into the fluorescence
measurement, and the corrected trace shows a small NADH oxidation.
In some animals where the reflectance changes were smaller, we saw
an NADH oxidation even in the uncorrected fluorescence trace.

The recovery of the corrected fluorescence trace from spreading
depression is much earlier than that of the EEG. The recovery of
the reflectance and of the uncorrected fluorescence trace are very
close to that of the EEG. It seems that the response to spreading
depression begins in a short vasoconstriction response, followed by
a longer vasodilation, as suggested also by van Harrenveld and Ochs
(9). It is also apparent that EEG activity in the contralateral side
of the brain (left side) was unaffected by the spreading depression
on the right side. The blood pressure was stable during this interval. We assume that the response to spreading depression contains
changes in blood flow or volume as well as changes in oxidation-
reduction state of NADH in the brain. That the oxidation of NADH
is due to an increase in oxygen consumption is in agreement with
other findings in relation to the energy change during spreading
depression. Bures (10,11) found an increase in oxygen consumption
during spreading depression, and Davies and Remond, using the oxygen electrode (12) showed an increase in oxygen consumption during
convulsions. Rosenthal and Jobsis reported that direct electrical
stimulation of the cortex led to NADH oxidation (13) and Brauser
et al. (14) showed that stimulating the isolated rat ganglion led
to oxidation of NADH.

In summary, we have presented here a new method which enables
us to measure the oxidation-reduction state of the brain. One can
use this method in chronic operated rats as well as in acute ones.
It also permits measurements on an awake animal.

ACKNOWLEDGEMENTS

We thank Allen Bonner for his help in developing the cannula,
and Norman Graham, John Sorge, and Michael Mason of the Electronics
Shop for their intensive and helpful aid.

REFERENCES

1. B. Chance, P. Cohen, F. Jobsis, and B. Schoener. Science, 137
    449 (1962).
2. A. Mayevsky. Ph.D. Thesis submitted to the Weizmann Institute,1972.
3. B. Chance, N. Oshino, T. Sugano, and A. Mayevsky. This volume, p.
4. B. Chance, D. Mayer, and L. Rossini. IEEE Trans, BME-17,
5. F. Jobsis, M. O'Connor, A. Vitale, and H. Vreman. J. Neurophysiol.,
    34, 735 (1971).
6. K. Harbig and M. Reivich. Submitted to J. App. Physiol.
7. B. Chance and B. Schoener. Nature, 195, 956 (1963).
8. B. Chance and B. Schoener. In Oxygen in the Animal Organism (Ed.
    F. Dickens and P. Neil) Pergamon Press,
9. A. van Harrenveld and S. Ochs. Am. J. Physiol, 189, 195 (1957).
10. J. Bures. J. Neurochem., 1, 153 (1956).
11. L. D. Lukyanova and J. Bures. Physiologia Bohemsolvaca, 16, 499
    (1967).
12. P. W. Davies and A. Remond. Res. Publ., Assoc. Res. Nerv. & Ment.
    Dis., 26, 205 (1946).
13. N. Rosenthal and F. Jobsis. J. Neurophysiol., 34, 750 (1971).
14. B. Brauser, Th. Bücher, and M. Dolivo. FEBS Lett., 8, 297 (1970).

ACTIONS OF HYPOXIA AND HYPERCAPNIA ON SINGLE MAMMALIAN NEURONS

E.-J. Speckmann, H. Caspers and D. Bingmann

Institute of Physiology, University of Münster/Westf.

Fed. Rep. Germany

The actions of oxygen deficiency on the bioelectrical activity of single neurons have been described in a number of papers (1-7, 9, 12). In these studies rather complex and sometimes even controversial neuronal responses were observed. Since a critical lowering of the pO_2 evokes an insufficiency of circulation and consequently an increase of the pCO_2, it may be assumed that the complex neuronal reactions are due partly to interactions of hypoxia and hypercapnia. This assumption was tested by intracellular recordings from moto- and interneurons in anesthetized and artificially ventilated rats and cats. In the experiments at first the isolated effects of hypoxia and hypercapnia were examined under continuous control of pO_2 and pCO_2 in blood and tissue. Subsequently the interactions of both effects were studied.

1) Effects of Hypoxia

A stepwise lowering of tissue pO_2 led to a progressive depolarization of cortical and spinal neurons provided that the pCO_2 was kept constant (2). Especially in interneurons the decrease of membrane potential (MP) was superimposed with spontaneously occurring and long lasting EPSPs which were enhanced in amplitude and frequency. These neuronal reactions were associated initially with an increase of discharge frequency. With progressing hypoxia action potentials regularly showed an A/B-blockade before spike generation failed (Fig. 1). In this stage EPSPs could still be evoked or might occur spontaneously. As a whole, increasing hypoxia induced progressing depolarization of cortical and spinal neurons associated with biphasic changes of discharge frequency. In complex neuronal networks seizure susceptibility behaved like the firing rate (2).

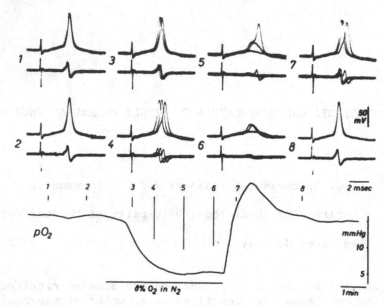

<u>Fig. 1</u>   Changes of intracellulary recorded action potential (AP) and their relation to pO₂ in surrounding tissue during hypoxia (horizontal bar). APs were elicited in a rat lumbar motoneuron (L₅) by weak dorsal root stimulation. Three tracings are superimposed. The lower traces in 1-8 represent the electrically differentiated records. Relation of curves 1-8 to pO₂ recording is indicated by corresponding numbers. As in following Figs. pO₂ in tissue was measured by a double microelectrode (from 12).

2) Effects of Hypercapnia

The actions of isolated hypercapnia on single neurons were tested by means of the so-called apnea technique (1, 12). Animals were ventilated with 100% oxygen for about 30 minutes. Then artificial respiration was interrupted with the respiratory tract kept connected to the oxygen container. With this procedure the pCO_2 was continuously enhanced, while the pO_2 in tissue did not fall beneath the initial value. Under this condition an increase of the pCO_2 evoked neuronal activity changes which can be devided into two types (12). Approximately 5-10% of lumbar interneurons classified as E-neurons showed a depolarization and an increase of discharge frequency. All cortical neurons and 90% of spinal neurons responded, conversely, with an increase of MP and a decrease in discharge rate (1,2,11,12. Cf. also 8). These cells classified as I-neurons were studied in more detail.

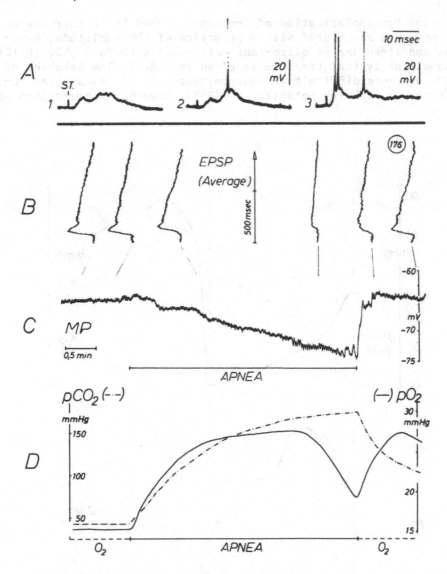

Fig. 2   Effects of CO_2 on membrane potential (MP) and on EPSPs of a motoneuron in the rat lumbar cord (I-neuron). A: EPSPs sequence elicited by single stimuli (ST.) applied to the sensorimotor cortex (1-3). B and C: Changes in EPSPs and MP evoked by increasing pCO_2 during apnea (horizontal bar). EPSPs represent average potentials of 20 responses following cortical stimulation. MP is traced by an inkwriter. D: Simultaneous variations in arterial pCO_2 and tissue pO_2 (from 2).

The hyperpolarization of I–neurons evoked by an increase of
the pCO_2 was associated with a reduction of the amplitude, duration and steepness of oligo- and polysynaptic EPSPs (1, 2, 10-12).
A sample of typical tracings is given in Fig. 2. The behavior of
IPSPs was more difficult to analyze since the MP was shifted toward the equilibrium potential of IPSPs. However, a comparison of

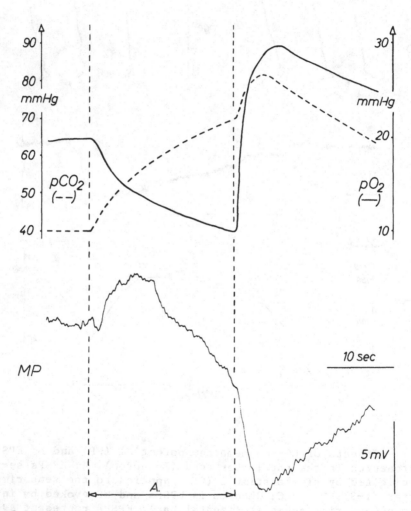

Fig. 3   Changes of membrane potential (MP) of a rat lumbar motoneuron (I–neuron) during asphyxiation (A). The curve was traced by
an inkwriter. Measures in the upper half of the Fig. show simultaneous changes of tissue pO_2 and arterial pCO_2 (from 12).

the affection of IPSPs by intracellular current injection with the actions of hypercapnia suggested that IPSPs were reduced, too. A marked increase in membrane input resistance during hypercapnia points in the same direction. Furthermore, antidromically evoked action potentials were blocked at CO_2 pressures exceeding 100 mmHg. Simultaneously the repetition rate of discharges elicited by intracellular current injection was reduced. This effect could not be attributed completely to the concomitant hyperpolarization. As a whole, these findings show that CO_2 depresses the activity of I-neurons both by direct actions on the cell membrane and via synaptic processes.

3) Interactions of Hypoxia and Hypercapnia

The interactions of hypoxia and hypercapnia were studied in asphyxiation experiments on I-neurons (1, 2, 12). An example is presented in Fig. 3. The tracings show an early depolarization of the neuron after the onset of respiratory arrest. The reduction of MP can be attributed to the developing oxygen deficiency. With continuing asphyxia the primary depolarization was followed by an intermediate re- and hyperpolarization which corresponded to an increase of the pCO_2. A reventilation in this period led to a further increase in MP associated with an additional rise in arterial pCO_2. If asphyxiation persisted, the intermediate re-increase in MP turned to a final depolarization which could be attributed to a critical decline of tissue pO_2. In spontaneously firing neurons spike activity ceased already in the peak range of the primary depolarization. EPSPs could still be evoked in the early section of the intermediate repolarization.

References

1) CASPERS, H. und SPECKMANN, E.-J. Gleichspannungsverschiebungen an der Hirnrinde bei Asphyxie. Ärztl.Forsch., 1971, 25: 241-255.

2) CASPERS, H. and SPECKMANN, E.-J. Cerebral pO_2, pCO_2 and pH: Changes During Convulsive Activity and their Significance for Spontaneous Arrest of Seizures. Epilepsia, 1972, 13: 699-725.

3) COLLEWIJN, H. and VAN HARREVELD, A. Intracellular recording from cat spinal motoneurons during acute asphyxia. J.Physiol. (Lond.), 1966, 185: 1-14.

4) CREUTZFELDT, O., KASAMATSU, A. und VAZ-FERREIRA, A. Aktivitätsänderungen einzelner corticaler Neurone im akuten Sauerstoffmangel und ihre Beziehungen zum EEG bei Katzen. Pflügers Arch.ges. Physiol., 1957, 263: 647-667.

5) ECCLES, R.M., LØYNING, Y. and OSHIMA, T. Effects of hypoxia
   on the monosynaptic reflex pathway in the cat spinal cord.
   J.Neurophysiol., 1966, 29: 315-332.

6) GLÖTZNER, F. Intracelluläre Potentiale, EEG und corticale
   Gleichspannung an der sensomotorischen Rinde der Katze bei
   akuter Hypoxie. Arch.Psychiat.Nervenkr., 1967, 210, 274-296.

7) KOLMODIN, G.M. and SKOGLUND, C.R. Influence of Asphyxia on
   Membrane Potential Level and Action Potentials of Spinal Moto-
   and Interneurons. Acta physiol.scand., 1959, 45: 1-18.

8) KRNJEVIC, K., RANDIC, M. and SIESJÖ, B.K. Cortical CO_2 tension and neuronal excitability. J.Physiol., 1965, 176: 105-122.

9) NIECHAJ, A. and VAN HARREVELD, A. Intracellular recording
   from cats spinal interneurons during acute asphyxiation.
   Brain Res., 1968, 8: 54-64.

10) PAPAJEWSKI, W., KLEE, M.R. and WAGNER, A. The action of
    raised CO_2 pressure on the excitability of spinal motoneurons.
    Electroenceph.clin.Neurophysiol., 1969, 27: 618.

11) SPECKMANN, E.-J. und CASPERS, H. Verschiebungen des cortica-
    len Bestandpotentials bei Veränderungen der Ventilationsgröße.
    Pflügers Arch., 1969, 310: 235-250.

12) SPECKMANN, E.-J., CASPERS, H. und SOKOLOV, W. Aktivitäts-
    änderungen spinaler Neurone während und nach einer Asphyxie.
    Pflügers Arch., 1970, 319: 122-138.

RESPONSE OF FELINE BRAIN TISSUE TO OSCILLATING ARTERIAL pO_2

W. J. Dorson and B. A. Bogue

Engineering Center, Arizona State University

Tempe, Arizona

BACKGROUND

An experimental system has been developed to investigate the transient response of tissue and cellular pO_2 to dynamic changes in perfusion. The in-vivo tissue transients resulting from short episodes of respirator-induced hypoxia were followed in the cerebral cortex of cats while simultaneously measuring tissue pO_2, total arterial pO_2 and flow rate, venous pO_2, and cell action-potential. The system was capable of producing, recording, and correlating oscillations induced by either respirator variations or a computer controlled exchange of venous and arterial blood.

The conceptual modeling of brain tissue metabolism and oxygen concentrations has been the subject of intensive efforts including the pioneering work of Krogh (1). The resultant geometric hypothesis of a modified tissue cylinder being supplied by nutrients from each capillary has been the basis of mathematical descriptions ranging from the early reports of Krogh and Erlanger (2) to the recent numerical computer solutions of Reneau, et. al. (3). The latter citation was successful in matching theory with data for steady-state changes in several physiological variables. Only short-term equilibrium variations could be measured for many years since researchers were restricted by macro analytical techniques. With the advent of ultra-micro polarographic oxygen electrodes, it has been possible to measure intercapillary tissue O_2 concentrations during episodes of varying arterial perfusion.

One of the early reports of transient brain tissue response to arterial O_2 changes demonstrated an overshoot of pO_2 upon

recovery from a 60-sec hypoxic episode (4). Inspired gases were
changed from air to nitrogen and then back to air. Both arterial
and tissue pO_2 were recorded. The recovery response of brain
tissue O_2 levels from hypoxia was verified by Metzger (5) in a
more detailed study of tissue pO_2 in the rat cortex. This overshoot phenomenon could not be directly predicted by first order
models (3). A compartmental approach with a delayed brain blood
flow response was subsequently proposed to explain this phenomenon
(6). However, simultaneous experimental flow measurements were not
available for incorporation into the model.

This prior work was restricted to the tissue response to step
changes in inspired O_2 concentrations. In addition to a more
complete documentation of transient behavior to such step changes,
the purpose of this work was to develop a dynamic experimental
system wherein the engineering tools of correlation and systems
analysis could be employed.

EXPERIMENT

The system employed in these studies of cat cerebral tissue
response is described in detail elsewhere in this volume. Four
types of experiments have been performed to date. Oscillations in
carotid artery pO_2 were obtained both by continuous variation in
respiratory gases and by a unique exchange system between venous
and arterial blood. The exchange system employed a multiple
chamber device in which arterial and venous blood was interchanged
with a computer-controlled pump. In order to accomplish this
mixing, both carotid arteries and jugular veins were cannulated.
Exit arterial pO_2 and entering venous pO_2 were monitored with micro
polarographic electrodes. Total exit arterial blood flow was
measured with a flow-through electromagnetic probe. All other
major vessels were clamped to establish a closed system. A schematic of the control scheme is shown in Figure 1, where constant
voltages, E_1 and E_2, were added to the sine and cosine functions
to avoid negative voltages. Step changes in respiratory gases were
also induced both with and without the exchange system in place.
In the step change and respirator cycling experiments without the
exchange system, a micro electrode was placed in one of the carotid
arteries and a wrap-around electromagnetic flow probe used in place
of the flow-through probe.

With the exchange bypass system in place, an estimate of total
O_2 consumption could be obtained. Serial samples were taken for
Hb, pO_2, PCO_2, pH, and percent saturation and these values correlated well with established saturation curves. Vital signs were
monitored during experiments including EKG, EEG, and blood pressure.
The tissue O_2 electrode was mounted on an automated microdrive

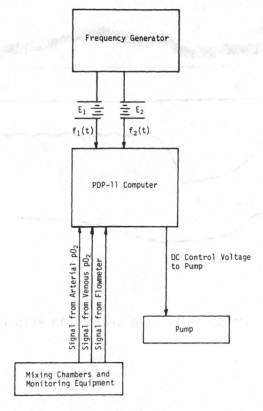

Figure 1. Schematic of the Exchange System Control

system which allowed position changes of 2.5 µ. This electrode
also measured cell action potentials.

RESULTS

A typical step change response is demonstrated in Figure 2
with the exchange system in place but not in operation. This
experiment was performed towards the end of extensive testing and
the cat's vital signs had deteriorated (note the low blood flow).
The tissue pO_2 overshoot follows an increased blood flow rate
during the recovery from hypoxia. In addition, increased blood
flow is sustained for several minutes. The observed tissue pO_2
cycles corresponded with respiration cycles (constant O_2 concentration).

The tissue response to respirator O_2 concentration cycling is
demonstrated in Figures 3 and 4 at two different frequencies with-

254

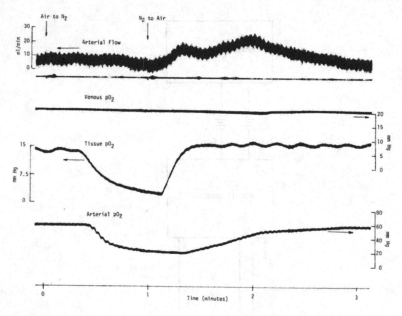

Figure 2.   Response to Step Changes in Respirator O$_2$

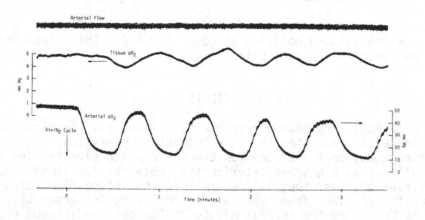

Figure 3.   Response to Oscillating Respirator Gas
Concentrations (no exchange system)

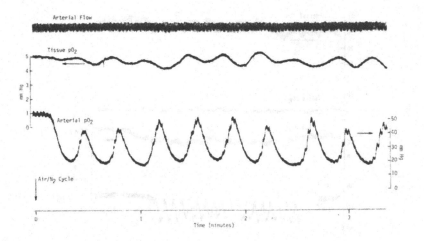

Figure 4.   Response to Oscillating Respirator Gas
           Concentrations (no exchange system)

out the exchange system in place. The wrap-around flow probe was
not as sensitive as the flow-through probe. The vital signs during
these two experiments were adequate but diminished compared to
normal values.

    One of the high frequency exchange system trials is shown in
Figure 5. Only low arterial pO_2 amplitudes were possible during
this particular experiment due to the small A-V oxygen differential.
Vital signs were normal. There was an oscillatory correlation of
both venous and tissue pO_2 with arterial pO_2 cycles which may not
be visibly obvious, but was proven with correlation analysis. This
is demonstrated by the cross-correlation of the same data in
Figure 5 which is shown in Figure 6. Even though the test duration
(and therefore sample collection) was not extensive, an excellent
correlation exists between venous, tissue, and arterial pO_2 values.
Phase lags between these values were due primarily to flow. As
examples of the flow induced time lag, tissue pO_2 phase lags varied
from $\sim$ 60° at 0.01 Hz to $\sim$ 32π + 290° at 1 Hz. The tissue to
arterial pO_2 amplitude ratios also varied from 0.45 to zero respectively. Under low flow conditions, the time lag between arterial
and tissue pO_2 was as high as 22 sec. with the exchange system and
18 sec. without the exchange system, the difference being due to
chamber and cannula delay. For the experiment shown in Figures 5
and 6, the arterial to tissue pO_2 lag was $\sim$ 11 sec., arterial pO_2
induced flow change was $\sim$ 14 sec., and arterial to venous pO_2 lag
was $\sim$ 29 sec.

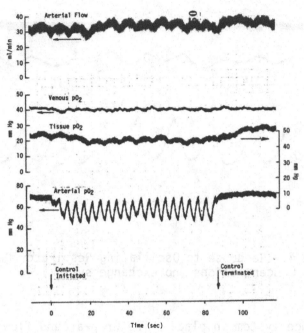

Figure 5.   Response to Oscillating Arterial pO$_2$ with
the Controlled Exchange System

The correlation of arterial pO$_2$ with itself (autocorrelation)
shown in Figure 6 demonstrates a good sine wave production from the
control system which, again, is not visibly evident from the data
shown in Figure 5. Cross-correlation is the product of two functions, one of which is delayed by the time τ shown in Figure 6.
This relation can be expressed as $f_1(t)f_2(t+\tau)$. Another benefit
of correlation techniques is the ability to separate any functional
dependence from signals which are affected by either noise or artifact. This is of particular importance since the goal of this
phase of the investigation is to provide a better understanding of
the dynamics of brain tissue oxygen and metabolic response during
physiological changes. The data can be compared to theoretical
models over a wider range of variables with the use of correlative
techniques.

Mathematical analyses done in conjunction with the experiments
included the simultaneous roles of autoregulatory and metabolic
contributions to tissue pO$_2$ response. The combined measurement
system allows detailed theoretical comparisons to be made and
various hypotheses to be tested. In this regard, the traverse of
the tissue pO$_2$ electrode showed less than a 2 sec. time lag difference between minimum and maximum response positions, which is
consistent with established diffusion models. The initial theoretical model developed during the course of this work is shown in

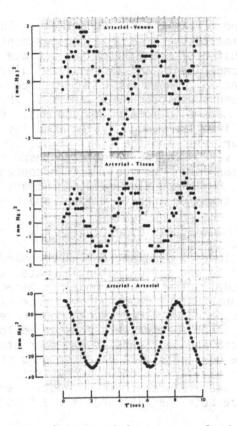

Figure 6. Auto- and Cross-correlations of the
Exchange System Data

Figure 7 as a multi-compartment approach with cellular O_2 metabolic
rates denoted by M_8 and M_9. The carotid artery perfusion flow
(Q, p_0, C_0) is delayed by a time Δt_1 which depends upon the flow
rate. Mixing between the exchange system and entrance to the

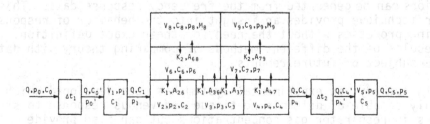

Figure 7. Compartment Model for Tissue Dynamic Response

capillaries is allowed for in the V_1 compartment. Capillary axial
gradients are approximated by three small compartments in series,
V_2, V_3, and V_4. Transfer of metabolites takes place between each
of the three blood compartments and two extracellular fluid chambers denoted by V_6 and V_7. These two chambers then exchange with
two cellular compartments depicted as V_8 and V_9. These latter two
compartments include metabolic models (M_8 and M_9). Blood exiting
from the capillaries into the venous system is delayed by Δt_2,
mixed in the V_5 compartment, and the final values (p_5 and C_5) can
be compared with the venous chamber electrode response. On Figure
7 the symbol definitions are: V = volume, C = concentration,
p = partial pressure, Q = blood flow rate, K = transfer coefficient,
A = intercompartment transfer area, t = time, and M = reaction rate.

Three metabolic models have been considered. The first is a
constant metabolic consumption of O_2, the second is a two term O_2
consumption which includes a constant cellular demand plus an O_2
reaction proportional to the action potential rate, and the third
is a total kinetic model. The kinetic model is based on a simplification of the elemental steps reported by Chance (7). Both
aerobic and anaerobic paths were reduced to four rate-limiting
reaction steps. All other species were considered to be in equilibrium with the products and reactants in the four steps. The
reported kinetic rate constants were based on step changes in
glucose and assumed elementary reaction mechanisms. Since the
metabolic scheme has been reduced to four reaction equations, it is
possible to generalize both the rate orders and constants.

With the simultaneous measurement of pO_2's and flow, autoregulation of perfusion can be incorporated directly into the
mathematical model. The remaining tissue dynamic response would
thus be due to either the kinetics of metabolism or concentration
dependent transfer. The increased range of variation made possible
with the described system along with the use of correlation techniques allows extensive testing of proposed metabolic mechanisms.
In this regard, the relative completeness of the experimental
measurements is mandatory. Proposed models can be compared directly
with the data, and through the use of systems analysis, transfer
functions can be generated from the frequency response data. This
latter technique provides an insight into the behavior of response
limiting processes without the need for their exact definition.
The results of the different methods of comparing theory with data
are the subject of future reports.

In summary, an experimental system has been developed which is
not only capable of determining tissue and venous response to step
changes in respirator gas concentrations but can also provide
oscillatory perfusion rates by several methods. Some examples are
presented of each type of response. With a true dynamic input,

several engineering analysis tools can be employed to help in the understanding of tissue O_2 response to varying physiologic conditions. With the simultaneous measurement of arterial, tissue and venous pO_2's along with total arterial flow and cell action potentials, detailed comparisons of proposed theoretical models with the data are possible. Also, autoregulatory and metabolic effects can be separated.

REFERENCES

1. Krogh, August, "The Anatomy and Physiology of Capillaries," Yale University Press, New Haven, Conn., 1922, 1 ed.

2. Krogh, August, "The Number and Distribution of Capillaries in Muscles with Calculations of the Oxygen Pressure Head Necessary for Supplying the Tissue," *J. Physiol.*, 52:409-415 (1918-19).

3. Reneau, D. D., Jr., D. F. Bruley and M. H. Knisely, "A mathematical simulation of oxygen release, diffusion, and consumption in the capillaries and tissue of the human brain," in *Chemical Engineering in Medicine and Biology*, ed. by D. Hershey, New York: Plenum Press, 1967, p. 135-241.

4. Bicher, H. I., and M. H. Knisely, "Brain tissue reoxygenation time, demonstrated with a new ultramicro oxygen electrode," *J. Appl. Physiol.*, 28:387-390, 1970.

5. Metzger, H., W. Erdmann and G. Thews, "Effect of short periods of hypoxia, hyperoxia and hypercapnia on brain O_2 supply," *J. Appl. Physiol.*, 31:751-759, 1971.

6. Reneau, D. D., Jr., H. I. Bicher, D. F. Bruley and M. H. Knisely, "A mathematical analysis predicting cerebral tissue reoxygenation time as a function of the rate of change of effective cerebral blood flow," in *Blood Oxygenation*, ed. by D. Hershey, New York: Plenum Press, 1970, p. 175-200.

7. Chance, B., D. Garfinkel, J. Higgins and B. Hess, "Metabolic control mechanisms. V. A solution for the equations representing interaction between glycolysis and respiration in ascites tumor cells," *J. of Bio. Chem.*, 235:2426-2439, 1960.

CHANGES OF OXYGEN SUPPLY TO THE TISSUE FOLLOWING INTRAVENOUS APPLICATION OF ANESTHETIC DRUGS

Wilhelm Erdmann and Stefan Kunke

Departments of Anesthesiology and Physiology

University of Mainz, Germany

The main function of the clinical anesthiologist is to make surgical treatment painless for the patient. For this purpose he uses drugs that severely interfere with the regulation of oxygen supply to the tissue. The same problem exists for the scientists working on animal experiments where he has to decide whether his experimental results were not changed by the anesthiological treatment.

The drugs used for anesthesia may induce a depression of spontaneous respiration and of blood pressure and a reduction of the heart minute volume. Blood pressure can be maintained very well within the normal range by pharmacological treatment and suffucient oxygenation of the blood by artificial ventilation of the lungs. Thus the oxygen supply of tissue is furthermore only dependent on

1.) the hight of capillary blood
   flow and
2.) the amount of oxygen consumption
   of the cells.

In the following study intravenous anesthetics have been examined for their effects on microcirculation and on intercapillary oxygen partial pressure.

Methods:

The experiments were performed with quickly producable ultra-microelectrodes (fig.1).

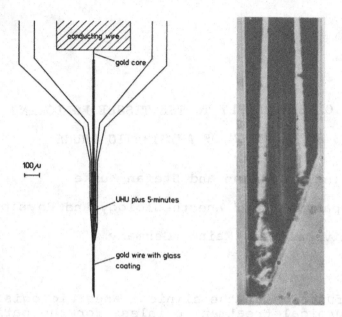

1a: Goldmicroelectrode
 b: ground tip of a goldmicroelectrode (tip dia-
    meter 4 /u).

The electrode tips were obliquely ground at one side.
This sharpened the electrode tip and at the same time
the surface of the oxygen measuring gold core was
well polished. To ensure partial pressure measurement
and to avoid poisoning of the metal surface in the
tissue the electrodes were covered with a special
plastic (Primal Ac-35, Decryl-Chemie, Frankfurt/Main,
Germany). When H_2-clearance measurements were to be
performed, the gold surface was platinized before use
by the procedure described previously (3,5).
Calibration was performed in o,2 molar KCl.

Experimental procedure: The experiments were performed in the frontal cortex of the brains of Albino
rats with mono- and multimicroelectrodes (4). The
animals were initially anesthetized with ether for
tracheotomy and vessel canualation. Analgesia was
maintained by $N_2O - O_2$ (7,9:2,1) led through a

T-shaped canula inserted into the trachea. The animal
was fixed in a stereotactic holder (LPC Co., Paris,
France) and the electrodes were inserted into the
brain through small holes drilled into the skull cap.

H_2-clearance-measurement (5) was applied along with

continuous oxygen partial pressure registration in
order to know something about the changes of microcirculation. As we used the clearance method via an
externally applied indicator (H_2 instead of N_2 in the
inspired gas), only relative changes of microcirculation could be stated according to the changes of the
half time value of the H_2-clearance-curves.

The influence of the following intravenous anesthetics on tissue perfusion of the brain and oxygen partial pressure distribution in the brain cortex has
been studied.

1.) barbiturates Methohexital (3o mg/kg body weight)
                 Thiopental   (3o mg/kg body weight)
                 Hexobarbital (5o mg/kg body weight)
2.) Propaidid (3o mg/kg body weight)
3.) Ketamine (5o mg/kg body weight)

All experiments studying the changes of PO_2 and blood
flow following barbiturate application upon respiration (1). On the other hand artificial respiration
proved to be unneccessary in the case of Propanidid
and Ketamine anesthesia.

Results

Barbiturates have been tested using 12 grown up rats
under artificial ventilation. After intravenous application of thiopental (5o mg/kg body weight) tissue
PO_2decreases to lower values in about 3o - 6o seconds
(fig.2). At the same time blood pressure and heart
rate changes by about 15 % and thus do not leave the
autoregulative range of CBF.

These changes of tissue - PO_2 are seen with all examined barbiturates. The duration of tissue PO_2 depression is closely correlated to the time of anesthetic effect; for tiopental duration of PO_2-depression
amounts to 2o - 25 minutes, for methohexital as short
time acting barbiturate changes of PO_2 do not exceed
5 to 1o minutes of duration and for hexobarbital as a
long time acting barbiturate.

The amount by which tissue PO_2 decreases following
application of barbiturates depends very signifi-
ciantly on the initial value before introduction of
barbiturate anesthesia (fig.3) and at initial values
above 4o mm Hg the usual tendency of PO_2 changes to
lower values is not seen or even opposite with a
slight increase of tissue PO_2.

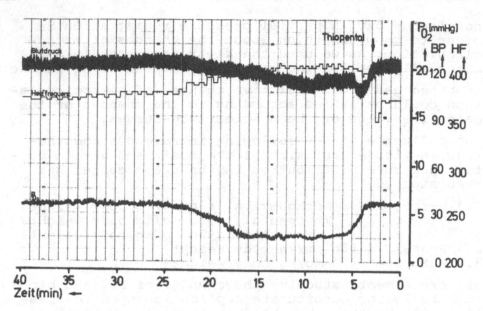

2: Tissue - PO_2 (PO_2) in the cortex of the rat brain
   during thiopental anesthesia.
   BP= arterial blood pressure   HF= heart rate

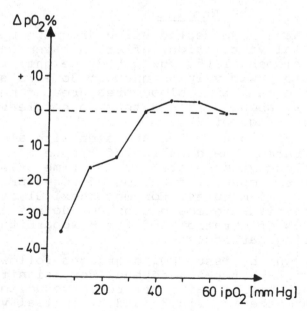

3: Changes of tissue-PO_2 percentagewise of initial
   PO_2.

All three drugs entering into the examination showed
a close correspondance to the dose applied. A typical
step phenomena is seen between 15 and 2o mm Hg according to the barbiturate injected (fig.4).

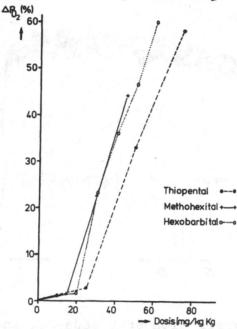

4: Dose related reaction of thiopental, methohexital
   and hexobarbital. Changes of tissue-PO_2 in percent
   of the initial value (ΔPO_2%). The graph shows a
   typical threshhold phenomenon for all the three
   barbiturates.

Propanidid has been studied in 12 rats. Shortly after
injection, blood pressure decreased by about 3o% while
heart rate increased by up to 2o%. These changes of
circulation values did not remain longer than one minute. Tissue PO_2 in brain cortex usually did not
change at all, sometimes a moderate decrease of some
seconds did occur correlated to the acute blood pressure reaction.

Ketamine has been examined for tissue-PO_2 reactive
effects in 12 rats. After intravenous application
blood pressure decreased, it recovers in 1o seconds
and then it remains above the original value for 1o-
2o minutes by about 2o-3o%. Heart rate increased at
the same time by 1o-2o%.
After quick injection tissue-PO_2 showed a short time
decrease which recovered in 1o-15 seconds. In the

following large oscillations of PO_2 were seen around the initial value (fig.5).

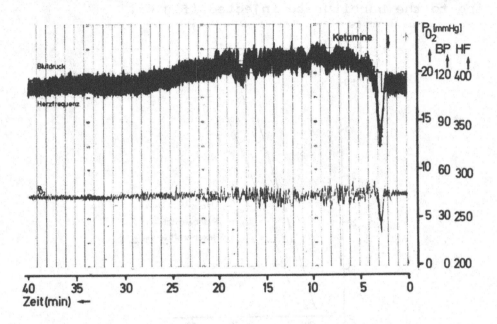

5: Original registration of tissue-PO_2 in the brain cortex during Ketamine anesthesia.
BP= arterial blood pressure   HF= heart rate

The slow large waves of tissue-PO_2 under Ketamine anesthesia permit disappearance of normal PO_2-rhythm completely. After 15-25 minutes the hight of the oscillation range diminuished and the rate rises until normal PO_2-rhythm is reached.
The PO_2-rhythm changing effect of Ketamine without significant alteration of mean tissue-PO_2 is seen in all parts of the capillary network at high and low initial values.

The relative changes of tissue perfusion have been studied by means of H_2-clearance curves following respiration of an H_2-O_2-gas mixture in the cortex of 24 rats.

B a r b i t u r a t e s : After injection of 3o mg/kg
body weight of thiopental half time value of H_2-clear-
ance curve amounts from 2 minutes to 2 minutes 4o seconds. The curve was registered when PO_2 changes had
reached their maximal deviation in the case of thiopental 2 minutes following injection. The original half
time value of H_2-clearance curve was reached 21 minutes
following thiopental injection (fig.6).

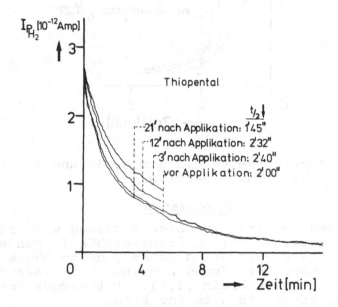

6: H_2-clearance-curve before induction with thiopental
   and following injection 3, 12 and 21 minutes afterwards.

Corresponding to the dose dependent effect of PO_2-de-
pression following barbiturate application, the
changes of time constants of the H_2-clearance curves
are correlated to the dosage as well.

P r o p a n i d i d : has no effect at all on tissue
perfusion rate.

K e t a m i n e : induced a significant diminuation of
H_2-clearance half time values. 21 minutes following
the Ketamine injection the initial value was reobtai-
ned (fig.7).

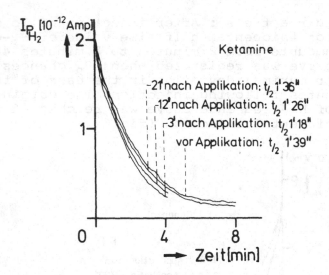

7: H$_2$-clearance-curve before and 3, 12 and 21 minutes
   following Ketamine injection.

Discussion

The described results have been obtained with rats.
We assume that this data is transferable to man as the
changes of tissue perfusion correspond to those results which have been found previously in measurements
for the whole human brain (1,2). Furthermore the pharmacological effect is also the same.

The experiments reveal different effects between the
examined anesthetics.

1. A PO$_2$-depression which occurs simultaneously to the
   reduction of H$_2$-clearance velocity in the brain
   cortex: This is seen during barbiturate anesthesia.
   The conclusion is approached in that reduction of
   tissue perfusion must exceed the amount which
   would be correlated to the known reduction of the
   oxygen consumption of the brain. Thus barbiturates
   severely interfere with the tissue-oxygenation regulating factors and changerable local ishemia
   might occur.

2. A change in PO$_2$-rhythm by superimposed large and
   relatively slow oscillations without changes of
   mean tissue PO$_2$: At the same time H$_2$-clearance-
   time constants become shorter, that means tissue
   perfusion is increased. The assumption can be

made that this increase of tissue perfusion is only a
compensation of the increased oxygen consumption
during ketamine anesthesia (2).

3. Other narcotics such as Propanidid do not interfere
   with the tissue oxygenation factors at all. As to
   the medical practicality of the described results
   it is once more revealed that the difficulties are
   variable which exist in the final conclusions when
   experiments are performed in anesthetized animals.
   On the other hand the performed experiments bring
   new aspects when weighing two anesthetics whether
   one is preferable to the other.

References

1. Betz, E.: Central Nervous System Depressants. In:
   International Encyclopedia of Pharmacology and
   Therapeutics. Pergamon Press, Oxford-New York-
   Toronto-Sydney-Braunschweig. Sect. 33,149-18o /1972.

2. Dawson, B., Michenfelder, J. and R.A. Theye: Effects
   of Ketamine on Canine Cevebral Blood Flow and Metabolism. Modification by prior administration of
   Thiopental. Anaesthesia and Analgesia 5o,443-447 /
   1971.

3. Erdmann, W.: A Quickly Produced Ultra Microelectro-
   de for Oxygen, H_2-clearance and Action Potential
   Measurement. Mount Sinai Prize of Anesthiology,
   Mount Sinai School of Medicine, New York / 1971.

4. Erdmann, W., Kunke, S. and Krell, W.: Tissue-PO_2
   and Cell Function. - An Experimental Study with
   Multimicroelectrodes in the Rat Brain. In: Oxygen
   Supply. Eds. Kessler Urban & Schwarzenberg,München-
   Wien / 1973.

5. Heidenreich, J., Erdmann, W., Metzger, H. and
   G. Thews: Local Hydrogen Clearance and PO_2-Measure-
   ments in Microareas of the Rat Brain. Expérientia
   26,257-259 / 1970.

LOCAL PO$_2$ AND O$_2$-CONSUMPTION IN THE ISOLATED SCIATIC NERVE

K. Kunze
Department of Clinical Neurophysiology
Neurological Clinical University of Giessen
Giessen, West Germany

Local oxygen pressure can be measured by means of Pt-micro-needle electrodes and this gives information about oxydative tissue metabolism. Under special conditions local oxygen consumption in tissue can be estimated with this technique too.

Therefore investigations in isolated sciatic nerves of chickens have been performed using a technique which has been described earlier (Kunze). Sciatic nerves of chickens, 3 weeks old, have been excised carefully and firstly stored for 20-30 minutes in mammalian Tyrode solution and gased with carbogen ($95\%O_2 + 5\%CO_2$). After this the nerves were mounted in a special chamber which could be equilibrated with different gases at $37^{o}C$. Before starting oxygen pressure measurements compound nerve action potentials were lead off after supramaximal stimulation of the nerve and conduction velocities were calculated.

The conduction velocity in 20 sciatic nerves was found to be $101,2 \pm 16$ m/sec. The survival times (time from starting anoxia until no response of the nerve to stimulation) of the nerves were 16 minutes in the mean. During anoxia the conduction velocity decreased to $78,0 \pm 0,2$ m/sec. These values were not influenced by a stimulation rate from 1-200/sec.

For studying local oxygen supply in the resting nerve the needles were inserted as perpendicularly as

With support of Deutsche Forschungsgemeinschaft

possible, thus measuring PO_2 in vertical direction by steps of 50 u. Calibrations were done in the nerve tissue itself, near the margin of the nerve. A gradual stepwise decrease was measured until the needle reached the axis of the nerve (fig.1).

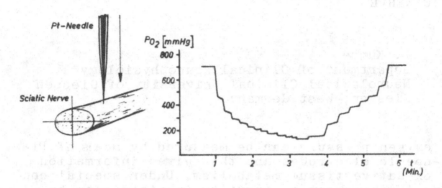

<u>Fig.1:</u>   Oxygen pressure measurements in the sciatic nerve. The procedure is shown on the left side schematically.

A plot of these readings against insertion depth is given in fig.2. Please notice that under these conditions PO_2 values at a chamber equilibration with 20,7%O_2 are very low and that the difference from the margin to the axis values is smaller than at an equilibration with carbogen, indicating insufficient supply conditions of the nerve.
From measurements of PO_2 at the margin and at the axis of the nerve, it is possible to calculate local O_2-consumption in this tissue which is supplied with oxygen from the periphery only. This is possible by using the formula of Thews for the tissue cylinder supplied from the periphery, which he has published together with Opitz in 1952 (calculations for 37°C, α = 2,2 x 10^{-2} cm^3 O_2/cm^3 Atm, K = 2,3 x 10^{-5} cm^3 O_2/cm min Atm
        The calculated mean value of 1,1x10^{-3} cm^3 O_2/g min is in agreement with those measured earlier by Gerard and Wright who used the Warburg technique.

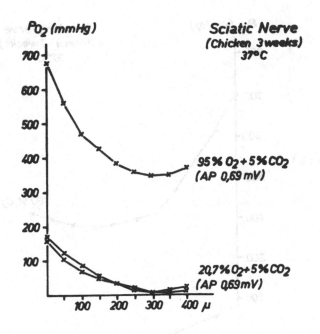

Fig.2:   PO$_2$measurements in the sciatic nerve equilibrated with addition of 5 %CO$_2$.

In these nerve preparations a storage cylinder and
nerve chamber equilibration with carbogen had been
used. This refers to early investigations of Adrian
who tried pure oxygen for equilibration and found the
nerve in a state of continuous firing and then undergoing deterioration. When using pure oxygen in these
experiments instead of carbogen, there was actually
no much influence on PO$_2$ readings. But when the nerves
were kept for a longer time in pure oxygen, that means
from dissection to measurements, the PO$_2$ differences
from margin to axis were smaller than those in carbogen atmosphere (fig.3). This could be shown in the
same nerve preparation too (fig.4).
Comparing a group of 10 nerves in carbogen and in a
pure oxygen atmosphere (fig.5) a statistically significant difference (p 0,01) could be proved. Besides
that a difference exists in carbogen atmosphere between nerves of 3 weeks old chickens and chickens of
1 year old. These differences refer to PO$_2$differences
from the margin to the axis as well as to calculated
O$_2$-consumption (fig.6).

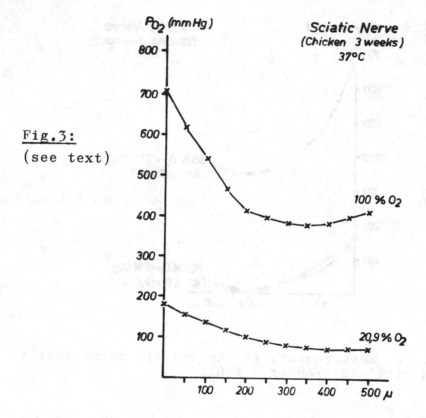

Fig.3:
(see text)

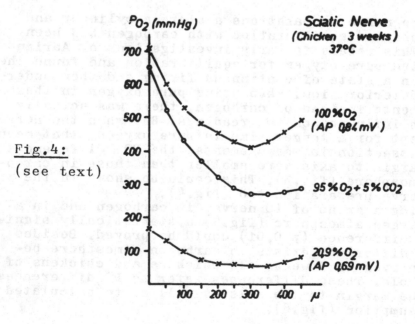

Fig.4:
(see text)

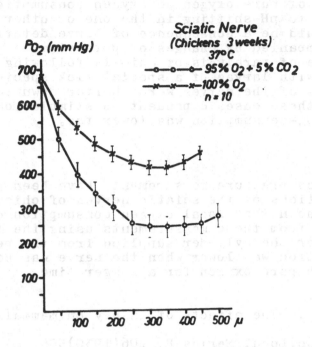

Fig.5: Oxygen pressure measurements in nerves equilibrated with carbogen and pure oxygen. 10 nerves in
each group with standard deviation for different PO_2
readings.

Sciatic Nerve		ΔPO_2	R	O_2 - Consumption (calculated)	
Chickens 3 weeks	Carbogen n = 10	454 ± 68 mmHg	345 ± 50 μ	1,1 ± 0,1	$10^{-3} \frac{ml\ O_2}{g\ min}$
	100% O_2 n = 10	276 ± 58 mmHg	335 ± 41 μ	0,7 ± 0,1	$10^{-3} \frac{ml\ O_2}{g\ min}$
Chickens 1 year	Carbogen n = 6	430 ± 76 mmHg	550 ± 45 μ	0,4 ± 0,08	$10^{-3} \frac{ml\ O_2}{g\ min}$

Fig.6: PO_2 differences (ΔPO_2) between margin and
axis (R) and calculated O_2-consumption (after Thews)
in nerves equilibrated in carbogen and pure oxygen.

The effect of pure oxygen on oxygen consumption which
is not due to pH-shifting in the one or other equilibration could be a consequence of nerve deterioration accompanied by changes of potassium.
In the case of paralysis of animals following in-
festation with larvae of a special tick species survival times of the nerves were shorter down to 4 minutes, in these cases dependent on stimulation rates,
and local O_2-consumption was lower too.

Summary:

Local oxygen pressure measurements have been performed
in preparations of the sciatic nerves of chickens. It
could be shown that local oxygen consumption can be
calculated from these measurements using the formula
of Thews for the cylinder supplied from the periphery.
O_2-consumption was lower when the nerve was equilibrated with pure oxygen for a longer time.

References:
Adrian,E.D.:   The effects of injury on mammalian nerve
fibres.
Proc.Roy.Soc.Lond. Series B. 106(1930)596

Gerard,R.W.:   The response of nerve to oxygen lack.
Amer.J.Physiol. 92(1930)498

Kunze,K.:   Action potential, conduction velocity and
oxygen pressure in the isolated sciatic nerve of the
chicken.
in: Oxygen Supply ed. by Kessler,M. et.al.
Urban & Schwarzenberg, München-Berlin-Wien 1973, p.175

Wright,E.B.:   A comparative study of the effects of
oxygen lack on peripherae nerve.
Amer.J.Physiol. 147(1946)78

Opitz,E. und G.Thews : Einfluss von Frequenz und Fa-
serdicke auf die Sauerstoffversorgung des menschlichen Herzmuskels.
Arch.f.Kreislaufforschg. 18(1952)137

BASIC PRINCIPLES OF TISSUE OXYGEN DETERMINATION FROM

MITOCHONDRIAL SIGNALS

B. Chance, N. Oshino, T. Sugano, and A. Mayevsky

Johnson Research Foundation, School of Medicine

University of Pennsylvania, Philadelphia PA 19104

The importance of measuring intracellular oxygen concentrations in tissues has, over the years, emerged as a basic parameter in the physiology and biochemistry of living tissues. The credibility of oxyhemoglobin determinations, even as refined A/V differences, is taxed especially in cases where inhomogeneous tissues with variable oxygen demands and oxygen supply are served. The formation of lactic acid in the venous blood is often used as a criterion of anoxia, but it also lacks credibility where inhomogeneous circulatory pathways are served and in addition, is questionable from the standpoint of whether the appearance of excess lactate is an unequivocal criterion of oxygen insufficiency. To indicate my empathy with polarographic techniques as they have been developed at the Johnson Foundation, I wish to recall the pioneering works of Bronk(1) Brink (2), Davies and Remond (3) that stand as landmarks in the exploration of tissue oxygen tension by microelectrode methods. I served my apprenticeship with them.

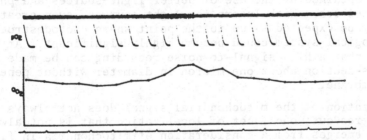

Figure 1. Illustrating the use of the platinum microelectrode to measure quantitatively the cortical oxygen tension during an epileptic seizure. Upper trace, electrocorticogram. Second, pO_2 shown as a series series of curves, each one giving oxygen tension as a function of time after local occlusion of the pial circulation. Third trace, Q_{O_2}, a plot of the linear portions of these curves as proportional to the rate of oxygen consumption. (From Davies & Remond, 1946 [3])

MITOCHONDRIAL INDICATION OF INTRACELLULAR pO_2

However, the organelles that surely exhibit the intracellular oxygen tension are the ones that are using the oxygen. These are the mitochondria. They do not need to be reached by electrodes; they emit spectroscopically detectable signals themselves. It is the purpose of this paper to show how these signals may be read.

The accumulation of evidence since the pioneer work of Otto Warburg on "atmungsferment"(4) and David Keilin on cytochromes (5) as the keystones of cellular oxygen utilization led us to a study of the redox states of electron carriers in isolated mitochondria as a function of oxygen concentration, and to develop techniques to measure the states of anoxia and normoxia in living tissues.

The morphology of the system is a primary consideration, and we shall begin by showing where the mitochondria are situated and what they may reveal on account of this location. The ubiquity of mitochondria in eukharyotic cells is due to their superlatively efficient energy conservation system. Often, one-third or more of the volume of an active tissue, such as mammalian cardiac tissue, may be filled with mitochondria. Similarly, the oxygen utilization of the brain as compared with that of the whole body stands as testimony to mitochondrial activity in that organ. Thus, there is no doubt that the readout of mitochondrial redox states takes us to the very source and furthermore, the cell membrane does not need to be penetrated in order to do so.

Granting that an intracellular indicator is thus available, the question remains as to how precisely it may be measured, i.e., how many mitochondria are required for a readable signal of their redox state? Fortunately, this has been determined by both microfluorometry and microspectrophotometry; using as experimental material a single large mitochondrion, that of the insect spermatid in meiotic telephase, we find signal-to-noise ratios of about 10 at bandwidths of a few cycles per sec(6,7). Somewhat improved performance has recently been obtained by the use of better light sources and photon-counting detectors. With lasers for light sources, even greater progress may be expected -- up to the point where photodestruction of the biological system could become highly significant. At least, one can say that a high signal-to-noise recording can be made from a tissue cross-section about one micron in diameter without penetrating the cell membrane.

Localization of the mitochondrial signal does not always require microscopic readout; one facet of localization that is not always appreciated emerges from a consideration of mitochondria in flight-muscle, where the repeat pattern of mitochondrial localization and function is sufficiently regular that averaging of the signal from many mitochondria nevertheless ensures that the recording can be referred to the intimate relationship of a single mitochondrion and its adjacent myofibril. It is not clear that this is the case with the brain, where the distribution of mitochondria in the cell bodies, the synapses, and the glia may well require microscopic techniques in order precisely to localize the mitochondrial response to a certain kind of process in a particular portion of a cell.

It is further appropriate to consider whether the mitochondrial redox state can be calibrated in terms of oxygen requirements. The oxygen requirements can be determined precisely by two general approaches, kinetic and steady-state. Considering first the kinetic method, we have a simple expression based on the assumption that the cytochrome oxidase system works on a mechanism that was demonstrated in detail in our early studies of peroxidase (8) according to modifications of the Michaelis-Menten theory:

$$K_m = k_3/k_1 \tag{1}$$

The quantity k_3, while a kinetic parameter, is most readily determined from the steady state rate of oxygen utilization at high oxygen concentration, as measured by the oxygen electrode, and may simply be identified from the turnover number, TN, of cytochrome oxidase:

$$k_3 = TN = \frac{4 \; dO_2/dt}{[a_3]} \tag{2}$$

The factor of 4 equates the number of oxidizing equivalents per mole of oxygen with the electron-handling capability of cytochrome $\underline{a_3}$. Thus, K_m is directly proportional to the turnover number or the respiratory activity of the mitochondria.

The denominator of the expression, k_1, the rate of combination of cytochrome oxidase with oxygen, generally requires the use of the rapid flow apparatus for its determination. An example of the measurement of this constant by laser photolysis of CO-inhibited cytochrome oxidase in a suspension of isolated mitochondria in the presence of 17 μM oxygen is shown in Figure 2. It is seen that the reaction time is very short, about one millisecond under these particular conditions. This value, which is appropriate to the reaction of roughly 10 mm oxygen with the cytochrome oxidase of the tissue, is indeed the parameter to which cytochrome oxidase owes its remarkably high oxygen affinity. The value of K_m for several sources of resting mitochondria is calculated to be 10^{-8} M oxygen (9), and for highly activated mitochondria, about ten-fold greater, 3×10^{-7} M,

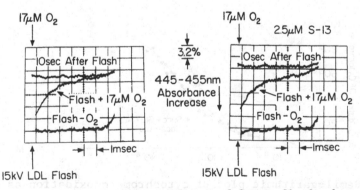

Figure 2. Illustrating the technique of laser flash photolysis for measuring the rate of reaction of oxygen (17 μM) with cytochrome oxidase in suspensions of CO-inhibited pigeon heart mitochondrial membranes in the coupled (left) and uncoupled (right) states. (127-8,9V; courtesy of Archives of Biochemistry and Biophysics [9]).

at 23°. The many identical properties of isolated and in situ mitochondria support the applicability of the in vitro data to the in
vivo conditions.

The steady state approach has the advantage that it is strictly
analogous to some of the procedures that are applicable to intact
tissues as well. What is needed in this case is an extremely sensitive and linear oxygen indicator. A variety of approaches are
available; we have preferred luminous bacteria (10) since they afford
the greatest dynamic range, from almost 1 μM downwards towards 10^{-10}
M. A calibration curve of the luminous bacteria system is shown in
Figure 3 (11).

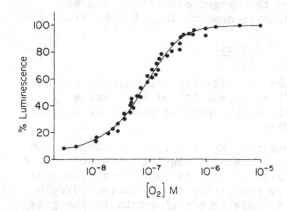

Figure 3. Calibration
curve of oxygen consumption
vs. luminescence in a suspension of Achromobacter
fischeri.   (NO-161)

The applicability of this method to the determination of the
oxygen affinity of the cytochromes of pigeon heart mitochondria is
illustrated in Figure 4, where p_{50} for cytochrome c has been evaluated. Plotted on a semilogarithmic scale, the cytochrome c response
is sigmoidal, corresponding to a rectangular hyperbola. The oxygen
concentration required for half-maximal oxidation of cytochrome c
varies with the turnover number; 6×10^{-7} M oxygen for the

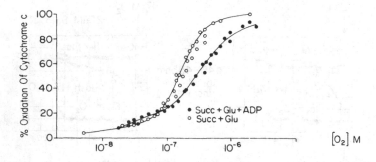

Figure 4. Semilogarithmic plot of cytochrome c oxidation as a
function of oxygen concentration for the rapidly respiring State
3 (●) and without added ADP (O).   (TS-N-5A)

rapidly respiring State 3 (12) in good agreement with the kinetic data. In the absence of ADP, a smaller K_m is observed but not as small as when the mitochondria are in a true resting State 4.

Relative Sensitivity to Anoxia of the Respiratory Components.

It is important to consider which component best represents the performance of the mitochondria. A synopsis of the components of the respiratory chain, roughly in order of increasing mid-potential, is shown in Figure 5. In an equilibrium system, the mid-potential of the respiratory components will determine their sensitivity to oxygen; the component at the most negative potential will respond most sensitively to oxygen, and that at the most positive potential, least sensitively. NADH, at approximately -300 mV, is at the extreme low potential end of the chain, and thus may be the oxygen indicator of choice in mitochondria and tissue as well; while one species of flavoprotein is also of a very negative mid-potential, the NADH fluorescence signal in the normoxic-anoxic transition is larger and less sensitive to artifacts. Cytochrome c, at +220 mV, is in the upper range of midpotentials and thus less sensitive to changes of oxygen concentration. From a kinetic standpoint, however, it is a more useful indicator of electron transport and energy coupling rates than is NADH.

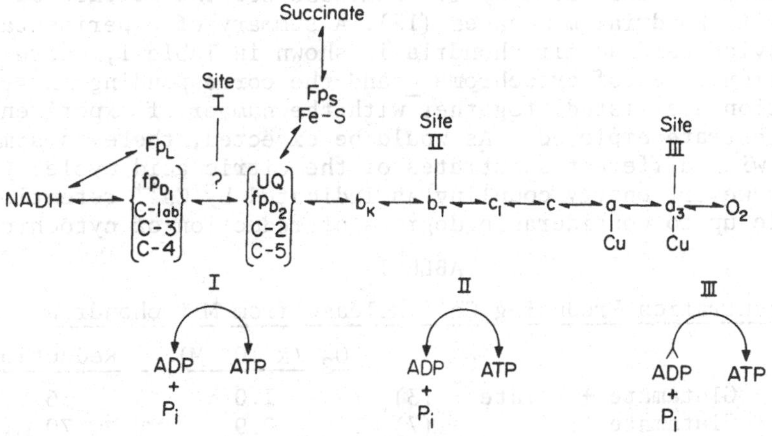

Figure 5. Schematic diagram of the respiratory components from the most negative (NADH) to the most positive (O_2) midpotential.

Figure 6 illustrates the relationship between the percent of maximal NADH oxidation and the corresponding value for cytochrome c in a suspension of rat brain mitochondria. Under these conditions, 50% oxidation of NADH occurs with only 10% oxidation of cytochrome c, as might be expected in view of their relative midpotentials. These levels of oxidation of the two components correspond to about 10^{-7} M oxygen, or 0.07 torr.

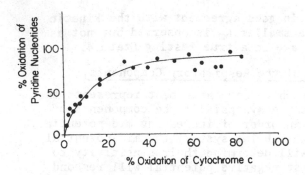

Figure 6. Relationship
between extent of NADH
oxidation and percent
of cytochrome c oxida-
tion, in the former
case taken as a fraction
of steady state values.
Rat brain mitochondria.
(TS-N-8A)

Oxygen Requirements for Energy Coupling

It is essential in order to evaluate cell function to know the
oxygen concentration at which energy coupling can be activated, and
for this purpose we have studied one of the several energy-linked
functions of mitochondria (13), the ability of the mitochondria to
accumulate divalent cations such as Ca^{++}. This ability is measured
with exquisite sensitivity by the jellyfish protein, aequorin (14)
kindly provided by Dr. F. H. Johnson. As the mitochondrial suspension is slowly rendered anaerobic, there is an oxygen concentration
-- and a corresponding oxidation-reduction level for cytochrome c --
at which aequorin indicates by its luminescence the release of $\bar{Ca}^{++}$
from the mitochondrial membranes (15). A summary of experimental
data for avian cardiac mitochondria is shown in Table I, where both
the reduction level of cytochrome c and the corresponding oxygen
concentration are listed, together with the number of experiments
and the substrate employed. As would be expected, there is some
variation with different substrates of the citric acid cycle. In
general, however, energy coupling as indicated by Ca^{++} retention,
is feasible up to considerable degrees of reduction of cytochrome c.

TABLE I

O_2 Concentration Producing Ca^{++} Release from Mitochondria

		O_2 (x 10^{-7}M)	% Reduction, c
Succinate + Glutamate + Malate	(3)	1.0	66
Succinate + Glutamate	(7)	0.9	70
Glutamate + Malate	(3)	1.1	58
Glutamate	(5)	0.6	47
β-hydroxybutyrate	(2)	0.9	41
Malate	(2)	0.4	75

Thus the oxidation-reduction state of cytochrome c is an effective
indicator not only of the electron transport rate through the respiratory chain but also of the capability of the mitochondria for
energy coupling. In metabolic state characteristic of living tissues,
the graph of Figure 6 gives the appropriate conversion from cytochrome
c to NADH oxidation.

SENSITIVE FLUOROMETRY OF TISSUE NADH

Having identified that NADH, being the most sensitive component
of the respiratory chain to oxygen, is most competent to serve as an
indicator of intracellular oxygen concentrations, and having determined the degree of NADH oxidation required for energy-linked function, we may consider how the oxidation-reduction state of NADH may
be measured.   This component is, in fact, a natural fluorochrome;
excitation in the range 340-370 nm gives rise to fluorescence emission of the reduced form with a peak centered around 450 nm.   Figure
7 shows the fluorescence change from the oxidized to the reduced
states in a suspension of rat liver mitochondria.   Excitation of
NADH fluorescence at 340 nm gives an approximately four-fold increase
of fluorescence intensity in the transition from the aerobic, sub-
strate-free state to the anaerobic state of the mitochondria.

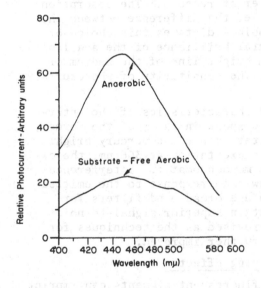

Figure 7. Comparison of the
intensity of fluorescence
emission from a suspension
of mitochondria in the anaerobic vs the aerobic, substrate free states.
(Courtesy of The Journal of
Biological Chemistry [16]).

This large fluorescence increase may not always be observed in situ,
where substrates are continuously supplied to the cell from the
bloodstream.   Fluorescence increases observed experimentally in
living tissue in the normoxic-anoxic transition are in the range
of 25% to 50%.

Sensitive fluorometry of tissue NADH has three requirements:
1) a high quantum yield of fluorescence; 2) a high rejection of
excitation light from the secondary filter; 3) a control of the
magnitude of artifacts due to absorption, reflectance, and scattering changes in the excitation and emission wavelengths.

Quantum Yield

The quantum yield of NADH is relatively low in solution --
approximately 0.1%. Our observations of NADH fluorescence in

the cell, however, indicate that this value is increased by a factor which may run as high as twenty-fold; thus one may expect a
quantum yield of approximately 2% for the bound fluorochrome in the
tissues. This relatively high quantum yield has three great advantages: first, that of ensuring that NADH will be selectively excited
and observed to emit on illuminating the tissue with a wide range of
wavelengths in the region from 330 nm to 370 nm; second, that the excitation and emission filters can be relatively simple; third, that
artifacts of reflectance and scattering may be minimal.

Filter characteristics

The design of the primary and secondary filters for the measurement of NADH fluorescence involves some fundamental considerations.
The first is the choice of wavelengths. 366 nm is appropriate for
the excitation of tissue NADH fluorescence and 450 nm for the measurement of its emission for a number of reasons. The absorption
of interfering pigments - for example, the difference between the
absorption of oxy- and deoxyhemoglobin - dictates this choice of
wavelengths. Furthermore, the natural brilliance of the available
light sources speaks for the 366 nm bright line of the medium or
high pressure mercury arc sources. The sensitivity of photosurfaces
is good in the region 440-460 nm.

The monochromatic or broad-band characteristics of the interference or dye filters theoretically speak in favor of the former,
but practically in favor of the latter; since the mercury bright
line gives essentially monochromatic excitation at 366 nm, the excitation filter does not need to be monochromatic. Interference
filters are capable of giving narrow-band response to the emitted
light. We have tended, however, to use broad-band filters for
emission measurement in order to obtain superior signal-to-noise
ratios, although this point may be revised as the techniques for
the detection of light signals are further improved.

Absorption, Reflectance, and Scattering Effects

Strong absorption bands of non-fluorescent pigments can imprint
their own spectra upon the excitation and emission spectra of fluoro-
chromes and their effects can thereby be readily recognized. In addition, reflectance and light-scattering changes can cause apparent
changes of fluorescence intensity, even when the cross between the
excitation and emission filters is "perfect" and none of the excitation light directly affects the emission photomultiplier. Reflectance and scattering changes in the sample would, however, have an
effect upon both the excitation effectiveness and the emission intensity. For example, increased reflectance of the tissue would
decrease the penetration of the exciting wavelength and decrease the
observed "fluorescence". Just the opposite effect would be expected
with increased light scattering, where the number of interactions of
the excitation and emission light-rays with the tissue cells would
increase and would therefore enhance the fluorescence emission.

Hemoglobin interference

One of the principal interferences would be expected to be in the oxy-deoxy hemoglobin transition. The spectra of these species for purified hemoglobin is shown in Figure 8, where it is seen that excitation of NADH fluorescence at 366 nm would be subject to an absorption difference in this transition, as would emission at 448 nm.

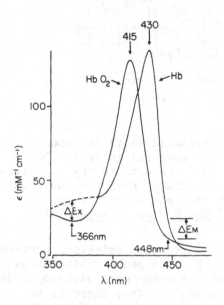

Figure 8. Difference spectrum of oxygenated and deoxygenated hemoglobin, indicating values at which absorption changes are equal and opposite. Thus these wavelengths are suitable for measuring excitation and emission changes.   (TA-211).

However, the effects are almost equal and opposite at the two wavelengths; $\Delta Ex \cong -\Delta Em$. Thus, a decrease of absorption of excitation is approximately corrected for by an increase of transmission at the emission wavelength.

Reflectance and emission spectra.

Figure 9 shows the changes of the reflectance spectrum of the rat brain cortex in the aerobic-anaerobic transition (air-nitrogen) in the wavelength region 700-400 nm. Such a curve is of most interest as a "difference" spectrum, since corrections for the properties of the detector are not included. It shows, however, the large change of reflectance in the red region at approximately 625 nm and the isosbestic point near 580 nm. The reflectance in the aerobic tissue in the region of measurement of the fluorescence emission (400-500 nm) is less in air than in the presence of nitrogen. The decrease of absorbancy at 625 nm can, in the air-nitrogen transition, be clearly attributed to hemoglobin (this is the "window" that is traditionally used in ear oximeters). At the shorter wavelengths,

the difference spectrum of oxy-deoxy hemoglobin is small and a generalized scattering change causes increased reflectance of the brain
in nitrogen as compared with air.

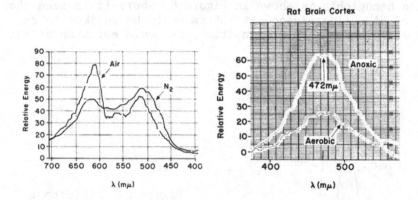

Figure 9. A, reflectance spectra of a normoxic (air) and anoxic
(N₂) rat brain cortex observed with a wide spectral interval (∿30
nm) and on a relative energy basis, as would be detected by a surface
fluorometer. B, fluorescence emission spectra of normoxic and anoxic
rat brain cortex observed through a similar optical system with a
similar spectral interval. (Courtesy of The Review of Scientific
Instruments [17]).

This result is consistent with the fluorescence emission spectrum
of the rat brain cortex shown in Figure 9B, obtained with 366 nm excitation. The sharp absorption bands of the hemoglobin-oxyhemoglobin
spectrum are not imprinted upon the emission spectra; there is no
evidence of the isosbestic points at 445 and 548 nm, or of the absorbancy changes of different sign above and below 445 nm. Thus, the
experimental data suggest a relatively minor screening effect of
hemoglobin vs. oxyhemoglobin. Figure 9A, however, indicates a reflectance or scattering change that may affect the fluorescence
emission measurements in the air-nitrogen transition.

The question of whether or not hemoglobin deoxygenation itself
causes a fluorescence emission change is further explored in Figure
10. In this case, a dual wavelength reflectance spectrophotometer
has been employed to measure hemoglobin deoxygenation and the usual
fluorometer (366 nm excitation, 450 nm measurement) to measure NADH
reduction and any associated artifactual response. The experimental
procedure is to proceed slowly from normoxia to anoxia so that the tissue passes through a series of steady states in which the hemoglobin
and pyridine nucleotide systems may separately reach their appropriate levels as the inspired oxygen is decreased from 20% to 10% to 6%
to zero. It is apparent from the record that a 60% deoxygenation of
hemoglobin occurs with only a 16% change of the uncorrected fluorescence intensity. Thereafter, the pyridine nucleotide is abruptly

reduced while the remainder of the hemoglobin is deoxygenated. Thus,
there is no proportionality between the hemoglobin deoxygenation and
the fluorescence increase, as would be expected for pure absorption
interference. It is apparent that not only is the effect small, but
the choice of a wavelength centered about the isosbestic point for
the hemoglobin-oxyhemoglobin transition largely removes the simple
absorption difference effect due to the normoxic-anoxic transition.

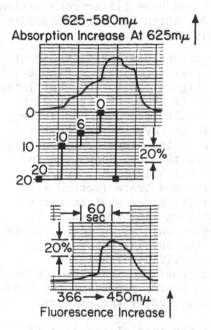

625-580mμ
Absorption Increase At 625mμ

366 ⟶ 450mμ
Fluorescence Increase

Figure 10. A comparison
of the dual wavelength absorbance changes at 625–
580 nm and the fluores-
cence emission changes at
450 nm, in response to 366
nm excitation, as measured
on the rat brain cortex
through the same optical
path and in response to
decreases of inspired oxygen of 20%–10%–6%–0.

Simultaneous Recordings of Reflectance and Fluorescence

In order, however, to estimate the reflectance change in a continuous manner during normoxic-anoxic-normoxic cycles, we record a
reflectance signal together with the fluorescence emission excited
at the same wavelength, as was done some time ago in electric stimulation of slices of the organ of the electric fish in experiments
together with R. D. Keynes and X. Aubert (18). Jobsis et al.(19) have
used 366 nm as a wavelength for monitoring reflectance for some
time while Kobayashi et al. (20) use 620 nm; in the latter case, a
computed function of the reflectance was used to correct the fluorescence trace. In this laboratory, Harbig has employed combined reflectance at 366 nm and 450 nm, based upon a modification of the
Ultropak apparatus employed by Chance and Schoener (21); these
results will appear elsewhere (22). The apparatus described in this
and the accompanying paper by Mayevsky and Chance (23) employs reflectance at 366 nm with a linear correction term at 1:1 gain.

The charts illustrate the current state of technology available
with a time-sharing fluorometer based upon an air turbine containing
the excitation and emission filters. The turbine employed in the

experiments of Figure 11 contains filters appropriate to 366 nm excitation and to reflectance measurements at 366 and 577 nm. The latter wavelength is also employed for excitation of electrochromic probes, results on which are reported elsewhere (24). The fluorescence is picked up by a separate photomultiplier containing a narrowband secondary filter at 445 nm (as close to the 448 nm wavelength indicated in Figure 9 above as feasible) of 5 nm half-bandwidth in Figure 11A, and in Figure 11B through a broad-band filter combination comprised of a Wratten 47 and a Wratten 2C, which has half-bandwidth points at 420 and 480 nm, with a peak near 450 nm.

The top trace represents reflectance traces similar to those of Figure 3 of the accompanying paper (21) corresponding, in Figure 11A to an "early" reflectance change, and in Figure 11B to somewhat later experiments on the same animal and similar to those of Figure 2, p. 279 . Due to reversed polarity changes in the recorder, the sense of all the traces is opposite to those of the Mayevsky and Chance paper; the time scales, however, and gain calibrations are identical. Thus, the 366 nm reflectance trace (next to the top) shows the characteristic initial decreased reflectance which is coincident with the increase of fluorescence in the uncorrected trace (second from the top). A 1:1 subtration of the two traces gives what is termed the "corrected: fluorescence trace. Additional information is provided by the 577 nm reflectance trace, which changes in the opposite direction from the 366 nm reflectance in the initial phase, but in the same way in the final phase. The sensitivities of all the reflectance and fluorescence traces are the same, and indicated to be 20% for two scale divisions. The next two traces represent the electrocorticogram at a scale of 500 μV, as indicated by the markers.

The experimental traces indicate that the initial decrease of reflectance at 366 nm is simultaneous with the fluorescence increase due to NAD reduction, and thus tends to obscure the initial phases of anoxia as measured on the uncorrected fluorescence trace. However, the late reflectance increase which occurs after the point "SN" (stop nitrogen) is nevertheless prior to the abrupt reoxidation of NAD due to the arrival of oxygen at the brain tissue. It should be noted that this secondary phase of reflectance is almost undetectable in Figure 11B, which represents a recovery from a late anoxia. In either case, the recovery from anoxia occurs at a time when the change of light reflectance at 366 nm is minimal. Observations of isolated mitochondria and perfused organs indicate that the "cycle" of normoxia-anoxia-normoxia is symmetrical, with equal amplitudes in both directions (25). This provides an external control over the efficacy of the compensation procedure by comparing the amplitude of the fluorescence decrease in recovery from anoxia with the fluorescence increase at the onset of anoxia; the two should be identical. Based on observations of perfused organs, a plateau at a constant level of fluorescence should be observed in the interval after reaching the steady state and prior to the recovery from anoxia. It is apparent that the compensated fluorescence traces are consistent with what is known of the performance of isolated organs.

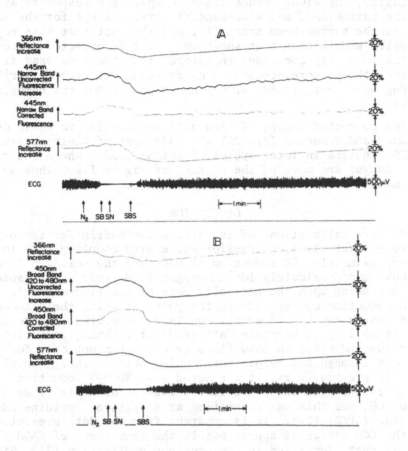

<u>Figure 11.</u> Combined reflectance and fluorescence measurements of
the rat brain cortex in cycles of normoxia-anoxia-normoxia. 11A
shows results obtained with the narrow-band filter (5 nm half-
bandwidth) centered at 445 nm and taken in the early interval of
experimentation, <u>i.e.</u>, with a fresh animal. 11B represents similar
data obtained later in the course of experimentation on the same
animal, but employing a wide-band emission filter of half-bandwidth
extending from 420 nm to 480 nm, and peaking at 450 nm. The calibrations appropriate to the eight traces are similar, as are the
calibrations for the ECG's. Note that increasing intensity is
indicated as an upward deflection in this figure, as contrasted
with Figures 2 - 4 of the accompanying paper, where increases are
indicated as downward deflections. Symbols: N_2, inspiration of
100% nitrogen; SB, stop breathing; SN, stop nitrogen; SBS, start
breathing simultaneously.

Lastly, the fluorescence traces compare the responses available with the narrow-band and wide-band filters. Except for the increased noise on the narrow-band trace (A), and the fact that this represents an earlier anoxia than that shown in (B), the corrected traces are identical. We may conclude, therefore, that the wide-band filter simulates the performance of the narrow-band filter by distributing wavelengths on either side of 445 nm to cancel out the hemoglobin changes.

The corrected traces of Figure 11 are similar to those obtained by Chance and Schoener (21, 26) who made most of their observations of NADH kinetics in later cycles of animal study, where the reflectance changes are more of the pattern of Figure 11B. Thus we find confirmation and extension of their results.

DISCUSSION

Precise calibrations of isolated mitochondria for the oxygen requirement for electron transfer and energy coupling (27) indicate that approximately 50% reduction of NAD from the normoxic level corresponds to approximately 10^{-7} M oxygen (0.07 torr), with some variation depending upon the metabolic rate of the tissue. This degree of NAD reduction corresponds to the point at which the mitochondria are no longer capable of energy coupling, as discussed here in terms of their ability to maintain Ca^{++} gradients. Thus, reduction of NAD beyond 50% indicates an insufficiency of oxygen not only for electron transport through the respiratory chain, but for energy coupling as well. In previous work, it was noted that 80-90% reduction of NADH was associated with the cessation of electrical activity as measured by the ECG, and this was identified as a critical pyridine nucleotide reduction (CPNR) (21). It is apparent from the data presented here that the ECG ceases at approximately the same level of NADH fluorescence as that identified in the previous publication (21). Since the mitochondrial calibrations indicate that roughly 50% reduction of NAD from the normoxic level corresponds to the cessation of energy metabolism, we find a close correlation between the in vitro data and the in vivo data on cessation of the ECG in relation to increased NAD reduction in brain tissue. Presumably the difference between the two values corresponds to the time required for depletion of energy reserves in the brain in terms of creatine phosphate and ATP.

SUMMARY

Problems of precise fluorometry of NADH on the brain cortex have been described, and the conclusions are applied to the design of a time-sharing fluorometer which permits the illumination of the brain with appropriate wavelengths of light, and measurement of both fluorescence emission and reflectance signals via ultraviolet transmitting light guides from the anesthetized animal. This paper examines the appropriateness of these wavelengths and the desirable degree of monochromaticity of both excitation and emission wavelengths and the problem of measuring NADH fluorescence changes in spite of significant changes of absorbancy and reflectance on the brain cortex during normoxic-anoxic-normoxic cycles. It is concluded that an appropriate choice of wavelengths and spectral intervals substantially removes the absorption of hemoglobin as a disturbing parameter, and leaves mainly reflectance and scattering changes consequent to hemodynamic and cell volume changes in the metabolic transitions. These changes, measured as reflectance on the brain at appropriate wavelengths, are entered as a correction term to the observed fluorescence changes, with the result that normoxic-anoxic-normoxic cycles are obtained which exactly simulate those to be expected on the basis of studies of isolated mitochondria and perfused organs.

The previous conclusion on the correlation between the degree of NAD reduction and the disappearance of the ECG is substantiated and extended by these data, and the critical pyridine nucleotide reduction (CPNR) remains a valid criterion for energy metabolism in the brain cortex. The present data show how these results can be obtained by compensated fluorometry in the fresh animal that exhibits reflectance artifacts in the fluorescence traces. Furthermore, data on isolated mitochondria show that the CPNR level corresponds almost exactly to the degree of anoxia at which the mitochondria are no longer competent in bioenergetic function. The exact pO_2 at which this occurs depends upon the metabolic flux but is generally in the range of 10^{-7} M oxygen or 0.07 torr.

ACKNOWLEDGEMENTS

The authors wish to acknowledge the contributions of Victor Legallais to the mechanical design of the time-sharing units and of Norman Graham, John Sorge, and Michael Mason to the electronic circuitry. They are also grateful for the collaboration of other members of the Johnson Research Foundation and the Department of Neurology, es.pecially Drs. Klaus Harbig, Martin Reivich, and Arisztid Kovach. The research was supported by NINDS-10939-01.

REFERENCES

1. D. W. Bronk. The American Scientist, 34, 55 (1946).
2. P. W. Davies and F. Brink. Rev. Sci. Instr., 13, 524 (1942).
3. P. W. Davies and A. Remond. Res. Publ. Assoc. Res. Nerv. & Ment. Dis., 26 205 (1946).
4. O. Warburg. Heavy Metal Prosthetic Groups and Enzyme Action. (Trans. A. Lawson). Clarendon Press, Oxford, 1949.
5. D. Keilin. The History of Cell Respiration and Cytochrome. Cambridge University Press, Cambridge, 1966.
6. B. Chance and V. Legallais. Rev. Sci. Instr., 30, 732 (1959).
7. B. Chance, R. Perry, L. Åkerman, and B. Thorell. Rev. Sci. Instr., 30, 735 (1959).
8. B. Chance. J. Biol. Chem., 151, 553 (1943).
9. B. Chance and M. Erecinska. Arch. Biochem. Biophys., 143, 675 (1971)
10. F. Schindler. Ph.D. Dissertation, University of Pennsylvania, 1964.

11. R. Oshino, N. Oshino, M. Tamura, L. Kobilinski, and B. Chance. Biochim. Biophys. Acta, 273, 5 (1972).
12. B. Chance and G. R. Williams. J. Biol. Chem., 217, 409 (1955).
13. Energy-Linked Functions of Mitochondria (B. Chance, Ed.) Academic Press, New York, 1963.
14. O. Shimumura, F. H. Johnson, and Y. Saiga. J. Cell. Comp. Physiol., 59, 223 (1962).
15. G. Loschen and B. Chance. Nature New Biology, 233, 273 (1972).
16. B.Chance and H. Baltscheffsky. J. Biol. Chem., 233, 736 (1958).
17. B. Chance, V. Legallais, and B. Schoener. Rev. Sci. Instr., 12, 1307 (1963).
18. X. Aubert, B. Chance, and R. D. Keynes. Proc. Roy. Soc., B-160, 211 (1964).
19. F. F. Jöbsis, M. O'Connor, A. Vitale, and H. Vreman. J. Neurophysiol., 34, 735 (1971).
20. S. Kobayashi, K. Kaede, K. Nishiki, and E. Ogata. J. App. Physiol., 31, 693 (1971).
21. B. Chance, B. Schoener, and F. Schindler. In Oxygen in the Animal Organism (F. Dickens and F. Neil, Eds.) Pergamon Press, Oxford, 1964. p. 367.
22. K. Harbig and M. Reivich. Submitted to J. Appl. Physiol.
23. A. Mayevsky and B. Chance. This Volume, p.239.
24. B. Chance. Proc. Am. Philos. Soc., in press.
25. B. Chance, J. R. Williamson, D. Jamieson, and B. Schoener. Biochem. Z., 341, 357 (1965).
26. B. Chance, P. Cohen, F. Jöbsis, and B. Schoener. Science, 137, 499 (1962).
27. N. Oshino, T. Sugano, R. Oshino, and B. Chance. Federation Proc., 32, 344Abs (1973).

SELECTIVE VULNERABILITY OF THE CENTRAL NERVOUS SYSTEM TO HYPERBARIC OXYGEN

J. Douglas Balentine, M.D.

Medical University of South Carolina

Department of Pathology, Charleston, S.C.   29401

The adverse effects of hyperoxia on the central nervous system (CNS) have been well known since the 19th century writing of Paul Bert. Acute CNS oxygen toxicity is manisfested by grand mal convulsions and may result in death following status epilepticus. Bean and Seigfried[2] reported a delayed or chronic type of oxygen poisoning in rats subjected to repeated brief intermittent exposures to hyperbaric oxygen (HO), which resulted in permanent limb paralysis. The paralyses observed in this type of oxygen toxicity usually affect the forelimbs bilaterally with the animals assuming a kangaroo-like posture. Rigidity of the paralyzed limbs is common. Animals capable of locomotion are ataxic. A few rats become quadriplegic.

Balentine and Gutsche found bilaterally symmetrical and selective CNS lesions in rats paralyzed by repeated 1 hour exposures on consecutive days to 5 atmospheres of pure oxygen.[3] Usually 4 exposures were required to produce paralysis. The lesions demonstrate a vulnerability of selected neurons to hyperbaric oxygen exposure and consist of either random necrosis of neuronal cell bodies within otherwise preserved nuclear regions (Fig. 1) or necrosis of entire nuclei (Fig. 2). The lesions were respectively classified as types A and B, because of their fundamental histologic differences and their predilection for different regions of the central nervous system. Type A lesions usually involve neurons in the spinal cord and hindbrain, whereas type B lesions affect the midbrain and forebrain.

(This work was supported by grant # NS09837 from the NINDS (USPHS) and by two research grants from the Medical University of South Carolina.)

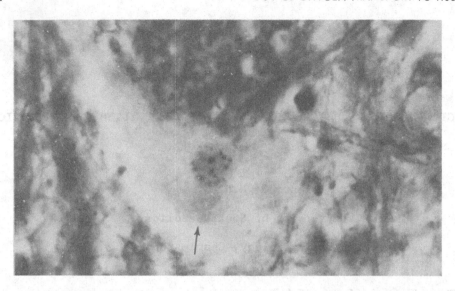

Fig. 1. Neuronal cell body (arrow) with karyorrhexis and homogeni-
zation of cytoplasm indicating necrosis. From spinal nucleus of
cranial nerve V in a rat paralyzed by repeated exposure to hyperbaric oxygen. H&E stain X 1337 (From Balentine and Gutsche[1]).

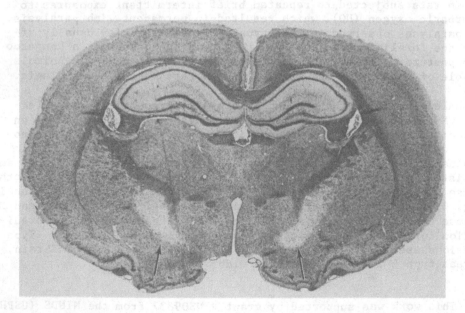

Fig. 2. Bilateral necrosis of globus pallidus (arrows) in a rat paralyzed by exposures to hyperbaric oxygen. Coronal section of forebrain. X9 (From Balentine, Am. J. Path. 53:1108, 1968).

Examination of the CNS lesions following hyperbaric oxygen exposure in young adult Osborne-Mendel, Sprague-Dawley, and Charles-River CDF rats has revealed a highly consistent and selective topographic pattern of involvement, illustrated in Figure 3.

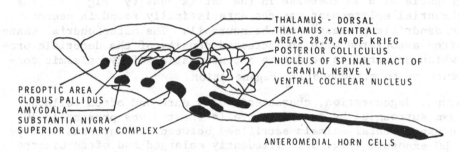

Fig. 3. Rat brain sagittal model illustrating regions of brain (in black) that are susceptible to necrosis following repeated exposures to 5 atmospheres of oxygen (From Balentine, Am. J. Path. 53:1100, 1968).

The anteromedial horn cells of the spinal cord, nucleus of the spinal tract of V, superior olives, substantia nigra, and globus pallidus are the most frequently affected areas. This pattern differs from the topography of CNS lesions induced in rats exposed to low oxygen tensions in a very significant way. The neocortex, hippocampus, and corpus striatum are the most common regions of the brain to become necrotic following hypoxia,[4] but are characteristically not affected by hyperbaric oxygen exposure.

In order to determine the cellular response to hyperbaric oxygen exposure in non-necrotic neurons, an ultrastructural investigation of cervical anteromedial horn grey matter was undertaken.[5] Thirty-four adult Sprague-Dawley female rats were subjected to a single 30 minute exposure to 5 atmospheres of oxygen and sacrificed in a time sequence varying from 30 minutes to 30 days thereafter. Chamber operations were similar to those previously reported except a Bethlehem #1836H small animal chamber was used, and no more than 10 rats were exposed simultaneously. No clinical abnormalities other than slight transient tachypnea were noted in any of the animals during or after exposure.

The animals were fixed by perfusion with 1% paraformaldehyde, 2% glutaraldehyde, and 2% osmuim in phosphate buffers. Tissue blocks from the cervical spinal cord were embedded in Epon and thin sections were double stained with lead citrate and uranyl acetate. Nine unexposed control rats were similarly prepared for electron microscopy.

The most characteristic finding within the first 72 hours in the experimental animals following HO exposure was an enlargement of mitochondria with an increase in the matrix density (Fig. 4). The mitochondrial enlargement was characteristically found in neurons within dendritic processes of the neuropil. The mitochondrial change was often associated with an increased density of the dendritic process which appeared to be due to a condensation of cytoplasmic constituents or to mitochondrial degeneration.

Axonal degeneration, characterized by dark and often collapsed axoplasm surrounded by an intact myelin sheath, was present in 70% of the experimental animals sacrificed between 24 hours and 30 days after HO exposure (Fig. 5). Frequently enlarged and often bizarre mitochondria were observed in the dark axoplasm of the degenerating axons.

Enlargement of terminal axons (boutons) with increased lysosomal structures and accumulations of neurofilaments was occasionally observed in three animals, sacrificed at 4 and 72 hours and 30 days post HO exposure. Light microscopic sections of the brain and spinal cords were prepared from the parts of the CNS of the animals in this study not processed for electron microscopy. No evidence of neuronal cell body necrosis was found in either the light or electron microscopy sections. None of the mitochondrial, axonal, or boutonal changes were found in the control animals.

The ultrastructural observations in this study suggests that there are intraneuronal patterns of selective vulnerability to oxygen toxicity. The cell processes of the neurons appear to be selectively involved in the presence of an intact neuronal cell body when the animals are exposed to oxygen doses insufficient to produce neuronal necrosis. The distinct mitochondrial abnormality within dendrites, seen in the early post HO exposure time period, suggests a pattern of selective vulnerability at the organelle level within the neuron.

It is apparent that the pathobiological theories of CNS oxygen toxicity have to consider the selective patterns of vulnerability of the nervous system at the regional, cellular, and subcellular levels of observations.

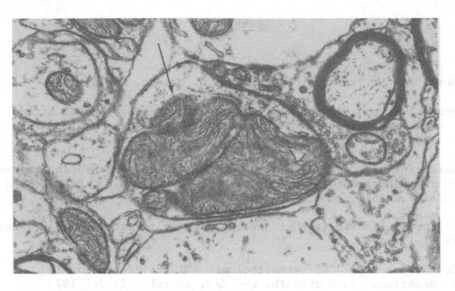

Fig. 4. Enlarged dark mitochondria of dendrite (arrow). Anterior
horn grey matter of rat 48 hours after a single 30 minute exposure
to 5 atmospheres of oxygen. X27,500.

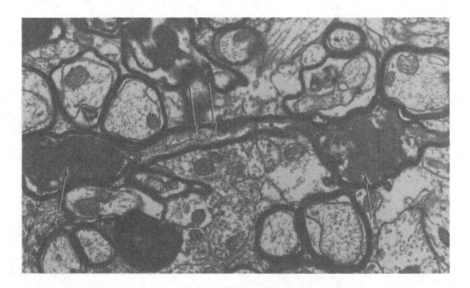

Fig. 5. Axonal degeneration in anterior horn grey matter of rat 48
hours after a single exposure to hyperbaric oxygen. Note dark (single
arrows) and collapsed (double arrows) axoplasm in presence of an intact myelin sheath. X15,400.

REFERENCES

1. Bert, P. La Pression Barometrique G. Masson, Paris, 1878.

2. Bean, J.W. and Siegfried, E.C. Transient and permanent after
    - effects of exposure to oxygen at high pressure. Am. J. Physiol.
    143:656:665, 1945.

3. Balentine, J.D. and Gutsche, B.B. Central nervous system lesions
    in rats exposed to oxygen at high pressure. Am. J. Path.   48:
    107-127, 1966.

4. Levine, S. Anoxic-ischemic encephalopathy in rats. Amer. J. Path.
    36: 1-17, 1960.

5. Balentine, J.D. CNS cytopathologic effects of hyperbaric
    oxygenation. J. Neuropath. and Exp. Neurol. 32:176, 1973
    (abstract).

OXYGEN TENSIONS IN THE DEEP GRAY MATTER OF RATS EXPOSED TO HYPERBARIC OXYGEN

Robert W. Ogilvie, Ph.D., and J. Douglas Balentine, M.D.

Department of Anatomy, Department of Pathology, Medical

University of South Carolina, Charleston, S. C., USA

Selective necrosis of neurons and nuclei consistently occurs within the central nervous system (CNS) of rats paralyzed by repeated 1 hour exposures to 5 atmospheres of oxygen.[1] The distribution of the lesions differs from those of hypoxia in the same animal species. Excessive oxygen inhibits many enzymes vital to cellular metabolism in the CNS and it is reasonable to hypothesize that the neuronal necrosis produced by hyperbaric oxygen exposure is related to elevated tissue oxygen tensions. However, hyperbaric oxygen notedly produces cerebral vasospasm and a reduction in cerebral blood flow, and regional ischemia has been a tenable hypothesis for the occurrence of the CNS lesions. This latter mechanism seems unlikely because unilateral carotid artery ligation protects the ipsilateral but not the contralateral cerebral hemisphere from the occurrence of the oxygen induced lesions.[2] (see Fig. 1)

The present investigation was undertaken to determine the oxygen tension in the globus pallidus of the rat brain which is susceptible to the selective necrosis utilizing the same conditions of hyperbaric oxygen exposure employed in the individual exposures of the experimental model which resulted in CNS lesions. Although cerebral cortical oxygen tensions have been measured under hyperbaric oxygen conditions[3], the cortex is not one of the sites where lesions are produced by hyperbaric oxygen.

Oxygen tension was recorded polarographically utilizing Transidyne General Corporation platinum wire glass insulated external referenced electrodes with tip diameters from 5 to 10 microns. The polarographic current produced by changes in oxygen tension was amplified with a Transidyne picoammeter and a permanent

record made using a Grass polygraph. Each electrode was calibrated
before and after the experiment by reading the current obtained
with the sensor cathode and reference anode immersed in a constant
temperature saline bath equilibrated with nitrogen, 5% oxygen: 95%
nitrogen, compressed air and oxygen.

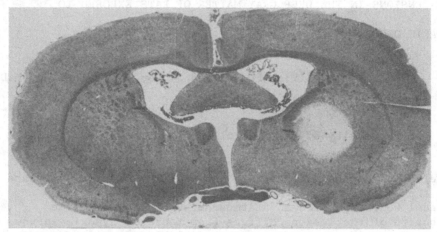

Fig. 1 Unilateral necrosis of globus pallidus following
contralateral carotid artery ligation and exposure to hyperbaric
oxygen. Coronal section of rat forebrain stained with luxol fast
blue-hematoxylin and eosin. X9 (from Balentine[2])

        Following calibration adult female Sprague Dawley rats were
anesthetized with sodium pentobarbital (40 mg/kg) or urethane
(1.5g/kg), a subtotal craniotomy was done over one hemisphere and
a thermistor probe was placed in the rectum for monitoring
temperature. The microelectrode was positioned stereotaxically
utilizing brain surface coordinates. A base line recording of
oxygen tension was obtained with the animal breathing room air.
The rat was then put into a Bethlehem small animal hyperbaric
chamber (Fig. 2). The chamber was flushed over a 10 minute period
with oxygen prior to compression. The outflow gas from the chamber
was measured with a Servomex oxygen analyzer to insure that the
chamber atmosphere was pure oxygen prior to compression.
Compression of the chamber with pure oxygen was staged over a four
minute period with periodic stops at 45, 30, 15, 7½, and 4 p.s.i.g.
Following decompression the polarographic determination was
continued in ambient air for 10-15 minutes. The animals were then
sacrificed by reclosing the chamber and flushing it with pure
nitrogen. Following the death of the animal the chamber was flushed
with oxygen and recompressed with 60 p.s.i.g. of pure oxygen in
order to control the polarographic determination by using the
deceased animal under hyperbaric conditions.

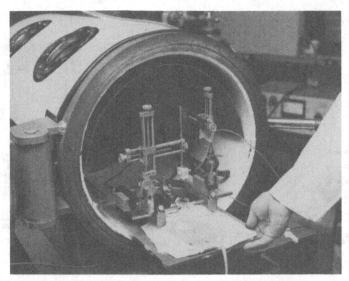

Fig. 2 Hyperbaric chamber with a rat in the stereotaxic apparatus and an oxygen electrode in place.

     At the end of each experiment the oxygen electrode was removed and a 25 gauge spinal needle was placed stereotaxically into the brain using the same coordinates as employed for the electrode, except that the depth was reduced by 1 mm to prevent obscuring the end of the track. The needle was filled with trypan blue and slowly removed allowing the dye to stain the track. The brain was removed and coronally sliced to locate the track and position of the electrode. The site of the electrode tip was estimated by measuring the depth used (5.5 mm) from the cortex in the direction of the stained track. In all experiments reported here the electrode was positioned in the globus pallidus.

     A total of six rat experiments were carried out with 3 rats anesthetized with urethane and 3 rats anesthetized with nembutal. Oxygen tracings from the globus pallidus were obtained using the same electrode in all rats except for Rat No. 12 (anesthetized with urethane).

     Base line oxygen tensions (animals breathing air) ranged from about 10-40 mm Hg. The oxygen level usually increased slightly while the chamber was being flushed. During compression up to 45 p.s.i.g. oxygen levels usually increased slowly compared to a more rapid increase which was observed from 45 to 60 p.s.i.g. The oxygen tension in the globus pallidus continued to increase for a few minutes after 60 p.s.i.g. of compression was achieved. This high level, which ranged from approximately 225 to 475 mm Hg depending upon the animal, was maintained usually for less than 10 minutes at which time the tension fell progressively to lower levels. The

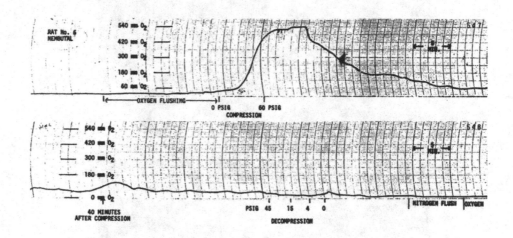

Fig. 3 Oxygen tension tracing obtained in the globus pallidus
of a rat anesthetized with nembutal.

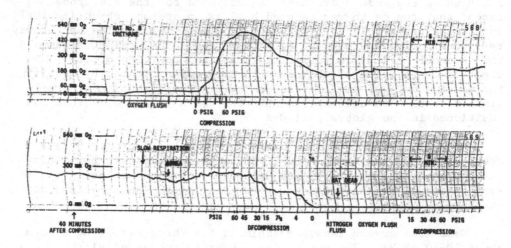

Fig. 4 Oxygen tension tracing obtained in the globus pallidus
of a rat anesthetized with urethane. Note that the oxygen level
remains higher during the period of compression than the animals
anesthetized with nembutal.

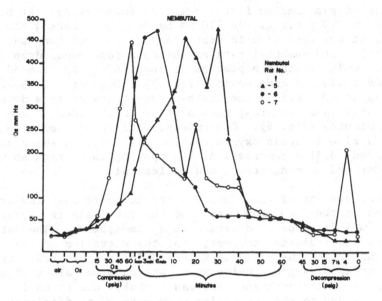

Fig. 5 Oxygen tensions obtained in 3 rats anesthetized with
nembutal using the same electrode.

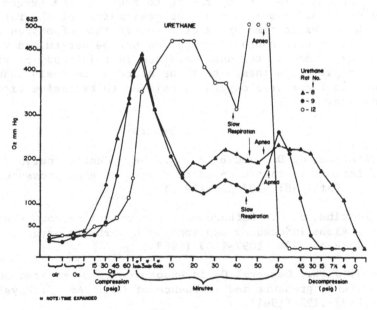

Fig. 6 Oxygen tension obtained in 3 rats anesthetized with
urethane. Note that each animal in this series suffered apnea
before 60 minutes compression at 60 p.s.i.g. of 100% oxygen.

average oxygen tension in the nembutal anesthetized rat brain at 40 minutes at 60 p.s.i.g. was 110 mm Hg (Fig. 3) whereas the average oxygen at the same time in urethane anesthetized rats was 225 mm Hg (Fig. 4). The nembutal rats exhibited a continuous drop in oxygen tension which reached a plateau at about 60 mm Hg from 50 to 60 minutes following compression (Fig. 5). However, at about 45 minutes at 60 p.s.i.g. the urethane anesthetized rats developed progressively slower respiration rates which ended in apnea between 49-57 minutes (Fig. 6). Concomitant with the slowed respiration and apnea a rise in brain oxygen tension was observed which usually persisted until decompression. Autopsy of these rats showed pulmonary edema congestion, and atelectasis.

The results of these experiments indicate that the oxygen tension in the deep gray matter of the rat brain is elevated when the animal is exposed to oxygen at 5 atmospheres. The data in these experiments indicate, however, that the elevation of the oxygen tensions is not sustained as reported for rat cerebral cortex.[3] The increased oxygen tension which was observed along with dyspnea and apnea in the urethane rats was probably due to an increase in brain CO_2 due to the increasing respiratory insufficiency. The fact that oxygen tension fell in both groups of rats and then rose in relationship to apnea is a strong indication that blood flow is one of the major factors operating to regulate the oxygen available to the neuronal tissue in the deep gray matter of the rat brain. Although the exact time or exact concentration of oxygen which is associated with neuronal damage cannot be determined with the present experiments, the data obtained in this study provide support to the original hypothesis that the neuronal necrosis induced by exposure to hyperbaric oxygen is related to excessive tissue oxygenation.

References

1. Balentine, J. D., and B. B. Gutsche. Central nervous system lesions in rats exposed to oxygen at high pressure. Amer. J. Path. 48: 107-127 (1966).

2. Balentine, J. D. Pathogenesis of central nervous system lesions induced by exposure to hyperbaric oxygen. Amer. J. Path. 53: 1097-1109 (1968).

3. Bean, J. W. Cerebral O_2 in exposures to O_2 at atmospheric and higher pressure and influence of CO_2. Am. J. Physiol. 201: 1192-1198 (1961).

THE INTERDEPENDENCE OF RESPIRATORY GAS VALUES AND pH AS A FUNCTION OF BASE EXCESS IN HUMAN BLOOD AT 37°C

Jürgen Grote and Gerhard Thews
Institute of Physiology, University of Mainz

The accurate estimation of the transport function of human blood for respiratory gases as well as the respiratory gas exchange in human body requires detailed knowledge of the respiratory gas partial pressures and the acid-base status in the blood. Because there is an interdependence between the different respiratory gas parameters described as Bohr and Haldane effect (3,4), it is possible to obtain a general picture of the whole transport system, if these interrelations are known.

After many investigations of the O_2 and CO_2 dissociation curve of human blood different authors were able to show the interdependence of respiratory gas values in the form of nomograms (5,6,7,8,11). The use of the nomograms, however, was limited for the conditions of base excess values within the normal range of BE = ± 2.5 mEq/l.

The purpose of this paper is to describe alignment nomograms which summarize the interdependence of respiratory gas values and pH in human blood at 37°C as a function of base excess. The nomograms are based on the results of investigations of the oxygen affinity at various CO_2 tensions (6) and the PCO_2-pH dependence at various degrees of oxygen saturation and varying buffer base concentrations in human blood at 37°C (6,9).

METHODS

The investigations were carried out on venous blood samples of about 120 young male and female subjects. The oxygen dissociation curve of the blood was determined at 37°C and at PCO_2

levels of 30, 40 and 50 mmHg after the method of Niesel and Thews
(10), using modified measuring equipment. Blood samples from
10 subjects were analysed for each of the 3 series of tests. In
each individual case, we determined the oxygen dissociation
curves 3 - 6 times, calculating the mean curve from separate
data (6).

The relationship between the pH value of plasma and the PCO_2
were determined using the Astrup micromethod (1,2) for 0 and
100% as well as for intermediate degrees of blood oxygen saturation at buffer base concentrations in the range of
BE = ± 10 mEq/l. The blood samples were equilibrated in Laue
tonometers, and, in a few cases in the Astrup tonometer, with
humidified gas mixtures of known PO_2 and PCO_2. The appropriate
plasma pH value was determined with the Astrup microelectrode
(AME 1, Radiometer, Copenhagen) after calibration with standard
NBS phosphate buffers. The various buffer base ranges were adjusted
by adding citric acid or $NaHCO_3$ to the blood samples (6,9).

RESULTS

The results of both series of tests were summarized on one
hand in mean blood oxygen dissociation curves for the different
PCO_2 levels and on the other hand in mean blood log PCO_2/pH
lines for the different buffer base concentrations and SO_2
levels. The determined oxygen dissociation curves and PCO_2-pH
dependences were summarized in O_2-CO_2 alignment nomograms
(Fig. 1 - 4). An additional scale for the total blood CO_2
content was inserted. The necessary data were derived from a
publication of Rahn and Fenn (11). The error that occured in
constructing the nomograms is, for every scale, smaller than their
smallest graduation.

Figure 1 shows the alignment nomogram which gives the interrelations between PO_2, SO_2, PCO_2, pH and total CO_2 content of
human blood at 37° C and base excess values between +10 and -15
mEq/l. If two of these values at different base excess levels are
known, the remaining three can be read at the points of intersection with the corresponding straight line. However, one of the
initial values to be measured should always belong to the CCO_2-
PCO_2-pH group, and the other to the PO_2-SO_2 group.

To facilitate the use of the nomogram special alignment
nomograms for the conditions of base excess values of +10, +5, 0,
-5 and -10 mEq/l were constructed (Fig. 2 - 4).

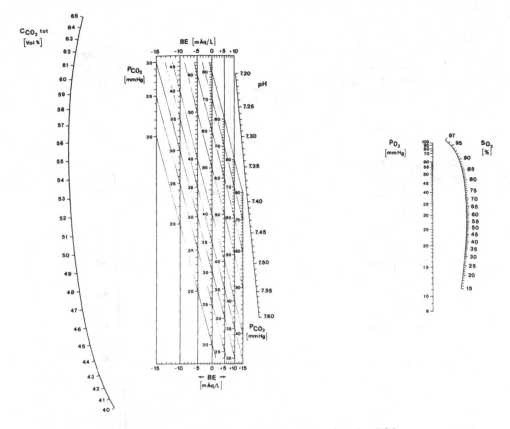

Fig. 1. Nomogram relating the total CO$_2$ content, PCO$_2$, plasma pII, PO$_2$ and SO$_2$ at 37°C for human blood with base excess values between +10 and -15 mEq/l and normal hemoglobin concentration.

The blood oxygen dissociation curves determined in vitro agree with in vivo oxygen dissociation curves found in anaero-bically-taken blood samples. There is a difference between the blood CO$_2$ dissociation curves determined in vivo and in vitro. However, the differences are small in the PCO$_2$ range between 20 - 60 mmHg. Therefore, the nomograms based on data measured in vitro can be applied with reasonable accuracy to the in vivo conditions (6). They enable us to estimate the transport function of the blood for respiratory gases under physiological and pathophysiological conditions. The nomograms may serve as a basis for the theoretical and experimental investigations of respiratory gas exchange in different organs for the conditions of normal acid-base status as well as for the conditions of respiratory and nonrespiratory disturbances.

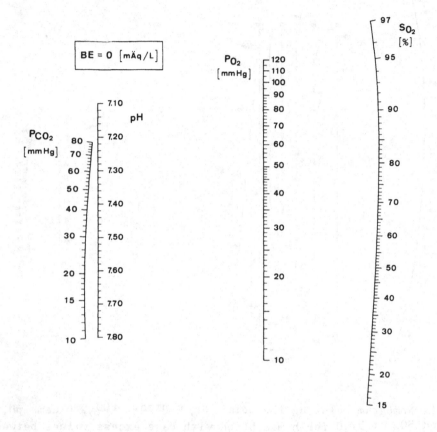

Fig. 2. Nomogram relating the total CO_2 content, PCO_2, plasma pH, PO_2 and SO_2 at $37°C$ for human blood with normal buffer base and hemoglobin concentration.

The nomograms cannot be used for the blood of children, for anaemic blood and in the case of diseases with accompanying shifts of the blood oxygen dissociation curve. An adequate degree of accuracy is furnished when the hemoglobin concentration is within the range of 12.5 – 17 g%.

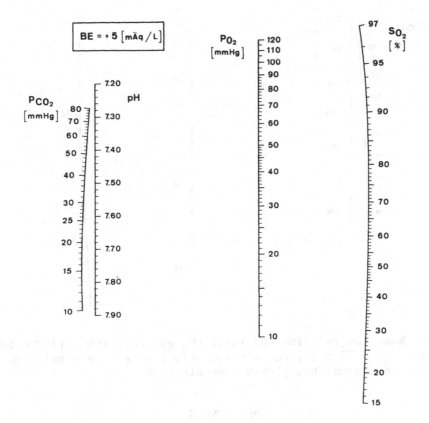

Fig. 3. Nomogram relating the total CO_2 content, PCO_2, plasma pH, PO_2 and SO_2 at 37 C for human blood with a base excess value of +5 mEq/l and normal hemoglobin concentration.

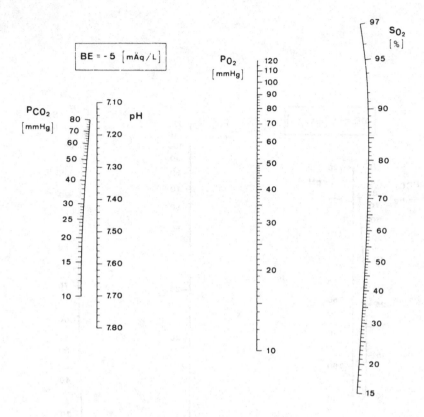

Fig. 4. Nomogram relating the total CO_2 content, PCO_2, plasma pH, PO_2 and SO_2 at $37^\circ C$ for human blood with a base excess value of -5 mEq/l and normal hemoglobin concentration.

REFERENCES

1. Astrup, P.: J. clin. Lab. Invest. 17, 33 (1956). 2. Astrup, P., Jørgensen, K., Siggaard-Andersen, O., and Engel, K.: Lancet i: 1035 (1960). 3. Bohr, C., Hasselbalch, K., and Krogh, A.: Scand. Arch Physiol. 16, 402 (1904). 4. Christiansen, J., Douglas, C.G., and Haldane, J.S.: J. Physiol. 48, 244 (1914). 5. Dill, D.B., Edwards, H.J., and Consolazio, W.V.: J. biol. Chem. 118, 635 (1937). 6. Grote, J.: In: Anaesthesiology and Resuscitation, vol.53, p.47, Berlin: Springer 1971. 7. Henderson, L.J.: Blood. A study in gen. physiol. New Haven: Yale Univ. Press 1928. 8. Lenfant, C., Ways, P., Aucutt, C., and Cruz, J.: Respir.Physiol. 7, 7 (1969). 9. Mengden, H.J.,v., Schultehinrichs, D., and Thews, G.: Respir. Physiol. 6, 151 (1969). 10. Niesel, W., and Thews, G.: Pflügers Arch. 273, 380 (1961). 11. Rahn, H., and Fenn, W.O.: A graphical analysis of the respir. gas exchange. Washington: Am. Physiol. Soc. 1955.

REGULATORY DYSFUNCTION OF MICROVASCULATURE AND CATECHOLAMINE

METABOLISM IN SPINAL CORD INJURY

N. Eric Naftchi, Edward W. Lowman, Maurice Berard,
G. Heiner Sell and Theobald Reich

Laboratory of Biochemical Pharmacology, Institute of
Rehabilitation Medicine, New York University Medical
Center, 400 E. 34th Street, New York, N.Y. 10016

INTRODUCTION

Since 1917 when Head and Riddoch (4) first described autonomic hyperreflexia in spinal cord injury, its attending neurophysiological symptoms have been well documented by other investigators. It is well known that the triggering mechanism may well be any noxious stimuli but most often autonomic hyperreflexia is caused by hyperirritability of the bladder due to formation of stones of calcium salts or infection of the urinary bladder; the common denominator being distension of the vesicular wall leading to increased intracystic pressure. The major symptoms during the so-called hyperreflexia are: pallor of the skin below in contrast to a histamine-like flush above the level of the lesion, vasodilatation in the head and neck accompanied by engorging pulsating corotid arteries. Moreover, the peak of hyperreflexia coincides with the height of intracystic and brachial blood pressures, headache, and piloerection. Guttmann and Whitteridge (3) were the first to observe that the hypertensive crises could be produced only in those subjects with lesions above the sixth thoracic dermatome (T6). The purpose of this communication is to shed more light on the etiology of these hypertensive episodes which occur spontaneously in human subjects with high level spinal cord injury and which are frequently the cause of cerebrovascular accidents.

METHODS

Digital blood flow was measured calorimetrically (6) in the fourth fingers and great toes of 30 normal, 15 paraplegic and 15

quadriplegic subjects. In seven quadriplegic subjects with complete transection of the spinal cord at the level of fifth and sixth
cervical dermatomes (C5-C6), the blood flow in fingers, toes, and
calves was also measured by venous occlusion plethysmography with
a Whitney mercury-in-rubber strain gauge, before, during, and after
hypertensive episodes induced by water loading during excretory
cystometry. Concomitantly, the brachial blood pressure was measured
by auscultatory or by intra-arterial strain gauge method and the
digital blood pressure by means of a Gaertner capsule using the
flush-throbe technique (6). Effective mean digital blood pressure
was measured by adding one-third of the pulse pressure to diastolic
pressure, e.g., 1/3 (systolic - diastolic) + diastolic. Digital
vascular resistance was calculated from the ratio of the effective
mean digital blood pressure and digital blood flow. The measurements were made with patients in the supine position in a temperature controlled room (27°C $\pm$ 1°C). Quadriplegic subjects with
complete physiologic lesions at the levels of fifth to seventh cervical dermatomes (C5-C7) and without any evidence of cardiovascular
or renal involvement were chosen during the chronic phase of the
injury (six months or longer after the onset). Normotensive control subjects showed no evidence of renal or peripheral vascular
disease and had no present or previous history of hypertension.
Experiments were started approximately one-half hour after equili-
briation in the temperature controlled room.

Twenty-four hour urine samples were collected from 35 quadriplegic subjects during the chronic phase of the injury. Aliquots
of these urine specimens were compared with those of 36 normal subjects for their content of catecholamine (CM) metabolites. Bidi-
mensional (2), column and gas-liquid chromatography (10) were used
for the analysis of CM metabolites: 4-hydroxy-3-methoxymandelic
acid (VMA), 4-hydroxy-3-methoxy-phenylacetic acid (HVA), 4-hydroxy-
3-methoxyphenylethyleneglycol (HMPG), and total metanephrines (TMN).
CM metabolites were also measured before, during, or just after
spontaneous hypertensive crises.

RESULTS

The blood flow in the fourth finger and the great toe of 15
paraplegic and 15 quadriplegic subjects is compared with that of 30
normal subjects in Figure 1. The blood flow in the finger of normal
and quadriplegic subjects was of the same order of magnitude, but
it was significantly higher than that in the finger of paraplegic
subjects (P<0.05). Despite the vasoconstriction in the fingers of
paraplegic subjects, the mean blood flow in their great toe was not
statistically different than that in the great toe of normal subjects. By contrast, the blood flow in the great toe of quadriplegic
subjects was significantly lower than that of normal subjects.

Effective mean brachial and digital blood pressures in para-

DIGITAL BLOOD FLOW IN 30 NORMAL, 15 QUADRIPLEGIC AND 15 PARAPLEGIC SUBJECTS.

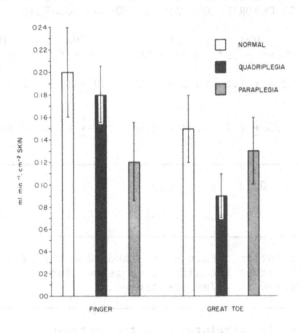

Figure 1.
Digital blood flow was measured calorimetrically. Note that the vasoconstriction in the fingers of paraplegic as compared with normal subjects is reversed in the hallus.

plegic subjects were significantly higher than that in quadriplegic and normal subjects (P<.05). Digital vascular resistance (mmHg·ml $^{-1}$·min^{-1}·cm^{-2}skin) in the fourth finger of paraplegic subjects was significantly higher than that found in quadriplegic and normal subjects (P<0.001).

Table I demonstrates that the mean excretion for each of the CM metabolites in 35 chronic quadriplegic subjects is greater than that in 36 normal subjects. The results of CM excretion in five untreated quadriplegic subjects who developed spontaneous hypertensive crises are shown in Table II. It is evident that despite higher output of CM metabolites just before the crises (autonomic hyperreflexia), the level of CM metabolites during or after hypertensive episodes was significantly higher than pre-crises concen-

TABLE I

COMPARATIVE EXCRETION OF URINARY CATECHOLAMINE METABOLITES
IN 35 QUADRIPLEGIC AND 36 NORMAL SUBJECTS

	VMA Mean ± SD*	HVA Mean ± SD*	TMN Mean ± SD*	HMPG Mean ± SD*
Quadriplegia 35 Subjects	2.4 ± 1.5	3.5 ± 2.2	1.9 ± 1.2	1.8 ± 1.3
Normal 36 Subjects	1.5 ± 1.1	1.4 ± 0.62	1.2 ± 0.68	0.86 ± 0.31
S.e.d.**	0.32	0.39	0.24	0.23
P***	<0.01	<0.001	<0.01	<0.001

*SD = standard deviation, **S.e.d. = standard error of the difference
***P = probability (that the difference is not due to chance)
Results are expressed in μg/mg creatinine.

trations and directly correlated with the increase in brachial
blood pressure. Moreover, in seven subjects in whom hypertension
was induced by means of water loading during excretory cystometry,
the height of intracystic pressure, and brachial and digital blood
pressures coincided with that of bradycardia, and with the lowest
level of blood flow in the fingers, great toes, and calves, which
was below detection limits. Maximum vasoconstriction in the fingers
and toes occurred in advance of that in the calves. These findings
were accompanied by headache, profuse flushing and diaphoresis in
the face and neck, and piloerection above and pallor of the skin
below the level of the lesion. Figure 2 represents a typical graph
of the experiments in which water intake was used to stretch the
urinary bladder during excretory cystometry, while recordings of the
brachial blood pressures, pulse rate, the blood flow in fingers,
toes, and calves and intracystic pressures were simultaneously
monitored.

DISCUSSION

The results indicate that during the resting state, when there
is no untoward side effects from sensory and/or autonomic stimuli,
there is a significant degree of vasoconstriction in the upper extremities of paraplegic and in the lower extremities of quadriplegic

TABLE II

ENHANCED EXCRETION OF CATECHOLAMINE METABOLITES IN QUADRIPLEGIA DURING SPONTANEOUS HYPERTENSION

SUBJECTS	BRACHIAL BLOOD PRESSURE mmHg		VMA µg/mg creatinine		HVA µg/mg creatinine		HMPG µg/mg creatinine	
	Before	After	Before	After	Before	After	Before	After
1	114/90	186/114	4.0	5.4	5.0	12.0	1.42	3.22
2	100/70	180/120	4.0	7.0	5.0	10.0	4.21	8.45
3	100/80	170/106	4.0	6.0	7.0	20.0	4.00	11.00
4	110/90	190/114	5.0	6.0	9.0	14.0	4.63	10.30
5	96/70	180/100	2.0	2.5	3.0	5.0	0.73	2.43
Mean $\pm$ SD	104/80 $\pm$ 7.6/10	181/111 $\pm$ 7.6/7.8	3.8 $\pm$ 1.1	5.38 $\pm$ 1.7	5.8 $\pm$ 2.3	12.2 $\pm$ 5.5	3.00 $\pm$ 1.79	7.08 $\pm$ 4.00
"t" test for significance of difference between paired samples			3.86		3.46		3.90	
Probability that the difference is not due to chance			$P < 0.001$		$P < 0.001$		$P < 0.001$	

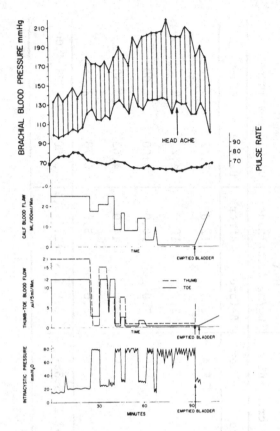

Figure 2. The increase in intracystic pressure is followed by the
increase in arterial blood pressure, a decrease in pulse rate, and
a concomitant reduction in blood flow of the finger, the great toe
and the calf.

subjects compared with normal controls (Figure 1). This vasoconstriction is reflected in greater excretion of catecholamine
metabolites in the urine of spinal cord injured humans during the
chronic phase (Table I). When spontaneous hypertensive crises
(Table II) occur in quadriplegic subjects, the excretion of CM
metabolites in urine is significantly increased (7). The greater
output of CM metabolites in chronic quadriplegia and paraplegia
may thus be due to several subclinical, undetected hypertensive
episodes which may occur because of fecal impaction, or more frequently, because of bladder overdistension, cystitis, or bladder
stones. During excretory cystometry, vasoconstriction in the upper
and lower extremities was anticipated because of the enhanced excretion of CM metabolites. One would expect compensatory vasodi-
litation in the calf muscle blood flow, but, instead, there was a
simultaneous decrease in the blood flow of calf musclature in all
seven subjects studied.

Roussan et al., (9) have shown that calf blood flow decreased during autonomic hyperreflexia. They implied that the gradual facilitation of the spinal cord was a primary cause for the reduced circulation of the calf musculator, and that the cause of, or increase in, hypertension was the result of sudden shifts of large blood volumes from skeletal muscle circulation to the capacitance vessels. In the light of our findings of intense peripheral vasoconstriction in the upper and lower extremities coincident with that of calf blood flow, the blood shift into the capacitance vessels must be of enormous magnitude.

In agreement with others (1,5), we have shown (8) that dopamine, norepinephrine, and serotonin disappear from the cord below the level of transection and accumulate proximally. The disappearance of these neurotransmitters suggests that one of these biogenic amines may be an inhibitory neurotransmitter. The loss of these neurotransmitters after spinal cord injury may cause facilitation of the cord below the level of the lesion. This permanent lack or curtailment of inhibition within the cord could be the primary reason why noxious stimuli easily produce such intense adrenergic response in spinal man. The stretch of the vesicular wall is accompanied by vasoconstriction in direct proportion to the amount of stretch and/or uninhibited detrusor contraction. It reaches its maximum when intracystic pressure has reached its peak, at which time the increased release of catecholamines causes a large blood volume transfer from peripheral blood vessels and those of the musculature into the capacitance vessels, causing a compensatory vasodilatation, profuse flushing, diaphoresis, and vasodilatation in the face and neck, headache and bradycardia. These manifestations are the reaction of the intact regulatory system; the hypertension sensed by the vasomotor center is transferred to carotid sinus, aortic arch, and sinuauricular node in order to reduce the hypertension. Without the removal of the stimulus or administration of ganglioplegic and/or sympatholytic drugs, these remaining regulatory mechanisms cannot appreciably lower the blood pressure.

SUMMARY

The blood flow, measured calorimetrically during the resting state, in the fourth finger and hallus of 15 quadriplegic and 15 paraplegic subjects was compared with that of 30 normal subjects.

There was a statistically significant reduction in the blood flow of the fingers and great toes of paraplegic and quadriplegic subjects, respectively.

In seven quadriplegic subjects (C5-7) simultaneous monitoring of the blood flow, measured by venous occlusion plethysmography during excretory cystometry, revealed an intense vasoconstriction in the thumb, the hallus, and the calf musculature. The reduction in blood flow coincided with that of heart rate and with the increase in arterial blood pressure and intracystic pressure.

The excretion of CM metabolites in 35 chronic quadriplegic subjects was found to be statistically increased compared with that of 36 normal subjects.

Occurance of spontaneous hypertensive crises in five cervical quadriplegic subjects was accompanied by enhanced elaboration of catecholamines. It is concluded that the higher excretion of CM metabolites in chronic quadriplegia may be due to many subclinical, undetected hypertensive episodes.

REFERENCES

1. Anden, N.E., Haggendal, E., Magnussen, T. and Rosengren, E.: The time course of the disappearance of noreadrenaline and 5-hydroxytryptamine in spinal cord after transection. Acta Physiol. Scand. 62:115-118, 1964.
2. Armstrong, M.D., Shaw, K.M.F. and Wall, P.E.: The phenolic acids of human urine. J. Biol. Chem. 218:293-303, 1956.
3. Guttman, L. and Whitteridge, D.: Effects of bladder distension on autonomic mechanism after spinal cord injuries. Brain 70:361-405, 1947.
4. Head, H. and Riddoch, J.: The automatic bladder, excessive sweating and some other reflex conditions in gross injuries of the spinal cord. Brain 40:188-263, 1917.
5. Magnusson, T. and Rosengren, E.: Catecholamines of the spinal cord normally and after transection. Experientia (Basel)19:229,1963.
6. Naftchi, N.E. and Mendlowitz, M.: Drug modification of digital vascular reactivity to vasoactive substances. Bibl. Anat. 10:133-144, 1969 (S. Karger, Basel, Switzerland).
7. Naftchi, N.E., Lowman, E.W., Sell, G.H., Demeny, M. and Rusk,H.: Hypertensive crisis associated with increased urinary catecholamine catabolites in spinal man. Fed. Proc.30:678, 1971.
8. Naftchi, N.E., Demeny, M., Kertesz, A. and Lowman, E.W.: The CNS and adrenal tyrosine hydroxylase activity and norepinephrine, serotonin, and histamine in the spinal cord after transection. Fed. Proc. 31:832, 1972.
9. Roussan, M.S., Abramson, A.S., Lippmann, H.I. and D'Oronzio, G.: Somatic and autonomic responses to bladder filling in patients with complete transverse myelopathy. Arch. Phys. Med. 47:450-456, 1966.
10. Wilk, S., Gitlow, S.E., Clarke, D.D. and Paley, D.H.: Determination of urinary 3-methoxy-4-hydroxyphenylethyleneglycol by gas-liquid chromatography and electron capture detection. Clin. Chem. Acta 16:403-408, 1967.

THE EFFECT ON CEREBRAL ENERGY METABOLITES OF THE CYANATE PRODUCED

SHIFT OF THE OXYGEN SATURATION CURVE

John Cassel, Kyuya Kogure, Raul Busto, Chang Yong Kim
and Donald R. Harkness

CVD Res. Ctr., Dept. of Neurol., Dept. of Med., Univ.
of Miami Sch. of Med., and Veterans Admin. Hosp., Miami,
Fla. USA

Cerami and Manning showed that cyanate inhibits the sickling
of red blood cells from patients with sickle cell anemia and suggested its use in the treatment of this disease (1). They further
showed that cyanate had no deleterious effects upon red cell metabolism (2) and that cells exposed to this compound in vitro and
reinfused into the patient had a prolonged survival (3). These
observations have stimulated considerable research into the biochemistry and pharmacology of cyanate and the mechanism by which
it inhibits sickling.

Cyanate reacts irreversibly with the α-amino groups of both
the α- and β-chains of hemoglobin and causes a remarkable increase
in affinity for oxygen (4). Presumably, it is this property of the
carbamylated sickle hemoglobin that retards sickling since only deoxy
sickle hemoglobin is capable of forming intermolecular aggregates(5,6).

Large doses of cyanate given to experimental animals leads to
sedation, seizures, and death (7,8). Chronic administration of sub-
lethal amounts produces sedation, weight loss, and hind limb paralysis. In man, oral doses of 30-40 mg/kg cause transient drowsiness
and diminished vision (10). These observations of apparent effects
of cyanate upon the central nervous system and the possibility of
inducing cerebral hypoxia when the blood oxygen dissociation curve
is shifted markedly to the left have prompted this study on the effects of relatively large doses of cyanate upon cerebral metabolism
in rabbits. The rabbit was chosen for these studies because of our
considerable prior experience with cyanate administration in this
animal (11).

METHODOLOGY

Male New Zealand white rabbits weighing from 1.7 to 2.3 kg. were obtained from a local animal dealer and maintained on Purina Standard Rabbit Chow. They were injected intraperitoneally with solutions of freshly prepared sodium cyanate in initial doses of 150 mg/animal on Mondays, Wednesdays, and Fridays. After two weeks the P_{50}'s had dropped from a normal value of 30.3 ± 2.4 mmHg to 15.0-17.5 mmHg. Thereafter the dose of cyanate was decreased and held constant at 75 mg/animal IP thrice weekly. This dose maintained the P_{50}'s at the same level and the animals began to gain weight, though at a slower rate than control animals. A P_{50} of 16 mmHg in the rabbit represents a carbamylation of 2.5 moles of cyanate per hemoglobin tetramer measured as valine hydantoin by the method of Manning, et al. (12). Our method for measuring and analyzing the whole blood oxygen dissociation curve has been described earlier (11).

After 3,5,7,8,11,12,13, and 14 weeks of treatment, each animal was anesthetized by intravenous injection of 1% Brevital Sodium. A tracheostomy and femoral arterial and venous cannulation were performed and the animal was paralyzed by intravenous injection of Flaxedil. Respiration and maintenance of anesthesia were then taken over by 80% nitrous oxide gas balanced with oxygen delivered by a Harvard Small Animal Respiration Pump. With the animal's head secured in a stereotaxic holder, the P_aO_2 and P_aCO_2 were adjusted by varying the respiration volume and concentration of oxygen in the respiration mixture. With the aid of the Radiometer microelectrode monitoring apparatus, P_aO_2 was regulated at 105 mmHg, P_aCO_2 at 40 mmHg, and pH at 7.4. The animal's temperature was kept near 37°C. and, when necessary, the blood gas values and pH were corrected to 37°C. Blood pressure was constantly monitored by a membrane type pressure transducer.

A midsagittal incision was made over the cranial vault and the skin and periosteum were reflected. A small bottomless plastic cup was then sutured into the wound. When the animal demonstrated good stability at the aforementioned values of blood gases and pH, simultaneous samples of arterial blood and cisternal CSF were anaerobically frozen in liquid nitrogen for subsequent metabolic analysis. A final arterial sample was also taken in order to measure final blood parameters and insure the steady state. The cranial vault was then frozen by pouring liquid nitrogen into the bottomless cup. The supratentorial cortex was then chiselled out and subjected to quantitative analysis for glucose (Glu), glycogen (Gly), pyruvate (Py), lactate (La), phosphocreatine (PCr), adenosine triphosphate (ATP), adenosine diphosphate (ADP) and adenosine monophosphate (AMP) (13). Total CO_2 was measured by the method devised by Pontén et al. (14). In a similar manner the frozen blood sample was analyzed for glucose, pyruvate, and lactate, and the CSF sample for glucose, pyruvate, lactate, and total CO_2.

CALCULATIONS

Intracellular bicarbonate $(HCO_3^-)_i$ and intracellular pH (pH_i) were calculated by the following equations (15):

$$(HCO_3^-)_i = \frac{(HCO_3^-)_t - 0.03(HCO_3^-)bl - 0.15(HCO_3^-)csf}{v_i}$$

In this equation v_i represents the intracellular volume.

$$pH_i = pK + \log \frac{(HCO_3^-)_i}{P_t CO_2 \times S}$$

The $P_t CO_2$ can be derived from the arterial CO_2 tension according to the relation described by Pontén and Siesjö (14).

Cytoplasmic $NADH/NAD^+$ ratio was obtained from the formula of Williamson et al. (16).

$$\frac{NADH}{NAD^+} = \frac{La_i}{Py_i} \times \frac{k}{(\overline{H^+})_i}$$

Energy reserve (E. Res.) was calculated by the equation suggested by Lowry et al. (17).

$$E.\ Res. = PCr + 1.4\ ATP + 2.0\ Glu + 2.9\ Gly$$

Energy charge potential (E. Ch.) was obtained from the formula of Atkinson (18).

$$E.\ Ch. = \frac{ATP + 0.5\ ADP}{ATP + ADP + AMP}$$

RESULTS

The effect of intraperitoneal cyanate upon the percent saturation curve of rabbit blood appears in Figure 1. The P_{50}'s of the treated animals decreased from a normal value of 30.3 ± 2.4 mmHg to 16.6 ± 1.3 mmHg while the hemoglobin concentration remained the same. No significant changes appeared in content of blood glucose, pyruvate, lactate, and lactate/pyruvate ratio. No changes appeared in brain tissue content of phosphocreatine, ATP, ADP, and AMP. Of the measured intermediate glycolytic metabolites, only pyruvate increased significantly. Mean values of these metabolic factors are shown in Table I. Directional changes in the analogous CSF concentrations paralleled the changes shown in the brain parenchyma.

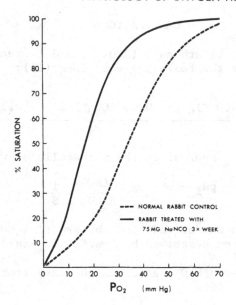

Fig. 1. Whole Blood Oxygen Dissociation Curve of Cyanate-treated and control Rabbits.

DISCUSSION

Availability of oxygen to brain tissue is a function both of P_{50} of the blood and cerebral blood flow. If the P_{50} is lowered significantly, oxygen availability from the blood to the brain tissue might be reduced unless the changes are compensated for by a concomitant increase in cerebral blood flow. Cerebral blood flow is thought to be regulated by hydrogen ion content in the muscle layer of the precapillary arteries (19) in addition to perfusion pressure (20) and neurogenic mechanisms (21). Therefore, cerebral blood flow becomes a function of P_aCO_2 (22,23), PO_2 (24) and possibly a function of metabolic activity of the brain paren-chyma (25) and CSF pH (26). In this experiment, the P_aCO_2 and P_aO_2 in the treated animals were adjusted to that of the normal animals, but neither CSF pH nor intracellular pH changed signi-ficantly. This suggests that there were no changes in cerebral blood flow.

Due to the decrease of P_{50} in the treated animals, the percent saturation of oxygen on the venous side increased as compared with the same P_vO_2 of the normal animal. Assuming that no change has taken place in cerebral blood flow, oxygen consumption of the brain should be reduced. From the metabolic analysis, however, it is no-ticed that no significant changes occurred with respect to oxidative metabolism. Therefore, the changes in oxygen availability to the brain were not great enough to produce tissue hypoxia.

Table I. Brain Metabolites in Treated and Control Rabbits

PCr		ATP		ADP		AMP	
C.	T.	C.	T.	C.	T.	C.	T.
4.42	4.18	2.46	2.51	0.32	0.34	0.02	0.01
±0.08	±0.13	±0.04	±0.04	±0.01	±0.01	±0.01	±0.01

Glu		Gly		Py		La	
C.	T.	C.	T.	C.	T.	C.	T.
2.69	2.66	4.22	4.30	0.08	0.12	1.24	1.43
±0.32	±0.45	±0.21	±0.37	±0.01	±0.00	±0.07	±0.16

E.Ch.		E.Res.		pH_i		$NADH/NAD^+$	
C.	T.	C.	T.	C.	T.	C.	T.
0.92	0.93	25.5	27.5	7.08	7.07	2.58	2.13
±0.01	±0.00	±0.6	±0.9	±0.04	±0.02		

Units are expressed as mmoles/kg.; C.=control, T.=treated

Since the tissue content of metabolic substrates gives no insight into the dynamic turnover rates, the changes in pyruvate, lactate/pyruvate ratio, and $NADH/NAD^+$ ratio may be indicative of the incipient stages of significant changes in one or another metabolic rate. For example, the rate of energy utilization can decrease in proportion to the reduced production rate.

It is possible that higher dose levels of cyanate will actually result in demonstrable tissue changes. Our most recent studies in rats (Table II) clearly demonstrate that higher doses of cyanate do in fact lower tissue content of phosphocreatine and ATP and increase glucose.

Table II. Brain Metabolites in Treated and Control Rats*

PCr		ATP		Glu		Py	
C.	T.	C.	T.	C.	T.	C.	T.
5.4	4.2	2.8	2.6	3.8	5.0	0.11	0.12
±0.1	±0.2	±0.0	±0.1	±0.0	±0.3	±0.00	±0.01

*Rats were treated with 100 mg/kg NaNCO IP daily for 10 days; units as in Table I.

In summary each of the rabbits treated chronically with IP sodium cyanate had P_{50}'s approximately one half normal. Cerebral energy metabolites were evaluated on these animals at controlled steady state. No evidence of brain tissue hypoxia was observed.

ACKNOWLEDGEMENTS

We are indebted to Miss P. Goldman, Mrs. S. Roth, Mrs. M.
Santiso, Mrs. E. Martinez, Mr. G. Marcos, and Mr. A. Montiel for
their expert technical assistance. This work was supported by
grants from the United Health Foundation, the Veterans Administration, the Meyergold Research Fund and HEW Grants NINDS-NS058 20-08
and AM-09001-08.

REFERENCES

1. Cerami, A. and Manning, J.M.: Proc. Nat. Acad. Sci. U.S.A.
    68:1180, 1971.
2. de Furia, F. G., Miller, D.R., Cerami, A. and Manning, J.M.:
    J. Clin. Invest. 51:566, 1972.
3. Gillette, P.N., Manning, J.M. and Cerami, A.: Proc. Nat.
    Acad. Sci. U.S.A. 68:2791, 1971.
4. Kilmartin, J.V. and Rossi-Bernardi, L.: Nature 222:1243, 1969.
5. Diederich, D.: Biochem. Biophys. Res. Commun. 46:1255, 1972.
6. May, A., Bellingham, A.J., Huehns, E.R. and Beaver, G.H.:
    Lancet I:658, 1972.
7. Birch, K.M. and Schütz, F.: Brit. J. Pharmacol. 1:186, 1946.
8. Cerami, A., Allen, T.A., Graziano, J.H., de Furia, F.G.,
    Manning, J.M. and Gillette, P.N.: J. Pharmacol. Exp. Therap.
    In press.
9. Gillette, Peter: Personal communication.
10. Schütz, F.: Experientia 5:133, 1949.
11. Harkness, D.R., Roth, S., Goldman, P., and Goldberg, M.:
    Adv. Exper. Med. and Biol. 28:415, 1972.
12. Manning, J.M., Lee, C.K., Cerami, A., and Gillette, P.N.:
    J. Lab. Clin. Med. In press.
13. Hohorst, H.J., Kreuz, F.H. and Bucker, T.: Biochem. Z. 332:
    18, 1969.
14. Pontén, U. and Siesjö, B.K.: Acta Physiol. Scand. 60:297, 1964.
15. Siesjö, B.K.: Acta Physiol. Scand. 55:325, 1964.
16. Williamson, D.H., Lund, P. and Krebs, H.A.: Biochem. J. 103:
    514, 1967.
17. Lowry, O.H., Passonneau, J.V., Hasselberger, F.X. and Schulz,
    D.W.: J. Biol. Chem. 239:18, 1964.
18. Atkinson, D.E.: Biochemistry 7:4030, 1968.
19. Shinohara, Y.: Neurology 23:186, 1973.
20. Harper, A.M.: J. Neurol. Neurosurg. Psychiat. 23:398, 1966.
21. Meyer, J.S., Teraura, T., Sakamoto, K. and Kondo, A.:
    Neurology 21:247, 1971.
22. Reivich, M.: Am. J. Physiol. 206:25, 1964.
23. Severinghaus, J.W., and Lassen, N.A.: Circ. Res. 20:272, 1967.
24. Kogure, K., Scheinberg, P., Reinmuth, O.M., Fujishima, M., and
    Busto, R.: J. Appl. Physiol. 29:223, 1970.
25. Ingvar, D.H. and Risberg, J.: Exper. Brain Res. 3:195, 1967.
26. Skinhøj, E.: Acta Neurol. Scand. 42:604, 1966.

ON THE ACCURACY OF AN IMPROVED METHOD FOR THE MEASUREMENT OF O_2-DISSOCIATION-CURVES ACCORDING TO NIESEL & THEWS, 1961

Wolfgang Barnikol and Waltraud Wahler

Physiologisches Institut der Universität

6500 Mainz, Saarstr. 21, BRD

During the first part of its journey to tissue oxygen is carried by blood. The greatest part thereby is bound chemically to hemoglobin. The molecular mechanism of this binding gives the so-called O_2-dissociation-curve its typical, sigmoidal form. The O_2-dissociation-curve is the function between O_2-saturation and O_2-partial-pressure. This curve is of great importance for the O_2-supply of the tissues. It is important for practice as well as for formulating a theory in this field. Within the last few years it has been discovered, that the O_2-dissociation-curve is influenced by organic phosphates, e.g. 2,3-DPG (CHANUTIN, CURNISH, 1967; BENESCH, BENESCH, 1967). Because of this new discovery a correlation to metabolism and also new therapeutic possibilities have been found. The influence of a low molecular substance on the O_2-dissociation-curve could be deduced from a theoretical analysis of the O_2-hemoglobin-equilibrium, too (BARNIKOL, THEWS, 1969).

Perhaps because of this new discoveries new efforts to measure the O_2-dissociation-curve were began. Before I give a short survey upon the methods, I should clarify what is to be measured: that is, the in-vivo-O_2-dissociation-curve of the unaltered blood; if possible, with a continuously measuring micromethod. Now let me explain: the "in-vivo-O_2-dissociation-curve" - because metabolism continues after venipuncture, shifting the O_2-hemoglobin-equilibrium and "unaltered blood" - because perhaps we do not know yet all factors, which influence the O_2-dissociation-curve. According to our experience the measurement must be concluded two hours after the venipuncture, if one wants to obtain an in-vivo-dissociation-curve.

The oldest way to measure the O_2-dissociation-curve is perhaps the common known VAN SLYKE-method. It has the great advantage to be free from methodical errors. However it has the disadvantage, that one can determine the O_2-dissociation-curve only point by point.

In 1960 HAAB, PIIPER, and RAHN proposed a method in which venous and arterial blood (analysed by the VAN SLYKE-method) are mixed to a known O_2-content, and PO_2 is measured. This procedure is easier than the classical VAN SLYKE-method. It simulates the in-vivo arterial-venous mixture very well resulting in an effective O_2-dissociation-curve. But it seems not very easy to get the first part of the O_2-saturation-curve.

In 1962 another experimental approach was made to simplify the measurement of the O_2-dissociation-curve (CAROL, FRANCO, LONGMUIR, MC CABE, 1962; COLMAN, LONGMUIR, 1963). The O_2-content was linearly diminished with stated time by adding an appropriate amount of heart muscle tissue. In this method one has to take into account an altering of the blood sample and perhaps a spezific disturbance of the O_2-hemoglobin-equilibrium.

In 1970 DUVELLEROY and others published a new method for registration of the O_2-dissociation-curve. A fixed volume of deoxygenated blood (about 5 to 10 ml) is equilibrated with a fixed quantity of O_2. The saturation is measured as the decrease of O_2-partial-pressure in the gas phase. Both, the O_2-partial-pressure in the gas phase and the O_2-partial-pressure within the blood are measured with O_2-electrodes. Using this technique the method implies all complications caused by electrodes, e.g. drift, and it is no micro-method; and therefore it is not very suitable for small animals. In addition the earliest time one gets an O_2-dissociation-curve after venipuncture is approximately 1 1/2 hours. Repeated measurements are not possible without opening and re-filling the apparatus.

In 1972 KIESOW and others published a new photometric method. The O_2-saturation is measured with the aid of a dual-wave-length-photometer, to avoid the problems of optical inhomogeneity, and the O_2-partial-pressure is increased linear with time by catalytic decomposition of H_2O_2. The main objection to this method is that the blood must be altered; i.e. diluted.

The oldest of the newer methods for registration of the O_2-dissociation-curve is the micro-photometric technique of NIESEL and THEWS (1961). As this method is published in german and perhaps not yet generally known I will briefly describe it. In principle the O_2-saturation of a blood smear is determined photometrically, equilibrated with humidified gas of appropriate composition. For continuous registration the O_2-partial-pressure above the blood smear is raised continuously and proportionally to stated time after complete deoxygenation with O_2-free gas. The blood smear is placed in a chamber with optical windows, so that the extinction may be measured. The mentioned proportionality which is necessary between 0 and 100 mmHg is achieved by an

appropriate diffusion resistance. If the extinction is plotted against time, almost immediately one obtains the O_2-dissociation-curve. As the registration
takes only 10 minutes and one can begin with the measurement immediately
after venipuncture, it is possible to obtain the true O_2-dissociation-curve
from only one droplet of blood. So one must not be afraid, that the intracellular, ionic milieu, e.g. the concentration of organic phosphates will be changed.

As ingenious as the conception of NIESEL and THEWS may seem, it demands
extraordinary experimental skill. This can only be achieved with much experience. One must take into account many failures. There are two reasons for
this: firstly a 10 μ thick blood smear, which is subjected to a flow humidified
gases produces a very unstable system. With slight under saturation the blood
smear dries out and with slight over saturation it is diluted. Secondly, it requires special precautions to avoid the steaming up of the optical windows,
which means the necessity to avoid an over saturation of the equilibration
gases.

That is why the method of NIESEL and THEWS has been improved
(BARNIKOL, DÖHRING, THEWS, 1971):

Firstly the blood smear was sheltered by an extremely thin teflon membrane
of about 0,5 μ. This idea was already realized in 1969 by SCHMIDT and
HEUSER with commercial membranes. But commercial membranes are unquali-
fied for more than one reason. So in conjunction with DÖHRING and DIEFEN-
THÄLER (1971) we developed a new way of producing an extremely thin teflon
membrane. This already has been reported on the last symposium in Dortmund
in connection with the construction of a very fast electrode. Secondly a special equipment for humidification of the gases was developed, which enables
a constant and optimal H_2O-saturation. Now the gas no longer bubbles through
the water, but is spread on a water surface with the aid of porous glass. Third-
ly the upper optical window of the apparatus was doubled to achieve a better
thermal isolation. The next picture shows an original registration.

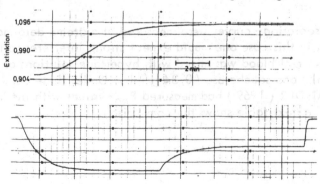

Fig. 1 : Original registration with the improved apparatus

One can see, in which way the time axis is calibrated in O_2-partial-pressure: after complete registration of the O_2-dissociation-curve the chamber is equilibrated with a gas of known O_2-content. Now the recorder indicates any O_2-saturation between 0 and 100 %. A horizontal line is drawn, which intersects the O_2-dissociation-curve at a time corresponding to the known O_2-partial-pressure.

With the help of the improved method it is possible to repeatedly register the O_2-dissociation-curve from one blood layer, and it is possible to get the O_2-dissociation-curve from hemoglobin solutions. The mean reproducebility for PO_2 is about 1,6 mmHg, and 2 % for the saturation. Such measurements show that a blood layer remains stable for 2-3 hours. Within this time the registrated O_2-dissociation-curve do not systematically differ from each other. Shifting of the O_2-dissociation-curve would suggest changes in the blood layer. The constancy with time is also a strong indication, that the true O_2-dissociation-curve is measured.

A very sensitive indicator for the stability of the blood layer is a constant extinction in a distinct state of oxygenation: each change in the blood layer, e.g.movements of erythrocytes, causes a drift of the extinction. Within the stated time the extinction has the same drift as the photometer itself. Microscopically the erythrocytes show no visible deformations. After this time, however, the drift increases.

Because the O_2-saturation using this method is determined indirectly, i.e. photometrically, and it is an inhomogeneous medium, it is necessary to check the accuracy of the method against another. When measuring micro-photometrically the O_2-saturation of a single erythrocyte one has to face great methodical errors, which are caused by form variations leading to undefined light scattering. But when measuring photometrically the O_2-saturation of 1 million erythrocytes in a monocellular layer, there is a good chance that these errors are compensated by averaging out. For checking the accuracy of the new method the VAN SLYKE-analysis seems quite suitable, as it is almost free from methodical errors.

Firstly O_2-dissociation- curves were measured at extreme deformation of the erythrocytes as in this case one would expect strong interference from light scattering. Normal blood was mixed with hypertone solutions of sodium-chlorid (0,03 g/ml) and saccharose (0,34 g/ml). Under these conditions WALDECK and ZANDER (1969) had measured P_{50}-values with the VAN SLYKE-method. The next table shows the comparison.

Table 1 : Comparison of P_{50}-values (mmHg) of normal blood
in hypertone solutions

	VAN SLYKE 2 persons	this method 1 person
Blood–NaCl 1 : 2	28,7/32,1	31
Blood–Saccharose 1 : 2	9,6/10,8	10

One can see, that within the range of error the P_{50}-values measured by both methods are identical.

In another series of experiments, we kept the normal geometric form of the erythrocytes, but we produced an extreme shift of the O_2-dissociation-curve taking P_{CO_2} as zero. Under these conditions the O_2-dissociation-curve of one person was measured with both methods. The next figure shows the results:

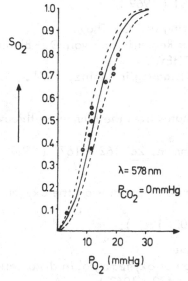

Fig. 2 : Comparison of the improved method with the VAN SLYKE-method.

The continuous line represents the measurements with the new chamber. The single points belong to the VAN SLYKE-measurements. As we have only single measurements from the VAN SLYKE-method, it is logical to compare the whole

range of variation and not the standard deviation. Therefore the broken line
gives the range of variation from 8 measurments with the new method. And
one can see, that the single points lie within this range. No systematic deviation is be found.

Although these are preliminary results we may conclude from them, that
the new chamber-method shows no systematic error as compared to the VAN
SLYKE-method.

This work was supported by Deutsche Forschungsgemeinschaft (Th 14/10).

Literature

W.K.R. Barnikol, G. Thews
Zur Interpretation der O_2-Bindungskurve des Human-Hämoglobins
Pflügers Arch. 309, 232 - 249 (1969).

W.K.R. Barnikol, G. Thews
Zur Dissoziation des Human-Hämoglobins
Pflügers Arch. 309, 224 - 231 (1969).

W.K. R. Barnikol, W. Döhring und G. Thews
Eine verbesserte Methode zur Registrierung von O_2-Bindungskurven nach dem
Verfahren von NIESEL und THEWS
4. Atmungsphysiolog. Arbeitstagung in Mainz, 1971.

R. Benesch, R.E. Benesch
The effect of organic phosphates from the human erythrocyte on allosteric pro-
perties of hemoglobin
Biochem. Biophys. Res. Commun. 26, 162 - 167   (1967).

A. Chanutin, R. Curnish
Effect of organic and inorganic phosphates on the oxygen equilibrium of
human erythrocytes
Arch. Biochem. 121, 96 - 102(1967).

C.H. Colman, J.S. Longmuir
A new method for registration of oxyhemoglobin dissociation curves
J. Appl. Physiol. 18 , 420 - 423 (1963).

W. Döhring, K. Diefenthäler und W.K.R. Barnikol
The production and application of 0,2 to 1,0 μ thick polytetrafluorethylene
membranes to continuous polarographic measurement of oxygen tension in the
gas phase.
Oxygen Supply, Urban und Schwarzenberg S. 86 - 91 (1973).

M.A. Duvelleroy, R.G. Buchles, S. Rosenhaimer,C.Tung, and M.B. Laver
An oxyhemoglobin dissociation analyzer
J. Appl. Physiol. 28, 227 – 233 (1970).

C.H. Franco, I.S. Longmuir, and M.Mc Cabe
New methods for the continuous registration of oxyhemoglobin dissociation
curves
J. Physiol. (London) 161, 54P – 55P (1962).

P.E. Haab, J. Piiper, and H. Rahn
Simple method for rapid determination of an O_2 dissociation curve of the blood
J. Appl. Physiol. 15, 1148 – 1149 (1960).

L. A. Kiesow, J.W. Bless. D.P. Nelson, and J.B. Shelton
A new method for the rapid determination of O_2 dissociation curves in
small blood samples by spectrophotometric titration
Clin. Chim. Acta 41, 123 – 139 (1972).

W. Niesel und G. Thews
Ein neues Verfahren zur schnellen und genauen Aufnahme der Sauerstoff-
bindungskurve des Blutes und konzentrierter Hämoproteidlösungen.
Pflügers Arch. 273, 380 – 395 (1961).

K. Schmidt und K.H. Heuser
Methodischer Beitrag zur Aufnahme der Sauerstoff-Dissoziationskurve an ein-
lagigen Erythrozytenschichten
Respiration 26, 16 – 34 (1969).

F. Waldeck, R. Zander
Lageveränderungen der Sauerstoffbindungskurve in Abhängigkeit von den
intraerythrozytären Kationen – und Hämoglobinkonzentrationen.
Klin. Wschr. 47, 1068 – 1078 (1969).

Chairmen: Dr. Ian A. Silver, Dr. Goran M. Kolmodin and
           Dr. Britton Chance

DISCUSSION OF PAPER BY H. I. BICHER

Chance: Your last slide did not show the extra oxygen consumption
due to the increased electrical activity as determined in 1947 by
Davis and Remond. Why is there a discrepancy of your results?

Bicher: We are aware of their data, that constitutes one of the
basis of our theory. The lack of a pO_2 drop in the contralateral
side could be explained either because of the short time of the
response or a blood flow compensation.

Song: I suppose you have induced a driving reflex by a chemical
means lowering pO_2 level. Is it true that you can observe a
generalized decrease of CNS activity (action potentials) by lowering PaO_2 level in cerebral arteries? For example, in respiratory
centers or cardiovasomotor centers, etc.?

Bicher: pO_2 is depressed all through the brain during nitrogen
breathing. However, in short anoxic anoxia periods, no major
changes in vital center activity is observed.

Zielinski: (1) Do you have any statistical evidence of the correlation between pO_2 of the nervous tissue and neuronal activity
in your records?
        (2) How do you identify precise structure of your records in
the brain?

Bicher: (1) No, the action potentials recorded through an oxygen
electrode are deformed and do not lend themselves readily to detailed
analysis. What we are recording are mainly "all or none" responses.
        (2) We recorded from the ventral horn motoneurons in the spinal
cord, as Prof. Kolmodin described yesterday, or, in most experiments,
in the prefrontal motor areas.

Whalen: We have performed some similar N_2-breathing experiments on
cats and find that the pO_2 goes to near zero (0-2 mm Hg) nearly
always. In one of the five cats, pO_2 did not go to zero. Its body
temperature was low and it had been given considerable amounts of
barbiturate. What were the body temperature and barbiturate doses
in your experiments?

Bicher: I agree that the anesthetic may have an influence. Body temperature and vital functions (blood pressure, heart rate) were maintained and only experiments considered from animals with functions within "normal" limits. You may need a longer experimental series.

Kovach: What was the response time of your microelectrodes? How did you measure flow? Were flow, electrical activity and pO_2 measured on the same place? On your presented slide, I did not see parallel changes of tissue pO_2 and arterial pO_2. To the sensing element, not the smooth muscle itself, I think on the experiments of Honig. Activation of CNS activity must lower the pO_2 in the tissue.

Bicher: The response time is less than one second. We measured flow at the carotid artery, pO_2 and electrical activity through the same microelectrode. Arterial pO_2 dropped before the change in flow. Activation of CNS activity changes tissue pO_2 if there is no concomitant change in flow or ApO_2.

DISCUSSION OF PAPER BY I. A. SILVER

Duling: How long does it take the tissue to recover from one of these brief hypoxic episodes? You show incremental responses, but if you only do one, then how long is it until you get a usual response again?

Silver: If you do one 30-second or 60-second hypoxia, you can do them about once an hour. After about three hours, at that interval, you begin to get an increase in potassium. We have tried one or two animals which we have kept long term and have exposed them at intervals of three or four days and then repeated it, and we do not get any change then. If we just give a brief hypoxic episode, the animal recovers and then you repeat it 3 or 4 days later and do it over 2 or 3 weeks, there is no change then. But if you do it at intervals of half an hour, it builds up just as badly as if you do it every ten minutes.

Panigel: The difference in ultrastructural changes of various cellular elements reacting to hypoxia, is indeed very interesting. Pericytes are usually poor in mitochondria contrary to fibroblasts. They are particularly rich in rough endoplasmic reticulum. Did you observe changes in lysosomes or lysosome-like organelles in response to hypoxia?

Silver: Yes, we have seen lysosomal damage as a result of hypoxia but it is much more obvious in dividing or synthesizing cells than in quiescent cells. There is no structural damage in macrophages even during long-term shock. Endoplasmic reticulum became swollen in synthesizing or dividing fibroblasts, but not in pericytes.

In brain we saw no evidence of fine structural damage after multiple short periods of hypoxia even when severe potassium leakage was occurring. We did not see the microvacuolation reported by Brierly and Brown in "Brain Hypoxia" 1970.

Coburn: Have you considered comparing effects of brief anoxia in your preparation with brief exposure to ouabain? You postulate that deterioration of neurons may be due to exposure to extracellular K^+ "leaking" out of glial cells. Use of ouabain might separate "membrane" effects of hypoxia from effect of decreases in energy production in neuronal cells.

Silver: We have not tried ouabain as yet on our brain preparation, but I agree that it would be a useful approach. We have produced potassium leakage from glial cells in culture by applying local hypoxia to monolayers by means of 'large' microelectrodes, but do not yet know if the same thing happens in the brain.

Kovach: I was very impressed by your pK leakage results during hypoxia in the CNS. We have found that during hemorrhagic and tourniquet shock the CNS is releasing potassium. The sagittal sinus blood potassium is elevated. I think that your idea about the glia, instead of neurone, is of interest. We have found elevated CO_2 levels in the hypothalamus and frontal cortex during hemorrhagic shock; that means the pH was very strongly lowered. Maybe that is related to potassium leakage. Did you see potassium leakage with your microelectrode studies also in hemorrhagic shock in the same way as in hypoxia?

Silver: Yes, we have found increase of extracellular potassium during hemorrhagic and endotoxic shock in liver, brain, and wound tissue. The change of K^+ concentration was more rapid in liver and slower in brain but these are very preliminary results. Intracellular pH changes in shock are very obvious and in liver and wound cells, correlate well with fine structure changes. In brain, there appear to be more extracellular pH changes than intracellular at first. We have not been able to correlate ultrastructural changes in brain with functional changes.

DISCUSSION OF PAPER BY U. SCHINDLER, E. GARTNER AND E. BETZ

Miller: (1) Since you found a decrease in pH as a result of the hypercapnic treatment, I wondered if you have tried to adjust pH to normal levels? We have done this with THAM in experiments using lower percentages of CO_2.

(2) I wonder if the increased utilization of oxygen by the brain in the hypercapnic animals might be related to increased blood

supply to the brain which would result from the elevated CO_2 content
of the blood?

Schindler: (1) We tried to adjust the pH with THAM too, but with
our high CO_2 concentrations the infusion volume was very great and
we could not reach the initial pH.
    (2) When measuring the increased oxygen utilization, we found
concomitantly a decreased cerebral blood flow in the cortical area.
We cannot exclude that in other regions there was a higher blood
supply caused by the high pCO_2.

Kovach: Congratulations to you on your very important contributions.
Some remarks: Were there any cerebral regional differences in your
studies with high CO_2 concentration? We have found that during
hemorrhagic shock in dogs, regional changes occur in cerebral CO_2
content. The hypothalamic and frontal cortical CO_2 elevated 3 times.
It was shown in our carrier studies, that the cerebral total ATP and
CP decreased only in the terminal stages of shock. In the same time
ATP and CP resynthesis was strongly depressed. Total ATP or CP
changes can cover local ATP or CP changes. We have found elevated
cerebral oxygen consumption in the brain tissue of hemorrhagic and
tourniquet shock rats and dogs. In baboon, the cerebral O_2 consumption during hemorrhagic shock was decreased.

Schindler: Until now we have only investigated the metabolism of
the cerebral cortex during hypercapnia.

DISCUSSION OF PAPER BY A. MAYEVSKY AND B. CHANCE

Kessler: I am really impressed by your beautiful results, but I
have one question concerning your reflectance measurements. Why
do you think that the reflectance corresponds to blood flow? According to our experience, you measure both local concentrations
of erythrocytes and relative changes in blood flow.

Mayevsky: I agree that the measurement of the reflectance is affected not only by the blood flow and may be more affected by blood
volume (Klaus Harbig, personal communication).

Lübbers: I would also like to stress that you should not talk about
blood flow, since you are measuring blood volume at the same time, a
value which is not easily correlated to flow. We have seen, in similar experiments, the same reverse action of fluorescence caused by
hemoglobin or blood flow. Did you see a shift of the maximum? We
have observed that the maximum fluorescence was shifted during the
hypoxia or anoxia phase and later on came back to the same level.
Could you comment on this?

The other thing is, if you give some quantitative data on this, it is always very difficult to have an idea how much of the light you really get back in the different state. Is the relight scattering or reflectance change in the whole system? Did you try to quantify these things in any way?

Mayevsky: Not yet.

Chance: We have measured emission spectra on the brain cortex and published them and have mentioned, just yesterday, that Lipton took a cortical slab and measured reflectance and scattering changes. We have not integrated them all to explain exactly the nature of in vivo data.

Kovach: It is of great importance that we can measure fluorescence changes for a long time, and I hope it will be possible to do measurements also in anesthetized animals in the future. It would be very important to clear up what the reflectance measurement means. I do not think that you can speak about blood flow and even blood volume without controlling it with flow measurements. Maybe it would be possible to adapt to your experiments the heat clearance method.

Mayevsky: I agree that we did not measure the blood flow in parallel to the reflectance measurement, but as it had been shown by K. Harbig, there is a good correlation between blood volume and the reflectance measurement.

Harbig: How did you determine the effect of different blood volumes on the fluorescent and the reflected light? How big is the blank fluorescence of your instrument?

Mayevsky: In some pilot experiments, we used your method of flashing saline into the carotid artery, so the blood volume was changed. The effect of this flashing was that increases in reflectance and fluorescence were obtained. The ratio was about 1:1 or 1.5:1. The blank fluorescence in our instrument was very low (about 20% from the brain).

DISCUSSION OF PAPER BY E.-J. SPECKMAN, H. CASPERS AND D. BINGMANN

Song: Can you show any difference between autonomic neurons and synaptic neurons responses? I wonder whether you tried different types of neurons, like autonomic neurons in a sympathetic nerve or a vagus nerve or something like that?

Bingmann: These experiments were done in the CNS and spinal cord and in the cortex of the brain, and these experiments do not review to the sympathetic system.

Lübbers: I congratulate you on your very beautiful experiments, but there is one thing I really do not like so much. If we are talking about critical oxygen tension, then we just found that we have to go to a very low level, at least below one mm Hg. You had, on your figures, values which are almost 20, 25 and 15 mm Hg, and that is far above what we would expect if the whole story depends on energy. Could you comment on this?

Bingmann: No, I cannot. I know the discrepancy, but point to the fact that Dr. Kolmodin has figures with the same values at about 15 mm Hg. His activity was abolished and perhaps it is a question that here the respiratory chain is affected by another mechanism, but I have no explanation for this.

Bicher: I really have to congratulate you for your beautiful experiments. From all the neurophysiology that I have seen associated with oxygen, yours are far superior to any. What I especially like is that your figures coincide so well with ours. During hypoxia you get first an increase and then a decrease of EPSP's. Now, what do the IPSP's do?

Bingmann: I do not know the answer at this time.

Zielinski: Did you perform your experiments on buffered animals or not, with cut fibers from chemoreceptors and baroreceptors?

Bingmann: No, the chemoreceptors were not cut, but we did these experiments in the cortex of the brain by stopping the connection.

Zielinski: The animals were decerebrated?

Bingmann: No, but sometimes there was a reversal between the connection of the spinal cord and the cortex which was stopped by cooling it locally at C One. Also, in spinal cord and cortex, we saw the same reactions. The chemoreceptor efferents were going to the brain, and the neurons in the spinal cord were reacting as well as before.

Zielinski: Excuse me, but chemoreceptor and barareceptor information is not going through the spinal cord.

Bingmann: No. If neurons are impaired in the spinal cord and I stop the connection between brain and spinal cord at C One, I have stopped the connection between chemoreceptors and baroreceptors.

Zielinski: It concerns the records taken from spinal cord, but it does not concern records taken from cortex?

Bingmann: They are from spinal cord and from cortex, and both cells show the same behavior. In spinal cord, also after stopping the connection between brain and spinal cord by cooling at C One.

DISCUSSION OF PAPER BY W. J. DORSON, JR. AND B. A. BOGUE

Chance: At the termination of the sinusoidal drive, one would have expected sustained oscillation in view of the natural oscillatory properties of the system. Indeed, spontaneous oscillations might well be a more appropriate drive for the system.

Dorson: We have not, as yet, observed sustained tissue pO_2 oscillations after terminating the induced variations. There were occasional spontaneous oscillations in tissue pO_2 of 0.08 Hz which were not directly related to experimental or respiratory conditions (See Fig. 2). These occurred generally under or after hypoxic conditions and may well have been due to the expected metabolic instability. We hesitate to categorize the manner by which these are obtained until many more improved experiments are performed.

In answer to your second comment, it is axiomatic in the theory of systems analysis that the input signal be varied as the independent parameter. The natural oscillations to which you refer represent part of the response which we wish to determine, and therefore could not be utilized as the drive for the system.

Lübbers: The following of the tissue pO_2 to the arterial pO_2 and consequently also the reaction of the venous pO_2, we have seen in mostly what we call bad animals. In better animals, mostly the tissue has its certain own activity so total circulation is not connected in such a clear way with the microcirculation anymore. You get special local reactions, and the trouble is, with pure locally positioned pO_2 electrodes, you can look in a very small spot so, in normal animals, I wonder if you have any idea if you could get the same good correlations.

Dorson: That last slide was as normal as we have achieved, to date. The preparation problems are quite severe, and we are trying to eliminate as much of the electronics as possible. I really do not know how to answer your question because I do not think we have achieved a perfectly normal cat in this operation.

Lübbers: What was the narcosis you used, the anesthesia?

Dorson: Sodium pentabarbitol. There are a lot of things to be investigated if we are to perfect the system.

Bicher: Your results coincide with ours. On the other hand, I noticed that the waves (tissue and artery pO_2) seem to be 180° out of phase. Can you explain it?

Dorson: Our step responses were similar. These studies also included total flow for theoretical model comparisons. For the oscillations shown, the major lag between tissue and arterial pO_2 was due
to flow. At different flow rates and frequencies, the phasic relation varied from 180°. In tissue traverse experiments, the largest
lag within the tissue was approximately 2 seconds which corresponds
with diffusion models. The cross-correlation would be zero if tissue
(or venous) response was unrelated to the arterial pO_2 wave.

Bruley: Have you considered using pulse testing rather than direct
frequency forcing to obtain the frequency characteristics of the
system?

Dorson: Yes, we have several techniques available to determine
system response independent of model development. We considered
pulse response but felt there might be too many deficiencies with
our experimental procedures, especially in subsequent model comparisons with the data.

DISCUSSION OF PAPER BY W. ERDMANN

Shapiro: Your findings showing a decrease in the tissue oxygen
levels are of some concern when you try and match this to the known
metabolic effects. The barbiturates which are depressant and similar hypothermia have been shown (hypothermia with much more evidence)
actually to protect the brain against anoxia or ischemia, and there
is evidence although scattered over the years, and quite intermittent,
showing that barbiturates might have this effect. I wonder if you
would comment on that.

In addition, I am a little concerned about the fall in blood
pressure that you showed with thiopental. Although it does not go
below the so-called autoregulatory range in unanesthetized patients,
we have here an agent that causes cerebral vasoconstriction. With
the drop in blood pressure, if that agent can override the hypoxic
drive to the vessels, then you may be getting lower pO_2 levels than
you would obtain in another kind of instance.

Thermann: What about your initial values? How deep was the
anesthesia?

Erdmann: We prepared our animals in ether narcosis, then we gave
them a continuum of the anesthesia. We gave only N_2O anesthesia, and
we think that this is the most harmless anesthetic you can give. We
do not know really the effects of N_2O. That is the problem, but I
told you that the problem is the anesthesia.

Chance: The barbiturates, of course, are all respiratory inhibitors at site one in the mitochondria. Yet, we certainly do a number of controls to insure that the anesthetic levels are far below those levels. I would really like to check with Dr. Shapiro as to whether or not you were referring to such high levels of barbiturate, that they were inhibiting the mitochondrial respiration.

Shapiro: Neilson has done the only work with that, and his levels are not high enough to inhibit.

Chance: We usually do choline controls to insure that the anesthetic does not alter the mitochondrial steady state.

DISCUSSION OF PAPER BY K. KUNZE

Lübbers: The calculation of the oxygen consumption brings with it a certain problem, because the direction of the puncture does not always hit exactly the center of the fiber. For such direction, you should have correct calculations. How can you avoid such errors?

Kunze: That is quite an important question. All measurements have not been taken in the single fibers. If you are in a whole bundle of fibers, and not in the center vertically going through, you would not get this rise of oxygen pressure coming through the axis of the nerve. Because we used only measurements in which we could find this rise of oxygen pressure, I have a certain confirmation for this calculation. And the other point is the agreement with former measurements taken by another method.

Buerk: Did your oxygen profile correspond closely to a theoretical profile based on your calculated oxygen consumption?

Kunze: Yes, it did.

DISCUSSION OF PAPER BY B. CHANCE, N. OSHINO AND T. SUGANO

Bingmann: You found that the EEG was abolished at very low pO_2 levels. In our experiments, the pO_2 in the immediate surrounding of the impaled neurons was found to be much higher when spike generation failed. The structures generating EEG and spikes seem to be not identical. We have to assume that these different structures show a different sensitivity to O_2-deficiency. This is thought to explain partly the discrepancy between both findings.

Chance: I thank you for your suggestions, but wish to point out my previous work with Schoener where we monitored metrazol-induced spiking on the brain cortex and found the same critical level of NADH as with the EEG. So, in spite of the differences of spiking and EEG from the physiological standpoint, they have the same critical O_2 requirements. Thus, it seems necessary to determine what the two methods are measuring. The intracellular location of mitochondria assures that we are measuring intracellular oxygen. The electrode measures extracellular oxygen and very probably the oxygen tension in a somewhat damaged tissue volume.

Lübbers: May I comment to the last question? The trouble is that the brain itself, if it is properly perfused, has gradients in the order of 15 to 20 Torr over a rather short distance. Thirty microns is a distance which easily can be covered by a cell with its dendrites, so it is difficult at the moment to see or look for a method which is able here to give clear-cut results. The microelectrode which was used by Speckman and his associates was a platinum electrode 5 or 10 microns distance from the tip of the recording electrode, so it is mostly sitting on the outside of the cell membrane. Measurements are very carefully done because the tip of the reference pO_2 electrode is very close to the measuring electrode so there is no error possible. It could be that the system itself has an indwelling gradient which you really cannot avoid. Thus, if your measurement has an intracellular indicator, you are integrating more of the cell, and you have a local measurement of pO_2 outside or close to these areas. This could explain some of the difference.

Chance: I agree that there can be quite significant gradients between where the electrode is and where the mitochondria area is. There is a large variety of these neurocyanin dyes. Dr. Larry Cohen has tried 80 of them and this particular one is the one that gives the best results in the squid axon. The data that I indicate here are first trials in cortical tissue and, as far as we can see, it is not extremely damaging to the tissue, but it is not innocent either. The animals 24 hours later, as Dr. Mayevsky shows, are not in as good condition as controls but can be used. They function.

DISCUSSION OF PAPER BY J. D. BALENTINE

Chance: There are two effects of hydrogen peroxide at the mitochondrial level that would be of interest to you; first, the inhibition of energy dependent NAD reduction with succinate as an electron donor; second, the increased generation of H_2O_2 by the mitochondria. These effects occur immediately upon increasing the O_2 pressure.

Balentine: Yes, the next phase of our work should be to determine
what the enlarged mitochondria are actually doing biochemically.
Others have reported similar mitochondrial changes in the liver
and lung following hyperoxia and have interpreted the changes as
"adaptive." However, I think that the enlarged, dense mitochondria
observed in this study of brain are probably undergoing a degenera-
tive alteration because they are being packaged into lysosomes by
autophagy as well as by phagocytosis. Phagocytes appear in the
tissue in 48-72 hours, and endocytose altered mitochondria which
have presumably been released by degenerating dendrites. I would
predict that, if these CNS mitochondria following hyperbaric oxygenation can be isolated and studied appropriately, that one would
find one or both of the effects that you mentioned.

Myers, R. E.: The pattern of pathology in the brain described by
Dr. Balentine as occurring with hyperbaric oxygen exposure has many
similarities to that seen after episodes of total oxygen deficiency
with survival. In both of these situations there occur prominent
lesions of inferior callicilus, nucleus of spinal V, superior olive,
thalamic nuclei, etc. (See Myers, R. E., Two Patterns of Brain
Damage and their Conditions of Occurrence, Am. J. Obstet. Gyncol.,
pg. 241, Jan. 15, 1972.). Thus, both high levels of oxygen and its
total lack lead to about the same damage. In looking at the pattern
of pathology after anoxia there seems to be a relation between the
patterns of pathology generated and the general relative normal
blood flow rates of the various brain regions. That is, the inferior
callicilus, the most vulnerable to injury with total anoxia (in newborn monkeys) is also that brain structure which shows the highest
blood flow rate. Those working with flow rates assume a relation
between flow rates and metabolic rates. If this assumption be true,
then there would seem to be a relation between the relative metabolic
rates of different brain loci and the occurrence of brain injury with
anoxia (and hyperbaric oxygen exposure).

Balentine: In most of the regions of the rat brain that are susceptible to oxygen induced necrosis, the relative oxygen consumption
under normal conditions and the enzymes of oxidative phosphorylation are relatively low (Friede, Topographical Brain Chemistry, Acad.
Press), as compared to the areas susceptible to hypoxia. However,
one would not be surprised if hypoxia and hyperoxia have common
pathophysiologic effects, especially in view of the many enzyme
alterations and the varied vascular effect of both conditions. One
cannot compare, though, lesions in newborn animals with those of
adults, because there are different patterns of selective vulner-
abilities to hypoxia and hyperoxia as a function of age, which is
probably a function of different rates of metabolism and/or different
enzyme systems (i.e., newborn brain is more capable of utilizing
anaerobic metabolic pathways than adult).

Penneys: Apropos of Dr. Chance's comment on the effect of hydrogen
peroxide with hyperbaric oxygen, we found a citation in the literature several years ago when we were considering administering hydrogen peroxide intra-arterially in patients with arterial disease of
the extremities, that hydrogen peroxide could be toxic in some
species of mammals because of differences in their catalase systems.
Could this be a pertinent factor in your animal experiments?

Balentine: Yes, catalase could be a factor, but the problem is
complicated by the fact that over 40 enzymes are inhibited by
hyperbaric oxygen. I do not know what the catalase content of the
rat brain is.

DISCUSSION OF PAPER BY R. W. OGILVIE AND J. D. BALENTINE

Holness: Administration of GABA is known to protect against oxygen-
induced convulsions. Has GABA administration ever been considered
in your experiment and in the previous experiment by Dr. Balentine?

Balentine: I have not planned to do any GABA studies at the present.
We are still trying to understand the fundamentals of the basic lesions in the brain as they occur and things like GABA really, I
think, will turn out to be a dose-related phenomenon. I probably
can give enough atmospheres of oxygen to overcome any protective
effect. We really have not gotten into manipulation of the model
with these various protective effects of GABA and a whole host of
other things.

Chance: Did you carry out any experiments under conditions where
you could measure the brain oxygen or the incidence of convulsions?
This would mean lighter anesthesia or electrical recording.

Ogilvie: No, the only time we saw the incidence of convulsions
correlate with the oxygen level changes was just by chance when
we were observing and noticed the seizure and the oxygen going up
simultaneously. We are tuning up for respiratory measurements
and pressure and EEG, and as yet we have not done those.

Silver: The electrodes in your study with tip diameters of 5-10
microns are likely to cause obvious tissue damage and might affect
your results slightly.

Ogilvie: Admittedly, there may be some injury caused by the electrode. As you know, injury is present in almost all biological
experiments but can be relatively reduced and must be judged in
relationship to what one is measuring. We feel, in these experi-

ments, since we were interested in the oxygen tension of a considerably larger area than a single cell or small groups of cells,
that the size of the electrode tip was appropriate. In one experiment done recently, using chloralose as an anesthetic, the oxygen
tissue remained elevated during the entire period of compression.
The different results obtained with nembutal, methane and chloralose
strongly suggest that blood flow is changing in the presence of the
electrode and that factors other than the electrode are responsible
for the change.

DISCUSSION OF PAPER BY J. GROTE AND G. THEWS

Ditzel: It is a very interesting paper and I assume that you have
made this alignment for the clinician. Is that correct?

Grote: That is correct. We did this on the one hand for the clinician, but on the other hand, we have used these nomograms as a basis
for our theoretical calculations of the oxygen partial pressure distribution in different organs.

Ditzel: What should the clinician use this for?

Grote: At first, he is able to get good information about the different respiratory gas parameters in a very short time. He has to
measure two of the five different parameters and can take all the
others from the nomogram.

Wissler: Have you prepared a digital computer program which one
can use instead of the nomograms?

Grote: We plan to do this in the near future. Dr. Bruley and his
co-workers prepared a computer program for the interdependence of
respiratory gas parameters for the conditions of normal base excess
values using the nomograms we published previously (Grote, Anaesthes-
iologic and Wiederbelebung, Vol. 30, 1969.).

Clark, J.: I am confused as to exactly how this differs from the
figures and your nomogram. Is there any difference in information
content between the two?

Grote: There is a difference because at that time we did not know
the correct interrelation between pH and pCO_2 at different base
excess levels. At this point there is a difference, but the oxygen
saturation curve will agree very well with the normal oxygen dissociation curve we all know for pH 7.4; however, there is a little
difference. The oxygen dissociation curve we measured was at con-

stant pCO_2 levels of the different values, but all the other oxygen dissociation curves are measured or are calculated for constant pH, and there is a little difference. The data you will get from the nomogram agrees completely with the so-called normal oxygen dissociation curve of the different pH values.

DISCUSSION OF PAPER BY N. E. NAFTCHI, E. W. LOWMAN, M. BERARD,
     G. H. SELL AND T. REICH

Gelin: I think this was a very beautiful presentation and a very important one. Have you examined the tissue, the bladder tissue, or any tissue below the transected score?

Berard: At present we are in the process of doing this. Most other patients, particularly the quadriplegics, do wind up having TUR's, transurethral receptions, in the process. This tissue has been analyzed in the past and we find that there is a hypertrophy of the ditrusive muscles.

Gelin: I am asking because Dr. Santin and Dr. Dostram in our department have studied the bladder muscle. In that muscle, there is rapid growth of fibers containing a lot of catecholamines. That might be, expecially if it is present also in tissue other than bladder.

Berard: We also feel that the prostate, in the case of the male, may be involved. We have noticed prostate hypertrophy in the rat, for instance, and also to some extent in the human. We are in the process of looking into this area.

DISCUSSION OF PAPER BY J. CASSEL, K. KOGURE, R. BUSTO AND
     D. R. HARKNESS

Lübbers: I did not understand if you have measured the blood flow. The effect of the changed position of the oxygen binding curve can be abolished by increasing the blood flow. Also I would like to know if you have seen any signs of electrical activity.

Cassel: We did not measure the blood flow. But cerebral blood flow is thought to be regulated by hydrogen ion content in the muscle layer of the capillary arteries in addition to the oxygen pressure. Cerebral blood flow becomes a function of arterial pCO_2 tension and oxygen and may be a function of intravascular pH. Those measured and calculated parameters are not changing in our experimental animals. We assume that there is no change in blood flow.

Lübbers: But if the blood flow has changed, then it could explain all your data. With changing blood flow, the oxygen transfer capacity increases, and then you could have, even with the changed oxygen binding curve, perfect tissue oxygenation.

DISCUSSION OF PAPER BY W. K. R. BARNIKOL AND W. WAHLER

Gatz: It has been reported that there are some problems involved in the use of nucleated red blood cells in an apparatus such as you describe (Wood and Moberly, Respir. Physiol., 1971.). Have you used your apparatus to determine the oxygen-hemoglobin dissociation curve on nucleated blood samples such as frog and if so, have you compared your results to those obtained by Van-Slyke techniques?

Barnikol: No, we have not yet used our apparatus to determine the oxygen dissociation curve of nucleated blood samples.

Mochizuki: (1) Did you use only one wavelength or two?
     (2) How did you control the thickness of the blood sample?

Barnikol: (1) We used only one wavelength.
     (2) With this technique, it is not necessary to control the thickness of the blood sample; it must be guaranteed that the thickness remains constant during the measurement. This is controlled by the registration of the extinction.

Subsession: ABDOMINAL ORGANS

Chairmen: Dr. Manfred Kessler, Dr. Jürgen Grote
and Dr. James A. Miller, Jr.

HOMEOSTASIS OF OXYGEN SUPPLY IN LIVER AND KIDNEY[+]

M. Kessler, H. Lang, E. Sinagowitz, R. Rink, and J. Höper
with the technical assistance of
B. Bölling, K. Hájek, K. Horak, D. Schmeling, R. Strehlau,
and U. Tlolka
Max-Planck-Institut für Systemphysiologie
Dortmund, West Germany

Local oxygen supply of liver, pancreas, duodenum and skeletal muscle has been investigated in our laboratory. The histograms of oxygen tension which result from these measurements are relatively uniform and very similar to one another (see also Kunze 1966). Fig. 1 shows a typical histogram of the liver of the anaesthetized, spontaneously respiring rat (Görnandt et al. 1973). The histograms of the other organs mentioned above do not differ substantially. In contrast to these Po_2-distribution curves the histogram of the outer cortex of kidney (Sunder-Plassmann et al. 1973) lies within a higher range of oxygen tension (Fig. 2). This is due to the high functional perfusion rate of kidney.

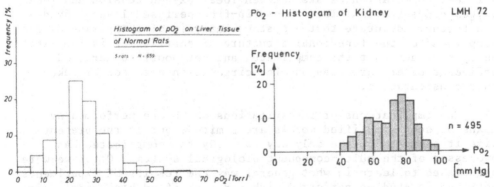

Fig. 1 and 2: Po_2-histograms of liver and of kidney

[+] Supported by Grant of the Landesamt für Forschung of Nordrhein-Westfalen.

When the histogram of Fig. 1 is plotted as a continuous curve (Fig. 3), and when this curve is compared to the dissociation curve of hemoglobin, it becomes evident that under physiological conditions hemoglobin is one of the important factors which greatly influences the oxygen distribution field in tissue (Kessler et al. 1973).

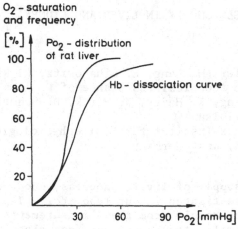

Fig. 3: Comparison between Po_2 distribution curve of rat liver and hemoglobin dissociation curve

In order to eliminate the non-linear part of the slope of oxygen tension which is seen when hemoglobin containing medium passes through the sinusoid, we developed a new model of a hemoglobin-free perfused rat liver. In the hemoglobin-free model a linear correlation exists between local oxygen tension and local oxygen concentration. The hemoglobin-free perfused liver provides the further advantage that a systems analysis of the tissue oxygen supply and of the functional structure of capillaries is facilitated by the fact that the complicated and yet poorly understood influence of erythrocytes on microcirculation need not be taken into consideration.

The implications of investigations which are performed by means of such simplified models are limited, but at the present time it seems to be the only way to study the complicated basic processes of the multi-component biological systems. Often we were astonished to learn in what general way the results of experiments obtained in studies performed with our simplified biological model can be applied for the interpretation of in situ measurements.

In our first investigations on the isolated and hemoglobin-free perfused rat liver we obtained distribution curves of tissue oxygen tension which indicated that microcirculation was disturbed (Fig. 4). The Po_2 distribution curves were very irregular and showed many low values. The group between 0-25 mmHg and between

0-5 mmHg (black pillars) increased drastically when the flow was
decreased below 2.2 ml/g/min. An increase of perfusion flow to
3.0-3.4 ml/g/min did not cause a significant shift of the distribution curve to the right, as was expected, but only induced an
increase of venous Po_2.(The little triangles mark the venous Po_2).

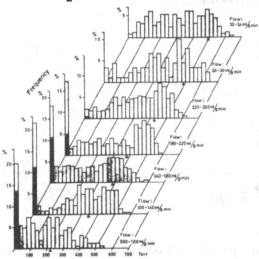

Fig. 4: Po_2 distribution of hemoglobin-free perfused rat liver
        (27 g/l albumin)

Consequently we tried to improve our perfusion model by
modifications of several parameters which are listed in Table 1.
The Po_2 distribution curve which results from the improved perfusion model demonstrates the benefit of these modifications
(Fig. 5).

Hemoglobin-free liver perfusion

	27 g/l	35 g/l
albumin	27 g/l	35 g/l
perfusion pressure	20 cm H_2O	14 cm H_2O
equilibration with CO_2	0 %	5 %
$NaHCO_3$	12 mM/l	35 mM/l

The Po_2 distribution curve became much more regular, and the
low Po_2 values disappeared. It was surprising, however, that the
venous Po_2 remained high.

This improved model can be perfused over a period of five
hours without causing appreciable damage. After five hours of
perfusion all functional tests are unchanged and the morphological
analysis which was performed by means of electron microscopy

shows only slight edema of the Golgi apparatus (Schäfer et al. 1972).

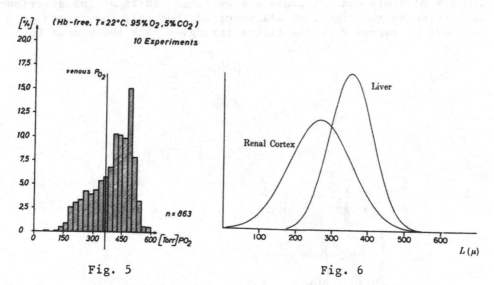

Fig. 5   Fig. 6

Fig. 5: Po_2 distribution of perfused rat liver after improvement of technique

Fig. 6: Distribution curve of capillary length of liver and of renal cortex

By means of morphometric measurements we tried to determine whether a diffusion shunt from influent to effluent vessels could occur. The distances between 200-500 u which we found (we appreciate the kind help of Dr. Seidl of our Institute) indicate that only a small amount of oxygen can pass by direct diffusion shunt from the influent to the effluent. During our morphometric studies we realized that the length of the hepatic sinusoids differs very much. Our observations were confirmed by the careful investigations of Suwa and Takahashi (1971). In various organs such as liver and kidney they found an inhomogeneous distribution of capillary length (Fig. 6).

When we analyze the oxygen supply of various organs (liver, pancreas, small intestine, and skeletal muscle) under physiological conditions, we always observe that the venous Po_2 bears no relation to the low oxygen tensions in tissue. Usually more than 50 % of the Po_2 values which are measured in the tissues are considerably lower than the venous Po_2. These observations suggested the hypothesis that the inhomogeneous distribution of capillary length in tissues might cause an inhomogeneous distribution of the flow pattern in the capillaries. Consequently, this would mean that the venous oxygen tension, or the venous oxygen saturation, might be a mixed value.

In a first step we tried to calculate the sinusoidal flow of
our perfused model as a function of the sinusoidal length. For our
calculations, which were based on the law of Hagen and Poiseulle,
we used the frequency distribution of sinusoidal length of Suwa
and Takahashi. Fig. 7 shows that under these assumptions the
microflow in the very short sinusoids is higher by a factor of
2.5 than in the very long sinusoids. Subsequently, we tried to
estimate the venous Po_2 of the different types of sinusoids. We
assumed that the Po_2 at the venous end of the longest sinusoids
corresponds to the lowest values of the Po_2 histogram. Then a
ΔPo_2 of A = 475 mmHg results (Fig. 8). As we know the length of
the longest sinusoids, the ΔPo_2 and the venous Po_2 of the others
can be calculated too.

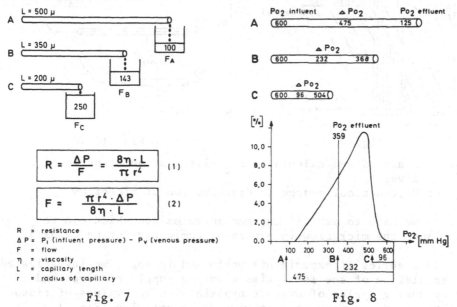

$$R = \frac{\Delta P}{F} = \frac{8\eta \cdot L}{\pi \, r^4} \quad (1)$$

$$F = \frac{\pi \, r^4 \cdot \Delta P}{8\eta \cdot L} \quad (2)$$

R = resistance
ΔP = P_i (influent pressure) – P_v (venous pressure)
F = flow
η = viscosity
L = capillary length
r = radius of capillary

Fig. 7   Fig. 8

Fig. 7: Microflow as a function of the length of sinusoids
Fig. 8: Calculated venous Po_2 of different sinusoids

When we combine the calculated venous Po_2 values and the
calculated values of microflow, we are able to estimate a mixed
venous Po_2 of 370 mmHg as compared to an experimentally determined
value of 359 mmHg. In a similar way the Po_2 histogram of the
hemoglobin-free perfused liver was calculated. Fig. 9 shows the
curves which were determined experimentally and theoretically, and
it is surprising how close the relation is between the two curves.

Summarizing these results we come to the conclusion that in
partial hypoxia and anoxia a very uneconomic situation would exist,
if the distribution of microflow could not change. Practically, it
would mean that in short sinusoids a luxurious flow would exist,

whereas at the end of the long sinusoids the cells would suffer
from oxygen deficiency (Fig. 10).

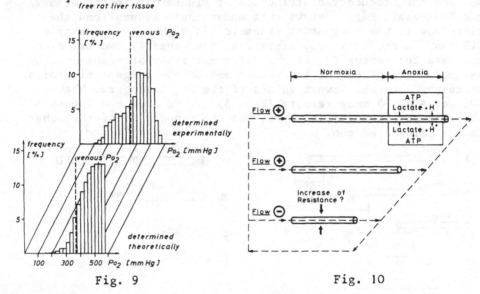

Fig. 9   Fig. 10

Fig. 9: Measured and calculated Po$_2$ distribution of perfused rat
        liver.
Fig.10: Hypothetical change in distribution of microflow

So we have to ask, if any mechanism exists which can re-
distribute the microflow in a more economic way during hypoxia.

    In a series of experiments performed in dogs, we investigated
the regulation of the local tissue oxygen supply of liver and of
kidney during cycles of hypoxic hypoxia. The Po$_2$ values of tissue
were recorded by means of multiwire Po$_2$ electrodes (Fig. 11). It
can be seen that after a change to 10% oxygen which corresponds to
an altitude of about 16,500 feet, a rapid decrease in Po$_2$ results,
and oscillations of mean arterial pressure begin to appear. Fig. 12
shows an evaluation of these Po$_2$ measurements. As was mentioned
above, the hemoglobin causes a non linear slope of oxygen tension
along the sinusoids. In order to produce a more linear relation
for our analysis, we used the local Po$_2$ values of tissue and tried
to estimate the local oxygen saturation by means of the dissociation curve of the dog (Bartels et al. 1959). As the local Po$_2$
gradient from the capillary to the tissue was unknown, it was not
taken into consideration. Therefore, the evaluation contains a
systematic error which can produce an absolute deviation between
the single values of about 10%. Nevertheless, we think that these
first results are very informative. In fact, they show that in
liver there is no parallel shift of the local values when arterial

oxygen saturation is decreased from 98 to 74 %. This indicates
that the distribution of microflow probably changes in the sinusoids
under the conditions of hypoxic hypoxia. In this context it should
be mentioned that in liver no flow dependant oxygen uptake can be
observed unless the blood flow falls short of its critical value.

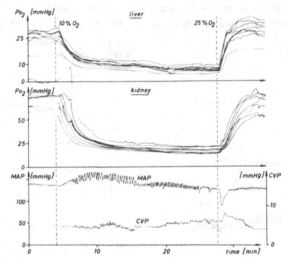

Fig. 11: Cycle of hypoxic hypoxia in dog

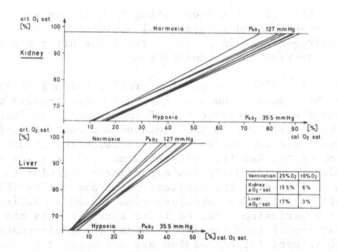

Fig. 12: Correlation between arterial saturation and calculated
         local hemoglobin saturation

In kidney the situation is less clear than in liver. When the
animal is respired with 10% oxygen the renal blood flow (RBF)
starts to oscillate and can increase as well as decrease during

the initial period of hypoxia (Fig. 13). In contrast to this,
deeper hypoxia (5% O_2) always causes a distinct decrease of RBF.
Since it is well known that the oxygen uptake of the kidney is
greatly influenced by RBF, it is not yet possible to define the
meaning of the shift of local Po_2 and of local oxygen saturation
which can be observed in the kidney during a hypoxic episode.
Further investigations with measurements of local oxygen uptake
and of local microflow will enable us to solve this problem.

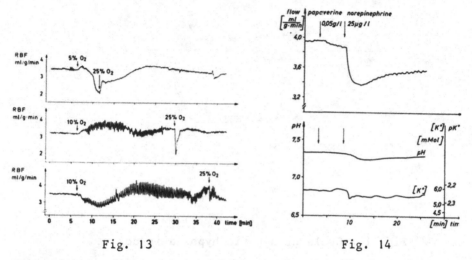

Fig. 13   Fig. 14

Fig. 13: Blood flow of dog kidney during hypoxic hypoxia
Fig. 14: Flow reaction and interstitial activity of potassium and
         of hydrogen ions in perfused rat liver after application
         of papaverine and norepinephrine

        Changes in the distribution of microflow which seem to be
initiated in the hepatic sinusoids during hypoxic hypoxia may be
partially caused by the contraction of smooth muscles. Investigations which were performed in the isolated and hemoglobin-free
perfused liver indicate, however, that cellular reactions of the
hepatocytes or of the Kupffer cells also may induce changes in the
pattern of microflow. In perfusion experiments vascular smooth
muscles were inhibited by the application of papaverine (Fig. 14).
The subsequent injection of norepinephrine caused a distinct
decrease of the perfusion rate. As it is shown in this example,
small oscillations of flow can appear under these circumstances.
Very often these oscillations of flow are accompanied by oscillations
of intracellular NADH fluorescence. We also found changes in the
interstitial activity of potassium and hydrogen ions. All these
observations indicate that cellular reactions are induced by
norepinephrine in spite of the application of papaverine or of
other vasodilating drugs. Consequently, there is some evidence
that the microflow of liver is influenced by cellular factors. A

conceivable mechanism which might influence the microflow could
be the active shift of water into the cells caused by ionic gradients.
Of course, the latter would be an energy consuming process. An
ionic gradient of 0.5-1.0 mM between the cell and the extracellular
space would cause a difference of the osmotic pressure of about
10 mmHg.

SUMMARY

1. The variation in the length of the sinusoids causes an
inhomogeneous distribution of microflow in the liver.
2. In experiments in dogs we have obtained some preliminary
evidence that in hypoxia a change in the distribution of microcirculation may occur.
3. Investigations in isolated perfused rat livers indicate that
not only the contraction of vascular smooth muscles but also
cellular reactions may effect sinusoidal microflow.

REFERENCES

1. Bartels, H. and Harms, H.: Sauerstoffdissoziationskurven des
   Blutes von Säugetieren. Pflügers Arch. ges. Physiol. 268,
   334 (1959).

2. Görnandt, L. and Kessler, M.: Po$_2$ histograms in regenerating
   liver tissue. In: Oxygen in tissue, ed. by M. Kessler,
   D.F. Bruley, L.C. Clark, D.W. Lübbers, I.A. Silver and
   J. Strauss, p. 288. Urban & Schwarzenberg München-Berlin-Wien
   1973.

3. Kessler, M., Görnandt, L. and Lang, H.: Correlation between
   oxygen tension in tissue and hemoglobin dissociation curve.
   p. 156. Ibid.

4. Kunze, K.: Die lokale kontinuierliche Sauerstoffmessung in der
   menschlichen Muskulatur. Pflügers Arch. ges. Physiol. 292,
   151 (1966).

5. Sunder-Plassmann, L., Sinagowitz, E., Rink, R., Dieterle, R.,
   Meßmer, K. and Kessler, M.: The local oxygen supply in
   tissue of abdominal viscera and of skeletal muscle in extreme
   hemodilution with stromafree hemoglobin solution.
   This Symposium.

6. Schäfer, D., Höper, J., Starlinger, H. and Kessler, M.:
   Influence of different perfusion media on ultrastructure and
   function of perfused liver. Pflügers Arch. ges. Physiol.
   335 (Suppl.), R 34 (1972).

7. Suwa, N. and Takahashi, T.: Morphological and morphometrical
   analysis of circulation in hypertension and ischemic kidney.
   Ed. by F. Büchner. Urban & Schwarzenberg München-Berlin-Wien
   1971.

TISSUE PO_2 LEVELS IN THE LIVER OF WARM AND COLD RATS ARTIFICIALLY RESPIRED WITH DIFFERENT MIXTURES OF O_2 AND CO_2

James A. Miller, Jr. and Manfred Kessler with assistance of Dietgard Schmeling

Tulane University, School of Medicine and Max-Planck-Institut für Systemphysiologie, Dortmund, West Germany

INTRODUCTION

Studies by Giaja, Andjus, Smith and others demonstrated clearly that when animals are cooled in sealed vessels while being exposed to decreasing oxygen and increasing CO_2 levels, they can be reanimated in 90-100% of the cases from body temperatures near $0^{\circ}C$. Both hypoxia and hypercapnia were found to contribute significantly to the success of the technique (3). Lewis, using artificial respiration with 95% O_2+5% CO_2 or 90% O_2+10%CO_2 concluded that it was impossible to resuscitate mammals at $10^{\circ}C$ or less unless CO_2 was used (2).

In addition, newborn animals which had been cooled in the presence of hypoxia and hypercapnia were more tolerant of asphyxia than were littermates which had been cooled to the same temperature while breathing air (5). Hypoxia-hypercapnia largely counteracted the generalized arterial vasoconstriction found in animals cooled to less than $20^{\circ}C$. In puppies, which had been cooled to $15^{\circ}C$ while breathing air, there was a 50% reduction in blood volume of the heads whereas no reduction was seen in littermates that had been cooled while breathing 10% O_2 and 5% CO_2 (5). These and other data all indicate that high blood O_2 levels tend to produce vasoconstriction whereas elevated CO_2 levels tend to increase blood flow to tissues. However, there has never been a complete analysis of the relative rôles of O_2 and of CO_2 in this situation.

With the development of multiple oxygen electrode units (1) it was possible to measure actual tissue Po_2 levels on the surface of intact, undamaged livers of rats which were artificially respired with different mixtures of O_2 and CO_2 while coenothermic[+] or hypothermic (to $15^{\circ}C$).

[+] (Coenothermic = normothermic or euthermic, but is the preferred term, (4)).

RESULTS IN COENOTHERMIC RATS

Figure 1, from our first experiment, shows the results of breathing 100% O_2, 95% O_2+5% CO_2 and 92.6% O_2+7.4% CO_2 on the mean tissue Po_2 of the liver of a rat. As seen on the graph, increasing the CO_2 percentages caused increasingly high liver Po_2 levels. This type of result was seen in all experiments including those in which CO_2 levels were increased to 30% or higher.

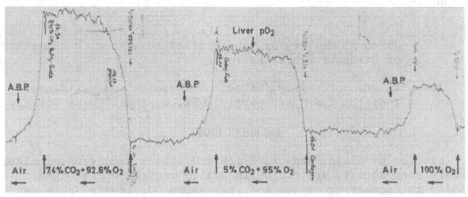

Fig. 1

Table I summarizes the entire experiment and illustrates the fact that 10% CO_2 (+ 90% O_2) increased the Po_2 levels four times more than did breathing 100% O_2. The final re-exposure to 95% O_2 + 5% CO_2 with a two times increase, demonstrated that there had been no change in responsiveness of the animal during the experiment.

Table I
Effects of CO_2 on Rat Liver Po_2

Gas	Increase (Torr)	% of Increase by 100% O_2
100% O_2	10.8	100%
5% CO_2+95% O_2	21.1	195%
7.4%CO_2+92.6%O_2	33.8	313%
10%CO_2+90%O_2	43.4	402%
5%CO_2+95%O_2	21.7	201%

In Figure 2 are seen the effects of alternating 10 minute pulses of air and of 10%, 15%, 20%, 25%, 30%, 35%, 40% and 50% CO_2, with the remainder of the gas being O_2. Variations in O_2 between 90% and 60%, appeared to have little influence on liver Po_2; however, regular stepwise increases were seen with CO_2 increases up to 40% CO_2.

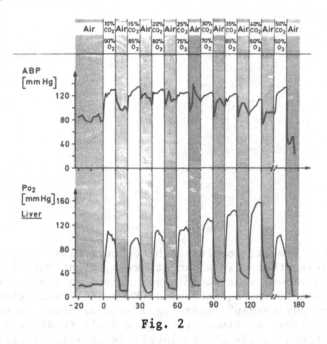

Fig. 2

The blood pressure records showed a rapid drop in blood
pressure in each case immediately after the onset of air breathing. This was followed by a rapid recovery which, in the period
following the exposure to 25% CO_2, produced a large overshoot.
Heart rate varied between 300 and 500 excepting as indicated below.
It rose each time the high O_2+CO_2 mixtures were used and fell during air breathing. Cardiac irregularities were seen during air-
breathing following 25% CO_2 and following each of the higher exposures also. In two instances cardiac massage was administered.
Upon reexposure to an O_2+CO_2 mixture these cardiac problems resolved themselves. When, in later experiments, blood pH was controlled
with infusions of THAM, the cardiac problems likewise were
controlled.

In this experiment oxygen in the inspired air decreased with
each increase in CO_2. In the next experiment the O_2 levels in the
mixtures were kept at 70% and only CO_2 was varied. Thus the rat was
artificially respired alternately with 15 minute pulses of air and
of 70% O_2 mixed either with 0% CO_2+30% N_2, 10% CO_2+20%N_2, 20% CO_2+
10% N_2 or with 30% CO_2. The tissue Po_2 readings were recorded
separately for each electrode. Figure 3 illustrates the possible
locations of the electrodes with reference to the source of the
oxygenated blood in the liver lobules. The records of electrodes
No 1 through 8 on Figure 3 are similarly numbered on Figure 4.

From several points of view the most interesting results were
obtained when the individual electrodes were recorded separately.

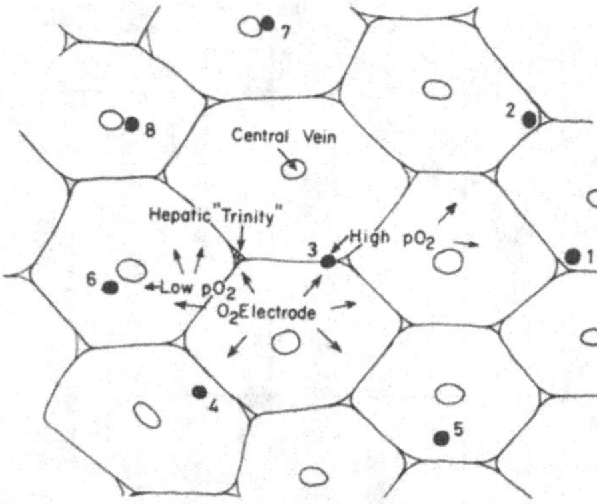

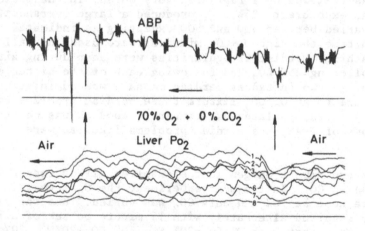

Fig. 3

These showed that several lobules might be controlled by a single
mechanism, whereas others, in adjacent areas, might vary independently. They also showed that the highest recording electrodes responded first when liver Po_2 increased (Figs.5+6). This observation
tends to confirm our concept regarding electrode position with reference to liver lobules. Since, in Figure 3 electrode No 1 is the
closest to the blood supply of its lobule (a hepatic "trinity"),
it would be the first to receive any increase in blood flow that
might occur.

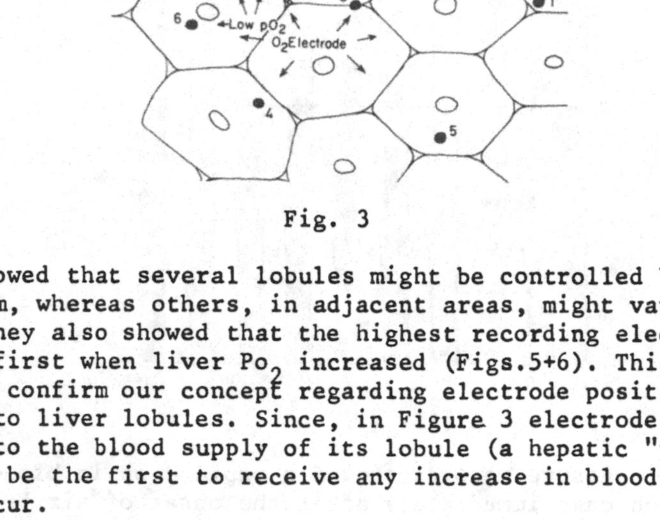

Fig. 4

Figure 4 shows that 70% O_2 alone caused a moderate increase
in tissue Po_2 in the sites which were better oxygenated while breathing air. However, site 7 showed little and site 8 showed no response. The rising record for arterial blood pressure suggests
that progressive vasoconstriction was taking place. With the re-

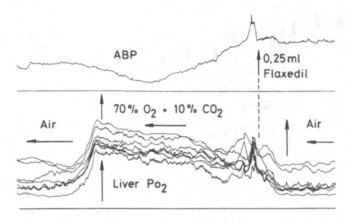

Fig. 5

introduction of air the blood pressure fell. The diminished amplitude of the oscillations suggests that vasomotor activity also decreased during air breathing.

The addition of CO_2 to 70% O_2 produced striking changes in
liver Po_2 (Figs. 5,6 and 7). There was a prompt, rapid increase
at all sites to levels which depended upon the CO_2 concentration.
In addition, the rates of oscillations in the individual records
increased markedly and blood pressure first fell but later regulated. The initial fall is evidence for generalized vasodilation in
response to high CO_2 of the inspired air.

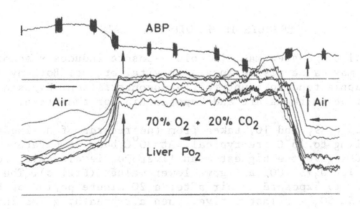

Fig. 6

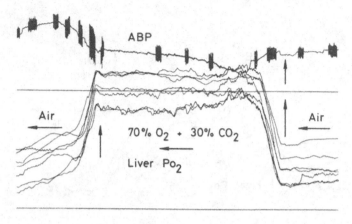

Fig. 7

When flaxedil was given in sufficient quantities to paralyze spontaneous respiration, the tissue Po_2 was not reduced. This shows that the elevated liver Po_2 levels were not related to respiratory effort.

Breathing CO_2 lowered blood pH levels, however, when acid-base disturbances were controlled by infusion of THAM, the tissue Po_2 levels remained high. Thus, elevating blood pH levels did not change tissue Po_2. We have no information on tissue pH levels in these experiments. The results of the THAM treatment suggest that the Bohr effect played a minor role in our results. If it had been significant there would have been a drop in tissue Po_2 with the rise in pH during the THAM infusion; instead it remained unchanged.

RESULTS IN HYPOTHERMIC RATS

In well oxygenated mammals cold exposure induces vasoconstriction which may cause tissue anoxia in vital organs. Both hypoxia and hypercapnia tend to counteract vasoconstriction. Hypoxia is more effective in the heart and hypercapnia for the brain.

Figures 8, 9, and 10, taken from the records of a single rat during cooling to $15^{\circ}C$ are typical. At $30^{\circ}C$ body temperature 15% O_2+5% CO_2 gave the highest mean liver Po_2 levels. Air, 20% O_2+ 5% CO_2 and 10% O_2+5% CO_2 all gave lower values (Fig. 8). The response of liver Po_2 to exposure to air after a 20 minute period of breathing 10% O_2+5% CO_2 was instructive. When air-breathing was introduced, there was a sudden increase in liver Po_2 in response to doubling the volume of oxygen. As CO_2 was blown off by the artificial

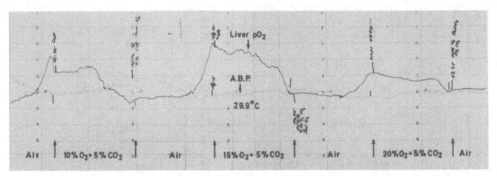

Fig. 8

ventilation, vasoconstriction developed, blood pressure rose and liver Po_2 fell steeply. At $21^\circ C$ liver temperature $10\%O_2+20\%$ CO_2 gave the highest liver Po_2 levels (nearly 30 Torr) in spite of very low blood pressure levels (25-40 mmHg) (Fig. 9).

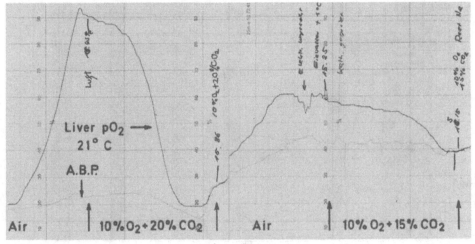

Fig. 9

At $15^\circ C$ body temperature even 10% O_2 mixtures failed to increase liver Po_2 levels but 5% O_2 when combined with high CO_2 levels again produced Torr values near 30 (Fig. 10).

When a rat is at $30^\circ C$ body temperature, the air contains too much O_2 and an inadequate supply of CO_2 for maintainence of liver Po_2 levels at or above 20 mmHg (Fig. 11). When the gas mixture was shifted to 10% $O_2+15\%$ CO_2, liver Po_2 levels rose to nearly 30 mmHg.

Then, upon exposure to circulating icewater, the liver Po_2 levels dropped steeply to near zero as cold-induced vasoconstriction

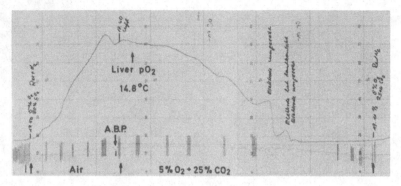

Fig. 10

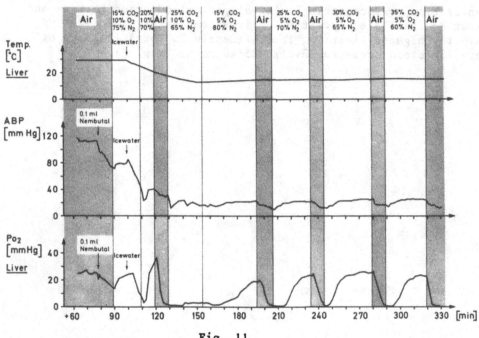

Fig. 11

developed. At this point the CO_2 in the inspired air was increased
to 20%, and liver Po_2 rose precipitously to over 30 mmHg. It fell
even more precipitously to less than 5 mmHg upon reintroduction of
air into the respirator. By this time the animal's body temperature
had reached 17°C and even 10% O_2+25% CO_2 was ineffective in elevating liver Po_2. By contrast 5% O_2+15% CO_2 restored liver Po_2 to
20 mmHg, and breathing air again caused a precipitous fall in Po_2.
By keeping the same level of oxygen (5%) in the inspired air it was
found that 25% CO_2 was more effective than was 15% and that 30% CO_2
gave the highest liver Po_2 readings. Again, each time air was used
there was a precipitous fall in liver oxygenation (Fig. 11).

Arterial blood pressure fell to low levels during cooling. Although it fell with each period of air breathing, and increased with exposure to low O_2 + high CO_2, it is important to appreciate the fact that the amplitudes of these changes were small, particularly when compared with the liver Po_2 changes.

The O_2 requirements of mammals are reduced to approximately 25% of normal by lowering body temperature to $15°C$. Accordingly, if liver Po_2 measurements are characteristic for other vital organs, there is no necessity for the maintenance of high arterial blood pressure at this temperature. If vasoconstriction is prevented, blood pressures in the range of less then 10 mmHg can give ample tissue oxygenation.

DISCUSSION

Since arterial blood is more than 95% saturated while breathing air, the opportunities for increasing tissue Po_2 levels by increasing the oxygen which is inspired are limited. Even 100% O_2 produces only a small increase in liver Po_2. In addition, O_2 has the unfortunate propensity of causing vasoconstriction which can produce disastrous sequelae, as was discovered when prematures were exposed to 100% O_2. CO_2, however, is the naturally occurring vasodilator, whose efficacy in increasing liver Po_2 has been demonstrated in these experiments. If tissue Po_2 levels should be raised, should not the CO_2 content of the inspired air be increased rather than merely the O_2 content?

There are a number of conditions in which central lobular necrosis may occur. Since the area around the central vein is exposed to the lowest Po_2 levels in the lobule, local hypoxia is a possible complication in these situations. Because elevated CO_2 increased Po_2 levels strikingly from all sites from which records were taken, this study suggests that pulses of CO_2 exposure might be of benefit in many conditions in which liver hypoxia or central lobular necrosis is threatened.

The studies during cooling and at $15°C$ body temperature show that artificial respiration with high levels of oxygen generates tissue hypoxia. During cooling, first 20% O_2 produces vasoconstriction, then 15% O_2, and finally, at $15°C$ body temperautre, even 10% O_2. At the same time, as temperature falls, CO_2 becomes less and less effective in counteracting vasoconstriction, until at $15°C$ 30% was required to increase the mean Po_2 in the liver to 20-30 Torr. It is suggested that some of the problems encountered during the clinical applications of hypothermia are related to O_2 excess during artificial respiration at reduced body temperatures.

SUMMARY

1. As measured in the liver, pulses of breathing mixtures with elevated CO_2 cause great increases in tissue Po_2 levels. This fact may have significance in the treatment of conditions involving liver hypoxia or central lobular necrosis.

2. During cooling the highest liver Po_2 levels are achieved by reducing the O_2 in the inspired air and increasing the CO_2. In the rat at $15^{o}C$ the maximal levels were found with 5% O_2 and 30% CO_2.

REFERENCES

1. Kessler, M., and Grunewald, W.: Possibilities of measuring oxygen pressure field in tissue by multiwire platinum electrodes. Progr. Resp. Res. 3, 147-152 (Karger, Basel-NewYork) (1969)

2. Lewis, F.J.: Hypothermia. Surg. Gynecol. & Obstet. 113, 307-336 (1961)

3. Miller, J.A.,Jr., and Miller, F.S.: Factors contributing to the successful reanimation of mice cooled to less than $1^{o}C$. Am. J. Physiol. 196, 1218-1223 (1959)

4. Miller, J.A.,Jr.: Coenothermia and mesothermia, two new terms for physiologists. The Physiologist 9, 123-125 (1966)

5. Miller, J.A.,Jr.: New approaches to preventing brain damage during asphyxia. Am. J. Obstet. Gynecol. 110, 1125-1133 (1971)

PRESERVATION OF ATP IN THE PERFUSED LIVER

Jens Höper, Manfred Kessler, Hilde Starlinger

Max-Planck-Institut für Arbeitsphysiologie Dortmund

In recent years we investigated anaerobic glycolysis in isolated perfused rat livers. For these experiments we used the perfusion model described by Kessler (2) and Lang (3). After a short initial ischemia associated with preparation of the organ we perfused the liver with an O_2-saturated medium for 30 min, then for one hour with a N_2-saturated medium.

The experiments showed that it was possible to perfuse an isolated rat liver with an oxygen free medium for one hour without development of edema and without significant release of intra-cellular potassium. ATP-determinations in these organs showed that during one hour of anoxia there was only a small decrease of ATP-level (Fig. 1).

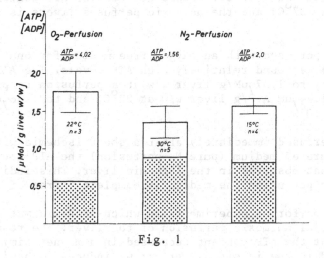

Fig. 1

371

In contrast to these results it is well known that during
ischemia the ATP-levels of liver tissue decrease rapidly. Krebs (1)
and coworkers as well as ourselves found that the ATP-levels decrease
in 4-5 min to 1/4 of the normal values (Fig. 2). The curve indicates
the results of our ATP determinations. The values which are desig-
nated by a circle were found by Krebs (1).

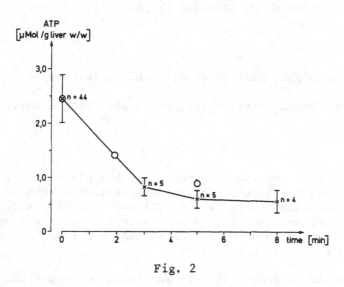

Fig. 2

Fig. 3 shows the results of ATP determinations under different
conditions. The values which are connected by straight lines were
found under similar perfusion conditions but at different perfusion
temperatures. The upper line connects the values we found under
normoxic conditions. The difference between the ATP content in the
in situ liver (37°C) and the normoxic perfused livers is caused by
temperature.

When we perfused with an oxygen free medium for one hour
(middle line) we found relatively high ATP levels. The ATP content
decreased only to 1.57 uM/g liver w/w at a perfusion temperature
of 15°C, to 1.44 uM ATP/g liver w/w at 22°C, and to 1.36 uM ATP/g
liver w/w at 30°C.

If we perfused immediately after a short ischemia with a
nitrogen saturated medium (pure N_2-perfusion) the ATP content was
similar to that observed in the ischemic liver. This indicates that
during anoxic perfusion the medium is completely free of oxygen.

We also performed experiments in which ischemia was induced
after an initial normoxic perfusion of the liver. The results
indicated that the ATP content decreased in a manner similar to
that observed in the in situ liver. If we induced ischemia in the

22°C normoxic perfused liver the ATP content decreased from 1.76 uM ATP/g liver w/w to 0.67 uM ATP/g liver w/w. When we induced ischemia at 30°C we found a similar value (0.57 uM ATP/g liver w/w, lower line). Note that there is a large difference between the ATP content after 1 hour of anoxia (middle line) and 10 min of ischemia (lower line).

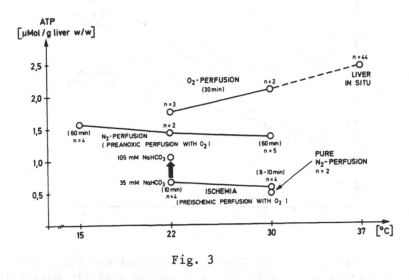

Fig. 3

During these experiments we also measured the pH of liver tissue with pH needle electrodes and with pH surface electrodes. We found that during anoxia, when a large amount of well buffered perfusate was used, the pH decreased only to 7.3. By contrast, it decreased during ischemia to about 7 when there was only about 2 ml medium in the vessels.

In consideration of a possible pH effect on the changes in ATP content we increased the bicarbonate content of the medium from 35 mM/l to 105 mM/l. With this medium the pH decreased only to 7.25, and the ATP content remained much higher (1.06 uM/g liver w/w) during 10 min of ischemia (22°C). The difference between the ATP-content under the conditions of a medium containing 35 mM NaHCO3 and a medium containing 105 mM NaHCO3 is more than 60 %.

From the results of our pH-measurements and ATP determinations we suspected that the acidosis had caused a depolarisation of the cell membranes. In order to test our assumption we measured interstitial potassium ion activity with a valinomycin electrode and sodium ion activity with an orion sodium electrode. During ischemia we found an increase in interstitial potassium ion activity and a decrease in sodium ion activity. Fig. 4 shows the increase of potassium ion activity in two typical experiments. If we used a medium containing 35 mM NaHCO3/l (continuous line) the potassium

ion activity increased from 5.5 mM/l to 13.9 mM/l. If we used a
medium containing 105 mM/l bicarbonate it increased only to 9.2 mM/l
(dashed line). In both cases the decrease of the sodium ion activity
was the reciprocal of the changes in potassium.

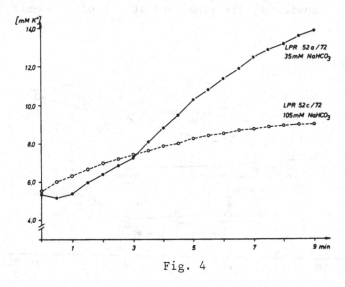

Fig. 4

From the results of the ATP determinations and the measurements of
the ionic changes we suggest that the severe acidosis during ischemia
causes an increase in membrane permeability. This induces a shift
of sodium and potassium ions. The ionic changes produce an
acceleration of the sodium potassium pump which rapidly utilizes
ATP.

From additional experiments we suggest that there is another
unknown factor which influences the membrane permeability during
ischemia. When the pH of the medium of an oxygen free perfused
organ is decreased to 6.5 no significant change in interstitial
potassium ion activity or in the ATP content is observed. This
indicates that disturbances which are found during ischemia cannot
be caused only by the increase in interstitial hydrogen ion activity.

During anoxic perfusion we suggest the metabolism is partially
inhibited by reduction of the hydrogen transferring coenzymes.
Under these conditions the relatively smaller energy requirement
is compensated by anaerobic glycolysis. Because we have a large
amount of well buffered medium there is only a very small degree
of acidosis and the permeability of the cell membranes is not
influenced. These results show that it is possible for the isolated
rat liver to maintain its integrity under conditions of insufficient
oxygen supply if the organ is well perfused with a medium buffered
sufficiently to prevent severe acidosis.

It seems possible that organs in situ are also able to tolerate a short period of local anoxia (4,5). During the latter state, when lactate and other acids are eliminated by the circulating blood, anaerobic glycolysis is a benefical mechanism to compensate the energy requirement. By contrast, in ischemia when the acids accumulate the cells are destroyed by their own products.

REFERENCES

1. Brosnan, J.T., Krebs, H.A., Williamson, D.H.: Effects of ischemia on metabolite concentrations in rat liver. Biochem. J. <u>117</u>, 91-96 (1970).

2. Kessler, M.: Normale und kritische Sauerstoffversorgung der Leber bei Normo- und Hypothermie. Habilitationsschrift, Marburg/Lahn, 1968.

3. Lang, H.: Die Regulation der Lactat- und Pyruvatkonzentrationen durch die hämoglobinfrei perfundierte Leber bei unterschiedlichen CO_2- und O_2-Drucken. Dissertation, Bochum 1970.

4. Schmahl, F.W., Betz, E., Dettinger, E., Hohorst, H.J.: Energiestoffwechsel der Großhirnrinde und Elektroencephalogramm bei Sauerstoffmangel. Pflügers Archiv. <u>292</u>, 46-59 (1966).

5. Schindler, U., Gärtner, E., Betz, E.: Energy-rich metabolites and EEG in hypoxia and in hypercapnia. This Symposium.

Acknowledgement

These studies were performed with the excellent technical assistance of Miss U. Tlolka and Mrs. H. Sauerwald.

INFLUENCE OF HEMOGLOBIN CONCENTRATION IN PERFUSATE
AND IN BLOOD ON FLUORESCENCE OF PYRIDINE NUCLEOTIDES
(NADH AND NADPH) OF RAT LIVER

Herbert Rahmer and Manfred Kessler
with the technical assistance of Karin Hájek

Max-Planck-Institut für Arbeitsphysiologie
Dortmund, West Germany

Measurements of pyridine nucleotide fluorescence (NADH and
NADPH) provide information about changes in intracellular redox
state as we know from Chance and other investigators (1,2,3,7,8,9).
In vivo measurements are greatly influenced by light absorption of
hemoglobin which produces a filter effect in tissue (2,5,6). In
order to quantify this effect we used the isolated perfused rat
liver as a model. The hemoglobin concentration was changed by
addition of washed bovine erythrocytes to the perfusion medium. Our
technical equipment enabled us to investigate changes of the
fluorescence of pyridine nucleotides and changes of the local
hemoglobin concentration and the local oxygenation in tissue by a
simultaneous fluorescence and reflectance measurement.

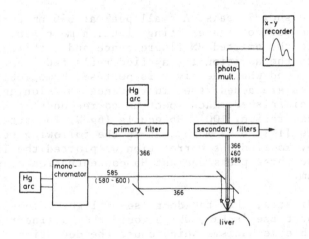

Fig. 1. Schematic diagram of fluorometer.

Methods: Fig. 1 shows our technical equipment (4). PN fluorescence in liver is excited by a mercury arc lamp and a Schott interference filter with maximal transmission at 366 nm. For reflectance measurement of relative hemoglobin concentration and oxygenation we applied light in the range of 585 nm. This light was produced by a second mercury arc lamp and a monochromator. Both lights were coaxially guided to the organ surface by an ultropac objective. The combined spectrum of the emitted fluorescence and the reflected light is scanned by Schott interference filters and recorded by an X-Y recorder. The spectra we obtained with this method are shown in Fig. 2.

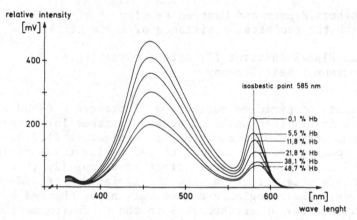

Spectra of emitted fluorescence light and of reflected light at different hemoglobin contents measured in rat liver perfused with erythrocytes.
PN fluorescence is excited at 366 nm; reflected light is used at 580-600 nm.

Fig. 2

The spectra show 3 peaks. A small peak at 366 nm corresponding to the reflected part of the exciting light, a mean peak at 460 nm corresponding to the emitted PN fluorescence and a third peak corresponding to the additionally applied reflected light. The upper spectrum is obtained when the liver is perfused hemoglobinfree. When erythrocytes are added, the fluorescence emission and also the reflectance is diminished. Each spectrum corresponds to a certain hemoglobin concentration. 100 % Hb equals 16g %. The attenuation of light at 0 to 11 % Hb is more than in the following steps from 11 % to 48 % Hb. To find the correlation we plotted the light intensity at the three peaks against Hb concentration of the perfusion medium.

Fig. 3 indicates, that the decrease of light intensity does not follow Lambert Beer's Law, which would show a linear relationship. The possible mechanisms which cause the deviation are changes in the depth of light penetration and the nonhomogeneous distribution of the hemoglobin in the tissue as was pointed out by

Lübbers and Wodick (10) and the light scattering (5,6). The diagram suggests also that shorter wavelengths are less diminished than longer wavelengths. The effect of deoxygenation of hemoglobin on fluorescence is shown in figure 4.

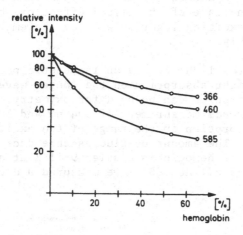

Intensity of reflected light in the perfused rat liver at different hemoglobin contents in logarythmic scale. 100 % = 16 g / 100 ml perfusion medium.

Fig. 3

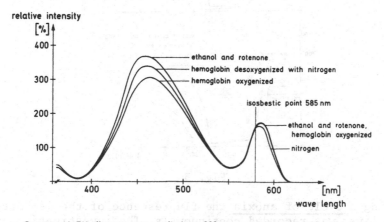

Spectra of PN-fluorescence excited at 366 nm and reflected light at 580-600 nm in liver perfused with erythrocytes. Hemoglobin content 48,7 %.

Fig. 4

Here we first reduced the PN by addition of ethanol (4 mM) and
rotenone (25 uM) and recorded an increase of fluorescence. Then
the hemoglobin was desoxygenized by switching to nitrogen. Subsequently a decrease of the emitted light instead of the expected
increase of PN fluorescence was observed. This reaction seems to
be paradoxical. It is caused by the desoxygenation of hemoglobin
which induces an increase of the filter effect of the tissue.
Consequently, the exciting light as well as the emitted light are
quenched considerably.

In the reflected light we see an isosbestic point at 585 nm
and an increased light absorption on the longer wavelength side.
This change of absorption can be used for oxymetry. It is
performed as difference measurement of 594 nm and 585 nm. The
increased light absorption in the range of the exciting light is
recorded at 366 nm. The amount of fluorescence decrease caused by
the desoxygenation of hemoglobin equaled 9-11 % at an hemoglobin
concentration of 7-9 g%. At 366 nm we measured a decrease of 12-14%.

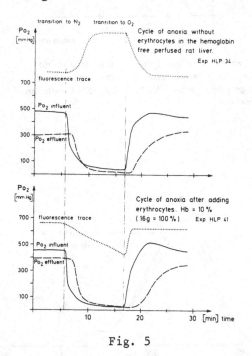

Fig. 5

During a cycle of anoxia the fluorescence of the isolated
perfused liver was recorded continuously. The investigations were
performed in organs which were perfused with a hemoglobinfree
medium (upper part of figure 5) and with a medium containing
bovine erythrocytes (lower part of figure 5). Po_2 in the influent
and effluent medium was concomitantly recorded. In the hemoglobin-

free perfused liver the fluorescence shows the well known PN reduction indicated by the fluorescence increase (1,7,8,9) during anoxia. In the liver perfused with erythrocytes we see a decrease after switching to nitrogen. Also the reoxidation shows different kinetics in both livers.

Figure 5 shows that the conditions of the liver perfused with erythrocytes are not optimal for the fluorescence measurement. The reason may be that the sinusoids are dilated maximally. By contrast, in situ conditions are better because the sinusoids are not dilated, and the hemoglobin containing compartment in the measured field is relatively small compared with the fluorescence emitting compartment.

SUMMARY

The influence of both Hb concentration and oxygenation was quantitatively investigated using the perfused rat liver as a model. The increase of Hb concentration as well as the desoxygenation attenuated the fluorescence. A method which enabled us to measure both parameters simultaneously was demonstrated.

REFERENCES

1. Bücher, Th.: The state of DPN system in liver. In: Pyridine Nucleotide Dependent Dehydrogenases. Springer Verlag 1969.

2. Chance, B., Jöbsis, F.: Intracellular oxidation-reduction states in vivo. Science 137, 499 (1962).

3. Chance, B., Leyallis, O.: A spectrofluorometer for recording of intracellular oxidation-reduction states, IEE Trans. Biol.-Med. Electron. 10, 40-47 (1963).

4. Kessler, M., Olech, K.-H., Schnase, G.: Microscopic photometer for simultaneous measurement of intracellular fluorescence (NADH and FAD) and of local hemoglobin concentration and oxygenation of the tissue. In preparation.

5. Kobayashi, S., Nishiki, K., Kaede, K., Ogata, E.: Optical consequences of blood substitution on tissue oxidation-reduction state microfluorometry. J. appl. Physiol. 31, 93 (1971).

6. Kobayashi, S., Kaede, K., Nishiki, K., Ogata, E.: Microfluorometry of oxidation-reduction state of the rat kidney in situ. J. appl. Physiol. 31, 693 (1971).

7. Lübbers, D.W., Kessler, M., Scholz, R., Bücher, Th.: Cytochrome reflection spectra and fluorescence of the isolated perfused hemoglobin free rat liver during a cycle of anoxia. Bio. Z. 341, 346 (1965)

8. Schnittger, H., Scholz, R., Bücher, Th., Lübbers, D.W.: Comparative fluorometric studies on rat liver in vivo and on isolated, perfused hemoglobin free liver. Biochem. Z. 341, 334 (1963)

9. Scholz, R., Thurman, R., Williamson, J., Chance, B.: Flavine and pyridine nucleotide oxidation-reduction changes in perfused rat liver. J. Biol. Chem. 244, 2317 (1969)

10. Wodick, R.: Neue Auswertverfahren für Reflexionsspektren und spektren inhomogener Farbstoffverteilung dargestellt am Beispiel von Hämoglobinspektren. Inauguraldissertation, Marburg 1971

STUDIES OF OXYGEN SUPPLY OF LIVER GRAFTS

M. Thermann, O.Zelder,F.Hess,C.R.Jerusalem,
H.Hamelmann
Dept.Surg.Univ.Marburg/L.,Lab.Cyt.and
Hist.R.K.Univ.Nijmegen

Oxygen supply of the grafts is of considerable interest in transplantation surgery. By means of a Clark-type Pt-surface electrode of KESSLER and LÜBBERS (2) we measured local oxygen pressures on heterotopic auxiliary liver grafts in rats.

METHODS

1. Materials:

The transplantations were performed in Wistar rats of 250-300 g body weight using the method of HESS, JERUSA-LEM and v.d.HEYDE (1). The animals were anesthetized with ether and breathed room air spontaneously.

2. Transplantation procedure:

Donor operation: Ligation of the hepatic artery, preparation of portal vein and inf.vena cava.
host operation: right nephrectomy, preparation of portal vein and inf.vena cava. During preparation of the host the graft remained in situ and was perfused by portal inflow. After finishing preparation of the host the two caudal lobes (about 30 % of the liver parenchyma) were removed from the donor and perfused with 4°C cooled Ringer-Lactate-solution. Implantation of the graft.Resection of 50 % of the host liver parenchyma. After finishing the procudure the graft (30 % of normal rat liver parenchyma) was supplied with portal blood, the remaining host liver (50 % of parenchyma) was supplied with hepatic arterial blood only, the common bile duct of the host liver was ligated.

3. Electrode and measurement technique :

For local PO_2 measurement we used a Clark-type Pt-surface electrode of KESSLER and LÜBBERS (2). The 16 wires
of the electrode (diameter 15 /u) gave a common signal,
a mean value of 16 different points of parenchyma.
In every phase PO_2 was measured on 96 - 160 different
points, measuring range of every point of tissue 50 -
70 /u.
We measured PO_2 of liver parenchyma in the course of 6
transplantations in the following phases:
a) after opening the abdomen
b) 2-3 min after ligation of the hepatic artery
c) after preparation of graft and host liver
d) during extracorporal hb-free hypothermic perfusion
   and implantation
e) 3-6 min after revascularisation of the graft.

We performed sham experiments. After ligation of hepatic artery we stopped further manipulations for the
time used for preparation of the graft. Then ligation
and resection of 70 % of the parenchyma followed. The
circulatoric conditions of the remaining two caudal
lobes were equivalent to those of the graft.
Furthermore we measured PO_2 in 14 animals of our Marburg
and Nijmegen group, surviving transplantation till 12
month.

RESULTS

During preparation (fig.1,phase A) we see a strong drop
of PO_2 after ligation of the hepatic artery. In the
following 45 min PO_2 remains low. During extracorporal
perfusion and implantation the organ is anoxic.
(Phase C). After revascularisation with portal blood only (Phase D) PO_2 of parenchyma rises to initial values.
Note the difference of PO_2 in Phase B and D, althougt
blood supply of portal vein is equal.
In Fig. 2 you will see PO_2-values during control experiments. Low oxygen pressures result after ligation of the
hepatic artery. After ligation of 70 % of liver parenchyma the whole portal blood supplies only the two caudal lobes. PO_2 of these lobes rises within 3 min to
values found in normal rat livers with arterial and portal blood supply.

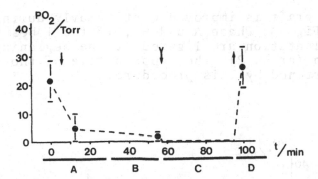

Fig. 1:   Oxygen pressures during transplantation
            (n = 6). Mean values and S.D. of mean
            values of single experiments

Phase A: Preparation of donor hepatectomy with liga-
         tion of hepatic artery (↓)
Phase B: Preparation of the host. The graft remains in
         situ and is supplied by portal blood
Phase C: Hepatectomy of the donor and implantation, be-
         ginning with ligation of lobes not used for
         transplantation (↓)
Phase D: Revascularisation (↑)

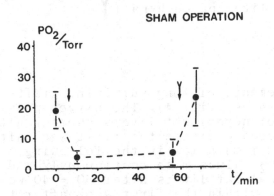

Fig. 2:   Control experiments
PO$_2$ values after ligation of hepatic artery (↓) and
ligation of 70 % of liver parenchyma (↓)

PO_2 of the graft is improved distinctavly during preparation (Fig. 3, Phase A und B), if the lobes not used
for transplantation are ligated at the beginning of the
preparation (arrow 2). The hypoxic time of the graft
may be shortened by this procedure.

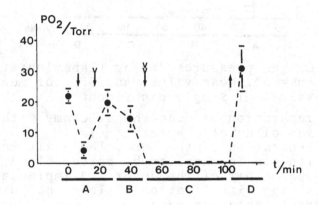

Fig. 3:

PO_2 values corresponding to Fig. 1, but early ligation of 70 % of liver parenchyma ( )

Oxygen measurements of long surviving grafts show
remarcable changes (Fig. 4). The oxygen pressures
reach values of normal rat livers shortly after trans-
platation. Decrease within the first week after transplantation and remain low in the following 4 weeks.
Furthermore PO_2 values rise continuously and reach
values of normal rat livers after 30 - 40 weeks.
These decrease within the first week after transplantation period. They remaind low in the following four
weeks.

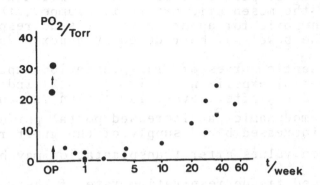

Fig. 4: PO₂ of grafts after transplantation

On the left initial values and values after revascularisation resp., taken from Fig. 3
The following values are mean values of single animals, 160 different points of tissue. S.D.ranging
from 0,3 - 4,9 (weeks 1 - 5) and 1,6 - 7,0 (weeks
5 - 60) Torr.

DISCUSSION

The low PO₂ after ligation of the hepatic artery can
not be explained by loss of arterial blood supply only,
but by an additional reduction of portal blood flow,
perhaps by irritation of splanchnic nerves, liberation
of catecholamines or early phase of shock. After revascularisation of the graft PO₂ rises to initial
values or exceeds, although the graft is supplied with
portal blood only.
The following causes may be reasonable:
1) The whole portal blood volume supplies only 30 % of
   liver parenchyma. Therefore the perfusion rate of
   parenchyma in elevated, an increased PO₂ results.
2) reduced oxygen utilisation, caused by hypoxic tissue
   damage and reduced tissue respiration.

3) elevated PO_2 of portal blood. During implantation of
the graft the mesenteric artery is clamped, the
bowel is hypoxic for about 30 min, tissue respiration of the bowel may be reduced by hypoxic damage.

The nearly identic curves of transplantation experiments and control experiments (Fig. 1 and 2) indicate
that increased PO_2 after revascularisation is caused
by changed hemodynamics, an increased portal perfusion
rate and an increased blood supply of the graft result.

The low oxygen values after transplantation may be
caused
a) by increased tissue respiration rate of the regenerating parenchyma
b) by increased capillary length . The diameter of the
hepatons increases in the first phase of regeneration.

Normalisation of PO_2 after 30 - 40 weeks coincidences
with normalisation of microarchitectonic structure,
apperently by dichotomy of central veins, an additional oxygen supply by ingrown arterioles may be
discussed.

SUMMARY

Using the method of HESS, JERUSALEM and v.d.HEYDE (1)
we performed auxilliary heterotopic liver transplantations in rats. By means of local oxygen measurements
we got the following results:

1) During preparation a strong drop of PO_2 from 21.4
± 7.4 (S.D.) torr to 4.8 ± 4.7 (S.D.) torr results
2) PO_2 of the graft increases to 25.3 ± 7.2 (S.D.) torr
after revascularisation although the graft is
supplied by portal inflow only. The cause is an elevated portal perfusion rate, for only 30 % of donor
liver is used for transplantation and supplied with
the whole portal blood volumen.

After transplantation we find very low oxygen values
within the first weeks with gradual increase to normal
PO_2 values for rat livers after 12 month.

References:

1) Hess,F., C.R.Jerusalem, N.v.d.Heyde:
Arch.Surg. 104., 75 (1972).
2) Kessler,M.,: in: LÜBBERS,D.W., U.Luft:
Oxygen transport in blood and tissue
Thieme Stuttgart 1967.

A CONTRIBUTION CONCERNING THE UNSETTLED PROBLEM OF INTRASPLENIC MICROCIRCULATION

W.Braunbeck, H.Hutten, P.Vaupel

Institute of Physiology, Johannes Gutenberg-

University, Mainz, Saarstr. 21, W.-Germany

From morphological studies it is well known that the vascular bed of the spleen consists of at least two different compartments. Figure one schematically shows how the splenic microcirculation can be subdivided. One compartment corresponds to the white pulp (pathways number 1 and 2), the other compartment to the red pulp, for which the existance of either an open or a closed type of terminal vascular bed is discussed. Futhermore

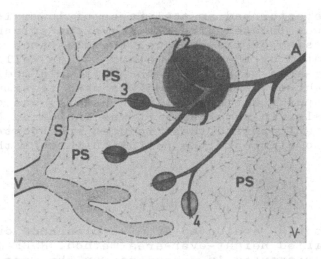

Fig.1. Schematical arrangement of the different types of the intrasplenic microcirculation STUTTE (3)

there are references that the microcirculation in the
red pulp is not homogeneous but composed of both types,
as illustrated by the pathways marked by number 3 and 4.

However, there is a great variety in morphology
and function of the spleen with regard to different
types of animals. The human spleen as well as the
rabbit's spleen belong to the so called metabolic type
of spleen and are characterized by considerable
morphological similarities.

METHODS

In 11 rabbits, anesthetized with Ketamine, the regional
splenic blood flow (rSBF) was measured by means of the
85-Krypton-(ß)-clearance technique. The rabbits were
placed on her right hand side. The spleen was exposed
by an abdominal incision and fixed with the aid of
Histoacryl^R tissue glue on an insulated copper plate,
thermostabilized at 38.5°C. Blood pressure was measured
in the femoral artery by means of a Statham transducer
and usually recorded as mean arterial blood pressure
(MABP). The indicator, dissolved in physiological
saline solution, was injected through a catheter into
the aorta thoracica as a slug injection.

The detector had an active area of 16 mm in diameter and was located directly above the spleen without compression of its surface. The clearance curves
were evaluated by the slope-method (2) as well as by
height-over-area method (5). In addition a modification
of the height-over-area method was used to simulate
a better input function (4). MABP usually was changing
spontaneously, in some cases it was increased by injection of epinephrine. Heat induced spherocytes (1)
were used to eliminate the perfusion through the pulp
cords.

RESULTS

Fig.2 shows rSBF evaluated from 46 clearance curves
by the modified height-over-area method. RSBF (dotted
line) is represented in dependance on the mean arterial
blood pressure. Over a wide range it linear depends on
MABP. Only for very high values of MABP the mean rSBF
is increased more than linear. Mean rSBF for normal
MABP amounts to 110 ml/100g/min. When the mean arterial
blood pressure is within a range of 50-70 mmHg, the

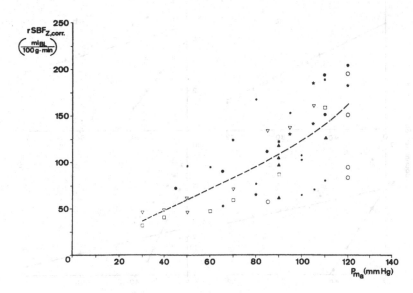

Fig.2. Relationship between rSBF, evaluated by the modified height-over-area method, and mean arterial blood pressure (Pm_a). Dotted line: average rSBF

clearance curves show typical monoexponential shapes, as it is demonstrated in fig. 3a. This is a clear evidence for homogeneous perfusion of the spleen. It is not possible to recognize the two mentioned compartments of the white and the red pulp; rSBF amounts to 73 ml/100g/min. However, raising the mean arterial pressure to approximately 100 mmHg causes the clearance curves to change their shapes and to become biexponential. This fact can be interpreted by an inhomogeneous perfusion, which is composed of two compartments. In fig. 3b, rSBF in the faster compartment amounts to 200 ml/100g/min, whereas in the slower compartment rSBF is decreased slightly to 40 ml/100g/min. The biexponential shape of the curve is more pronounced if the mean arterial blood pressure is still increased. rSBF in the faster compartment is enlarged to 232 ml/100g/min as to be seen in fig. 3c and to 338 ml/100g/min in fig. 3d. In contrast, rSBF of the slower compartment nearly remains independent upon mean arterial blood pressure.This behaviour becomes more evident in some experiments, in which the fast compartment showed an autoregulative reaction.

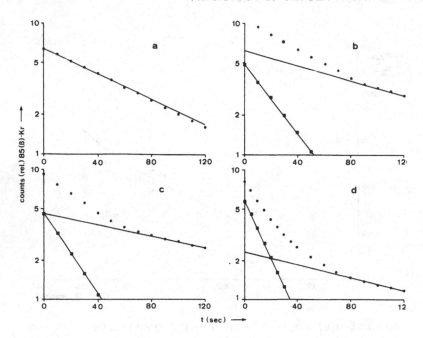

Fig.3. clearance curves dependend on different MABP

Fig 4a shows the biexponential shape of clearance curves, which is typical for a normal arterial blood pressure of 90 mmHg. One minute after injection of heat-induced spherocytes, the curve represented in fig 4b was measured. During this time the spherocytes are captured in the pulp cords. The shape of the clearance curve is already nearly monoexponential. Ten minutes after application of the spherocytes the curve of fig. 4c was recorded. The fast compartment had completely disappeared. Only the slow compartment, which can already be seen in fig. 4a, remained unchanged. After raising mean arterial blood pressure by injection of epinephrine, and after the vasoactive reaction in in splenic vascular bed had ceased, the clearance curve of fig. 4d was measured. Again a fast compartment is evident, however, the flow through the slow compartment is significantly decreased.

                          DISCUSSION

Raising the mean arterial blood pressure the regional blood flow in the fast compartment increases, as well as the mean regional blood flow. This phenomenon can only be explained if the following assumptions are made:

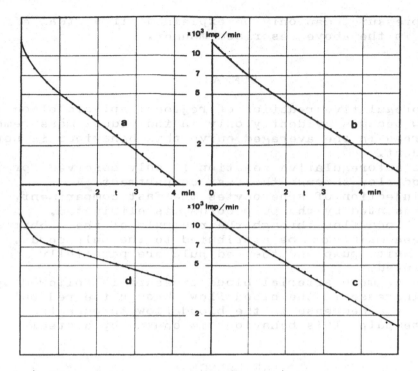

Fig. 4a):Clearance curves before, b):one minute after
c):ten minutes after injection of spherocytes, and
d):after raising the MABP by epinephrine.

Both compartments are parallelly perfused, and when
perfusion of the fast compartment is enlarged, blood
flow in the slow compartment is reduced by a steal
effect.

      The mean regional blood flow is mainly determined
by the fast compartment. It completely disappears.after
injection of spherocytes, because they are captured in
the pulp cords. So it must be concluded, that nearly
all red pulp blood flow is passing through the pulp
cords, which represent the open circulation. It must be
assumed, in addition, that the vascular bed of the slow
compartment, represented by the white pulp, is not at
all influenced by the spherocytes. After raising the
mean arterial blood pressure, the fast compartment becomes obvious again. It cannot be decided whether
additional pathways through the pulp cords are opened or
whether pathways, which had been choked by spherocytes,
are re-opened. Again the reduction in rSBF through the
slow compartment, following the rise in mean arterial

blood pressure, can only be explained, if a steal effect
exists in the above described manner.

SUMMARY

1. Autoregulative reaction of regional splenic blood
   flow becomes evidently only in individual measurements,
   whereas in the averaged curve this behaviour is not
   evident.
2. This autoregulative reaction is only observed for the
   blood flow through the fast compartment.
3. By injection of spherocytes the fast compartment,
   represented by the pulp cords, is eliminated.
4. The blood flow through the red pulp of the rabbit's
   spleen mainly can be attributed to the pulp cords.
5. The white pulp and the red pulp are parallelly
   perfused.
6. Rise of mean arterial blood pressure is followed by
   an increase in the blood flow through the red pulp
   and by a decrease in the blood flow through the
   white pulp. This behaviour is caused by a steal effect.

REFERENCES

(1) Fischer,J.:Klinik und Diagnostik der Milzerkrankungen,
             Verh.dtsch.Ges.inn.Med.69,798,(1963).
(2) Ingvar,H.,and N.A.Lassen: Regional blood flow of the
             cerebral cortex determined by krypton 85.
             Acta physiol.,scand., 54, 325 (1962).
(3) Stutte,H.J.: Zur Pathogenese des Hypersplenismus,
             Dtsch.Med.Wschr. 98, 388, (1973).
(4) Waldeck,F.,H.Hutten,J.Grote: Die Messung der Leber-
             durchblutung bei Ratten im Entblutungs-
             schock mit der Kr-85 Clearance.
             Pflügers Arch.ges.Physiol. 294, 201 (1967).
(5) Zierler,K.E.: Equations for measuring blood flow by
             external monitoring of radioisotops.
             Circulat.Res. 16, 309 (1965).

THE LOCAL OXYGEN SUPPLY IN TISSUE OF ABDOMINAL VISCERA AND OF SKELETAL MUSCLE IN EXTREME HEMODILUTION WITH STROMAFREE HEMOGLOBIN SOLUTION

L.Sunder-Plassmann,E.Sinagowitz,R.Rink,R.Dieterle,
K.Meßmer and M.Kessler
Institut f. Surgical Research, University Munich,
Max-Planck-Inst. Apllied Physiology, Dortmund, W.Germany

Stromafree, non nephrotoxic hemoglobin solutions have become a subject of great interest in recent years, since in all cases where a rapid normalization of a disturbed oxygen transport to tissues is required, the theoretical advantages of hb-solution, as compared to whole blood or conventional plasma substitutes are obvious: Unlimited supply and storage, no risk of serum hepatitis, chemical O_2binding, and low viscosity. To evaluate its effectiveness in vivo the changes in tissue PO_2 of various organs have been investigated in extreme hemodilution with hb-solution.

METHODS

Four splenectomized dogs, anaesthetized with sodium pentobarbital were subjected to a stepwise decrease in hematocrit (hct) by repeated exchanges of 10 ml/kg whole blood for 20 ml/kg of a 6 % stromafree hemoglobin solution[*]. Two multiwire platinum electrodes (KESSLER,1) were attached to each of the surface of liver, pancreas, kidney, small intestine and skeletal muscle. Thus continuous registration of tissue PO_2 could be made as arithmetic mean as well as from all single values. In addition cardiac output

---

[*] BIOTEST SERUM INSTITUT, FRANKFURT

blood pressure and blood gases were determined at hematocrit 30 %
20 %, 10 % and following a 60 min postdilutional period where the
animals were kept without further infusion. O_2-dissociation curves
were established manometrically (van SLYKE) and plotted according
to HILL's equation. At the end of the experiments the animals were
sacrificed for zero reference of the PO_2 electrodes.

RESULTS

Changes   in   hemoglobin   concentration ,   blood O_2-
capacity   and   hemo-dynamics   are   summarized   in   Fig.1.
Plasma hemoglobin at extreme dilution (hct 11%) was 4.9 g% corresponding to a plasma O_2-capacity of 5.9 Vol%. Cardiac output in-

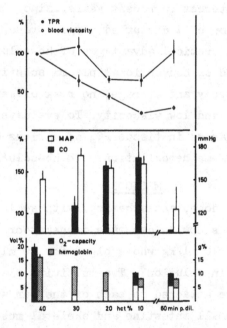

Fig.1: Total hemoglobin and O_2-capacity (white parts of the columns indicate plasma-hb and plasma-capacity), arterial blood pressure (MAP), cardiac output (C.O.), peripheral resistance (TPR)
and blood viscosity in relation to hematocrit (hct) in extreme
hemodilution with hb-solution.

creased to 167 % with extreme dilution and decreased to 80 % of
control within the postdilution period. Peripheral resistance was
reduced to 69 % but increased again within the following 60 min
period.

Throughout the dilution procedure a slight decrease in $AVDO_2$ was
noted from 6.4 to 5.2 Vol% with however a rise to 6.5 Vol% in the
postdilution period, corresponding to an increase in 65 % a-v saturation difference. Central-venous PO_2 consequently dropped from
43 at control to 13 mm Hg at the end of the experiments.

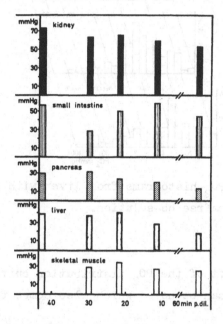

Fig.2: Mean tissue PO_2 of abdominal viscera in relation to the decrease in hematocrit in extreme hemodilution with hb-solution.

Mean values of tissue PO_2 from a total of 6653 single measurements
were nearly maintained in liver and skel.muscle in limited dilution (hct = 20%), but decreased continuously in pancreas and kidney (see Fig.2). In contrast PO_2 in small intestine decreased from
56 to 28 mm Hg after the first dilutional step but improved with

further dilution. Local tissue oxygen supply is shown in the PO_2-
histograms of the liver in Fig.3

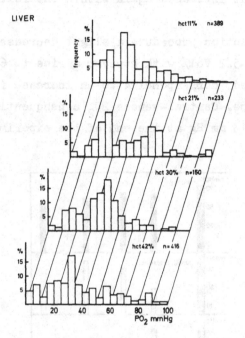

Fig.3: Changes in PO_2-histograms from liver with progressive hemodilution with stromafree hb-solution.

A gradual left shift of the PO_2 distribution curve with progressive hemodilution can be noted which also comes true for the pancreas and kidney.
With increasing amounts of free plasma hemoglobin the oxygen dissociation curve of whole blood is more and more shifted to the left
(Fig.4), the DPG concentration decreasing from 14 to 8 µMol/gHb
simultaneously.
Correlating P_{50} and DPG concentration yielded a linear relationship with a correlation coefficient of 0.83.

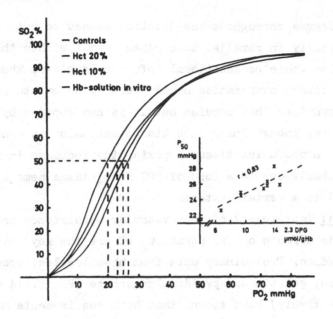

Fig.4: Changes in O_2-dissociation curve from whole blood in hemodilution with hb-solution. O_2 DC of hb-solution is given for comparison. Curves from right to the left: Control, hct 20 %, hct 10%,
hb-solution in vitro. All values corrected for a Serum-pH of 7.4.

DISCUSSION

In <u>normovolemic</u> hemodilution the decrease in blood viscosity has
been shown to produce an increase in both total and local blood
flow which compensates for the decreased O_2-capacity thus maintaining tissue oxygen supply (2). For hemoglobin recent studies
using 131-J bound hemoglobin have shown a dissapearance half time
of 95 min. In agreement exchanging whole blood for hb-solution in
an 1:1 ratio produced significant hypovolemia (3). It follows
that the flow increasing effect of a lowered viscosity is counteracted in vivo by a lack in blood volume and thus venous return.
This is confirmed by the fact that tissue PO_2 is maintained to a

tolerable degree throughout the dilution procedure but deteriora-
tes dramatically in parallel to cardiac output within the postdilution period where no additional infusion is given. Thus, on
principle, tissue oxygenation could probably be maintained by hb-
solution, provided that cardiac output is not impeded by a lack in
venous return. Though inadequate tissue perfusion is considered as
key factor in producing tissue hypoxia, the increase in Hb-O_2 affinity, probably due to a loss of DPG from plasma hemoglobin, has
contributed to a certain extent.

Conclusions: Improvement of intravascular persistence and elimination of side effects on the normal O_2 DC are the key points of
further studies. Preliminary data from hb-molecules, cross linked
with albumin, gelatin and pyridoxalphosphate (P_{50} 5, 14 and 30
mm Hg respectively) have shown, that both requirements may be met
in the future.

SUMMARY

A 6 % hemoglobin solution was exchanged in a 2:1 ratio for whole
blood in anaesthetized dogs to produce a decrease in hematocrit
to 10 %. Tissue PO_2 of abdominal viscera decreased gradually at
first but deteriorated significantly within a 60 min postdilution
period. Tissue hypoxia was primarely due to inadequate tissue perfusion and accentuated by a left shift of the oxygen dissociation
curve of the dogs blood. The significance of blood volume effect
of hemoglobin solutions is discussed as main cause of insufficient
blood flow rate.

REFERENCES

1. KESSLER,M., GRUNEWALD,W. Progr.Resp.Res.3: 147-152 (Karger,
    Basel/New York 1969).

2. MESSMER,K.,LEWIS,H.D.,SUNDER-PLASSMANN,L.,KLÖVEKORN,W.P.,MEND-
    LER,N. and HOLPER,K. Europ.Surg.Res. 4: 55 (1972).

3. SUNDER-PLASSMANN,L.,JESCH,F.,GROHMANN,W.,SEIFERT,J. and
    MESSMER,K. Proc. 7th Conf. Microcirculation, Aberdeen (Karger
    Basel) in press .

RESPIRATORY GAS EXCHANGE AND pO_2- DISTRIBUTION IN SPLENIC TISSUE

P.Vaupel, W.Braunbeck, G.Thews

Institute of Physiology, Johannes Gutenberg-

University, Mainz, Saarstr.21, W.-Germany

Little attention has been paid to physiological aspects of O_2 supply to splenic tissue. Studies are performed to examine the factors determining the supply conditions for the rabbit's spleen, which has little reservoir function and, therefore, it is very similar to the human spleen. Previous studies on respiratory gas exchange, applying the arterial and spleno-venous blood gas values, have shown a mean arterio-venous O_2-difference of 0.5 Vol.% (2). Taking into account a mean splenic blood flow of 110 ml/100g/min (12), the O_2 consumption of splenic tissue amounts to 0.6 ml/100g/min.

The present study examines 1.the intrasplenic oxygen tension distribution in the microstructure, and 2.the influence of vaso-active drugs, of heat-induced spherocytes and of short periods of hyperoxia on pO_2-distribution in splenic tissue.

METHODS

All experiments were performed on adult male rabbits (n=31), weighing 2.0-2.7 kg, and anesthetized with ketamine (40 mg/kg, anociation with atropine 0.04 mg/kg, both intraperitoneally). The animals were breathing spontaneously and subsequently given small maintenance doses of ketamine as necessary. Catheters were placed in the abdominal aorta via a femoral artery for blood presure measurements, using a Statham transducer, and in the contralateral femoral vein. Drugs and infusions were given through the femoral vein catheter. In our experiments, heart rate was controlled by means of a time-frequency converter (4).The spleen was exposed via an epigastric incision. After surgical preparation the spleen was carefully supported with a thermostabilized (38.5°C) manipulator.

Splenic tissue O_2 tensions in the microstructure were measured using gold-microelectrodes. The external diameter of the electrodes was 3-8 um, the diameter of the gold cathode 1 um. After capsulotomie the previously calibrated microelectrodes were lowered into the tissue 0.4 mm deep enough to avoid the influence of enviromental O_2 (2) and then pushed forward continuously. In order to confirm the mean pO_2 values measured polarographically, anaerobic and representative pulp samples were rapidly drawn from the pulp by tissue aspiration. The respiratory gas parameters in the pulp samples were measured by means of a blood gas analyzer.

In a second experimental group, at least two hours before anesthetizing the rabbits, venous blood (5-8 ml) was withdrawn from a margin ear vein. To avoid clotting ACD-Stabilisator* was added. After separating and washing, the erythrocytes were thermically alterated at 49.5°C during 20 min, according to FISCHER et al.(3), and thereby transformed into spherocytes. When the microelectrode was locked in position at a certain depth, the spherocytes were given i.v. (2-3 ml) and subsequent changes in tissue pO_2 were recorded.

To evaluate the influence of vaso-active drugs on pO_2 distribution in splenic tissue, the effects of some drugs were examined: epinephrine (15-20 ug/kg i.v.), norepinephrine (15-20 ug/kg i.v.), etilefrin (0.15 mg/kg i.v.), vasopressin (5 mU/kg i.v.), phentolamine (25 ug/kg i.v.), nylidrin (0.15 mg/kg i.v.), and hydergine (10 ug/kg i.v.).

In another experimental group we tried to analyze the change of the intrasplenic pO_2 distribution pattern during short periods of arterial hyperoxia by alteration in inspiratory gas concentration from air to 100 Vol.% O_2 with special regard to pO_2 pulses during spontaneous variations of the mean arterial blood pressure.

---

*Fa. Braun, Melsungen, GFR

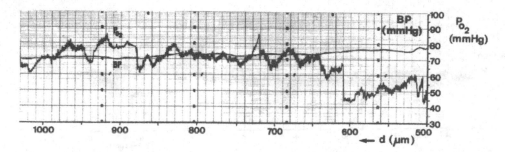

Fig.1. pO_2 profiles in splenic tissue and mean arterial blood pressure (BP). The original record is read from right to left.

RESULTS

When measuring intrasplenic O_2 tensions by means of polarographic O_2 microelectrodes, the pO_2 profiles were characterized by high mean O_2 tensions with flat gradients and missing very low O_2 tension values (fig.1).

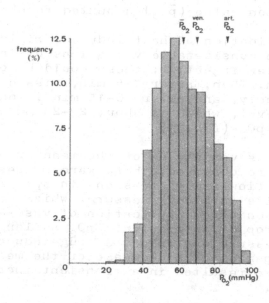

Fig.2. pO_2 histogram of splenic tissue. Result of 1054 measurements in 11 experiments. Markers indicate mean tissue O_2 tension ($\bar{p}O_2$), venous pO_2 (68.5 mmHg), and arterial pO_2 (86.5 mmHg).

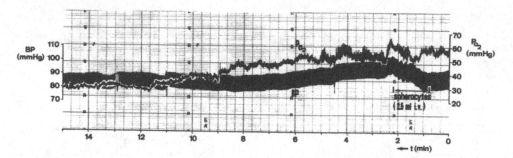

Fig.3. Changes of intrasplenic pO$_2$ distribution after
i.v.application of heat-induced spherocytes. Markers indicate the injection of spherocytes. The record is read
from right to left.

When locking the microelectrode in position, alterations
in tissue pO$_2$ could be observed in most of the experiments.
pO$_2$ histograms showed a marked variation of intrasplenic
O$_2$ tension values between 20 and 100 mmHg (fig.2). The
mean oxygen tension value ($\bar{p}O_2$) amounted to 63.5 mmHg.

     The i.v.application of heat induced, rigid sphero-
cytes resulted in considerable variations of intrasplenic
pO$_2$ instantly after injection; these could be observed
for about 3-5 min. Then, after 5-6 min, tissue pO$_2$ decreased continuously, and after 10-15 min it came up to
a steady state level, which is about 20-25 mmHg lower
than the initial pO$_2$ (fig.3).

     If spontaneous variations of the mean arterial
blood pressure were observed, there were corresponding
changes of blood flow and O$_2$ tensions in splenic tissue.
In contrast, a rise in blood pressure, which was caused
by vasoconstriction after application of vaso-active
drugs led to a drop of intrasplenic pO$_2$ as long as the
rise in blood pressure continued. A drug-induced vasodilatation accompanied by a decrease of the mean arterial blood pressure resulted in a transient increase of
intrasplenic pO$_2$.

     Short periods of arterial hyperoxia were followed
by an increase of local pO$_2$ in splenic tissue. The size
of the response of the tissue electrode and the time
till tissue pO$_2$ reached its maximum directly varied with
the mean arterial blood pressure, mean splenic blood
flow respectively, and with the resting tissue pO$_2$.

DISCUSSION

As a result of earlier investigations (2) we found a low O_2 uptake of splenic tissue. This minimal O_2 consumption can only be compared to the O_2 consumption of the myelinated nerv (7), to the O_2 uptake of the resting skeletal muscle (1), and to the limited O_2 uptake of tumors (11). Besides the high spleno-venous pO_2 (2), the polarographic measurements of intrasplenic O_2 tensions directly refer to a low O_2 consumption of splenic tissue. Low O_2 uptake of the spleen and a relatively high splenic blood flow of 110 ml/100g/min (12) can be regarded as the cause for the high mean tissue pO_2 of 63.5 mmHg and for the flat gradients. pO_2 measurements of the pulp after tissue aspiration aprove the high tissue pO_2.

On account of the considerable sensitivity of the terminal splenic vascular bed to temperature (9) we kept the temperature of the spleen in a constant balance of $38.5^{\circ}C$, in order to avoid a break down of the spontaneous sphincter actions. Besides the spontaneous splenomotoric waves, these sphincter actions must be the causes for spontaneous pO_2 alterations if the microelectrode is locked in position. In this connection single phenomena can only be explained according to the intrasplenic vascular regulations described by KNISELY (5,6).

Relatively rigid spherocytes are quickly accumulated selectively in the spleen, because they are captured by the red pulp. As a result there is an obstruction of the 'open' type of intermediary splenic circulation. In our experiments a decrease of tissue pO_2 can be observed as an immediate consequence of subsequent decrease of blood flow. From the inhibition of the blood flow in the red pulp may be concluded that there must exist an 'open' type of splenic circulation besides the 'closed' type in rabbit as well as in man (10).

Examining the effect of epinephrine, norepinephrine, etilefrin, and vasopressin, the momentary drop of tissue pO_2 must be attributed to vasoconstriction and emptying of blood stores, since there is concurrent disturbance of splenic blood flow and flow distribution(8). Accordingly,the changes in the tissue pO_2 pattern after administration of phentolamine, nylidrin, and hydergine may be the consequence of distinct dilatations and changes of the storage function.

Short periods of arterial hyperoxia are followed by a pronounced increase of local pO_2. The size of the

responses and the response times directly vary (similar
to many other organs) with the resting pO_2, and with the
mean arterial blood pressure, splenic blood flow resp..

SUMMARY

The investigations on respiratory gas exchange and pO_2
distribution in splenic tissue demonstrate
1. low O_2 uptake of the spleen of 0.6 ml/100g/min,
2. pO_2 profiles with high mean O_2 tensions, flat pO_2
   gradients and missing very low pO_2 values, the mean
   tissue pO_2 being 63.5 mmHg,
3. spontaneous variations of intrasplenic pO_2 as a possible consequence of rhythmic blood flow through the
   spleen, and corresponding alterations of tissue pO_2
   along with spontaneous variations of splenic blood flow,
4. a decrease of intrasplenic pO_2 values after injection
   of spherocytes as a result of the obstruction of the
   'open' type of intrasplenic circulation in the red pulp,
5. changes of the pO_2 pattern, if vaso-active drugs are
   given, in consequence of vasoconstriction, vasodilatation, storage function, and of blood stores being
   emptied,
6. marked increases of tissue pO_2 in response to alterations of arterial pO_2.

REFERENCES

(1)Asmussen,E.,E.H.Christensen,M.Nielsen : Scand.Arch.
Physiol.82,212,1939; (2)Braunbeck,E.,P.Vaupel,St.Kunke,
G.Thews:Pflügers Arch.339, R 35,1973; (3)Fischer,J.,
R.Wolf,H.Gamm:Dtsch.Ärztebl.70,401,1973; (4)Hutten,H.:
Pflügers Arch.297,27,1967; (5)Knisely,M.H.:Anat.Rec.65,
23,1936; (6)Knisely,M.H.:Anat.Rec.65,131,1936;
(7)Kunze,K.:Pflügers Arch.339,R 71,1973; (8)Lutz,J.,
E.Bauereisen:Abdominalorgane, in:Physiologie des Kreis-
laufs, Springer 1971; (9)Peck,H.M.,N.L.Hoerr:Anat.Rec.
109,479,1951; (10)Stutte,H.J.:Dtsch.med.Wschr.98,388,
1973; (11)Vaupel,P.,H.Günther,J.Grote,G.Aumüller:Zschr.
ges.exp.Med.156,283,1971; (12)Vaupel,P.,W.Braunbeck,
H.Hutten: Pflügers Arch.339, R 22,1973.

RENAL TISSUE OXYGENATION DURING PULSATILE AND NONPULSATILE LEFT HEART BYPASS

A. V. Beran, D. R. Sperling, A. Wakabayashi, and
J. E. Connolly

University of California, Irvine, College of Medicine
Irvine, California

Data favoring pulsatile over nonpulsatile left heart bypass are conflicting. To study this problem, renal cortical and medullary tissue oxygen availability (O_2a) and total renal oxygen flow was compared with total renal oxygen consumption during four hours of pulsatile and nonpulsatile bypass in dogs.

METHODS

Micropolarographic electrodes were constructed of glass insulated platinum wire (75 μ) encased in silver tubing as previously described (1). Cortical electrodes were 8 mm and medullary electrodes were 17 mm in length; the electrodes were calibrated in vitro and only those with a linear response were used.

Eighteen mongrel dogs (20-30 kg) were used in the study. The left kidney was exposed extraperitoneally under sterile conditions. Two cortical and two medullary electrodes were inserted through four punctures on the lateral surface of the kidney. Electrodes were secured by suturing the plastic sheet to the renal capsule, care being taken not to traumatize kidney parenchyma. The microprong connector was then made water-tight with a silicone rubber cover (Dow Corning) and placed subcutaneously. Ten to 14 days were allowed for the animals to recover after which time the left heart bypass was performed.

Following usual anesthesia procedures, the implantation incision was reopened, the subcutaneous microprong connector exposed and connected to the polarography system. Twenty minutes were

allowed to obtain a baseline recording of the tissue O_2a before
further procedures. Electrode response was tested by allowing
the animals to breathe 100% oxygen. Of the four electrodes implanted in each animal, one cortical and one medullary electrode
with the best response were used during the study.

Through a left pararectal incision, the left renal artery and
vein, and the left internal spermatic or ovarian vein were isolated.
An electromagnetic flow probe (Micron, 2-3 mm) was placed around
the renal artery and a vascular occluder made of teflon-coated
wire (2) was used to obtain zero flow level. For blood sampling
the renal vein was cannulated via the internal spermatic vein. The
left iliac artery was isolated for the insertion of an arterial input cannula (Bardic #20) and placement of flow probe (Micron, 3.5 mm).
The right femoral artery and vein were cannulated for pressure monitoring and blood sampling.

The chest was opened through the left fourth intercostal space,
the dogs were heparinized (3 mg/kg) and the left atrial output
cannula (Bardic #36) was inserted. Left heart bypass was started
at a low flow rate and the descending thoracic aorta was then
cross-clamped. Flow rate was gradually increased to equalize blood
pressures above and below the clamp. Bypass was conducted for four
hours, nonpulsatile in nine animals and pulsatile in nine animals.
The bypass system consisted of an open reservoir and a roller pump
for nonpulsatile flow and a pneumatically driven ventricular pump
with heat exchanger (Brunwick) for pulsatile flow.

                              RESULTS

Cortical O_2a during cross-clamping of the descending aorta and
establishment of left heart bypass is seen in Figure 1. With both
pulsatile and nonpulsatile left heart bypass renal cortical O_2a
never returned to control level.

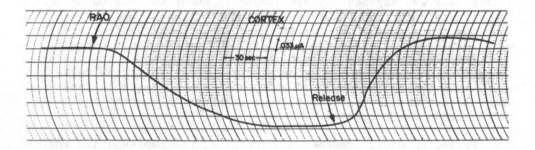

Figure 1.   Cortical O_2a following clamping of aorta and beginning
            of bypass.

During pulsatile (P) and nonpulsatile (NP) prefusion, the mean and standard deviation for renal blood flow (RBF), hematocrit (Htc), hemoglobin(Hb), arterial oxygen content (CaO_2), renal vein oxygen ($CrvO_2$), total renal oxygen flow (RO_2F), renal oxygen consumption (VO_2), and cortical and medullary O_2a at 1,2,3, and 4 hours are contained in Table 1. Data were analyzed using the analysis of variance method to find the point at which changes in physiological variables became statistically significant as related to the control levels.

Renal blood flow decreased steadily during the bypass in both groups. The decrease was greater in the nonpulsatile group, and it occurred during the third hour of bypass. In the pulsatile group it occurred during the fourth hour of bypass. Hematocrit decreased in both groups even though supplemental blood was given. A statistically significant decrease occurred in the nonpulsatile group during the third and fourth hour of bypass. Hemoglobin did not change appreciably during the four hours of pulsatile bypass; during nonpulsatile bypass there was a significant decrease during the third and fourth hour. Central arterial and renal vein oxygen content was maintained at control values during the entire four hours of pulsatile bypass; during nonpulsatile bypass it decreased significantly during the third and fourth hour. Renal oxygen flow and total renal oxygen consumption decreased in both groups, but the significant decrease was greater and occurred earlier in the nonpulsatile group. Cortical and medullary O_2a (Figure 2) decreased similarly in both pulsatile and nonpulsatile groups during the first two hours of bypass; however, at the end of four hours the decrease was greater in the nonpulsatile group. During pulsatile and nonpulsatile bypass the decrease in O_2a in the cortex was always less then in the medulla.

The relation between renal oxygen flow and total renal oxygen consumption is seen in Figure 3. Statistical analyses were carried out on 117 independent determinations of renal oxygen flow and consumption (63 in nonpulsatile and 54 in pulsatile bypass groups). The slope for the pulsatile bypass group is .323 and for the nonpulsatile group is .086. The regression coefficient is .72 and .59, respectively. The slopes for the pulsatile and nonpulsatile data were tested using the analysis of variance method and were found to be significantly different at the 99% level ($F = 34.47$, $p < .001$). These statistical data provide further evidence that at a given renal oxygen flow, renal oxygen consumption is greater with pulsatile than with nonpulsatile bypass.

Table I. Effect of four hours pulsatile (P) and nonpulsatile (NP) left heart bypass on physiological variables. NS = no signifigance; t value of 2-4 indicates a signifigance of 5% level (P < .05); t value of >4 indicates a signifigance at 1% level (P < .01)

VARIABLES	UNITS	CONTROL C P	CONTROL C NP	BY PASS (HOURS) 2.0 P	BY PASS (HOURS) 2.0 NP	BY PASS (HOURS) 4.0 P	BY PASS (HOURS) 4.0 NP
Ca_{O_2}	ml/100 ml	17 ± 4	17 ± 2	18 ± 3	17 ± 4	17 ± 2	14 ± 3
	%	100	100	109 ± 19 NS	99 ± 21 NS	100 ± 21 NS	83 ± 13 t=3.63
$C_{rv_{O_2}}$	ml/100 ml	15 ± 3	14 ± 2	14 ± 2	14 ± 3	14 ± 2	12 ± 3
	%	100	100	93 ± 11 NS	95 ± 20 NS	98 ± 24 NS	82 ± 19 t=4.16
RO_2F	ml/min	24 ± 8	31 ± 1	22 ± 8	24 ± 10	17 ± 7	15 ± 6
	%	100	100	89 ± 15 NS	81 ± 37 NS	69 ± 13 t=2.06	52 ± 17 t=9.62
$\dot{V}_{O_2}$	ml/min	4.1 ± 2.6	4.2 ± 1.5	4.9 ± 2.2	3.6 ± 1.8	3.3 ± 1.8	2.4 ± 1.3
	%	100	100	141 ± 33 NS	86 ± 27 NS	79 ± 24 NS	59 ± 29 t=2.45
CORTEX O_2a	%	100	100	70 ± 9 t=83.76	62 ± 4 t=137.44	58 ± 5 t=164.17	40 ± 5 t=331.85
MEDULLA O_2a	%	100	100	58 ± 5 t=77.49	56 ± 6 t=83.94	53 ± 5 t=97.03	30 ± 5 t=216.12

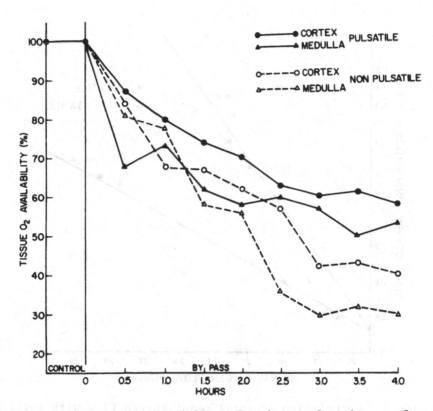

Figure 2.   Cortical and medullary O_2a during four hours of
            pulsatile and nonpulsatile bypass.

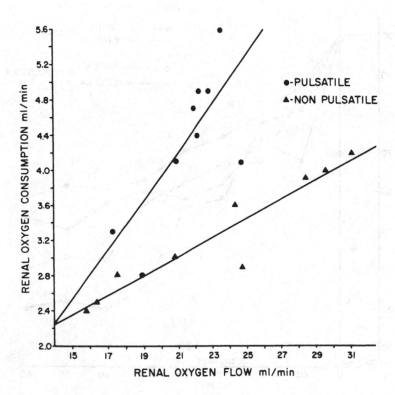

Figure 3.   Correlation of total renal oxygen flow with total renal
oxygen consumption.   Each point represents the mean
obtained at a specific time during bypass.

DISCUSSION

Conclusions of the investigators working in this field of
research fall into two categories: those who find no advantage of
pulsatile over nonpulsatile perfusion, and those who find definite
advantage of pulsatile perfusion. Investigators who found no advantage of pulsatile over nonpulsatile perfusion based their conclusion on the observations that mean renal blood flow was unaffected by 15 minutes of depulsation (3) and that there was no difference in renal function with pulsatile and nonpulsatile perfusion when the flow was maintained at 130 cc/kg/min. (4,5)

Investigators who found definite advantage of pulsatile perfusion based their conclusion on the observations that oxygen consumption (6,7), effective capillary blood flow (8), vasomotor control (6), tissue acid-base status (6), blood pressure (6), and survival rates (9) were better with pulsatile perfusion.

To study further the efficacy of pulsatile and nonpulsatile
bypass, renal cortical and medullary O_2a and total renal oxygen
flow and consumption were determined. During four hours of bypass
cortical and medullary O_2a decreased steadily. The decrease was
greater with nonpulsatile perfusion, and the medullary decrease in
O_2a was always greater than cortical. This preferential decrease
in medullary O_2a has also been observed during hemorrhagic shock
(10,11).

While the mean arterial blood pressure was maintained between
90 and 110 mm Hg, renal blood flow steadily decreased during bypass in both groups. The percentage of decrease was greater with
nonpulsatile than with pulsatile, suggesting that vascular tone
is less disturbed.

Renal oxygen consumption was maintained at pre-bypass levels
during the first two hours of pulsatile perfusion and then decreased
during the next two hours, but to a lesser degree than with nonpulsatile perfusion.

Hematocrit and hemoglobin were also better maintained with pulsatile than with nonpulsatile perfusion. This is probably due to
decreased hemolysis, decreased heparin requirements, and the minimum priming volume of the ventricular pulsatile system.

The concept of total renal oxygen flow has been introduced to
eliminate the effect of independent variables (hematocrit, pH,
pO_2, oxygen content, and renal blood flow) on total oxygen supply
to the kidney. When total renal oxygen flow was plotted against
total renal oxygen consumption (Figure 3), the regression line for
pulsatile bypass is significantly steeper than that for nonpulsatile

bypass, proving that oxygen utilization is more efficient with pulsatile perfusion. It should be emphasized that this difference exists even when renal blood flow and hematocrit were maintained at high levels during the first two hours of pulsatile and nonpulsatile bypass.

These data, along with the maintenance of higher level of cortical and medullary O_2a with pulsatile flow, provide additional evidence for the superiority of pulsatile perfusion.

Possible explanations for this superiority of pulsatile perfusion are: better flow distribution and fewer intrarenal shunts.

REFERENCES

1. Beran, A.V., Mukherjee, N.D., Taylor, W.F., Wakabayashi, A., and Connolly, J.E. Decrease in renal tissue oxygen following placement of magnetic flow probe around the renal artery. To be published.

2. Beran, A.V., Strauss, J., Brown, C.T., and Katwich, N. A simple arterial occluder. J. Appl. Physiol. 24:838, 1968.

3. Many, M., Soroff, H.S., Birtwell, W.C., Wise, H.M., and Deterling, R.A. The physiologic role of pulsatile and nonpulsatile blood flow. Arch. Surg. 97:917, 1968

4. Wesolowski, A.A. Role of pulse in maintenance of systemic circulation during heart-lung bypass. Trans. Amer. Soc. Artif. Intern. Organs 1:84, 1955.

5. Wesolowski, S.A. and Welch, C.S. Experimental maintenance of the circulation by mechanical pumps. Surgery 31:769, 1952.

6. Clowes, G.H., Jr. Extracorporeal maintenance of circulation and respiration. Physiol. Review 40:826, 1960.

7. Shephard, R.B. and Kirklin, J.W. Relation of pulsatile flow to oxygen consumption and other variables during cardiopulmonary bypass. J. Thorac. Cardiovasc. Surg. 58:694, 1969.

8. Ogata, T., Ida, Y., Nonoyama, A., Takeda, J., and Sasaki, H. A comparative study of the effectiveness of the pulsatile and of nonpulsatile flow in extracorporeal circulation. Arch. Jap. Chir. 29:69, 1960.

9. Dalton, M.L., McCarty, R.T., and Woodward, K.E. The army artificial heart pump II. Comparison of pulsatile and nonpulsatile flow. Surgery 58:840, 1965.

10. Strauss, J., Beran, A.V., Katurich, N., and Brown, C.T. Renal regional O_2 consumption under "normal" and hemorrhagic shock conditions. Intern. Congr. Nephrol., 4th, Stockholm, 1969.

11. Strauss, J., Beran, A.V., Baker, R., Bovdston, K., and Reyes-Sanchez, J.L. Effect of hemorrhagic shock on renal oxygenation. Amer. J. Physiol. 221:1545, 1971.

NEW ASPECTS ON THE MECHANISM OF AUTOREGULATION OF BLOOD FLOW

Christoph Weiss and Volker Thiemann

Physiologisches Institut der Universität

Kiel, Germany

The term autoregulation as used here denotes the ability of an isolated organ to keep the blood flow relatively constant in spite of changes of perfusion pressure. In previous communications pertaining to a system theory analysis of autoregulation (1,2,3,4,5, 6) we reported observations on periodic spontaneous fluctuations of the perfusion flow ($\dot{V}$)of isolated rat kidneys, isolated rat hearts, isolated hind limbs and isolated mesentery showing periodicities in the range of 25 sec. (6). These fluctuations which were only observed when the arterial pressure was maintained at values higher than 80-100 mm Hg (i.e. in the range of autoregulation) did <u>not</u> appear as proper sinusoidal oscillations with defined shapes and constant periodicity. Instead, irregular increases and decreases of the flow ($\dot{V}$) of varying periodicity were observed (fig.1). A more detailed study of these irregular periodic changes seemed to promise information on the nature of the underlying process. Especially so since similar periodicities were previously reported from other circulatory areas and from smooth muscle preparations (3, 7-13). For this purpose we have applied the method of time series analysis consisting in the determination of autocorrelation

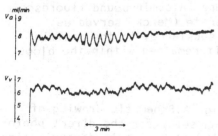

Fig.1 Time histories of total organ flow at a perfusion pressure of 100 mm Hg in an isolated rat hind limb. Upper curve: arterial registration; lower curve: venous registration.

417

and power spectral density functions.

Fig. 1 shows arterial and venous flow curves from an isolated rat hind limb recorded at a perfusion pressure of 100 mm Hg. Identical curves were obtained from the other organs studied. Visual inspection of these records indicates that the periodicity of flow waves varies between about 10 and 30 sec. Fig. 2 contains a plot of autocorrelation versus time displacement for the arterial flow curve. It indicates a periodicity of about 30 sec.

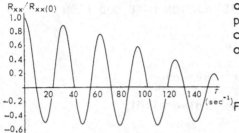

Fig. 2 Autocorrelogram of the arterial flow curve of fig. 1

Fig. 3 shows the corresponding power density spectrum which has a distinct maximum at a frequency of 0.03 Hz. In order to correlate the observed periodic changes of flow with changes of vascular diameter a photomicrofluorimetric method for the continuous direct measurement of the diameter of single arterioles was elaborated.

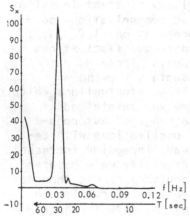

Fig. 3 Power density spectrum of the curve of fig. 1

Fig. 4 shows the principle. For the excitation filtred light of 350 - 400nm wavelength was used. A daylight sensitive photomultiplier served as photoelectric transducer. Signals were recorded on tape. Albumin-bound fluorescein -iso-thiocyanate (Merck) served as fluorescing substance. In the protein bound form it remained within the blood vessels.

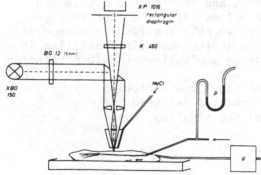

Fig. 4 Schematic drawing of the setup for the direct photomicrofluorometric determination of the diameter of single resistance vessels.

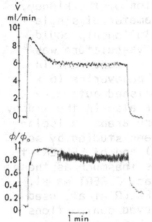

Fig. 5 Time histories of total organ flow (upper curve) and of the diameter of a single resistance vessel (lower curve) after an upward pressure step from 0 to 120 mm Hg perfusion pressure.

In fig. 5 the time histories of the total organ flow (upper curve) and of the diameter of a single arteriole in a perfused rectus abdominis muscle are depicted after an upward pressure step from 0 - 120 mm Hg was applied. Following an initial steep rise of flow to 9 ml/min. within the ensuing 60 sec. the flow decreases to 6 ml/min. 30 sec. after the pressure step fluctuations of flow and diameter of gradually rising amplitude occur.

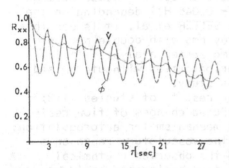

Fig. 6 Autocorrelograms of the two curves of fig. 5.

Fig. 6 shows the autocorrelograms of flow and diameter. Periodicities of 3 sec. duration can be seen in both curves. The corresponding power density spectra show peaks in the range of 0.03 Hz, and – since in the meantime we increased the time resolution of our equipment – a large maximum for the diameter and a smaller one for the flow in the range of 0.35 Hz. (fig. 7).

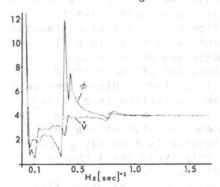

Fig. 7 Power density spectra of the two curves of fig. 5.

While the amplitude of the periodic flow changes increased with rising pressure the frequency of the periodic changes of flow and diameter was not significantly affected by changes of pressure within the range of autoregulation (80 - 200 mm Hg).

In all isolated organs studied, with the exception of the kidney, periodic changes of total organ flow, of the diameter of single vessels, and an autoregulatory pressure-flow relationship could only be observed if a minimum basal tone of the vasculature was provided by the addition to the perfusion fluid of noradrenalin $(0.5 \times 10^{-6}\text{g/ml})$ or of vasopressin. Addition of papaverine (6 $\times$ $10^{-6}\text{g/ml})$ to the perfusion fluid reversibly abolished autoregulation and periodic changes of flow and diameter also in the kidney.

Rhythmic activities of different circulatory areas in isolated organs as well as in organs in situ, have been studied by several authors. The findings of GEBERT et al. (7) and of SELLER et al. (12) are especially pertinent to our studies inasmuch as these authors have also used isolated circulatory areas. GEBERT et al. used isolated bovine facial arteries, whereas SELLER et al. used isolated skin areas of dogs. GEBERT et al. observed contractions of the arteries with a periodicity of 15 $\pm$ 8 sec. (corresponding to a frequency range between 0.043 and 0.14 Hz), and KOEPCHEN et al. (11) a periodicity of (12 - 30 sec.)(or 0.033 - 0.038 Hz). An average length of 22 - 25 sec. (0.04 - 0.046 Hz) depending on the perfusion medium was also reported by SELLER et al. It is possible that these authors would have found rhythms with double periodicity as we did, if they had used the time series analysis. It is very difficult to detect two close periodicities without the aid of the mathematical tools used in this study.

On the basis of these and earlier results of studies (1;2;3; 4;5;6) on the dynamics of pressure induced changes of flow resistance we tentatively propose a model mechanism for autoregulation: Provided the longitudinal tension of the vasculature represents the adequate stimulus for contraction the observed rhythmical changes of vascular diameter, i.e. of flow resistance could be explained by the following sequence of events.

1. A rise of the transmural pressure gradient provides an increased tangential tension in the vascular wall which elicits a contraction and thereby a diminution of the vascular diameter.
2. As described by LAPLACE the diminution of the vascular diameter at constant transmural pressure gradient leads to a diminution of the tangential tension and thus to a decrease of the stimulus to subthreshold values resulting in a relaxation of the vasculature.
3. The vessel is passively dilated until the longitudinal tension threshold is reached again, and another contraction is elicited. It seems plausible that the described sequence of events leads to a reduction of the (time integrated) mean diameter of the oscillating vessels. Since the flow resistance is inversly proportional to the square of the diameter, relatively small changes of the latter cause significant changes of the former.

However, the observed periodic changes of total organ flow presuppose the existence of a synchronising mechanism which leads to (nearly) simultaneous changes of vascular diameter in the whole organ, or at least in large parts of it.

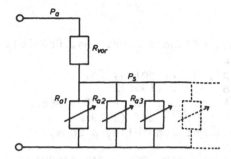

Fig. 8 Diagrammatic representation
        of the series and parallel
        flow resistances in an organ
        (see text for further expl.).

In fig.8 the artery (Pa), its series
resistance (Rvor), and four variable
resistors in parallel (Ra1;Ra2;
Ra3 ....), standing for individual
resistance vessels, are schemati-
cally representing the arterial and arteriolar vascular bed of an
organ. If, by a rise of blood pressure (at Pa), the tension threshold for the constriction of Ra1 is reached, and its resistance
consequently increased, the ensuing further rise of pressure at
Ps will excite the vasculature of Ra2 and lead to a rise of its
resistance which in turn will raise again pressure at Ps, thus
exciting the vasculature of Ra3.... and so forth.

      Though electrical spread of excitation between adjacent cells,
or - in some instances - synchronisation by sympathetic activity
may occur, the described hydro-mechanical events alone would explain the observed synchronisation.

      Largely based on theoretical considerations FOLKOW (14) has
proposed a model mechanism for autoregulation the explanatory
principle of which is centered on a periodic changing of the vasculature between the states of excitation and relaxation. Our
findings contain new and more direct evidence in support of this
model mechanism. However, while FOLKOW expected the frequency of
the periodic contractions to increase with the extent of the
pressure induced passive muscular distension, we find no correlation between pressure and frequency. Furthermore, FOLKOW discussed the possibility that strong stimuli, i.e. high transmural
pressure gradients, could lead to a tetanus like, sustained constriction of the vasculature. In our experiments, even at perfusion pressures of 180 -200 mm Hg, total organ flow and single
vessel diameter always showed the described periodic changes.

      On the basis of our results and the evidence so far available
little doubt remains as to the validity of BAYLISS' myogenic
hypothesis of autoregulation. The extension of the mere static
original concept to a dynamic model adds no complexity but rather
reduces the minimum requirements for the model mechanism. The
only prerequisites being the well established stretch receptor
properties of smooth muscle cells, and the applicability of the
laws of OHM, KIRCHHOFF and POISEUILLE.

      The proposed model does not preclude the superimposition on
the basic autoregulatory mechanism of such modifying factors as
changes of basal vascular tone, pCO_2, pO_2, pH, the concentrations
of lactic acid or of other metabolifes.

References

1. Basar, E., Tischer, H., Weiss Ch.: Pflügers Arch. ges. Physiol. 299, 191 - 213 (1968).
2. Basar, E., Ruedas, G., Schwarzkopf, H.J., Weiss, Ch.: Pflügers Arch. 304, 189 - 202 (1968).
3. Basar, E., Weiss, Ch.: Pflügers Arch. 304, 121 - 135 (1968).
4. Basar, E., Weiss, Ch.: Kybernetik 5, 241- 247 (1969).
5. Bendat, J.S., Piersol, A.G.: New York: John Wiley & Sons, Inc. 1967.
6. Basar. E., Weiss, Ch.: Pflügers Arch. 319, 205 - 214 (1970)
7. Gebert, G., Konold, P., Seboldt, H.: Pflügers Arch. 299, 285 - 294 (1968).
8. Golenhofen, K. in Smooth muscle, chapt.: Slow Rhythms in smooth muscle. ed. Bülbring, E., A.F. Brading, A.W. Jones, T.Tomita. Edward Arnold Ltd.London 1970.
9. Johannson, B., Ljung, B.: Acta physiol. scand. 70, 299 - 311 (1967).
10. Johnson, P.C., Wayland, H.: Am. J. Physiol. 212, 1405 (1967).
11. Koepchen, H.P., Polster, J., Langhorst, P.: Pflügers Arch. 278, 24 (1963).
12. Seller, H., Langhorst, P., Polster, J. Koepchen, H.P.: Pflügers Arch. 296, 110 - 132 (1967).
13. Stolp, W., Thiemann, V., Weiss, Ch.: II. Internat. Sympos. Biokybernetik, Leipzig 1969.
14. Folkow, B., Circulation Res., Suppl. 1, XV, 279 - 285 (1964).

SYMPATHETIC NERVOUS CONTROL OF INTESTINAL O_2 EXTRACTION

A. P. Shepherd, D. Mailman, T. F. Burks, and H. J. Granger

Programs in Physiology and Pharmacology, The University of

Texas Medical School at Houston, Houston, Texas   77025

All three of the functionally defined series-coupled elements within the intestinal microcirculation respond to sympathetic nerve stimulation: the *resistance* vessels, the precapillary sphincters which govern the *exchange* vessels, and the *capicitance* vessels(1). In our computor model of the intestinal circulation (2,3), oxygen delivery to the intestinal tissues is regulated by arteriolar resistance to blood flow while the precapillary sphincters determine the number of open perfused capillaries; thus they control the diffusion parameters for oxygen (*i.e.,* capillary surface area and mean capillary-to-cell diffusion distance). The model predicts that sympathetic-induced reductions in the density of the perfused capillary bed will depress intestinal oxygen extraction. Therefore, the purpose of this work has been to test that prediction in an animal model. Since oxygen delivery is the product of the arteriovenous oxygen difference (A-V ΔO_2) and blood flow, we have studied the effects of norepinephrine infusion and sympathetic stimulation on intestinal oxygen extraction under constant-flow conditions in order to eliminate blood flow as a variable.

METHODS

In fasted mongrel dogs, which were anesthetized with sodium pentobarbital (30 mg/kg), a midline laparotomy was performed, and a segment of the small bowel was selected which was supplied by a single mesenteric artery and vein. This loop of gut was exteriorized and placed on saline-soaked gauze on the abdomen. The mesenteric artery and vein were dissected free of the mesentery; then the perivascular nerves were also dissected free and cut proximally. Heparin was administered (10 mg/kg i.v.), and the mesenteric vein was cannulated. When the venous drainage was established, the artery was cannulated. The ends of the intestinal loop were ligated tightly with umbilical tape, and vascular perfusion of the isolated loop was begun. The isolated loop was covered with saline-soaked gauze and plastic wrap and its temperature was maintained at 37°C with infrared lamps.

423

Constant-rate perfusion of the loop was accomplished by drawing arterial blood from a femoral catheter or from a reservoir by means of a peristaltic pump (Cole-Parmer, Model #7545). From the pump the blood passed through a heater and the arterial cuvette of a photometric arteriovenous oxygen difference analyzer before entering the gut loop. On leaving the loop, the blood passed through the venous cuvette of that instrument and then into a cyclinder for timing and flow determination or into counting tubes for the isotope determinations. The orifice of the venous outflow was set at the appropriate hydrostatic level to produce zero pressure at the mesenteric vein. On the arterial side, provision was made for infusing drugs with a syringe driver. Perfusion pressure was monitored with a pressure transducer connected to the arterial catheter. The arteriovenous oxygen difference analyzer provided a continuous, direct record of A-V ΔO_2 (4). Perfusion pressure and arteriovenous oxygen difference were monitored on a direct-writing recorder.

In the first series of experiments the effects of norepinephrine (NE) infusion were studied. The norepinephrine (levarterenol bitartrate, Winthrop Laboratories) was diluted in physiological saline. Dosages were calculated as μg NE base/ml blood. The infusion of NE was carried out for seven minutes and 10 to 15 min were allowed between infusions. The problem of recirculation was avoided by collecting the venous effluent in a reservoir.

In the second series of experiments, effects of sympathetic nerve stimulation (SS) were studied. The perivascular sympathetic nerves were stimulated for a period of seven minutes with square-wave pulses (Grass Instrument Co., Model SD5). The stimulation parameters were as follows: frequency, 5 to 15 Hz; duration of pulse, 5 to 10msec; voltage, 5 to 20 V. Ten to fifteen min intervals were allowed between the seven min stimulation periods.This stimulation technique is essentially the same as that described earlier for isolated, perfused mesenteric artery preparations; and it has been shown to stimulate postganglionic sympathetic fibers (5,6).

In a third series of experiments blood-to-tissue extraction of ^{86}Rb was measured during sympathetic stimulation. The theoretical basis of the ^{86}Rb extraction technique has been developed by Renkin, and experimental work (7) has established Rb extraction as a useful index of the capillary surface area exposed to flowing blood. In our experiments 200 to 300 ml of blood were obtained from femoral arterial catheters. The blood was placed in a reservoir and stirred gently. Radioactive ^{86}RbCl (Amersham Searle) was added to the reservoir to produce an activity of 5,000 counts/min/gm blood. The isolated gut loop was subsequently perfused with the radioactive blood by switching the pump input from the femoral catheter to the reservoir. Sampling of venous blood was begun when the loop had been perfused long enough to wash out the non-radioactive blood and when the perfusion pressure and the arteriovenous oxygen difference had been stable for 10 to 15 min. During 30 sec of each min venous blood was collected in pre-weighted counting tubes. This sampling was continued for 3 min prior to nerve stimulation, during the 7 min stimulation period, and for 3 min during the post-stimulation period. Nerve stimulation was conducted as previously described. At the end of the experiment, each collection tube was reweighed and counted to at least 10,000 counts (Nuclear Chicago Autogamma Counter).

Capillary transport coefficients (PS, permeability times surface area) were calculated as follows: PS = -Q ln (1 - E) where Q is blood flow (ml/min x 100g) and E is the arteriovenous extraction ratio for ^{86}Rb. The present technique is essentially that of Renkin and Rosell (7); however, it has been modified for discontinuous sampling which allowed use of smaller amounts of radioactive label.

In all three studies, the gut loop was excised and weighed after each experiment. The gut segments in these experiments weighed 10 to 30 gm. Blood flow has been expressed in ml/min x 100 gm tissue. Resistance was calculated by dividing perfusion pressure (mm Hg) by blood flow (ml/min x 100 g).

RESULTS

In the first series of experiments, the effects of close intra-arterial infusions of norepinephrine on intestinal vascular resistance and oxygen extraction were studied. Table 1 shows the mean of five NE experiments with gut loops from five different dogs. The vascular resistance was calculated as previously described. Control data (mean ± SEM) for these experiments were as follows: perfusion pressure, 96.0 ± 6.9 mm Hg; blood flow, 37.3 ± 5.1 ml/min x 100 g; A-V ΔO_2, 4.10 ± 0.48 vol %; oxygen consumption, 1.47 ± 0.21 ml/min x 100 g. As Table 1 shows, the infusion of NE (0.65 μg/ml) caused marked increases in the calculated intestinal vascular resistance. These increases in resistance became statistically significant by the first minute of infusion and ceased to be significant one minute after the infusion was stopped. By contrast, the A-V ΔO_2's were significantly less than control throughout the infusion period. A tendency of A-V ΔO_2 to fall to a minimum level by the second minute of infusion and to "escape" thereafter can be seen; however, the variability of the time-course of the resistance responses obscures the "escape" phenomena in the pooled resistance data. Table 2 shows that the effects of norepinephrine on intestinal vascular resistance and oxygen extraction were dose-dependent.

In the second series of experiments, the effects of perivascular nerve stimulation on intestinal vascular resistance and oxygen extraction were studied. Table 3 shows the mean of five sympathetic stimulation experiments with gut loops from five different dogs. As Table 3 indicates, the stimulation of the perivascular nerves (10 Hz) caused marked increases in the intestinal vascular resistance. These increases in resistance became statistically significant by the first minute of stimulation and ceased to be significantly different from control when the stimulation was stopped. The maximum resistance was consistently reached by the end of the first or second minute of stimulation; and, as Table 3 also shows, the resistance vessels "escaped" somewhat from the initial vasoconstrictor effect of the stimulation. The arteriovenous oxygen difference fell rapidly with the onset of stimulation and the minimal A-V ΔO_2 was consistently reached by the end of the first or second minute of stimulation. The A-V ΔO_2 underwent considerable "escape" from the initial effect of the nerve stimulation. Nevertheless, the arteriovenous oxygen differences were significantly less than control throughout the stimulation period. Both parameters returned to control when the stimulation ceased. Table 4 shows that the effects of sympathetic stimulation on both resistance and oxygen extraction were frequency-dependent.

In a third series of experiments, the effects of sympathetic stimulation on the blood-to-tissue extraction of ^{86}Rb were measured along with resistance and oxygen extraction. In these experiments extraction of ^{86}Rb fell concomitantly with oxygen extraction during sympathetic stimulation. The changes in PS (calculated as previously described) and in A-V ΔO_2 were in the same direction and followed the same time-course. The relationship between PS and A-V ΔO_2 has been analyzed statistically and it is illustrated in Figure 1. Ten points from each of three experiments were used. As this graph indicates, the correlation between these two parameters was found to be highly significant.

DISCUSSION

Since earlier studies indicated that sympathetic stimulation may close mesenteric precapillary sphincters thereby diminishing the density of the perfused intestinal capillary bed (8,9), the purpose of this study was to determine whether such changes in the intestinal microvascular dynamics were sufficient to reduce the capillary-to-tissue oxygen flux, as our calculations indicated (2,3). To our knowledge the present findings, namely that norepinephrine and sympathetic stimulation do reduce intestinal oxygen uptake despite constant flow perfusion, have not previously been reported. Because the subject of this symposium is oxygen delivery to tissues, we will not discuss the present resistance data, but we will consider in detail the oxygen and ^{86}Rb extraction findings. In these experiments norepinephrine and sympathetic stimulation caused dose- or frequency-dependent reductions in intestinal oxygen extraction. In the experiments in which ^{86}Rb extraction was measured, changes in PS were synchronous with and directionally the same as the changes in oxygen extraction. The finding that norepinephrine and sympathetic stimulation depress intestinal extraction of oxygen despite constant-flow perfusion may be explained by at least three mechanisms which we will discuss separately: diminished tissue demand for oxygen, "true" or anatomical shunting, and "physiological" (capillary-to-capillary) shunting.

A decreased tissue demand for oxygen could explain the present oxygen extraction findings. Norepinephrine and sympathetic stimulation could possibly reduce intestinal tissue O_2 demand by relaxing visceral smooth muscle. This explanation seems unlikely because the visceral smooth muscle accounts for only 25-20% of the total intestinal oxygen consumption (Dr. Stanely G. Schultz, personal communication). Thus, the large reduction decreases in oxygen consumption are quantitatively inconsistent with this explanation. Also, the finding in this study and others (9) that norepinephrine and sympathetic stimulation reduce intestinal extraction of the non-metabolizable indicator, ^{86}Rb, makes this explanation extremely unlikely.

Although the opening of large-bore, impermeable A-V channels might be inconsistent with the large increases in vascular resistance observed, it is possible that the depressed extractions of both oxygen and Rb could be caused by the opening of anatomical shunts. However, there is little evidence which supports this possibility. The large submucosal A-V connections reported by Spanner (10) have not been confirmed. It is now accepted that no more than 3% of the total intestinal blood flow passes through channels larger than 20 micra in diameter (11). Finally,

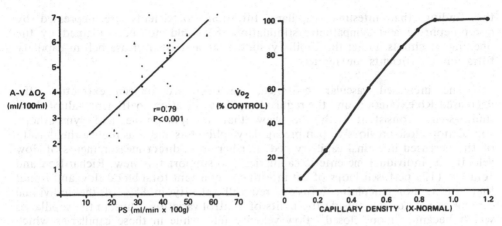

FIGURE 1.   Experimental results.   FIGURE 2.   Computor prediction.

TABLE 1.

N = 5		BEFORE	NOREPINEPHRINE INFUSION (0.65µg/ml)							AFTER NE	
		Min = 0	1	2	3	4	5	6	7	8	9
Resistance	x̄	274	589*	672*	702*	709*	689*	709*	714*	453	311
(mmHg/ml/											
min/100g)	SE	67.2	96.2	116.4	134.0	127.2	114.6	112.5	115.9	87.3	53.0
A-V ΔO₂	x̄	4.10	2.32*	2.14*	2.56*	2.48*	2.44*	2.52*	2.46*	3.26	3.54
(ml/100ml)	SE	0.48	0.32	0.34	0.27	0.34	0.38	0.42	0.36	0.36	0.33

*Indicates p<0.05 by paired t-test when compaired with time = 0

TABLE 2.

N = 5	DOSE OF NOREPINEPHRINE (µg/ml)			
	0	0.29	0.65	1.54
Resistance (% control ± SE)	100	165±21	280±42	368±50
A-V ΔO₂ (% control ± SE)	100	78.4±9.4	66.2±12.7	37.2±3.7

TABLE 3.

N = 5		BEFORE	SYMPATHETIC STIMULATION (10Hz)							AFTER SS	
		Min = 0	1	2	3	4	5	6	7	8	9
Resistance	x̄	100	281*	289*	260*	238*	234*	238*	226*	97	97
(%Control)	SE		29.6	38.8	54.8	59.4	59.5	55.0	51.2	5.1	4.2
A-V ΔO₂	x̄	100	70.2*	71.7*	76.8*	82.1*	84.7*	87.0*	85.7*	98.1	97.9
(%Control)	SE		2.20	3.58	4.64	4.90	4.81	3.26	3.00	2.87	1.91

TABLE 4.

N = 5	STIMULATION FREQUENCY(Hz)		
	0	10	15
Resistance (% control ± SE)	100	233±55.2	296±59.6
A-V ΔO₂ (% control ± SE)	100	85.8±3.4	73.5±5.4

the finding that intestinal capillary filtration coefficients are depressed by norepinephrine and sympathetic stimulation (8) could not be explained by the opening of shunts alone; the capillary surface area must decrease before capillary filtration coefficients are reduced.

The increased vascular resistance, the decreased oxygen extraction, the decreased Rb extraction, and the reduced capillary filtration coefficients--all of these findings--are consistent with the view that norepinephrine and sympathetic stimulation close previously open precapillary sphincters and thus reduce the density of the perfused intestinal capillary bed. Furthermore, direct measurements of flow velocity in individual mesenteric capillaries also support this view. Richardson and Johnson (12) perfused loops of cat intestine at constant total blood flow and found that during norepinephrine infusion, red cell velocity in 88% of the individual capillaries rose or fell outside the limits of control variation. Thus, in the capillaries which became "more closed" flow velocity fell, while in those capillaries which remained open flow velocity increased as they received blood flow from the capillaries undergoing closure. Also the same phenomenon that we find in the intestine (namely that sympathetic stimulation reduces oxygen uptake independently of its effects on blood flow) has been found in skeletal muscle. Renkin and Rosell (7) have reported that both oxygen and rubidium extraction are reduced in skeletal muscle by sympathetic stimulation. Finally, the computor simulation (Figure 2) shows that even if blood flow is held constant, simply reducing the number of perfused capillaries will lower oxygen extraction sharply once the density of the perfused capillary bed falls below a critical level.

In conclusion, the results support the view that sympathetic microvascular control of oxygen delivery to intestinal tissue operates by a dual mechanism: arteriolar regulation of blood flow and precapillary sphincter control of the diffusion parameters which determine oxygen extraction.

REFERENCES

1. Mellander, S., and B. Johansson. *Pharm. Rev.* 20:117-196, 1968.
2. Granger, H. J., and A. P. Shepherd. *Microvascular Research* 5:49-72, 1973.
3. Shepherd, A. P. and H. J. Granger. *Gastroenterology* (In Press).
4. Guyton, A. C., C. A. Farish, and J. W. Williams. *J. Appl. Physiol.* 14:145-147, 1959.
5. Rogers, L. A., R. A. Atkinson, and J. P. Long. *Am. J. Physiol.* 209:376-382, 1965.
6. Malik, K. U. *Circ. Res.* 27:647-655, 1970.
7. Renkin, E. M., and S. Rosell. *Acta Physiol. Scand.* 54:223-240, 1962.
8. Cobbold, A., B. Folkow, O. Lundgren, and I. Wallentin. *Acta Physiol. Scand.* 61:467-475, 1964.
9. Dresel, P., B. Folkow, and I. Wallentin. *Acta Physiol. Scand.* 67: 173-184, 1966.
10. Spanner, R. *Morph. Jahrb.* 69:394-454, 1932.
11. Delaney, J. P. *Am. J. Physiol.* 216:1556-1561, 1969.
12. Richardson, D. R., and P. C. Johnson. *Am. J. Physiol.* 219:1317-1323, 1970.

DISCUSSION OF SESSION II   SUBSESSION: ABDOMINAL ORGANS

Chairmen: Dr. Manfred Kessler, Dr. Jürgen Grote and
           Dr. James A. Miller, Jr.

DISCUSSION OF PAPER BY M. KESSLER, H. LANG, L. GOERNANDT,
   E. SINAGOWITZ, R. RINK AND J. HÖPER

Song: (1) How did you perfuse the liver--through both portal vein
and hepatic artery--or only one of those?
    (2) How about pO_2 gradient in the kidney from cortex to medulla
due to the countercurrent system in medullary blood flow and urine
flow. Have you observed any pO_2 difference or gradient in the renal
tissue?

Kessler: (1) The isolated rat liver was perfused through the portal
vein only. Our investigations showed that a sufficient local oxygen
supply can be provided when a perfusion rate of about 3.5 ml/g/min is
maintained and a critical temperature of 29-30°C (in hemoglobin-free
perfusion) is not exceeded.
    (2) The question of pO_2 gradients in the kidney was investi-
gated by Leichtweiss, H. P., et al., Pflügers Arch. ges. Physiol.,
309, 328 (1969) and by Baumgärtl, H. et al., Microvascular Res., 4,
247 (1972). In our own experiments, we only measured the local
oxygen supply in the outer cortex of kidney. Steinhausen, M.,
Pflügers Arch. ges. Physiol., 318, 244 (1970) was able to show that
in this part of kidney a countercurrent system may exist. As it is
shown in Fig. 2 of my paper, we observed a maximal pO_2-gradients of
60 mm Hg in the outer cortex. Measurements with pO_2 needle electrodes
under the control of vital microscopy have provided preliminary
indications that a countercurrent system as described by Steinhausen
may exist.

Coburn: I want to question the concept that the variations in tissue
pO_2 in your histograms necessarily mean nonuniform flow in the microcirculation. Could you not get variation in the presence of a homogeneous microcirculation as a result of sampling at different points
along a pO_2 gradient between capillary sites of O_2 consumption?

Kessler: In our analysis of homeostasis of tissue oxygen supply, we
took into consideration the pO_2 gradient along the capillary (Fig. 8
of my paper). The pO_2 gradient between capillaries amounts to only
2.0 - 2.5 mm Hg (at 22°C) and was not used for this reason. I agree
completely with your comment that the inhomogeneous pO_2 distribution
which we find in all tissues does not necessarily mean nonuniform
flow in the microcirculation. However, we can use the local pO_2
distribution as one parameter for the systems analysis, as we have
done it.

Van Liew: One way of testing whether the pO_2 differences are due to blood flow heterogeneity is to study pCO_2.

DISCUSSION OF PAPER BY J. A. MILLER, JR. AND M. KESSLER

Shapiro: CO_2 may also exert an effect on oxygen delivery via the pore effect. Do you have any idea as to what that might have been, especially in that you did correct for pH in one of your experiments?

Miller: Beyond that, I cannot offer you any data. This is one of the aspects of the study that I hope to continue when I return to Germany.

Shapiro: Did you see any difference between your pH corrected and non-corrected in terms of the relative gain in oxygenation?

Miller: No, it remained constant, so we do not think that the lowered pH was really reducing the oxygen utilization appreciably.

Shapiro: So you would think most of it was flow-dependent.

Kunze: Looking at one of your slides that was a record of surface pO_2, you had an increasing baseline after each increasing pCO_2, and I would like to know how long this effect lasted. The second question is, did you see any influence of the CO_2 to your pO_2 calibration curves, especially in the higher concentrations of CO_2?

Miller: These experiments represented a six-months period, and we have not really gotten to analyze all the aspects of the situation yet. I do not know precisely the significance of the change in baseline which sometimes was up and often went down. I do not know what that meant as a result of these treatments. Using short pulses of elevated CO_2 breathing probably does not sufficiently interfere with the physiology of function of the liver as to be a serious problem. I think the elevated oxygen levels may be of greater significance for some clinical conditions.

DISCUSSION OF PAPER BY J. HÖPER, M. KESSLER AND H. STARLINGER

Chance: Would you explain a little bit what the energy source was, and also comment upon the fact that the ADP level was considerably elevated? Actually, one could only tell from your bar graphs how high it went, but maybe some attention should be focused upon this. What was the energy source, in other words, what was the likely substrate for the anaerobic condition?

Kessler: The energy source was glycogen because we used fed rats. The glycogen content of these livers was after one hour of anoxia. We calculated that, in our experiments, the anaerobic glycolysis produced 8-10% of the quantity of ATP which is normally produced by oxidative phosphorylation. The ADP levels increased from 0.56 μmol/g liver w/w to 0.89 μmol/g liver w/w at 30°C and to 0.82 μmol/g liver w/w at 15°C.

Lübbers: Did you control the histological pattern or picture of your liver after the different ischemia or after the perfusion experiments?

Höper: Not after ischemia, but after anoxic perfusion, we made an experiment on some of the perfusions. The respiration of the tissue was in a normal range, and also in the liver.

Kessler: The morphological integrity seems to be fine. We did first electronmicroscopic studies, and as far as we can see, after one hour there is no severe damage.

Panigel: I wonder how, under the electron microscope, the morphological evaluation was done on different organelles? The liver cells are very rich in lysosomes and in dense bodies and I wonder what happened to the organelles in the liver after even a short perfusion. What was the exact duration of the perfusion in these experiments?

Höper: As I mentioned in my presentation, after five hours of normoxic perfusion, we have only very slight edema of the Golgi apparatus. Of course, when you have anoxia and severe acidosis, you will also get severe changes in morphological integrity. But, under these conditions, when the medium is well buffered and no severe acidosis happens, then it is very astonishing that the organ remains very fine over a period of one hour. We cannot know what happens over longer times.

DISCUSSION OF PAPER BY H. RAHMER AND M. KESSLER

Chance: Congratulations on your nice experiments. In the brain, it is possible to make simple corrections, as described by Mayevsky today, and Kobayeshi and Ogata have made such corrections for the kidney. Can you correct for the effects? Do you get the same results in situ or do they differ from the results obtained on liver in situ with Schoener?

<u>Rahmer</u>: For a correct interpretation of the fluorescence trace we postulate a calibration curve because in our experiment on rat liver we found no linear relationship. The correction of Kobayeshi is based on a linear relationship. It is also very difficult to establish the isolated effect of hemoglobin deoxygenation <u>in situ</u>.

<u>Kessler</u>: The calibration can be done by hemodilution if it is performed in a way that microcirculation is not disturbed: Messmer, K. et al., <u>Res</u>. <u>exp</u>. <u>Med</u>., <u>159</u>, 152 (1973). We found a large scattering of the values when different organs were compared. So each organ will need an individual calibration curve.

Our results of cycles of ischemia in liver, which were obtained by a similar method as used by Schoener, showed the same fluorescence increase. The isobestic measurement of changes in the local hemoglobin concentration, which was performed as reference measurement at 585 nm, showed that most of the fluorescence increase was due to the decrease of local hemoglobin concentration.

<u>Harbig</u>: (1) You mentioned that a change in blood volume and a change in hemoglobin oxygenation cause absorption artifacts. Do you have any idea on the relative importance of both in N_2-anoxia?

(2) Is it possible that the intensity of your ultraviolet light source was not high enough to penetrate the liver tissue deep enough? Under this consideration in anoxia the exciting light would be absorbed by the increasing blood volume already without reaching the NADH.

<u>Rahmer</u>: (1) In nitrogen anoxia <u>in situ</u>, we recorded both a decrease of the local hemoglobin concentration and an increase of NADH fluorescence. Thus, at least part of the fluorescence increase is due to the decreased blood content. As we were able to show, there is no linear relation between local hemoglobin concentration and extinction at 366, 460 and 585 nm. Furthermore, light scattering causes different absorption at different wavelengths. This has to be taken into consideration when the recorded signals are corrected.

(2) Our measurements, after giving ethanol and rotenone, showed that the NADH was excited because of the very constant response to the inhibitors.

<u>Lübbers</u>: Together with Schwikardi, we obtained the same effect in brain tissue. In anoxia, the local blood volume change can reverse the flrorescence signal for NADH.

DISCUSSION OF PAPER BY M. THERMANN. O. ZELDER, F. HESS,
    C. R. JERUSALEM AND H. HAMMELMANN

Huch: Did you take care that your measurements were made under
constant conditions, that means a constant arterial pO_2? Have you
measured correlations between PaO_2, pO_2 in the vena portae on one
side and surface pO_2 on the other side?

Thermann: Continuous measurements of arterial or portal pO_2 are
rather difficult in such a small animal as the rat. We have not
measured these values.

Messmer: Since Dr. Jerusalem, a well-known pathologist for the
evaluation of liver grafts is on your paper, it would be of interest
to have your comment on the liver's ultrastructure. How do histological changes correlate with the low pO_2 values observed over a
five-weeks period?

Thermann: In the first period of regeneration of the graft, we find
hypertrophy and hyperplasia of liver cells. The number and the size
of liver cells increases but the amount of hepatons remains equal.
The distance of the hepatic trinity to the central vein, normally
about 350 microns in the mean, increases to mean values of about 450-
500 microns. This increase of capillary length leads to an increase
of oxygen utilization and may be the cause of low oxygen pO_2. After
approximately two months, a dichotomy of central veins takes place,
and the amount of hepatons increases. The result is a decrease of
capillary length to normal values.

Panigel: I think that the use of radioactive microspheres may bring
an answer to the question of the cause of the low pO_2 during the
first weeks after liver transplantation. Scanning by isotropic
scintography is difficult in such a small organ as the rat liver,
but observation of the distribution of the microspheres by microscopic techniques may give a precious clue to hemodynamic changes
if they take place after transplantation.

Thermann: It would be very interesting to measure circulation rates
of the graft. We were not able to perform these investigations.

DISCUSSION OF PAPER BY W. BRAUNBECK, H. HUTTEN AND P. VAUPEL

Groom: (1) On what basis are you able to postulate that your slow
compartment represents blood flow through the white pulp only?

(2) I am a bit unhappy that in an organ where the hematocrit
can be 90%, you are relying on the use of only a plasma label (Kr^{85})
to measure what you term "blood" flow. Can you defend this?

<u>Braunbeck</u>: (1) We contribute the blood flow through the white pulp
to the slow compartment because the fast compartment completely disappears after injection of spherocytes, and if the red pulp is not
perfused, rSBF reveals values which correspond to that of the white
pulp.
        (2) The flow rates obtained by the Kr^{85} technique are not
depending on the hematocrit because the partition-coefficient of
Kr between plasma and red cells amounts to 1.0.

DISCUSSION OF PAPER BY L. SUNDER-PLASSMANN, E. SINAGOWITZ, R. RINK,
        R. DIETERLE, K. MESSMER AND M. KESSLER

<u>Murthy</u>: I must congratulate you for this very interesting study
with stroma-free hemoglobin solution. We are investibating the
use of stroma-free hemoglobin solution as a blood substitute. Our
studies on coronary vascular bed show very well maintained cardiac
contractility with hematocrit values as low as 20 vols % when
exchanges are carried out with hemoglobin solution.

<u>Sunder-Plassmann</u>: We can confirm your measurements on myocardial
contractility even in more extreme hemodilution down to a hematocrit of 10%. As published earlier, measurements of different contractility parameters, as deduced from the catheter-tip manometer
technique, have failed to demonstrate any detrimental effect on
cardiac performance of hemoglobin solution.

<u>Strauss</u>: This excellent work certainly opens new ways to the man-
agement of hemorrhagic shock. Your stated plans of binding hemoglobin to larger molecules should facilitate use of this solution.
From the clinical point of view, concern is expressed as to the
deleterious effects of free hemoglobin at levels higher than those
needed for renal excretion of hemoglobin. With the very high levels
which you attained in plasma, did you observe any renal functional
or histological changes?

<u>Sunder-Plassmann</u>: Special functional studies of the kidney have not
been made in these experiments. However, there seems to be conclusive evidence from the work of different laboratories (Rabiner,
Litwin, Relihan) that stroma-free preparations do not interfere with
normal kidney function even in dehydrated animals. Kidney damage,
as reported to occur when blood hemolysates are infused, or when
blood is hemolyzed <u>in</u> <u>vivo</u>, seems to be due entirely to the red
cell stroma.

<u>Duhm</u>: Do you think that this loss of hemoglobin from the solution
is probably because of the emission of hemoglobin dimers? Is it
possible that the hemoglobin is breaking down into dimers and getting

lost from the circulation into extracellular space?

Sunder-Plassmann: We have no evidence for that, but it could well be. On the other hand, if you collect the urine of these dogs and put it in the Van Slyke apparatus, measurements of oxygen capacity give exactly what you would expect from a normal hemoglobin molecule in tetrameric conditions. I think we can decide that definitely.

DISCUSSION OF PAPER BY A. V. BERAN, D. R. SPERLING, A. WAKABAYASHI
    AND J. E. CONNOLLY

Lübbers: I wonder if the oxygen flow has anything to do with the oxygen consumption. I know it is the blood flow which regulates the oxygen consumption. As a matter of fact, the perfusion rate and the reabsorption of the kidneys depends on the blood flow. Also, the oxygen consumption of the kidney depends on the flow; so for establishing your results, you should have changed the hemoglobin content of your blood really to establish or to make the conclusion for sure that it is the oxygen flow which you can relate on. I am not convinced it is just the blood flow. If you do not change hemoglobin content, you cannot decide between flow and transport, or oxygen which the blood has transported. The oxygen is not secreted and has nothing to do. For drawing this conclusion, you must give data on the variation of hemoglobin content.

Tepper: (1) Did the pulse generated in the aorta by your pump have a shape similar to that created by the natural heart?
    (2) If your graph of oxygen availability vs. oxygen consumption is extrapolated to zero oxygen availability, your curve does not read zero oxygen consumption. How do you explain this in terms of your use of a linear regression analysis?

Beran: (1) The pneumatically driven ventricular pump used in these experiments produced an aortic pulse wave form similar to the normal aortic form.
    (2) At higher and lower values for renal oxygen flow, the renal oxygen consumption curve flattens thus forming an "S" shape curve. Values depicted in Fig. 3 represent the middle portion of this curve.

Song: Could you give the reason that the pulsatile flow is better than non-pulsatile flow for renal tissue oxygenation? Perhaps in terms of hydrodynamical viewpoint, such as Wamersely's α coefficient?

Beran: From the nature of our data, we can only at best speculate that the reason for superiority of pulsatile perfusion is better flow distribution and fewer intrarenal shunts.

DISCUSSION OF PAPER BY CH. WEISS AND V. THIEMAN

Duling: As you know investigators have used elevations of venous
pressure as a means of separating the myogenic and metabolic hypotheses for autoregulation. Have you tested the responses of your
preparation to elevations in venous pressure?

Weiss: Yes, however, I think others have shown that the renal responses are consistent with a myogenic response. The skeletal muscle and heart appear to function quite differently and may be regulated by metabolic feedback. The metabolic hypothesis assumes that
an increase in perfusion pressure increases either the supply of
some substance or perhaps the washout of a metabolically linked
material. The substance is assumed to be vasoactive and an alteration in concentration causes a vasoconstriction of the vascular
smooth muscle and thus stabilizes flow.

DISCUSSION OF PAPER BY A. P. SHEPHERD, D. MAILMAN, T.F. BURKS
     AND H. J. GRANGER

Messmer: First of all I would like to congratulate you on your
very nice study. To which degree is the redistribution of flow
dependent upon the intraluminal pressure of the bowel segment?
Furthermore I would like to know if you have any evidence as to
where this redistribution of flow would take place in the bowel
wall.

Shepherd: I am afraid I really cannot answer that question. I
have not studied the effects of intraluminal pressure yet, and I
have myself no data about the relative distribution of one anatomical layer of the intestine or another. There are some Scandinavian
studies that have not yet been published in full regarding the
effects of norepinephrine infusion, but in the case of those experiments they were performed under constant pressure conditions, and
I would not dare to extrapolate from them to tell you which layer
of the intestine is more affected than another.

Rink: We have some information in rat that during bleeding, the
oxygen distribution along the mucosal surface drops very early during successive hemorrhages whereas it remains relatively high along
the serosal surface so at least in this animal perhaps there is
some indirect evidence of these AV shunts, perhaps located in the
submucosa.

Shepherd: I do not think we can made a very good case for submucosal AV shunts. The early report by Schponer in 1932 has been

discredited by most investigators. The microsphere data would indicate that no more than three per cent of the total intestinal
blood flow goes through channels larger than 20 microns in diameter
and furthermore this three per cent is not affected by vasoactive
agents.

Subsession: MUSCLE

Chairmen: Dr. Manfred Kessler, Dr. Jürgen Grote

and Dr. James A. Miller, Jr.

OXYGEN AUTOREGULATION IN SKELETAL MUSCLE

Thomas K. Goldstick

Chemical Engineering Dept., Northwestern University and
Research Laboratories, Evanston Hospital
Evanston, Ill., 60201 U.S.A.

Almost 100 years ago SEVERINI [1878] discovered that local
changes in PO_2 altered the caliber of small blood vessels. To this
day, however, we still do not understand this phenomenon [DULING,
1972] now referred to as oxygen autoregulation. Two major
questions remain to be answered. What exactly are the local
circulatory changes? And how are these changes mediated? Oxygen
autoregulation can be defined as the active, rapid adaptation of
the tissue oxygen supply system to changes in the availability or
utilization of oxygen. It occurs in all tissues, to a greater or
lesser extent, and involves both systemic and local adjustments.
In order to separate oxygen autoregulation from other phenomena,
such as pressure autoregulation, oxygen must be the only variable.
The objective here was to study the intensity and dynamics of the
response within an intact skeletal muscle (canine gracilis) to
changes in oxygen availability, with all other systemic parameters
constant, and, from the observed dynamics, to model the local
circulatory changes in oxygen autoregulation. An input-output
method identical to the one already employed to study tissue oxygen
transport [GOLDSTICK et al., 1969; WAGNER, 1971; GOLDSTICK et al.,
1973] was used here to study oxygen autoregulation. Its great
advantage was that it left the muscle as intact as possible. To
keep all other systemic parameters (such as blood pressures,

The research summarized here was supported by Evanston Hospital grant 3565 and N.I.H. grants GM-874, GM-17115, and GM-46231.
I gratefully acknowledge this support and also the advice, guid-
ance, and technical assistance of DRS. J. A. CAPRINI, W. A. FRY,
L. ZUCKERMAN, and MR. J. E. MITTERLING, all of Evanston Hospital.

gracilis muscle blood flow rate, and muscle oxygen consumption rate) constant, all tests were conducted with the animal euoxic, i.e., at or above normal PO_2.

METHOD

Animal Preparation

Adult mongrel dogs (18 to 25 kg) were anesthetized with sodium pentobarbital, intubated, and respirated under positive pressure (Harvard Apparatus Co., Millis, Mass.). Initially, the minute volumes were adjusted to give normal pHa values, 7.31 to 7.42 [ALTMAN and DITTMER, 1971], and then pHa was adjusted, by hyperventilation or hypercapnic gas mixtures, to give the desired value. Somewhat larger than normal tidal volumes were used to speed lung washout.

For withdrawal of blood samples and for pressure measurements, one femoral artery and vein were cannulated. Oxygen electrodes were placed in the primary gracilis blood vessels of the un-cannulated limb (Figure 1), after first heparinizing (1000 to 2000 U) to prevent clotting around the electrodes and litigating the small veins draining into the gracilis vein. The smaller gracilis blood supplies were left intact. The arterial electrode was inserted via a side branch into the femoral artery with its tip close to the gracilis artery. The venous electrode was inserted through a puncture hole into the femoral vein so that its tip projected into the mouth of the gracilis vein. The gracilis muscle itself was left virtually intact.

Electrodes and Data Reduction

Specially constructed [WAGNER, 1971], CLARK-type membrane-covered, needle oxygen electrodes (Figure 2) were employed to monitor continuously PaO_2 and PvO_2 in the gracilis vessels. The electrode, modified from the design originated by Instrumentation Laboratories (Lexington, Mass.), consisted of a 0.001-inch diameter, enamel-coated platinum cathode (Secon Metals, White Plains, N.Y.) embedded in water-resistant epoxy resin (Microcast 200, Electro-Science Laboratories, Philadelphia) inside a 30-gauge silver-plated hypodermic needle which served as the anode. The needle was encased in a tight, gel-filled, polypropylene membrane shaped like the finger of a glove (Instrumentation Laboratories).

Just before each experiment the electrodes were polarized for several hours at 0.8 V and then tested for responsiveness, stability, and linearity using gases of known PO_2. During an experiment the electrodes were checked <u>in situ</u> using blood samples. Only electrodes which were insensitive to stirring, had 90% response times of<10 sec, exhibited negligible drift, and were linear with PO_2 were used.   The electrode currents were amplified (Model 414S, Keithley Instruments, Cleveland, Ohio), recorded on a standard FM tape recorder, converted from analog to digital form at 3 points/ sec [WAGNER, 1971], and processed on the Northwestern University CDC 6400 computer with displays on a Calcomp plotter.

Experiment

The input-output method used here consists of rapidly changing gracilis PaO_2, continuously measuring gracilis PvO_2, and based on what is in the output transient and not in the input inferring what is happening in the muscle itself. During the PO_2 transient the femoral vein blood flow distal to the gracilis muscle was temporarily occluded so that only blood from the gracilis vein drained into the femoral vein at the point of the venous electrode. PaO_2 changes were made by changing the breathing gas between room air and 100% O_2 or between 5% CO_2 21% O_2 in N_2, and 5% CO_2 in O_2. Transients were always measured between gases of the same PCO_2 but different PO_2.

RESULTS

Typical experimental transients are shown in Figure 3 from the work of WAGNER [1971] in this laboratory. In a separate set

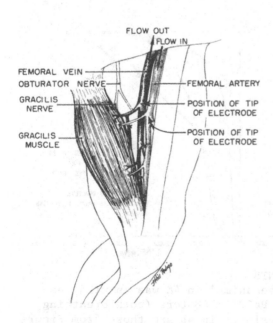

FIGURE 1: MUSCLE PREPARATION

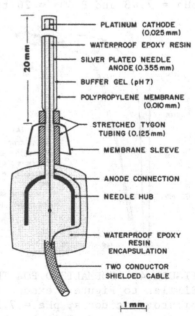

FIGURE 2: OXYGEN ELECTRODE

of experiments also in this laboratory, ELLWEIN [1972] found that during all types of PO_2 transients the gracilis muscle blood flow (QT) and pressure remained practically constant throughout the

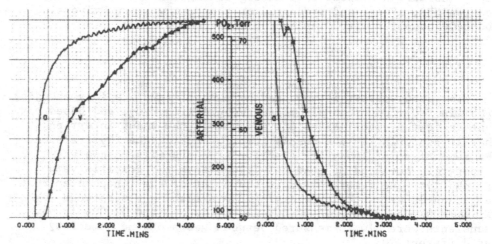

FIGURE 3:   ARTERIAL AND VENOUS PO_2 TRANSIENTS
At t = 0 the breathing gas was changed from room air to 100% O_2 (left) or from 100% O_2 to room air (right). These computer plots are essentially continuous (3 points/sec) with symbols for identification only. This animal was in mild respiratory alkalosis, pHa = 7.48 and $PaCO_2$ = 26 torr.

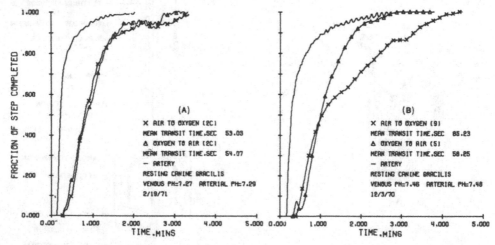

FIGURE 4:   NORMALIZED PO_2 TRANSIENTS
Similar to Figure 3 except that the animal in 4A was in mild respiratory acidosis, pHa = 7.29 and $PaCO_2$ = 48 torr (both breathing gases contained 5% CO_2). The transients in 4B are those from Figure 3 normalized. Only one of the PaO_2 transients is shown in each case.

transient, approximately 3 min. Also pH, PCO_2, and muscle a-v O_2 difference have always been found to remain constant during PO_2 transients.

Although the PaO_2 transients were always practically identical for all gas changes, on occasion it was found that the shape of the PvO_2 transient depended upon the direction of the PaO_2 change. They were different for upward and downward steps. These shape differences which can be seen more easily if the curves are normalized and superimposed (Figure 4) are measures of the system nonlinearity and thus, vida infra, are detectors of oxygen auto-regulation.

In addition to the visual comparison of transients possible in Figure 4, it might have been instructive to calculate the actual residence time distribution functions by converting from normalized PO_2 to normalized concentration and then deconvolving to eliminate the effect of the imperfection in the arterial step. This is now being done and preliminary results suggest that conversion to concentration has little effect on the venous curves, perhaps because the blood-oxygen saturation curve is straight in this region, and also that the arterial curves, which were usually more than three times faster than the venous, were probably fast enough to be considered perfect steps by comparison. As a first approximation then the mean transit time, t, was calculated [WAGNER, 1971] by considering the venous response to be the concentration transient corresponding to an arterial step change occuring at the arterial appearance time. Although the absolute values of t̄ contain in-accuracies, the differences in t indicate differences in the venous

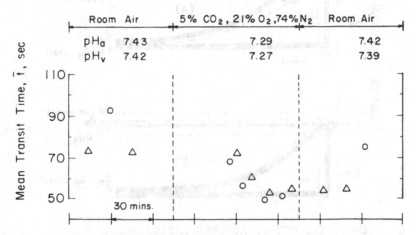

FIGURE 5:   OXYGEN MEAN TRANSIT TIMES
The lower PO_2 breathing gas compositions are listed above. For the higher, the N_2 was replaced by O_2. Circles are for increasing PaO_2 and triangles for decreasing.

response curves, i.e., nonlinearities in the muscle oxygen transport system. Figure 5 shows the $\bar{t}$'s for a series of transients on
the same animal with different sets of breathing gases.

DISCUSSION

Figure 4A illustrates an occasion when the normalized PvO_2
transients were identical whichever the direction of the PaO_2
change. In this case the gracilis muscle oxygen transport system
was linear as it invariably was with $pHa < 7.32$. Since the system
was linear it could not have been autoregulatory oxygen. Although
the value for $\bar{t}$ can really only characterize a linear, non-
regulating system, even for nonlinear systems (Figure 4B) $\bar{t}$ differences can still be used to quantitate the nonlinearity and thus the
intensity of autoregulation. Figure 5 shows by comparing the $\bar{t}$'s
for upward and downward steps that the system nonlinearity could be
reversibly and reproducibly suppressed by mild hypercapnic acidosis.
Furthermore, the extent of nonlinearity was found to increase progressively with increasing pHa. In the normal range of pHa, 7.31
to 7.42 [ALTMAN and DITTMER, 1971], the shapes of the PvO_2
transients evolved from those of Figure 4A close to those of
Figure 4B, but they never exhibited a hump [GOLDSTICK et al.,
1973].

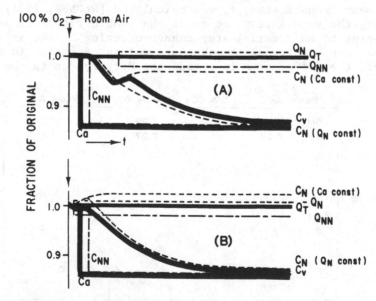

FIGURE 6:   SIMPLIFIED OXYGEN AUTOREGULATION MODEL
The two compartments are non-nutritional, NN, and nutritional, N.
C = oxygen concentration, Q = blood flow rate, T = total.

In mild hyperventilation-induced alkalosis, with pHa>7.47, the muscle oxygen transport system was not only nonlinear but invariably exhibited a characteristic hump in the downward PvO_2 transient (Figure 3, right). Since the muscle was always adequately supplied with oxygen, changes in PaO_2 had a minimal effect on the other parameters of the system external to the muscle. The nonlinearities, therefore, must have been related to an internal rearrangement of oxygen pathways. PAPPENHEIMER [1941] proposed just such a rearrangement between subsystems of high and low oxygen consumption. Figure 3 provides the data necessary to study the dynamics of this internal rearrangement. The hump of Figure 3 could only occur in a system with time varying elements. Although these elements could be modelled in many different ways, it seemed appropriate at this early stage of the study to utilize the simplest possible model capable of explaining the data, i.e., a two compartment PAPPENHEIMER-type model. Figure 6 illustrates the transients which result from such a model. For ease of presentation, oxygen concentration (C) is used rather than PO_2. The muscle oxygen transport system of Figure 6 is composed of two subsystems, a pure lag (NN) and a lag plus a first order term (N). The N subsystem has a constant oxygen consumption while the NN has zero. The NN circuit may be thought of as a blood shunt with the distribution of flow between it and the N circuit being the time varying element in the oxygen transport system. All changes except in PvO_2 are considered to be perfect steps.

This model is obviously a gross oversimplification. There are probably many more than two subsystems in a single muscle, no pure lags, no perfect steps, nor, according to SPENCE et al. [1972], any anatomical non-nutritional shunts. However, even with many multiordered subsystems each with a different oxygen extraction, with imperfect step changes, and with diffusional shunts like those found by SEJRSEN and TONNESEN [1972], the modelled transients would still be basically the same as shown in Figure 6, so long as the distribution of internal pathways for oxygen remained the time varying element.

Figure 6 was constructed by considering the effect on a downward Cv transient of an increase in QN, a decrease in QNN, and as observed experimentally, a constant QT. The flow redistribution was considered to occur either before or after the step in Ca (Figure 6B or 6A respectively). Cv is the smoothed sum of CNN and CN where the latter has a hump corresponding to the change in QN. The small step in Cv corresponding to the step in CNN would have been smoothed by our measuring system. According to Figure 6, a hump in Cv could have been observed in the transient records only if QN had increased after Cv started to decrease (Figure 6B). The hump of Figure 3 thus appears to be an autoregulatory redistribution of flow occurring after the PvO_2 transient has started. This is

suggestive of locally rather than centrally mediated circulatory
changes in oxygen autoregulation.

It is well known that the total blood flow to skeletal muscle
depends upon $PaCO_2$. This effect is both locally and centrally
mediated [BLAIR et al., 1960]. In unanesthetized humans, hypercapnic acidosis depresses muscle blood flow [BLAIR et al., 1960]
while hyperventilation enhances it [JUNG et al., 1971]. Similar
effects were observed here with anesthetized dogs. Hypercapnia
with pHa < 7.32 (the region of linearity and suppressed autoregulation) led to a decrease in gracilis muscle blood flow to approximately 70% of the normal resting value and hyperventilation with
pHa > 7.47 to an increase to approximately 150% of normal [ELLWEIN,
1972]. It was therefore, unfortunately, impossible to separate the
effects of pH, PCO_2, and QT. It remains to be determined which of
these three parameters controlled the observed changes in intensity
of oxygen autoregulation. Also, "black box" experimental preparations and models can rarely determine whether oxygen autoregulation
is mediated by local or central effects. Whatever the stimulus and
mechanism, autoregulation appears to be accomplished by an internal
rearrangement of oxygen pathways.

SUMMARY

Autoregulatory changes in oxygen pathways have been studied
within an intact, euoxic, resting skeletal muscle (canine gracilis)
following changes in PaO_2. This was done by analyzing the PvO_2
transient corresponding to the PaO_2 change. Shape differences between PvO_2 transients corresponding to increasing and to decreasing
PaO_2, when all other system parameters such as blood pressure,
total muscle blood flow, and oxygen consumption rate remained
constant, are thought to represent active internal rearrangement of
oxygen pathways and thus oxygen autoregulation. This rearrangement
could be reproducibly and reversibly suppressed by mild hypercapnic
acidosis (pHa < 7.32) and progressively intensified by increasing
pHa until, with mild respiratory alkalosis (pHa > 7.47), downward
PvO_2 transients became non-monotonic unlike any other transients
observed. The hump which was found confirmed the presence of time
varying elements within the oxygen transport system and permitted
the development of a simple model of the dynamics of the rearrangement. This model has two compartments, one a pure lag (non-
nutritional) the other a lag plus a first order term (nutritional).
From the present experiments, the effects on autoregulation
intensity of pH, PCO_2, and muscle blood flow could not be separated
because changes in these parameters always occurred together.
Also, the present data are not adequate to allow us to decide
whether the non-nutritional pathway represents a blood or gas shunt
nor whether oxygen autoregulation is centrally or locally mediated.

REFERENCES

ALTMAN, P. L. and DITTMER, D.S. (1971). "Respiration and Circula-
    tion." Federation of American Societies for Experimental
    Biology, Bethesda. p. 225.

BLAIR, D. A., GLOVER, W. E., McARDLE, L., and RODDIE, I.C. (1960).
    The mechanism of the peripheral vasodilatation following
    carbon dioxide inhalation in man. Clin. Sci. 19: 407-423.

DULING, B. R. (1972). Microvascular responses to alterations in
    oxygen tension. Circ. Res. 31:481-489.

ELLWEIN, R. W. (1972). "Flow Response of Skeletal Muscle to Hyper-
    oxia, Hypercapnia, and Hyperventilation." M.S. Thesis,
    Northwestern University, Evanston, Ill.

GOLDSTICK, T. K., ALLEN, B. J., and FRY, W. A. (1969). Oxygenation
    of tissue studied by an input-output technique. Proc. Int.
    Conf. Med. & Biol. Engineering. 8:1.2.

GOLDSTICK, T. K., FRY, W. A., CAPRINI, J. A., WAGNER, E. P., Jr. and
    ELLWEIN, R. W. (1973). Study of oxygen transport in skeletal
    muscle using an unsteady state method. In Proc. 7th Europ.
    Conf. Microcirculation, Aberdeen, 1972. (J. Ditzel and
    D. H. Lewis eds.). Karger, Basel.

JUNG, R. C., WALSH, J. A., and HYMAN, C. (1971). Response of human
    forearm muscle blood vessels to hyperventilation. Cardiovasc.
    Res. 5:347-352.

PAPPENHEIMER, J. R. (1941). Vasoconstrictor nerves and oxygen con-
    sumption in the isolated perfused hindlimb muscles of the dog.
    J. Physiol. 99:182-200.

SEJRSEN, P. and TONNESEN, K. H. (1972). Shunting by diffusion of
    inert gas in skeletal muscle. Acta Physiol. Scan. 86:82-91.

SEVERINI, L. (1878). "Richerche sulla Innervazione dei Vasi
    Sanguigni." Instituto Fisiologico, Perugia. pp. 94-102.

SPENCE, R. J., RHODES, B. A., and WAGNER, H. N., Jr. (1972).
    Regulation of arteriovenous anastomotic and capillary blood
    flow in the dog leg. Am. J. Physiol. 222:326-332.

WAGNER, E. P., Jr. (1971). "Investigation of the Response of
    Skeletal Muscle to Hyperoxic Changes in PO_2 at Different
    Levels of Blood pH." M.S. Thesis, Northwestern University,
    Evanston, Ill.

INTRINSIC METABOLIC REGULATION OF BLOOD FLOW, O_2 EXTRACTION AND TISSUE O_2 DELIVERY IN DOG SKELETAL MUSCLE

Harris J. Granger, Anthony H. Goodman, and D. N. Granger

Dept. Physiology & Biophysics, University of Mississippi

School of Medicine, Jackson, Mississippi, 39216

INTRODUCTION

In a recent systems analysis of intrinsic microvascular control of tissue oxygen delivery[1], we proposed that O_2 delivery to skeletal muscle cells was autoregulated in accordance with their metabolic requirements through local metabolic control of blood flow and O_2 extraction. We also suggested that blood flow is regulated through feedback regulation of arteriolar tone, and O_2 extraction is modulated through precapillary sphincter control of capillary surface area and capillary-to-cell diffusion distance. Our analysis, which includes as a major feature the assumption that precapillary sphincter sensitivity to metabolic control is greater than that of the arterioles, suggests that: 1) When the venous oxygen reserve is large, increased extraction is the major mechanism by which tissue oxygen delivery is maintained in accordance with cellular requirements, whenever the O_2 availability-to-demand ratio is reduced. Under these conditions, the contribution of local flow regulation is minimal. 2) As the prevailing venous oxygen reserve decreases, the contribution of the arteriolar flow control system increases and the importance of the precapillary sphincter control of O_2 extraction diminishes. Indeed, at a venous oxygen saturation of 25 per cent, blood flow responses account for over 90 per cent of the total compensation. 3) Thus, as metabolic stresses become greater, the major locus of intrinsic microvascular control of tissue oxygen delivery moves from the normally more sensitive sphincters to the upstream arterioles. In this manner, adequate tissue oxygenation is maintained over a wide range of metabolic stresses, the relative contribution of blood flow and O_2 extraction to the regulation of tissue oxygen delivery being determined by the prevailing venous oxygen level. The data presented in this paper represent the experimental basis of our analysis.

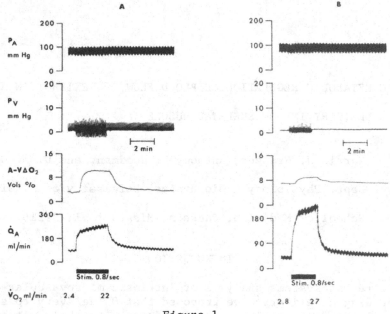

Figure 1

METHODS

The experiments were conducted on large mongrel dogs and the following variables were monitored: iliac artery pressure, iliac vein pressure, iliac artery flow, and hindlimb arteriovenous oxygen difference. To assure that the response of the monitored variables to a pertubation was intrinsic in nature, we eliminated nervous control loops by alcohol destruction of the spinal cord and decapitation. Positive-pressure respiration was used and normal vascular tone was maintained by constant infusion of epinephrine.

A blood reservoir was connected to the arterial system via a carotid catheter. The reservoir was suspended from the ceiling and arterial pressure could be controlled by adjusting the height of the reservoir. The metabolic and hemodynamic responses in the dog hindlimb to the following changes were studied: 1) direct stimulation of the thigh and calf muscles at frequencies ranging from .2 per second to 3.2 per second; 2) graded arterial hypoxia utilizing 10 per cent O_2, 8 per cent O_2, and 6 per cent O_2 mixtures; 3) arterial occlusion of 5 seconds to 5 minutes duration; and 4) step decreases in arterial pressure. To study the effect of the prevailing venous oxygen level on the metabolic and hemodynamic responses to these pertubations, we altered the venous oxygen concentration over a wide range in each dog in the following manner. The initial A-V O_2 difference was raised by increasing the rate of infusion of epinephrine, which caused a reduction in blood flow

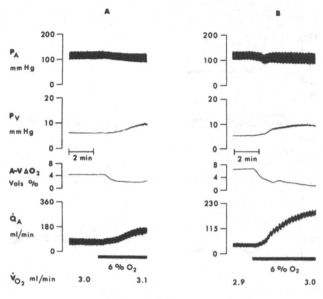

Figure 2

and an increase in A-V O_2 difference. Tissue oxygen delivery, however, was not significantly altered. In some experiments the venous oxygen content was lowered by other means as discussed below.

RESULTS AND DISCUSSION

The intrinsic responses to direct muscle stimulation at .8 per second are shown in Figure 1. Panel A shows the hemodynamic and metabolic response to muscle stimulation when the venous oxygen reserve is large. In this case, the contraction induces a three-fold increase in blood flow and a threefold increase in oxygen extraction, thereby producing a ninefold increase in hindlimb oxygen consumption. Panel B shows the response of the same preparation to the same stimulus after the initial A-V O_2 difference has been increased to 6.8 volumes per cent by increasing the epinephrine infusion rate. In contrast to the response obtained at a prevailing A-V oxygen difference of 3.3 volumes per cent, the functional hyperemia accounts for more than 70 per cent of the increase in tissue oxygen delivery, and O_2 extraction increases by less than 40 per cent.

In similar experiments we found that at lower and normal A-V O_2 differences, increased extraction of oxygen from flowing blood is the most important mechanism for incrasing tissue oxygen delivery when the hindlimb is stimulated to contract at low frequencies. At higher stimulation rates, the contribution of functional hyperemia increases. If, on the other hand, the initial venous oxygen

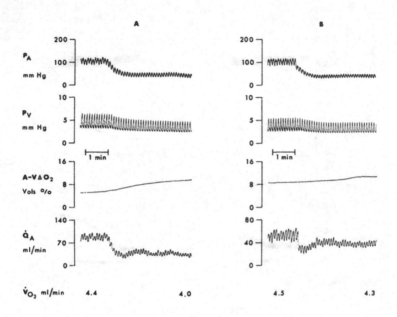

Figure 3

content is decreased by infusion of vasoconstrictors, then oxygen delivery is increased mainly by a large increase in blood flow, even at low stimulation frequencies.

The intrinsic metabolic control mechanisms can also maintain adequate tissue oxygenation when O_2 availability is reduced by decreasing arterial oxygen saturation. The metabolic and hemodynamic responses to 6 per cent oxygen breathing at two different initial A-V oxygen differences in the same preparation is shown in Figure 2. Blood flow doubled when hypoxia was induced at an initial A-V difference of 4.2 volumes per cent (Panel A), but increased fourfold when the initial A-V difference was set at 6.5 volumes per cent. Yet, in both cases, the combined contributions of changes in blood flow and changes in O_2 extraction were sufficient to maintain tissue oxygen delivery at the normal level. In similar experiments, we have found that in the lower normal venous O_2 ranges the blood flow response to arterial hypoxia does not become significant until the arteriolar Po_2 falls below 40 mm Hg. If, however, the initial venous oxygen content is decreased by infusion of vasoconstrictors, subsequent arterial hypoxia results in large increases in blood flow even at arterial Po_2 levels as great as 70 mm Hg.

The ability of the intrinsic control mechanisms to maintain adequate tissue oxygenation following a reduction in O_2 availability by reducing arterial pressure from 100 mm Hg to 45 mm Hg is demonstrated in Figure 3. At an initial A-V oxygen difference of 5

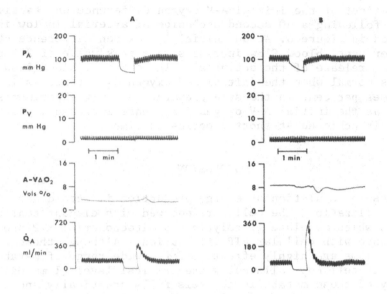

Figure 4

volumes per cent (Panel A), tissue oxygen delivery is maintained
within 10 per cent of control in the face of this step reduction of
arterial pressure primarily by the twofold increase in oxygen extraction. Although a small degree of blood flow autoregulation
occurs under these conditions, it accounts for less than 15 per cent
of the total compensation required to maintain tissue oxygen delivery
near the normal level. When the prevailing A-V oxygen difference
is artifically increased in the same preparation (Panel B), tissue
oxygen delivery is maintained primarily by an autoregulatory return
of blood flow to 75 per cent of control flow following the same step
decrease in arterial pressure. In contrast to the previous experiment, O_2 extraction contributes only 15 per cent. Thus, when A-V
oxygen difference is low or within normal range, blood flow autoregulation in the hindlimb of the dog following a step decrease in
arterial pressure is absent or weak, and tissue oxygen delivery is
maintained equal to cellular demand by increased O_2 extraction.
When the initial A-V O_2 difference is increased by infusion of vasoconstrictors, the return of oxygen delivery to normal following a
step decrease in arterial pressure is brought about mainly by a
high degree of blood flow autoregulation while the contribution of
increased oxygen extraction is reduced. We have obtained similar
results in experiments in which venous oxygen levels were decreased
by muscle stimulation. In addition, in two of three experiments we
found a greater degree of blood flow autoregulation when the venous
oxygen concentration was reduced by mild arterial hypoxia. In all
but the most extreme cases, tissue oxygen delivery was maintained
within a few per cent of control.

The effect of the initial A-V oxygen difference on reactive hyperemia following a 30 second occlusion of arterial inflow is illustrated in Figure 4. At an initial A-V oxygen difference of 4 volumes per cent, blood flow increases to a peak value of 2.5 times normal upon release of the occlusion. In contrast, blood flow rises to 7 times normal when the initial A-V oxygen difference is increased to 9 volumes per cent in the same preparation. Our experiments also show that as the initial A-V oxygen difference increases, peak hyperemic flow is achieved at shorter occlusion times.

CONCLUSION

To assure regulation of energy production in accordance with cellular utilization, the cells are endowed with elegant control mechanisms which modulate glycolytic and mitochondrial ATP production in accordance with cellular ATP utilization. Although these regulatory mechanisms are highly effective for a wide range of metabolic stresses, if cell Po_2 falls below the critical level (1 mm Hg) the efficiency of these metabolic controls falls drastically and cellular dysfunction may ensue. Our analysis and experimental data suggest that the intrinsic microvascular control mechanisms serve to prevent deleterious cellular hypoxia and, therefore, we propose that oxygen delivery to skeletal muscle cells is regulated by metabolic feedback to arterioles and precapillary sphincters. The function of the arteriolar control systems is to minimize changes in capillary Po_2 following alterations in the oxygen availability-to-demand ratio. This is achieved by feedback adjustment of blood flow in relation to tissue oxygen requirements. On the other hand, precapillary sphincters maintain tissue oxygenation by actively modulating diffusion parameters through changes in effective capillary density. In addition, a third protective factor against intracellular hypoxia is provided by the extent to which intracellular Po_2 exceeds the critical oxygen tension, i.e. the Po_2 below which O_2 availability limits cellular oxygen utilization. Thus, by working in concert, the arteriolar and precapillary sphincter control mechanisms and the oxygen buffering capacity of hemoglobin maintain intracellular Po_2 above the critical level and, therefore, ensure the highly efficient aerobic production of ATP.

Supported by USPHS grants HL 11678 and TW 1818 and a grant from the Mississippi Heart Association.

1. Granger, H. J. and A. P. Shepherd, Jr. Intrinsic microvascular control of tissue oxygen delivery. Microvas. Res. 5:49-72, 1973.
2. Whalen, W. J. and P. Nair. Skeletal muscle Po_2: effect of inhaled and topically applied O_2 and CO_2. Am. J. Physiol. 218:973-980, 1970.

REGIONAL HETEROGENEITY OF P_{CO_2} AND P_{O_2} IN SKELETAL MUSCLE

Hugh D. Van Liew (Technical Assistance by B. Rodgers)

Department of Physiology, School of Medicine,

State Univ. of N.Y. at Buffalo, Buffalo, N.Y.

Gas pockets in the peritoneal space and subcutaneous tissue have been used for estimation of oxygen and carbon dioxide partial pressures in tissue (Campbell, 1931; Van Liew, 1968). Inside of soft tissue it is difficult to form and later retrieve a gas bubble, so a special technique was devised whereby gas is retained inside a piece of hollow glass capillary tubing (Van Liew, 1962). Gasometric techniques have the major advantage that both P_{CO_2} and P_{O_2} are measured simultaneously.

This communication presents preliminary results of a study (in preparation) of tissue gases in skeletal muscle in rats.

Methods. Figure 1 illustrates the method. The glass capillary tube or microprobe has been sealed at one end. Inside the tissue, the gas expands due to increase of temperature, and entrance of water vapor and CO_2. Oxygen and CO_2 diffuse across the gas/tissue interface so that P_{O_2} and P_{CO_2} approach equilibrium with their counterparts in the surrounding tissue. At the end of the equilibration time, the external bubble can be knocked off, and a seal of tissue fluid enters the neck of the probe (bottom of the figure). The length of the trapped gas is measured with a micrometer and then CO_2 absorbing solution is put into the sealing drop. The change of length due to CO_2 absorption is a measure of CO_2 fraction of the sample. Oxygen fraction is analyzed in a similar manner by putting oxygen absorber into the sealing drop. Details on filling the probes with special gases and on handling the probes during analysis appear in the original publication (Van Liew, 1962).

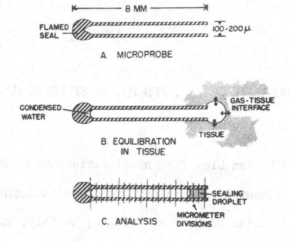

Fig. 1. Principle of the gasometric technique for measuring P_{CO_2} and P_{O_2} in tissue. (Reproduced from Van Liew, 1962.)

Figure 2 shows that microprobe analyses of gases of known composition were reliable over a wide range. The squares show means of several analyses of a particular known gas. Standard deviations of such a group of analyses are about 1% or 7 mm Hg.

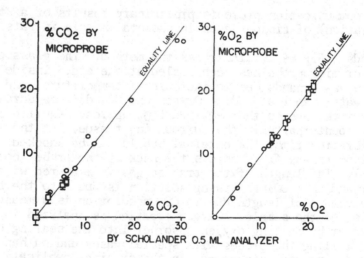

Fig. 2. Validation of microprobe analyses. (Reproduced from Van Liew, 1962.)

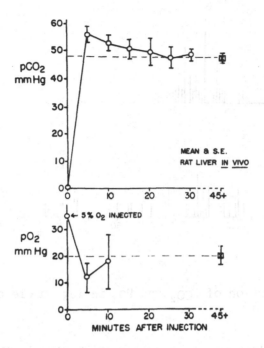

Fig. 3. Time-course of equilibration in liver tissue. (Reproduced from Van Liew, 1962.)

Figure 3 shows time relationships found previously in liver tissue of anesthetized rats. Microprobes withdrawn after 5 minutes in the tissue have a higher P_{CO_2} than microprobes that are left in place longer (top graph). The lower graph shows that when gas having P_{O_2} of 35 mm Hg was injected, there was an initial drop of P_{O_2} followed by a rise to the level that was found after about 3/4 hr. The interpretation of Fig. 3 is that in liver, the injection of the glass capillary causes an early transient vascular reaction which apparently subsides after about 15 minutes. We do not yet know whether such a transient reaction occurs in other tissues.

It is apparent that because of the size of the glass capillary tubes and the time necessary for equilibration, the microprobe method gives a space and time average for P_{O_2} and P_{CO_2}.

Results in skeletal muscle. Figure 4 shows frequency distribution of 41 analyses of microprobes that had been in place for 15 minutes or longer in exposed leg muscles of anesthetized rats. The figure is essentially a conventional histogram except that the class intervals are only 1 mm Hg, so many of the individual analyses stand alone.

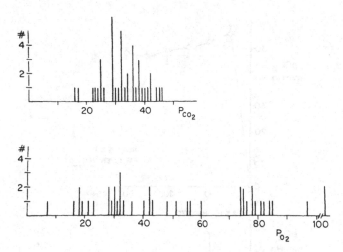

Fig. 4. Distribution of P_{CO_2} and P_{O_2} in leg muscle of anesthetized rats.

The P_{CO_2} values (top) are unexpectedly low in this particular
group of rats; on the basis of blood-gas analyses or large gas
pocket analyses, the values are expected to be 40 or 50 mm Hg
(Van Liew, 1968). Possible reasons for the low CO_2 could be acid-
base status or respiratory center excitability of the anesthetized
rats, or inadvertant loss of CO_2 by diffusion through the exposed
surface of the tissue.

The P_{O_2} data at the bottom of the graph range from 7 to over
100 mm Hg. There is a group of 11 analyses around 80 mm Hg, which
are probably close to arterial blood values. It seems therefore
that for O_2 there is a tissue group averaging about 33 mm Hg, and
an arterial group at 80. The three values near 100 are probably
errors.

Discussion. Because of the rapid diffusion of CO_2 in tissue,
the gradients for CO_2 within a single capillary domain must be
very small. Therefore variability of several mm Hg, such as that
shown in Fig. 4, can be ascribed to heterogeneity of local perfusion, or more specifically, to heterogeneity of the ratio of perfusion to CO_2 production.

Heterogeneity of the ratio of blood perfusion to metabolism
is further suggested by the observation that high P_{CO_2} tended to
be associated with low P_{O_2} (indicating regions with relatively low

perfusion), and low P_{CO_2} tended to be associated with high P_{O_2} (high perfusion regions). The slope of the regression line of P_{CO_2} and P_{O_2} was -.3, which is what one would expect on the basis of gas-carrying characteristics of rat blood. That is, the $Hb\text{-}O_2$ dissociation curve and the CO_2 dissociation curve of rat blood give a ratio of -.3 between P_{CO_2} and P_{O_2} if the variability of values is due to heterogeneity of perfusion.

If one assumes that all the P_{O_2} variability was due to heterogeneity of perfusion, one can quantitate the amounts of flow involved. Figure 5 shows a theoretical curve, drawn from known information on gas carriage of rat blood (Van Liew, 1968). The P_{O_2} of venous blood (on the x axis) depends on the perfusion-to-oxygen consumption ratio ($\dot{Q}/\dot{q}$) (on the y axis). The group of tissue P_{O_2} points from Fig. 4 is below the diagram. The projection off the curve shows the $\dot{Q}/\dot{q}$ ratio for each point. According to this treatment, the average $\dot{Q}/\dot{q}$ ratio for all the tissue points was about 12; that is, 12 ml of blood delivered one ml of O_2. On the low P_{O_2} side, the ratio was about 8 ml of blood per ml of O_2, and on the high side the ratio was 20 or 25 ml of blood per ml of O_2.

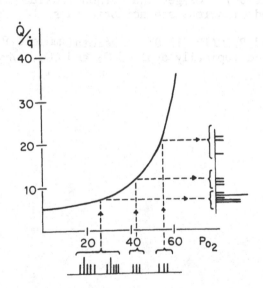

Fig. 5. Theoretical curve of perfusion-to-metabolism ratio ($\dot{Q}/\dot{q}$) vs. venous P_{O_2}. Data from the muscle analyses (below the graph) give estimates of $\dot{Q}/\dot{q}$ when projected off the curve.

The distribution of P_{O_2} values obtained by the 200 μ micro-probes appears to be similar to the distributions obtained with 1 to 5 μ electrodes (Kunze, 1968), but has median P_{O_2} about 30 mm Hg higher than the distribution obtained by Whalen and Nair (1970) with 1 or 2 μ electrodes. Perhaps the gasometric microprobes measure average extracellular P_{O_2}, whereas sometimes O_2 microelectrodes measure intracellular P_{O_2}.

(Supported in part by ONR Contract N00014-68-A-0216 and PHS Grant AM-08070.)

References

CAMPBELL, J. A. (1931). Gas tensions in the tissues. *Physiol. Rev.* 11: 1-40.
KUNZE, K. (1968). Normal and critical oxygen supply to the muscle. In *Oxygen Transport in Blood and Tissue*, edited by D.-W. Lübbers, U. C. Luft, G. Thews, and E. Witzleb. Stuttgart, Georg Thieme Verlag, pp. 198-208.
VAN LIEW, H. D. (1962). Tissue gas tensions by microtonometry; results in liver and fat. *J. Appl. Physiol.* 17: 359-363.
VAN LIEW, H. D. (1968). Oxygen and carbon dioxide tensions in tissue and blood of normal and acidotic rats. *J. Appl. Physiol.* 25: 575-580.
WHALEN, W. J., and P. NAIR (1970). Skeletal muscle P_{O_2}: effect of of inhaled and topically applied O_2 and CO_2. *Amer. J. Physiol.* 218: 973-980.

Chairmen: Dr. Manfred Kessler, Dr. Jürgen Grote and

Dr. James A. Miller, Jr.

DISCUSSION OF PAPER BY T. K. GOLDSTICK

Bingmann: Did you observe this hysteresis in the relation between the arterial pO_2 and the tissue pO_2 also during changes of the arterial pO_2 between normal levels and hypoxia?

Goldstick: No, we wished to maintain pCO_2 and pH constant during our transient and so our measurements were restricted to the hyperoxic region. Also, our measurement is not of tissue but rather of venous pO_2.

Kessler: Did you also analyze the situation in tissue such as by measuring local pO_2 or local microcirculation?

Goldstick: No, we did not. Judging from your data where you had to take so many points to get a histogram, I imagine a dynamic histogram would be beyond our reach at any rate.

Kessler: I think that one of your cases is really in the tissue, and maybe you should take it into consideration. The only way is to do the measurements there. I think it is not so difficult, but, of course, it is a big job, but it is possible.

Rakusan: There is a "black box" between your input and output data. Do you have any information about local changes in the oxygen consumption?

Goldstick: No, but we did measure the overall oxygen consumption $(Q \times AV\Delta O_2)$ and found no change in it following the PaO_2 change. The muscle was at or above normal pO_2 throughout.

DISCUSSION OF PAPER BY H. J. GRANGER, A. H. GOODMAN AND
     D. N. GRANGER

Goldstick: It appeared from your slide that the venous pO_2 must have been very low. What was it?

Granger, H.J.: We were not measuring venous pO_2. We were measuring

AV difference. With an initial AV difference of anywhere from 7
to 15 mm Hg which is higher than normal, we got very good autoregulation; whereas in the normal venous oxygen range where the AV
oxygen difference is normally anywhere from 3 to 5 mm Hg we obtained
very little autoregulation.

DISCUSSION OF PAPER BY H. D. VAN LIEW

Lübbers: (1) How can you control that one probe did not disturb
microcirculation during the experiment?
        (2) The histogram of the muscle you have shown is different
from the one published by Kunze for human skeletal muscle and
Schroder for frog skeletal muscle.

Van Liew: (1) We all have to worry about what our measuring
devices do to the tissue. This will be true for my glass capillaries
we well as for electrodes or mass spectrometer probes. I am encour-
aged by the close correspondence between the frequency distribution
of pO_2 in liver that we published in 1962 and the distributions
presented at this meeting by Kessler, et al. (autoregulation of
oxygen supply to liver and kidney).
        (2) Probably there are species differences. I would have to
scrutinize the methods and results of the studies mentioned before
trying to explain the differences any further. In general though,
it seems important to keep in mind that different kinds of measurement may give different values because they are operating at different levels. The finding that our variability of pO_2 was about
the same as the variability published by Whalen and Nair, even though
our average pO_2 was much higher, suggested to us that perhaps we were
sampling average extracellular pO_2 where as the microelectrode
studies were sampling intracellular pO_2.

Kessler: I would like to make a short comment. I am astonished
how close the values are which you get with your relatively thick
capillaries compared to the mean pO_2 values of the liver. This shows
that the method can give you a sufficient information on oxygen supply of liver tissue.

Van Liew: I would like to make one other comment that refers back
to Dr. Lübbers. When I inject these things into a tissue they can
move with the tissue. There is nothing holding them to anything
outside. So, I have the feeling that that may be better for the
tissue than to have something that has a long wire or whatever,
leading on off and as the tissue moves, have it re-stimulate the
microvasculature.

Gatz: What was the equilibration time of your microprobes and how
did you determine this time?

<u>Van Liew</u>: The data on pCO_2 and pO_2 vs. time of equilibration suggested to us that we should wait a half hour or more. However, it may be that less time is required in muscle. In liver, there seemed to be a vascular effect superimposed on the equilibration-time effect.

Subsession: SHOCK

Chairmen: Dr. Manfred Kessler, Dr. Jürgen Grote

and Dr. James A. Miller, Jr.

SIGNS OF HYPOXIA IN THE SMALL INTESTINE OF THE
RAT DURING HEMORRHAGIC SHOCK

R. Rink and M. Kessler with the technical assistance of
K. Hájek

University of Louisville School of Medicine, Louisville,
Kentucky, and Max-Planck-Institut für Arbeitsphysiologie,
Dortmund, West Germany

INTRODUCTION

The photometric measurement of fluorescence emitted by reduced
pyridine nucleotides upon ultraviolet stimulation (1,3) and the
polarographic measurement of Po_2 (5) in tissues and organs have
provided detailed information about the local effects of disturbances of O_2 supply and of microcirculation. Under experimental
conditions in which circulating blood is a factor it is also
necessary to measure absorbancy changes of hemoglobin by reflectance
photometry in order to accurately evaluate changes in reduced PN
fluorescence (6,9,11). In the present study both the photometric
and polarographic techniques have been focused on the small
intestine of urethane anesthetized rats subjected to periodic,
standardized hemorrhages.

METHODS

In one series of rats, during the 12-15 min interval between
hemorrhages (3.4 ml/kg), the fluorescence of reduced PN (366 nm
excitation) was measured at 465 nm. The reflectance of local Hb
concentration was measured at the isosbestic point of 585 nm and
of Hb oxygenation at 600 nm. The instrumentation was based on the
work of Chance et al. (1) and as modified by Kessler (fig. 1). In
another series, the Po_2 was measured by the Pt-multiwire surface
electrode (fig. 2) of Kessler and Lübbers (4). The protocol followed
allowed for the construction of O_2 histograms. Warming instruments
were used to maintain normal tissue temperatures in animals of
both series.

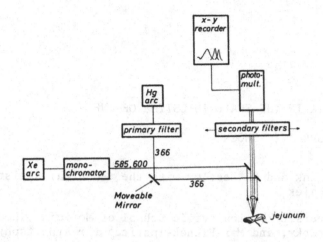

Fig. 1: Schematic diagram of photometric apparatus

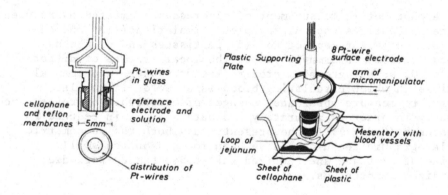

Fig. 2: Schematic diagram of the Pt-multiwire surface electrode
and its in situ application

RESULTS

Fig. 3 shows an oscillograph recording from an 8 Pt-wire surface electrode. Tissue Po_2 values declined with increasing hypovolemia and declining MAP. Rhythmic oscillations of the Po_2 became
prominent after the 1st hemorrhage. They tended to become less
uniform during late stages and began to disappear when blood
pressure was profoundly hypotensive. In the photometric measurements
oscillations of Hb concentration and emitted fluorescence were also
observed. Peristalsis was not a causative factor.

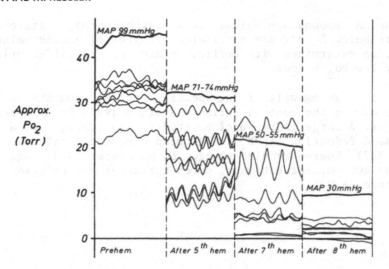

Fig. 3: Excerpts of an oscillograph recording of tissue Po_2 (Pt-
multiwire surface electrode) in the rat small intestine
following successive hemorrhages

Fig. 4 presents the O_2 histograms as derived from measurements
in 11 animals. Prehemorrhage control values ranged from 3-55 Torr
with a peak distribution in the range of 20-30 Torr. Following
early hemorrhages there were shifts of the range of maximum
distribution toward lower ranges, and after the 5th hemorrhage
values below 5 Torr increased slightly. The number of values in
the latter range increased sharply after the 6th and 7th bleedings
as the distribution curves shifted markedly to the left. At these

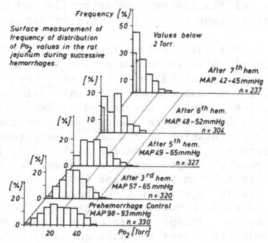

Fig. 4: Po_2 distribution in the rat small intestine following
successive hemorrhages

stages the MAP showed appreciably less post-hemorrhagic improvement.
The values below 2 Torr are considered as hypoxic. Anoxic values
could not be determined with sufficient accuracy to differentiate
from very low Po_2 values.

Fig. 5 is an example of the spectra recorded from the small
intestine during the control period and after death from successive
hemorrhages. A large increase of emitted fluorescence, indicative
of increased reduction of PN, is recorded when the local O_2 supply
fails (1,3,7). There are also changes of Hb content and oxygenation
at 585 and 600 nm, respectively, which influence the emitted
fluorescence (6,9,11).

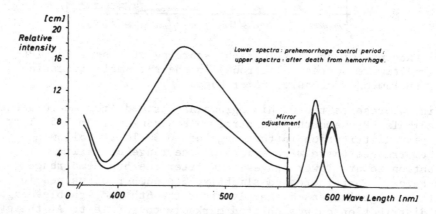

Fig. 5: Spectra of fluorescence emission (366 nm excitation) and
reflected light in the rat small intestine

Fig. 6 presents the combined results of photometric measurements in 11 experiments. The measurements were made at 4 intervals
between each bleeding. At 585 nm there are increases of intensity
of reflected light in association with increasing hypovolemia and
declining MAP. The increases are caused by decreases of local Hb
content (6,9). At 600 nm there are decreases of the intensity of
reflected light in relation to the 585 nm measurements. This is indicative of increasing disoxygenation of Hb (3,9) in association
with the hemodynamic changes mentioned above. The widening difference of intensity between the 585 and 600 nm measurements can be
plotted (fig. 7). It is evident that there is increasing disoxygenation with increasing volume of hemorrhage. Following the early
hemorrhages there are abrupt increases of disoxygenation which are
partially compensated before the subsequent bleeding. However,
after the 6th hemorrhage the increase is sustained. It was at a
similar point that the Po_2 values shifted markedly into the lowest
ranges.

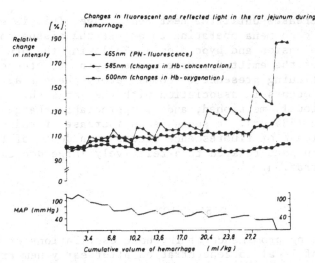

Fig. 6: Changes in fluorescent light (366 nm excitation) and
reflected light in the rat small intestine following
successive hemorrhages

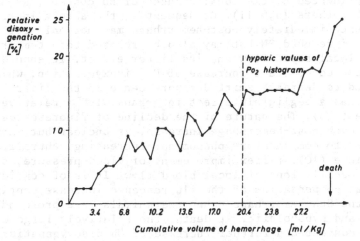

Fig. 7: Local disoxygenation of hemoglobin in the rat small
intestine following successive hemorrhages

At 465 nm (fig. 6) the general trend of emitted fluorescence
is one of increasing intensity, which is in part a result of
decreasing local Hb content and its filter effect (6,9,11). The
upward trend is marked by abrupt increases of intensity immediately
post-hemorrhage. This is concomitant to large increases of Hb disoxygenation (fig. 7). Consequently, the increases of fluorescence
may result from an alteration of the intracellular redox state with
increased PN reduction. However, the increases are temporary and

fluorescence decreases until the next hemorrhage. This is evidence
of compensatory phenomena operating to adjust the tissue to
progressive hypotension and hypovolemia. Following the 6th hemorrhage the slope of the emitted fluorescence begins to steepen
despite the continuing presence of compensatory phenomena. The
change of slope occurs in association with the large shift of Po_2
values, as previously mentioned, and no appreciable change of local
Hb concentration (585 nm). It suggests an increase of reduced PN.
The largest increase of fluorescence occurs upon death of the
animals and is in part related to a relatively large decrease of
local Hb concentration.

DISCUSSION

The increasing prominence of rhythmic oscillations of both the
Po_2 values and of local Hb concentration after early hemorrhages
is interpreted as resulting from rhythmic variations of local blood
flow. This activity may provide for a more effective distribution
of reduced blood volume. The intensity of emitted fluorescence was
inversely influenced by the local changes of Hb content, as has
been noted by others (6,9,11). Consequently, the abrupt increases
of fluorescence immediately post-hemorrhage may not only reflect
an increase of reduced PN but may also be related to a temporary
decrease of local blood flow and its filter effect. It should be
noted that the concomitant increase of Hb disoxygenation, which has
been observed to decrease emitted fluorescence in the liver (9),
most likely has a negligible effect in organs with a relatively small
Hb compartment (3). The nature of the decline of fluorescence,
relative to each post-hemorrhage increase, is unclear but thought
to be related to compensatory phenomena: increasing centralization
of blood volume (10), reflex improvement of blood pressure, and
perhaps the oscillations of local blood flow. It is of considerable
interest that compensation of the fluorescence increase continued
even after the 8th hemorrhage, when the animals were profoundly
hypotensive and hypovolemic. At death, the relatively large decline
of local Hb content and further increase of Hb disoxygenation
suggest that the microcirculation was continuing to a substantial
degree until that point. In view of the very low Po_2 values at which
mitochondria can continue to function adequately (2,8), the O_2
supply may still have been sufficient for much of the tissue until
death. It was only then that an uncompensated increase of emitted
fluorescence was recorded.

REFERENCES

1. Chance, B., Cohen, P., Jöbsis, F., Schoener, B.: Intracellular
   oxidation-reduction states in vivo. Science 137, 499-508 (1962).

2. Chance, B., Oshino, N., Sugano, T.: Cytochrome c and NADH as
   indicators of electron flow and energy coupling in mitochondria. International symposium on oxygen transport to tissue.
   April, 1973.

3. Chance, B., Schoener, B., Schindler, F.: The intracellular
   oxidation-reduction state. In: Oxygen in the animal organism,
   ed. by R. Dickens and E. Neil. New York, Pergamon 1963,
   pp. 367-388.

4. Kessler, M.: Normale und kritische Sauerstoffversorgung der
   Leber bei Normo- und Hypothermie. Habil.-Schrift, Marburg 1968.

5. Kessler, M., Bruley, D.F., Clark, L.C., Lübbers, D.W., Silver,
   I.A., Strauss, J.: Oxygen supply, theoretical and practical
   aspects of oxygen supply and microcirculation of tissue.
   Urban and Schwarzenberg, München-Berlin 1973.

6. Kobayashi, S., Nishiki, K., Kaede, K., Ogata, E.: Optical consequences of blood substitution on tissue oxidation-reduction
   state microfluorometry. J.Appl.Physiol. 31, 93 (1971).

7. Lang, H., Kessler, M., Starlinger, H.: Signs of hypoxia measured
   by means of Po_2 multiwire electrodes by NADH and NADPH fluorescence and determination of lactate and pyruvate formation.
   In: Oxygen supply, theoretical and practical aspects of oxygen
   supply and microcirculation of tissue. Eds. M. Kessler,
   D.F. Bruley, L.C. Clark, D.W. Lübbers, I.A. Silver, J. Strauss,
   München-Berlin: Urban and Schwarzenberg 1973.

8. Lübbers, D.W.: personal communication.

9. Rahmer, H., Kessler, M.: Influence of hemoglobin concentration
   in perfusate and in blood on PN fluorescence of rat liver.
   In: International symposium on oxygen transport to tissue.
   April, 1973.

10. Sapirstein, L.A., Sapirstein, E.H., Bredemeyer, A.: Effect of
    hemorrhage on the cardiac output and its distribution in the
    rat. Circulation Res. 8, 135 (1960).

11. Schnitger, H., Scholz, R., Bücher, T., Lübbers, D.W.: Comparative
    fluorometric studies on rat liver in vivo and on isolated,
    perfused hemoglobin free liver. Biochem. Z. 341, 334 (1965).

REFERENCES

BLOOD AND TISSUE OXYGENATION DURING HEMORRHAGIC SHOCK

AS DETERMINED WITH ULTRAMICRO OXYGEN ELECTRODES

Charles T. Fitts*, Haim I. Bicher**, and
Dabney R. Yarbrough III*

Department of Surgery* and Department of Anatomy**
Medical University of South Carolina
Charleston, South Carolina   29401

Recent clinical and laboratory observations in the field of shock have centered attention upon deficits in pulmonary function as one of the major causes of death and morbidity following shock and trauma.[1,2,3,4] Following the initial proposal that an oxygen debt was accumulated in hemorrhagic shock,[5] other investigators have found that an oxygen deficit indeed did occur in hemorrhagic shock and appeared to correlate with irreversibility.[6,7] Evidence in the literature is scanty concerning direct measurements of tissue pO_2 during hemorrhagic shock and is conflicting concerning arterial pO_2 measurements in the same condition. The experiments reported here utilize an ultramicro oxygen electrode to determine arterial pO_2 and renal and cerebral parenchymal pO_2 during a standard episode of hemorrhagic shock.

METHODS

Adult mongrel dogs were anesthetized with 30 mg. sodium pentobarbital per kg. of body weight intravenously and their tracheas intubated. The animals were then placed on a volume respirator utilizing room air for the remainder of the experiment. Using sterile technique one femoral artery was cannulated and used for monitoring arterial pressure, bleeding and reinfusing shed blood. The other femoral artery was exposed surgically using sterile technique and an ultramicro oxygen electrode placed. The right kidney was then exposed through a small flank incision and an ultra microelectrode was inserted into the cortex. The skull was then trephined, a dural flap carefully elevated and an ultra microelectrode fixed in a micromanipulator was lowered into the surface of the brain.

The head was rigidly held in a stereotaxic instrument. The ultramicro/ oxygen electrodes and the techniques for determining tissue pO_2 in brain and kidney and arterial pO_2 have been previously published.[8,9] Following a short period of stabilization the animals were given 5,000 units of heparin intravenously and bled into a sterile reservoir until a mean arterial pressure of 70 mm. Hg. was reached. This level was maintained for 90 minutes at which time further bleeding was permitted by lowering the reservoir until a mean arterial pressure of 30 mm. Hg. was reached. This level was maintained for 60 minutes. At the conclusion of this period all shed blood was reinfused. Following reinfusion each animal was given 50 mg. of protamine sulfate intravenously to reverse the heparin effect. Throughout this entire period of time pO_2 in kidney, brain and blood was monitored. Eleven animals were utilized in the experiments. In five animals the arterial electrode functioned throughout the entire experimental period while the renal electrode functioned similarly in four, and the brain electrode in three.

RESULTS

The data concerning arterial pO_2 is shown in Table 1. Compared to control levels there was a statistically significant drop in arterial pO_2 at the 75 mm. Hg. level of shock and at the 30 mm. Hg. level.

HEMORRHAGIC SHOCK
BLOOD pO_2 LEVELS

	Control	75mmHg	30mmHg
P1	138	104	50
P2	86	75	65
P6	113	88	46
P8	118	110	86
P9	108	83	55

*Control vs 75mm Hg: $p < .05$
*Control vs 30mm Hg: $p < .05$

TABLE 1. ARTERIAL pO_2 LEVELS IN FIVE ANIMALS
*t test for paired differences

HEMORRHAGIC SHOCK
KIDNEY pO_2 LEVELS

	Control	75mm Hg	30mm Hg
P2	52	42	24
P6	40	35	26
P8	44	40	30
P9	48	40	20

*Control vs 75mm Hg : $p < .05$
*Control vs 30mm Hg : $p < .05$

TABLE 2. RENAL pO_2 LEVELS IN FOUR ANIMALS
*t test for paired differences

The data concerning renal tissue pO_2 similarly revealed a statistically significant drop in pO_2 levels at the 75 mm. Hg. and 30 mm. Hg. levels when compared to control. (Table 2).

The cerebral tissue pO_2 did not differ from control at the 75 mm. Hg. level and there was still no significant decrease between the pO_2 levels when 30 mm. Hg. pressure had been reached as compared to control values. However, a slight but insignificant rise at the 75 mm. Hg. level (compared to control) coupled with the slight but insignificant decrease at 30 mm. Hg. (compared to control) combined to show a statistically significant decrease when the 75 mm. Hg. levels were compared with the 30 mm. Hg. levels. These results are shown in Table 3.

HEMORRHAGIC SHOCK
BRAIN pO_2 LEVELS

	Control	75mm Hg	30mm Hg
P6	20	33	26
P8	44	40	36
P9	54	50	46

*Control vs 75mm Hg : p > .05
*Control vs 30mm Hg : p > .05

TABLE 3. CEREBRAL pO_2 LEVELS IN THREE ANIMALS
*t test for paired differences

All animals revealed an increase in pO_2 levels in arterial
blood, renal and cerebral tissue upon reinfusion of the shed blood.
These levels moved toward but not back entirely to control levels.
It was interesting to note that protamine administered after
reinfusion to reverse heparinization was usually attended by a
transient but sometimes severe drop in blood pressure and
concomitant decreases in pO_2 levels in blood and tissue. (See
Figure 1). A graph of all the pO_2 levels throughout the experiment
is shown in Figure 2.

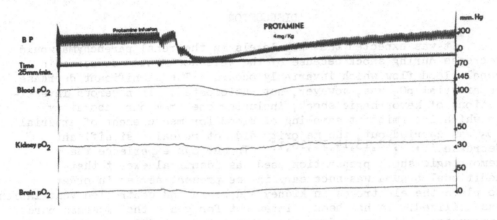

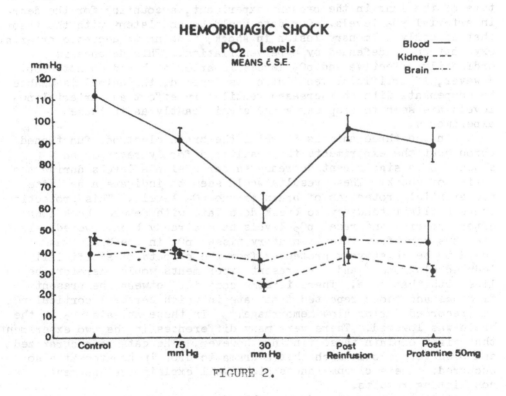

FIGURE 2.

DISCUSSION

It was expected that pO_2 levels in the renal parenchyma would decrease during shock because of the well documented decrease in renal blood flow which invariably occurs. The significant decrease in arterial pO_2 was, however, not anticipated. In numerous investigations of hemorrhagic shock, including one from our laboratory in which intermittent sampling of blood for measurement of arterial pO_2 was carried out, the majority did not reveal a significant decrease.[10,11,12,13,14,15,16,17] In our own experience the hemorrhagic shock preparation used was identical except that additional trauma was necessary in the present series in order to place the electrodes in kidney and brain and controlled ventilation was utilized. It has been pointed out for years that whereas pure hemorrhage will not produce microcirculatory sludging, addition of tissue damage such as crushing, cutting or burning will invariably do so.[18] It may be that such sludging occurred in the microvasculature of the lung in the present experiment, accounting for the decrease in arterial pO_2 levels. Our data would be consistent with the theory that an early pulmonary lesion in shock, tending to decrease arterial oxygenation is defended by hyperventilation. This defense is ordinarily effective and pO_2 levels in arterial blood do not drop. However, if artificial ventilation is imposed, the animal is unable to compensate with an increased ventilatory effort and arterial pO_2 levels are seen to drop early and significantly as in these experiments.

In the three animals in which the brain electrode functioned throughout the experiments the results uniformly revealed an absence of a significant decrease in cerebral pO_2 levels during the period of shock. These results would seem to indicate a definite preferential protection of brain tissue pO_2 levels. This protection shows a slight tendency to break down late with severe shock long after arterial and renal pO_2 levels have already been lowered. In previous work from this laboratory tissue pO_2 in the brain was found to be relatively protected from the effects of artificially induced sludging[19] and the present experiments would therefore be in line with that data. There is some conflict between the present findings and those reported from cats in which cerebral cortical pO_2 was recorded during slow hemorrhage.[19] In those animals pO_2 in the brain was lowered. There were many differences in the two experiments that might explain these findings however. The cats were curarized and bled very slowly such that a dramatic drop in hematocrit also occurred. These circumstances might well explain the apparent conflicting results.

The reason for the drop in blood pressure and concomitant decreases in blood and tissue pO_2 levels with protamine administration are not readily apparent. The rapidity with which the pressure drops tends to point toward a direct toxic effect on the circulatory system, but induced sludging from heparin reversal should also be considered. Direct observation of the microcirculation might resolve that problem.

SUMMARY

In a severe hemorrhagic shock preparation, with added tissue trauma secondary to placement of electrodes in brain, kidney and artery, the blood and renal pO_2 levels dropped significantly and early. Cerebral cortical pO_2 levels were relatively well protected throughout the shock episode. Protamine administration routinely administered to reverse the heparin effect was associated with a transient decrease in blood pressure and blood and tissue oxygen.

REFERENCES

1. Ashbaugh, D. G., Petty, T. L., Bigelow, D. B. et al.: Continuous positive pressure breathing (CPPB) in adult respiratory distress syndrome. J. Thorac. Surg. 57:31, 1969.

2. Collins, J. A.: Current research review: The course of progressive pulmonary insufficiency in surgical patients. J. Surg. Res. 9:685, 1969.

3. "Pulmonary Effects of Non-Thoracic Trauma." Proceedings of a conference conducted by The Committee on Trauma, Division of Medical Science, National Academy of Science-National Research Council. J. Trauma, Special Issue 8:1968.

4. McLaughlin, J. S.: Physiologic consideration of hypoxemia in shock and trauma. Ann. Surg. 173:667, 1971.

5. Bruner, H. and Butzengeiger, K.H.: Ueber experimentelle aenderungen der blutmenge-II, mitteilung; das verhalten des gasstoffwechsels bei entblutung. Arch. Kreislaufforsch 6:34, 1940.

6. Crowell, J. W. and Smith, E.: Oxygen deficit in shock. Amer. J. Physiol. 206:313, 1964.

7. Rush, B. F., Jr., Rosenberg, J. C. and Spencer, F. C.: Changes in oxygen consumption in shock. J. Surg. Res. 5:252, 1965.

8. Bicher, H. I. and Knisely, M. H.: Brain tissue reoxygenation demonstrated with a new ultramicro oxygen electrode. J. Appl. Phys. 28:387, 1970.

9. Bicher, H. I., Fitts, C. T. and Yarbrough, D. R. III: Effect of norepinephrine, blood sludging and respiratory gas change on blood and tissue oxygenation as determined with ultramicro oxygen electrodes. Surg. Forum 22:213, 1971.

10. Reich, M. and Eiseman, B.: Tissue oxygenation following resuscitation with crystalloid solution following experimental acute blood loss. Surgery 69:928, 1971.

11. Coran, A., Ballantine, T., Horwitz, D. and Herman, C.: The effect of crystalloid resuscitation in hemorrhagic shock on acid-base balance: A comparison between normal saline and Ringer's lactate solutions. Surgery 69:874, 1971.

12. Ehrlick, R. Kramer, S. and Watkins, E.: An experimental shock model simulating clinical hemorrhagic shock. Surg. Gynec. & Obs. 1174, December, 1969.

13. Vladeck, B., Bassin, R., Kark, A. and Shoemaker, W.: Rapid and
     slow hemorrhage in man: Sequential acid-base and oxygen transport
     responses. Ann. of Surg. 173:331, 1971.
14. Greenfield, L. McCurdy, W. and Coalson, J.: Pulmonary oxygen
     toxicity in experimental hemorrhagic shock. Surgery 68:662, 1970.
15. Moss, G., Siegel, D., Cochin, A. and Fresquez, V.: Effects of
     saline and colloid solutions on pulmonary function in hemorrhagic
     shock. Surg. Gynec. & Obs. 53, July, 1971.
16. Desai, J., Kim, S. and Shoemaker, W.: Sequential respiratory
     changes in an experimental hemorrhagic shock preparation
     designed to simulate clinical shock. Ann. Surg. 170:166, 1969.
17. Fitts, C. T. and Yarbrough, D. R. III: The evaluation of two
     different methods of resuscitation from hemorrhagic shock by
     restressing the survivors. J. Trauma 12:876, 1972.
18. Knisely, M. H.: Personal communication.
19. Bicher, H. I., Bruley, D. F., Knisely, M. H. and Reneau, D. D.:
     Effect of microcirculation changes on brain tissue oxygenation.
     J. Physiol. 217:689, 1971.

LOCAL AND WHOLE ORGAN RENAL OXYGENATION UNDER HEMORRHAGIC SHOCK

J. Strauss, R. Baker, A.V. Beran, and E. Sinagowitz

Dept. Ped., U. Miami, Miami, Fla.; Dept. Ped., Cal.
Col. Med., U.C., Irvine, Cal., U.S.A.; and Max-Planck
Institut für Arbeitsphysiologie, Dortmund, W. Germany

Reports of various authors on the use of different techniques
for assessing tissue oxygenation under a variety of hemorrhagic
shock conditions abound in this symposium and in the literature
(1,2). Undoubtedly these add to our knowledge of this exciting
and complex clinical and experimental state. Our hope is that
coordinated efforts will be undertaken to compare techniques and
experimental designs and thus facilitate interpretation of results.
In this way the role played by anesthesia, surgical trauma, temperature, and degree and duration of shock, among other variables, can
be evaluated. In addition, changes in results due to changes in
size, location, and type of electrodes as well as duration and
type of polarographic voltage can be identified. This report is
about one of our attempts in this direction: the comparison of
local renal oxygenation changes with those of the whole kidney
under hemorrhagic shock.

METHODS

Three experimental groups of male New Zealand rabbits were
studied to monitor three different sets of variables. The animals
from each group were prepared as follows:

A. The first group (I) had chronically implanted, oxygen-
sensitive bare wire electrodes, (Pt, active, negative; Ag-AgCl,
reference, positive) in four regions of the left kidney: cortex (C),
outer medulla (OM), inner medulla (IM) and papilla (P), (3, Fig. 1).
The Pt wire was 75-175 μ in diameter and insulated with epoxy resin
except for 1 mm at the tip; the Ag-AgCl wire was 500 μ in diameter
and uninsulated.

485

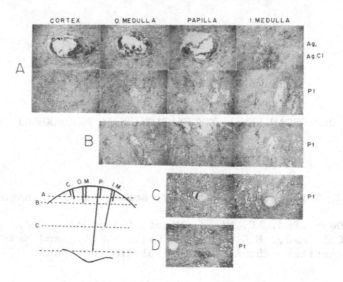

Fig. 1.   Histological sections showing tissue surrounding
          electrode canals and diagram showing intrarenal
          electrode locations.

Both wires were covered with silicone (Siliclad$^{(R)}$, Clay Adams) and
implanted with an arterial occluder (4) at least 10 days prior to
the experiment. These electrodes were used to monitor continuously
oxygen availability (O_2a) during experiments in unanesthetized
animals.

     Other variables monitored during these experiments were: (a)
central arterial blood pressure (CAP) and heart rate through a
catheter placed in the central earlobe artery or right femoral
artery and connected to a Statham pressure transducer (model P23AA);
(b) central venous blood pressure through a catheter placed in the
earlobe vein or right femoral vein and connected to a Statham pressure transducer (model P23BB); (c) respiration rate and expired CO_2
through a tube placed in a nostril and connected to a carbon
dioxide analyzer (N.V. Godart, model KK5802); (d) deep subcutaneous
temperature with a needle connected to a Yellow Springs Telether-
mometer (model 42SC); (e) arterial blood P_{O_2}, P_{CO_2}, pH were intermittently determined at each sampling period using a Radiometer
Blood Micro System (Type BMS 3b); and (f) hematocrit was measured
using microtubes centrifuged at 11,500 rpm for 5 min.

     B. In the second group (II), unanesthetized animals, a radio-
opaque catheter was introduced into the right jugular vein and
fluoroscopically placed into the left renal vein on the day of the
experiment. In addition, a catheter was placed in the right femoral artery. This allowed intermittent sampling of blood for P_{O_2},

P_{CO_2}, pH and hematocrit (as described above) for both left renal vein and central arterial blood. In this way the A-V O_2 content could be calculated for the left kidney using the Siggaard-Andersen Nomogram and the Severinghaus Blood-Gas Calculator. O_2 content $C_{O_2}T$ equals the sum of the physically dissolved $C_{O_2}d$ and the chemically bound (C_{O_2Hb}) where $C_{O_2}d$ = P_{O_2} (100 x 0.0231/760) and C_{O_2Hb} = S_{O_2} x O_2 cap. where O_2 cap. = g Hb x 1.34 ml O_2 at 100% saturation; Hb was calculated by the formula g Hb = Hct x 3.4 (5).

C. In the third group (III) an electromagnetic flow probe was placed around the left renal artery on the day of the experiment. Single kidney blood flow (SKBF) was monitored using a Micron flow-meter (RC 1000). The animals in this group were lightly anesthetized with Nembutal (R) throughout the experiment. The results of group II were combined with group III and single kidney $\dot{V}O_2$ (SK$\dot{V}O_2$) was determined for each sampling period using the following formula: SK$\dot{V}O_2$ = ($C_{O_2}a$ - $C_{O_2}v$) SKBF.

The same experimental design was used for all three groups (Fig. 2). This consisted of a 60 min control period followed by bleeding, 120 min of shock, reinfusion and then 60 min post-reinfusion ("recovery") period. Samples were taken at 30 min intervals during control, shock and post-reinfusion periods; bleeding and reinfusion were accomplished at the rate of 10 ml/5 min. Hemorrhagic shock was defined as 60 mm Hg systolic CAP. This pressure was maintained throughout the 120 min shock period by withdrawal or infusion of whole blood as needed.

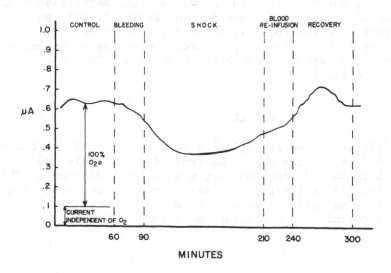

Fig. 2.   Diagram showing trend of composite O_2a levels during experiment.

RESULTS AND DISCUSSION

Previously we reported the effect of hemorrhagic shock on tissue oxygenation (6). As the systolic CAP of 60 mm Hg was reached a marked decrease in tissue O_2a was attained in all four renal areas monitored. After the 60 min of shock there was a gradual increase in O_2a of all areas with a proportionately greater increase in C and OM than in IM and P. C increased from 47% to 76%, OM from 39% to 75%, IM from 30% to 50%, and P from 32% to 56%. After reinfusion of shed blood, O_2a levels overshot and then returned to near control.

In studies regarding $SK\dot{V}O_2$, immediately after reaching shock there was a distinct fall in $SK\dot{V}O_2$ due to a decrease in SKBF; concomitantly the A-V O_2 content nearly doubled. However, this increase was insufficient to return $SK\dot{V}O_2$ to control levels. During shock SKBF remained relatively stable while $SK\dot{V}O_2$ fell, due mainly to a more rapid decrease in arterial O_2 inflow than in venous O_2 outflow. After reinfusion of shed blood, the $SK\dot{V}O_2$ returned to control while the SKBF remained below control.

There was a correlation between whole organ and local intrarenal oxygenation during the initial part of shock, but there was no correlation during the final part of shock, reinfusion and post-reinfusion. The reason for the lack of correlation during the final parts of the experiments is not clear from these studies. Local renal changes must have taken place which either were not measured or were not reflected in the whole organ determinations. These may include changes in blood and interstitial fluid pH, counter-current O_2 diffusion (7), shunting, blood flow (8), O_2 consumption, hematocrit, and temperature. Weiss has described a direct correlation between temperature changes and $\dot{V}O_2$ in isolated renal cells (9).

CONCLUSION

A multiplicity of physiological events including local tissue oxygenation and metabolism can be determined sensitively and reliably with implanted, continuously monitoring electrodes. This is to be desired in contrast to the direct measurement of a single whole body or organ variable such as blood flow, arterial or venous P_{O_2}, arterial blood pressure or a combination of these.

REFERENCES

1. Vladeck, B.C.; Bassin, R.; Slater, G.I.; and Shoemaker, W.C.: Oxygen availability to various organs during hemorrhagic shock. In: Oxygen Supply, Theoretical and Practical Aspects of Oxygen Supply and Microcirculation of Tissue (M. Kessler, D.F. Bruley, L.C. Clark Jr., D.W. Lübbers, I.A. Silver and J. Strauss, (eds.). Urban & Schwarzenberg, München, 1973. pp. 241-247.

2. Hartel, W.: The relationships between oxygen pressure at the renal surface and renal arterial flow in hemorrhagic shock. In: Oxygen Supply, Theoretical and Practical Aspects of Oxygen Supply and Microcirculation of Tissue (M. Kessler, D.F. Bruley, L.C. Clark Jr., D.W. Lubbers, I.A. Silver and J. Strauss, eds.). Urban & Schwarzenberg, München, 1973. pp. 248-251.

3. Strauss, J.; Beran, A.V.; Brown, C.T.; and Katurich, N.: Renal oxygenation under "normal" conditions. Am. J. Physiol. 215: 1482-1487, 1968.

4. Beran, A.V.; Strauss, J.; Brown, C.T.; and Katurich, N.: A simple arterial occluder. J. Appl. Physiol. 24: 838-839, 1968.

5. Beran, A.V.; Strauss, J.; Sperling, D.R.; Norton, A.C.; Garwood, V.P.; and Yamazaki, J.: Effect of Thalidomide on brain oxygenation. Pediat. Res. 5:199-205, 1971.

6. Strauss, J.; Beran, A.V.; Baker, R.; Boydston, L.; and Reyes-Sanchez, J.L.: Effect of hemorrhagic shock on renal oxygenation. Am. J. Physiol. 221:1545-1550, 1971.

7. Deetjen, P.: Normal and Critical oxygen supply of the kidney In: Oxygen Transport in Blood and Tissue (D.W. Lübbers, U.C. Luft, G. Thems and E. Witzleb, eds.). Georg Thieme Verlag, Stuttgart, 1968, pp. 212-226.

8. Aukland, L.; and Wolgast, M.: Effect of hemorrhage and retransfusion on intrarenal distribution of blood flow in dogs. J. Clin. Invest. 47:488-501, 1968.

9. Weiss, C.H.: Critical oxygen tension and rate of respiration of isolated kidney cells. In: Oxygen Transport in Blood and Tissue (D.W. Lübbers, U.C. Luft, G. Thems, and E. Witzleb, eds.). Georg Thieme Verlag, Stuttgart, 1968. pp. 227-237.

Supported by National Institutes of Health Grants HE-09351 and HE-14091.

FACTORS DETERMINING TOTAL BODY AND HIND LIMB
OXYGEN CONSUMPTION IN NORMAL AND SHOCKED DOGS

D. F. J. Halmagyi, J. Leigh, A. H. Goodman, and D. Varga

Gordon Craig Research Laboratory, Department of Surgery

University of Sydney, Sydney, Australia

O_2 uptake is determined by the relative
contributions of O_2 transport (=blood flow x art.O_2
content) and O_2 extraction. At constant metabolic
rate variations in O_2 transport produce inverse
changes in O_2 extraction (Fig.1), and with changes in
metabolic rate the resulting variations in O_2 extraction produce a feedback response of the autoregulatory
flow system (1). In addition to cellular metabolism,
O_2 extraction is also determined by the contractile
state of the precapillary sphincters (2): the inverse
variations in O_2 extraction with changes in blood
pressure (3) and arterial pCO_2 (4) (Fig.1) are presumably related to this function. In order to quantify
these complex interactions we submitted these parameters to multiple regression analysis with O_2 uptake
as the dependent variable.
METHODS. Seventy one greyhounds weighing 20-35
kg were used. The thiopentone-anesthetized and
intubated animals were bled into a hydrostatic
reservoir and 3 hours later the shed blood was
reinfused. Cardiac output, femoral arterial blood
flow, total body and femoral arterial O_2 uptake,
arterial, mixed venous and femoral venous O_2 contents,
arterial blood gases and core temperature were measured
before, during and after blood loss, as described in
previous papers (3,5). Variations in body temperature
were induced by surface cooling and shivering was
prevented by anesthesia; variations in O_2 transport
were induced by bleeding and by infusion of 5%

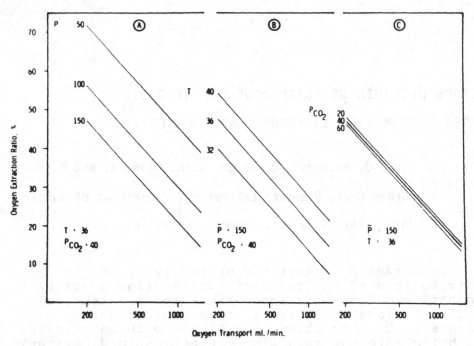

Figure 1. Dependence of total body extraction ratio on oxygen
transport in dogs, as affected by: A - blood pressure;
B - temperature; and C - arterial pCO_2.

dextran 70 in saline (Macrodex, Pharmacia). Regression analysis was carried out using a standard IBM
program. The log.of O_2 uptake was the dependent
variable, blood temperature, art.pCO_2 and log.O_2
transport were the independent variables. The effect
of hypotension was assessed by studying the bled and
reinfused (BP≠ 50±4 and 88±19 mm Hg, respectively)
dogs. The correlation matrices displayed in the
Tables are composed of the correlation coefficients
for each independent variable on the dependent variable
and on all other independent variables. The partial
regression coefficients indicating the regression of
each independent variable on the dependent variable,
after removing the effects of all other independent
variables, were also calculated and when significant
(P<0.02) were included in the regression equations
(reg.eq.) which were written in the following form:
$$Y_n = \beta_1 X_1 + \beta_2 X_2 + \ldots + \alpha$$

where Y_r = mean value of the frequency distribution
of Y for specified X_1, X_2, etc. The partial regression
coefficient β_1 measures the average or expected
change in Y when X_1 increases 1 unit, X_2, etc. remaining unchanged. A measure of the validity of the
regression equations was obtained by calculating the
F value. The regression lines were compared by a
standard test for parallelism and equality.

RESULTS AND DISCUSSION. As shown in Tables 1
and 2, with the parameters measured here O_2 uptake
in normal and shocked dogs can be predicted with
reasonable accuracy. Distinct from the total body,
hind limb O_2 uptake was not related to arterial pCO_2
suggesting that precapillary sphincters in the inter
nal organs are mainly responsive to this stimulus.

In all 3 groups total and femoral O_2 uptake was
closely related to O_2 transport suggesting that the
inverse changes in O_2 extraction associated with
variations in O_2 transport cushioned, but did not
abolish, the interdependence of these two functions.
In hypotension when O_2 extraction was more complete,
the relationship between O_2 transport and uptake was
even closer, the regression coefficient of O_2 uptake
on O_2 transport was higher, than in normotensive dogs.
This was consistent with the tendency of autoregulatory blood flow to increase at high arteriovenous O_2
difference (1), and accounted for the ability of
shocked dogs to maintain O_2 uptake when blood flow
was profoundly reduced.

The close correspondence between O_2 transport
and O_2 uptake is usually interpreted to suggest that
O_2 supply follows O_2 demand, despite repeated demonst-
rations (6,7,etc.) that varying muscle blood flow may
produce corresponding changes in O_2 consumption. When
testing this hypothesis Stainsby & Otis (8) reduced
blood flow through the resting muscle and found an
increase in the arteriovenous O_2 difference and no
change in O_2 uptake. However, they reduced blood
flow by lowering perfusion pressure, this probably
produced dilatation of the precapillary sphincters,
and created a situation similar to that prevailing
in our shocked dogs.

O_2 uptake of isolated muscle is reversibly
depressed by reduced pO_2 without altering other
measured cell functions suggesting that some oxidative
processes simply generate heat if pO_2 exceeds certain
minimal level (9). In intact animals hypoxia($10\%FIO_2$)
reduces total body O_2 uptake and abolishes non-shiv-
ering thermogenesis (10,11). In the resting muscle

T A B L E   1

Correlation matrices and regression equations for total body oxygen consumption

i n t a c t   (71 dogs, 89 observations)

	A	B	C	D	MEAN	SD
A	1.0000				2.1993	0.1512
B	0.6778*1.0000				36.8	2.4
C	0.8165*0.6201*1.0000				2.8846	0.1869
D	-0.2264*0.1163-0.2022 1.0000				41.8	8.7
r	....				0.86*	0.08

reg.eq.:A=0.0212B+0.4671C-0.0025D+0.1794 (F=77.8*)
        C=0.0482B+1.1121 (F=54.3*)

b l e d   (35 dogs, 105 observations)

	A	B	C	D	MEAN	SD
A	1.0000				2.1809	0.1605
B	0.5362*1.0000				37.7	1.4
C	0.8995*0.4442*1.0000				2.3478	0.1690
D	-0.0277 0.1764 0.1264 1.000				33.0	8.7
r	....				0.93*	0.06

reg.eq.:A=0.0225B+0.7917C-0.0031D-0.4241 (F=207*)
        C=0.0532B+0.3458 (F=25*)

r e i n f u s e d   (26 dogs, 98 observations)

	A	B	C	D	MEAN	SD
A	1.0000				2.2039	0.2027
B	0.8090*1.0000				35.6	3.0
C	0.5415*0.4295*1.0000				2.7666	0.2020
D	-0.3795*0.2157*0.0681 1.0000				36.7	10.3
r	....				0.86*	0.10

reg.eq.:A=0.0441B+0.2454C-0.0043D+0.1144 (F=93*)
        C=0.0287B+1.7424 (F=21.7*)
        D=-0.0736B+62.91 (F=4.7)

A= log.O_2 uptake, ml/min/m²BSA
B= temp.in inf.vena cava °C
C= log.O_2 transport, ml/min/m²BSA
D= arterial pCO_2, Torr
SD= standard deviation (continued next page)

T A B L E   2

Correlation matrices and regression equations for hind limb oxygen consumption

i n t a c t (42 dogs, 42 observations)

	A	B	C	D	MEAN	SD
A	1.0000				1.0028	0.1453
B	0.1222	1.0000			37.6	0.7
C	0.4820*	0.1027	1.0000		1.6768	0.1702
D	0.0899	-0.0333	-0.0512	1.0000	39.1	1.5
r	....				0.48*	0.13

reg.eq.: A=0.4115C+0.3128   (F=12.1*)

b l e d (26 dogs, 72 observations)

	A	B	C	D	MEAN	SD
A	1.0000				0.8875	0.3919
B	0.4080*	1.0000			37.9	1.2
C	0.9750*	0.4430*	1.0000		1.0433	0.3564
D	0.1479	0.2482*	0.1773	1.0000	33.5	9.6
r	....				0.97*	0.09

reg.eq.: A=1.0448C-0.2025 (F=1347*)
        C=0.1322 B - 3.9680 (F=16.9*)

r e i n f u s e d (17 dogs 46 observations)

	A	B	C	D	MEAN	SD
A	1.0000				1.0238	0.2741
B	0.7017*	1.0000			37.6	1.9
C	0.6675*	0.4055*	1.0000		1.4273	0.3494
D	0.1212	0.0180	0.1609	1.0000	32.2	8.7
r	....				0.82*	0.16

reg.eq.: A=0.0739B+0.3596C-2.2741 (F=43.2*)
        C=0.0740B-1.3603 (F=8.7*)

A=log.femoral O_2 uptake ml/min/m^2BSA
B=temp.in inf.véna cava °C
C=log.femoral O_2 transport, ml/min/m^2BSA
D= arterial pCO_2, Torr
r= multiple correlation coefficient and stand.error
*= level of significance below 1 per cent.

not all capillaries are perfused, mean tissue pO_2 is
low and is bound to rise steeply with increased perfusion. In other vascular beds with more homogenous
perfusion increased blood flow, if not called upon by
a rise in cellular metabolism, would also increase
tissue pO_2. Once tissue pO_2 exceeds a certain minimal
level more energy is produced. As opposed to the
basal oxygen consumption, this additional "luxury"
O_2 consumption may be partly converted to heat (9),
representing the fuel for chemical thermoregulation.
        Substances as thyroxin, dinitrophenol, and the
catecholamines increase O_2 uptake in vitro and a
similar effect observed in vivo is usually equated
with their direct cellular action. However, in vivo
these agents stimulate circulation, ventilation, and
raise body temperature: their "calorigenic" action is
likely to represent a combination of metabolic and
non-metabolic activities. Conversely, suppression
of thyroid function, severe sedation, and hypothermia
have an opposite effect on circulation and ventilation
and the lowered metabolic rate may again represent a
combination of metabolic and non-metabolic activities.
The equations developed here may facilitate the in
vivo assessment of interventions claimed to alter basal
tissue metabolic rate.

REFERENCES. 1. Shepherd,A.P.,H.J.Granger,E.E.Smith
and A.C.Guyton. Local control of tissue Oxygen delivery: the contributions of oxygen extraction and total
systemic autoregulation. In press. 2. Mellander,S.
and B.Johansson. Control of resistance, exchange and
capacitance functions in the peripheral circulation.
Pharmacol.Rev. 20:117,1968. 3. Halmagyi,D.F.J. and
M.Kennedy.: Dependence of oxygen consumption on
circulation in normovolemic and hypovolemic dogs.
J.Appl.Physiol. 29:440,1970. 4. Halmagyi,D.F.J.,
I.R.Neering and D.Varga.: Response to hemorrhage
during LO_2 breathing. J.Appl.Physiol. 28:465,1970.
5. Halmagyi,D.F.J.,A.H.Goodman and I.R.Neering.: Hind
 limb blood flow and oxygen usage in hemorrhagic
shock. J.Appl.Physiol. 27:508,1969. 6. Zierler,K.L.:
Skeletal muscle circulation. In: Mills,L.C. and J.H.
Moyer (ed): Shock and Hypotension. N.Y.,Grune &
Stratton,1965, p.170. 7. Beer,G.,and L.R.Yonce.:
Blood flow, oxygen uptake and capillary filtration
in resting skeletal muscle. Am.J.Physiol. 223:492,
1972. 8. Stainsby,W.N.,and Otis,A.B.: Blood flow,
blood oxygen tension, oxygen uptake and oxygen transport in skeletal muscle. Am.J.Physiol.206:858,1964.

9. Whalen,W.J.: Intracellular pO_2: a limiting factor in cell respiration. Am.J.Physiol. 211:862,1966. 10. Moore,R.E.: O_2 consumption and body temperature in newborn kittens subjected to hypoxia and reoxygenation. J.Physiol.(Lond),149:500,1959. 11. Hill,J.R.: The O_2 consumption of newborn and adult mammals. Its dependence on the O_2 tension in the inspired air and the environmental temperature. J.Physiol.(Lond). 149:346,1959.

OXYGEN TRANSPORT CHANGES AFTER TRANSFUSION WITH STORED BLOOD

IN A HEMORRHAGIC CANINE MODEL

C. E. Shields, M. G. Burns, A. Zegna, D. Meixner,

J. Bratton, D. Brooks, L. O'Malley, and G. Phillips

USA Medical Research Laboratory, Fort Knox, Kentucky

Transfusion therapy has the dual purpose of providing volume to replace shed blood and to provide red cells to replace the oxygen transport function.[1] Storage with the present collection solution, acid-citrate-dextrose (ACD), has been limited to 21 days because the red cell is undergoing continual deterioration during storage, with loss of many of its functions. One in particular, red cell oxygen transport as measured by the oxygen dissociation curve, decreased significantly. The intimate role of 2,3-diphosphoglycerate (2,3-DPG) with the oxygen function appeared involved, since the DPG level also decreased with storage. The clinical effect of these storage changes was reflected in the finding of lowered p50 values in the recipient after transfusion of the stored blood.[2-5]

Blood transfusion research has used other chemicals added to the collection solution to improve the preservation of the red cell function. One of these, adenine, was found to assist in providing stored cells that would be able to withstand longer storage periods and still survive in the circulation after transfusion as measured by isotope survival tests.[6,7]

The hemorrhagic canine model reported here was developed to study transfusion of blood stored under varying conditions. The emphasis of this phase was the effect on the oxygen curve, measured as a p50 shift, and DPG levels.

METHODS

A total of 50 healthy beagles, age 3-5 years, 8-14 kg,

were anesthetized and catheters placed. Each was bled over a
15-minute period until the mean arterial pressure (MAP) was 30 mm
Hg. The volume of blood removed averaged 50% of the initial estimated blood volume. MAP of 30 mm Hg was maintained over a 135-
minute period then ended by a transfusion equal to the volume removed during the bleeding and shock period. The transfusion was
given over a 30-minute period. Base line samples were drawn before the procedure and sampling repeated after bleeding, before
and after transfusion at 2, 10, and 120 minutes and 24 hours.
Oxygen determination tests used tonometer equilibration (5-8% O_2)
with readings (IL CO-Oximeter, Model #182, Corning pH and Oxygen
Digital 160 System meters) adjusted for temperature and pH to determine the oxygen dissociation curve, p50, and n value.[8,9] Other
tests included hematocrit and DPG testing by automated method
(Technicon AutoAnalyzer).[10]

The blood transfused had been stored in either ACD or ACD
with adenine (.5mM/500 ml whole blood) for periods of 14, 28, or
42 days. The control group received fresh blood. Of the 34 animals surviving the procedure, 17 received fresh, and 17 were given
the stored blood. Calculations and data were analyzed by statistical methods, primarily analysis of variance.

Table 1

Average Values for p50 for Fresh Control and Subjects Receiving Blood
Stored in ACD or ACD-Adenine for 14, 28 or 42 Days

	STORED						FRESH
	ACD			ACD-ADENINE			
	14	28	42	14	28	42	
Bag	27.3	20.5	18.3	26.4	19.9	18.5	32.0
Posttransfusion	31.1	25.6	27.5	29.7	31.6	25.8	34.2
10 min	31.8	27.0	27.4	31.0	31.6	27.2	--
120 min	29.0	27.2	26.1	29.5	28.2	25.1	35.6
24 hr	28.5	30.8	31.8	31.2	32.0	31.6	34.9

RESULTS

Oxygen curve shifts as indicated by the lower p50 was obvious in the stored blood (Table 1). The significantly lower level of the unit of stored blood influenced the posttransfusion values initially by depressing them, but by 24 hr, all subjects had normal values (Table 1). The time course of the return of the p50 value after transfusion shown in the graph (Fig. 1) did show a delay depending upon how low the bag value was.

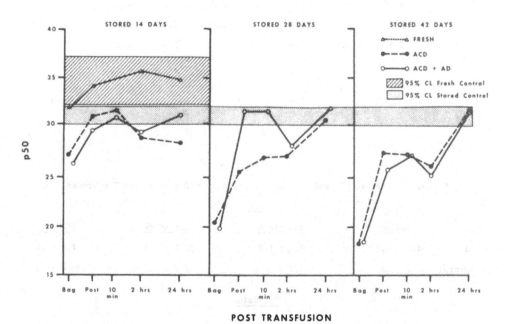

Fig. 1.   Average p50 values obtained at intervals after transfusion of fresh or blood stored in ACD or ACD + Adenine.

A difference was noted between the two collection solutions stored for 28 days, but this was not statistically significant. Changes in n values were not consistent, either in the bag or in the recipients before or after transfusion (Tables 2 and 3).

Table 2

Average Values for n for Fresh Control and Subjects Receiving Blood
Stored in ACD or ACD-Adenine for 14, 28 or 42 Days

	STORED						FRESH
	ACD			ACD-ADENINE			
	14	28	42	14	28	42	
Bag	2.10	2.13	2.38	2.32	2.28	2.41	2.20
Posttransfusion	2.12	2.40	2.18	2.35	2.15	1.85	2.04
10 min	2.32	2.30	2.22	2.39	2.58	2.39	--
120 min	2.63	2.50	2.20	2.71	2.06	2.05	1.97
24 hr	2.87	2.67	2.45	2.85	2.10	2.27	2.35

Table 3

Summary of Average p50 and n Values Prior to Transfusion of the Two Groups

	p50			
	Baseline	Post Bleed	Post Shock	24-Hour
Control	34.8 ± 1.1*	38.1 ± 1.0	39.0 ± 1.3	34.9 ± .6
Experimental	31.2 ± .4	33.5 ± .5	34.0 ± .6	30.8 ± .4

	"n" Value			
Control	2.50 ± .12	2.74 ± .23	2.22 ± .10	2.35 ± .18
Experimental	2.62 ± .10	2.55 ± .05	2.43 ± .08	2.54 ± .10

*Standard deviation of mean

Examination of the p50 values during the bleeding and shock periods revealed striking elevations (p < .01) (Table 3). Both control and experimental groups had been bled in the same manner, without transfusions during these periods; however, significant differences between the two groups were found based on technical procedures, so that the two groups could not be statistically combined. It should be noted that the trend was similar and significant in both.

DPG values were found to follow the same trends as the p50 findings with an elevation during the bleeding and shock period (p < .01), then lower levels in the stored blood and after transfusion (p < .05) (Table 4).

Table 4

Average DPG Values Obtained Before and After Transfusion of Stored Blood (mM/L Packed Cells)

| Baseline | Post Bleed | Post Shock | Bag | Posttransfusion | | | |
				2-min	10-min	120-min	24-Hr
5.42 ± .18*	10.02 ± .45	9.57 ± .78	2.34 ± .27**	3.87 ± .18	3.93 ± .18	3.93 ± .12	9.98 ± .21

*Standard deviation of mean

**Average for all stored units

DISCUSSION

With recent reports of a correlation between DPG and the oxygen dissociation response, storage with its damaging effects on cell metabolism would be expected to have an adverse effect on this metabolite which may be related to the adverse change in the oxygen dissociation curve. After transfusion, these lower levels of DPG and the curve shift in the stored blood depressed the values in the recipient. The model here involved transfusion of over 50% of the total blood volume and simple dilution might have caused the lowering of the p50 and DPG levels. Each subject's change from base line and after transfusion was related to the stored levels; however, the values did not appear to be from direct dilutional effects, because, generally, the recipient levels were higher than would be expected. The transfusion was given over a 30-minute period, and the sample drawn within 2 minutes after this, so that mixing of stored blood in the recipient during that period may have led to some physiological correction.

The sharp rise in p50 and DPG values following the bleeding
which was accomplished in 15 minutes appeared as an unusually
rapid response to this form of hemorrhagic hypoxia. Although
acidosis was encountered after the shock period, little change in
pH was noted during the bleeding period; hence, pH was not considered a major factor in causing the curve shift. The usual response of increased heart rate, respiration, and blood flow was
present during hemorrhage. Hence, the finding of the shift in the
oxygen curve and DPG levels may be indications of additional mechanisms used to compensate for loss of red cell mass and overall
oxygen transport function.

BIBLIOGRAPHY

1. Strumia, M. M., W. H. Crosby, J. G. Gibson, T. J. Greenwalt,
    and J. R. Krevans. *General Principles of Blood Transfusion*.
    Philadelphia: J. B. Lippincott Co., 1963.

2. Valeri, C. R., and N. M. Hirsch. Restoration *in vivo* of
    erythrocyte adenosine triphosphate, 2,3-diphosphoglycerate,
    potassium ion, and sodium ion concentrations following the
    transfusion of acid-citrate-dextrose stored human red blood
    cells. J. Lab. Clin. Med. 73:722, 1969.

3. Finch, C. A., and C. Lenfant. Oxygen transport in man.
    New Eng. J. Med. 286:407, 1972.

4. McConn, R., and L. R. M. Del Guercio. Respiratory function
    of blood in the acutely ill patient and the effect of ster-
    oids. Ann. Surg. 174:436, 1971.

5. Valtis, D. J., and A. C. Kennedy: Defective gas-transport
    function of stored red blood cells. Lancet 1:119, 1954.

6. de Verdier, C. H., L. Garby, M. Hjelm, and C. Högman.
    Adenine in blood preservation: Posttransfusion viability and
    biochemical changes. Transfusion 4:331, 1964.

7. Shields, C. E. Comparison studies of whole blood stored in
    ACD and CPD and with adenine. Transfusion 8:1, 1968.

8. Hill, A. V. Possible effects of the aggregation molecules
    on its dissociation curves. J. Physiol. (London) 40:IV, 1910.

9. Severinghaus, J. W. Blood gas calculator. J. Appl. Physiol.
    21:1108, 1966.

10. Powell, J. B., C. E. Emery, and G. A. Peyton. An automated
    procedure for the assay of 2,3-diphosphoglycerate by measur-
    ing the inorganic phosphorus released. Clin. Chem. 18:241,
    1972.

LOCAL OXYGEN SUPPLY IN INTRA-ABDOMINAL ORGANS AND IN SKELETAL MUSCLE DURING HEMORRHAGIC SHOCK*

E. Sinagowitz, H. Rahmer, R. Rink, L. Görnandt,
M. Kessler with the technical assistance of B. Bölling,
K. Hájek, K. Horak, D. Schmeling, R. Strehlau, and
K. Tlolka
Max-Planck-Institut für Systemphysiologie, Dortmund,
West Germany, and University of Louisville School of
Medicine, Louisville, Kentucky

Investigations of local oxygen supply and local hydrogen washout in tissue (Kessler et al. 1970, 1973a), as well as microphotometric studies in tissue (Lang et al. 1973) have shown that the measurement of local Po_2 is one of the most reliable methods for detecting tissue hypoxia or disturbances of microcirculation.

In previous investigations Kessler et al. (1970,1973a) found that during the development of hemorrhagic shock anoxic areas appear in the liver when the systolic blood pressure is still above 100 mmHg. These observations raised the question if there is a temporal sequence of disturbance of oxygen supply to intra-abdominal organs and the skeletal muscle during the development of hemorrhagic shock.

Using the same shock model as in previous experiments 5 splenectomized and anesthetized mongrel dogs were bled slowly and stepwise. Every 5 min we removed an amount of blood which corresponded to 0.1% of the dog's body weight. Bleeding was continued till a mean arterial blood pressure of 40 mmHg was reached. After keeping the pressure at this level for 30-60 min without any further external intervention, the withdrawn blood volume was replaced by a rapid infusion of a plasma expander.
Local Po_2 of liver, pancreas, duodenum, kidney and gracilis muscle was recorded continuously and simultaneously by means of platinum multiwire surface electrodes, according to Kessler (1968), of which two were placed carefully on each organ's surface. Fig. 1 shows the simultaneous recordings of the Po_2 in relation to the arterial blood

+ Supported by Grant of the Landesamt für Forschung Nordrhein-
Westfalen.

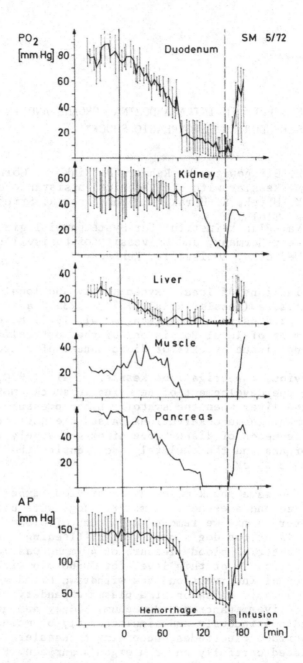

Fig. 1: Po$_2$ of different organs during the development of hemorrhagic shock

pressure. The blood pressure remains stable up to a blood removal
of 1.6% of body weight, then decreases sharply in a short time and
continues to decline slowly. After infusion blood pressure is reestablished rapidly.

The Po_2 on the surface of the pancreas decreases continuously,
beginning with the first bleeding step. When the systolic arterial
blood pressure is still above 60 mmHg, no oxygen tension can be
measured, indicating a relatively early pancreatic ischemia.
After an initial increase the Po_2 on the muscle decreases sharply,
and anoxia is found when the MAP is relatively high.
Anoxic areas are detected earliest in the liver. This indicates an
impairment of the microcirculation in the very early phase of
hemorrhagic shock.
In the outer cortex of the kidney almost normal values are measured
when the MAP is just below 60 mmHg, and the urine flow has already
ceased. When glomular filtration has stopped, the sodium reabsorption will cease also. Consequently, the energy requirement falls
drastically which may explain the high Po_2 values.
The Po_2 on the surface of the duodenum decreases continuously also,
but anoxic areas are found only in the very late phase of hemorrhagic
shock.

As mentioned above, the Po_2 of the muscle decreases in the
early phase of hemorrhagic shock. The comparison of the histograms
of skeletal muscle in the control period and during the period of
decreasing blood pressure (fig. 2 and 3) shows that a distinct
left shift of the histogram occurs very early.

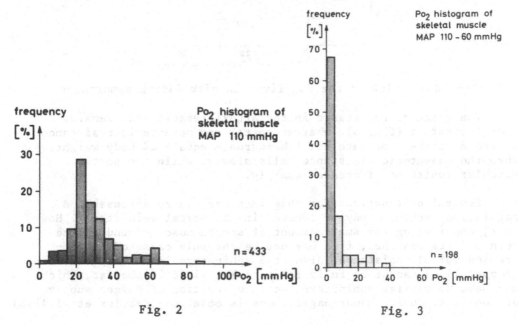

Fig. 2   Fig. 3

While the peak of the normal histogram lies in the range of 20 to 25 mmHg (Kunze 1966), nearly 70% of the Po_2 values are in the hypoxic order of 0-5 mmHg when the MAP decreases from 110 to 60 mmHg.

In order to investigate the blood flow and the resistance in the hepatic vascular bed another series of shock studies was performed on dogs (Sinagowitz et al. 1972). Vascular resistance was determined in the portal, the arteriohepatic and the mesenteric vascular bed. For this purpose blood pressure was measured in the aorta, the caval vein, and the portal vein, and blood flow measurements were performed in the hepatic artery and the portal vein by means of electromagnetic flowmeters.

During hemorrhage a distinct decrease in total hepatic blood flow occurs, which is almost completely due to the decrease in portal flow. By contrast, the arterial blood flow remains nearly stable (Fig. 4).

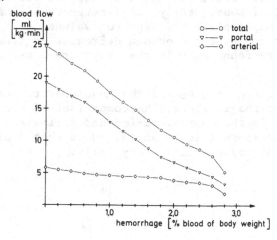

Fig. 4: Blood flow of the dog liver in situ during hemorrhage

The vascular resistance in the arteriohepatic area remains almost constant (fig. 5), whereas portal and mesenteric resistance increase at the same rate until hemorrhage equals 2% body weight. Then the mesenteric resistance falls slowly, while the portal vascular resistance increases sharply.

Several explanations for this increase can be discussed. A regulative mechanism may be located in the portal vein itself. However, considering the small amount of smooth muscle found in the vein and its branches, this may not be the only cause of the increased portal resistance. Also, the sphincters in the hepatic vein (Popper 1931) cannot be fully responsible, since in the rat, which may have no similar sphincters the same reaction of oxygen supply of the liver during hemorrhagic shock is observed (Kessler et al. 1973).

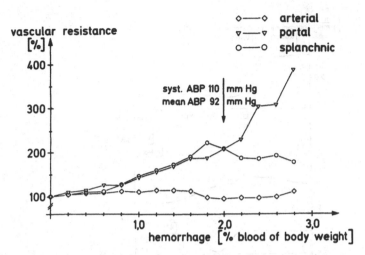

Fig. 5: Vascular resistance in the dog in situ during hemorrhage

Other regulating mechanisms are to be found in the sinusoids
themselves. Outlet and inlet sphincters are described by Knisely
et al. (1948) but their functional mechanism is not yet clear.

Presently, we assume that the increase of portal vascular
resistance is at least partially induced by mechanisms other than
contractions of vascular smooth muscle. Studies of flow in the
isolated, hemoglobin-free perfused rat liver have shown (fig. 6)
that after paralysing smooth muscle with papaverine the application
of norepinephrine in a high dose causes a decrease in flow of
about 70%. This is accompanied by marked changes in the interstitial activity of hydrogen and potassium ions. These findings
together with experiments with a lower dose of norepinephrine
suggest the presence of cellular factors acting to regulate the
intrahepatic microflow (Kessler et al. 1973b).

SUMMARY

During the development of hemorrhagic shock anoxic areas first
are found in the liver. Total anoxia develops first in the muscle
then in the pancreas, whereas an impairment of oxygen supply to the
duodenum and the kidney is observed in the late phase of hemorrhagic
shock. There is some evidence that the observed increase in portal
vascular resistance is at least partially caused by liver cells.

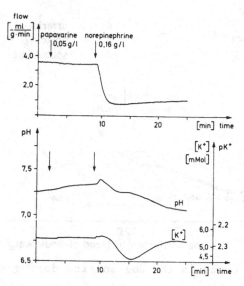

Fig. 6: Flow, pH, pK in the isolated perfused rat liver

REFERENCES

1. Kessler, M.: Normal and critical O$_2$ supply of the liver. In:
   Oxygen transport in blood and tissue ed. by D.W. Lübbers,
   U.C. Luft, G. Thews, E. Witzleb, pp. 90-99, Thieme,
   Stuttgart 1968.

2. Kessler, M., M. Thermann, H. Lang, W. Hartel, H. Schneider: O$_2$-
   Versorgung lebenswichtiger Organe im Schock mit besonderer
   Berücksichtigung der Leber. In: Schock, Stoffwechselver-
   änderungen und Therapie, ed. by W.E. Zimmermann, I. Staib.
   pp. 117-131, Schattauer, Stuttgart-New York 1970.

3. Kessler, M., L. Görnandt, M. Thermann, H. Lang, K. Brand, W.
   Wessel: Oxygen supply and microcirculation of liver in
   hemorrhagic shock. In: Oxygen supply, theoretical and practical
   aspects of oxygen supply and microcirculation of tissue, ed.
   by M. Kessler, D.F. Bruley, L.C. Clark Jr., D.W. Lübbers, I.A.
   Silver, J. Strauss, pp. 252-255. Urban & Schwarzenberg
   München-Berlin-Wien 1973.

4. Kessler, M., H. Lang, E. Sinagowitz, R. Rink, J. Höper:
   Homeostasis of oxygen supply in liver and kidney. In this
   book. Plenum Press New York 1973b.

5. Kniseley, M.H., E.H. Bloch, L. Warner: Selective phagocytosis I.
   Microscopic observations concerning the regulation of the
   blood flow through the liver and other organs and the mechanism
   and rate of phagocytic removal of particles from the blood.
   Kgl. Danske Videnskab. Selskab. Biol. Skrifter 4, 1-93 (1948).

6. Kunze, K.: Die lokale kontinuierliche Sauerstoffmessung in der
   menschlichen Muskulatur. Pflügers Arch. ges. Physiol. 292,
   151 (1966).

7. Lang, H., M. Kessler, H. Starlinger: Signs of hypoxia measured
   by means of Po_2-multiwire electrodes by NADH and NADPH fluores-
   cence and determination of lactate and pyruvate formation.
   In: Oxygen supply, theoretical and practical aspects of oxygen
   supply and microcirculation of tissue, ed. by M. Kessler,
   D.F. Bruley, L.C. Clark Jr., D.W. Lübbers, I.A. Silver,
   J. Strauss, pp. 193-198. Urban & Schwarzenberg, München-Berlin-
   Wien 1973.

8. Popper, H.: Über Drosselvorrichtungen an Lebervenen. Klin.
   Wschr. 10, 2129-2131 (1931).

9. Sinagowitz, E., L. Görnandt, M. Kessler, M. Thermann: Blood flow
   and vascular resistance in splanchnic, portal, and hepatic
   arterial systems during hemorrhagic shock. Pflügers Arch. 335,
   (Suppl.), R 24 (1972).

DISCUSSION OF SESSION II   SUBSESSION: SHOCK

Chairmen: Dr. Manfred Kessler, Dr. Jürgen Grote and
              Dr. James A. Miller, Jr.

DISCUSSION OF PAPER BY R. RINK AND M. KESSLER

Halmagyi: Is a rat, whose abdomen is opened and whose intestines
are spread out, normal at any stage of the experiment?

Rink: Certainly, simply anesthetizing the animal immediately alters
what is "normal." Beyond that, we believe there is a minimum of
insult to the intestine in relation to further manipulations. The
loop of intestine is not lifted out of the abdominal cavity, rather,
a plastic supporting plate is slipped beneath it to dampen motions
due to breathing. Then the dipping cone of the objective is applied
to the surface. Normal temperatures were maintained. The animals
were unheparinized and the laparotomy caused no blood loss.

Kessler: About Halmagyi's question: I think one very important
thing is to have the pO_2 measurements of tissue because these are
absolute measurements, and we always see when the animals are in
bad condition that the oxygen supply to tissue is disturbed.

Gibson: (1) Did you do non-bleeding controls?
      (2) Might you consider the oscillation in the pO_2 in the
intermediate phase of shock as similar to the 'hunting' phenomenon
seen in cold injury (i.e., apparent opening and closing beds)?

Rink: (1) In some of the experiments with the photometric apparatus
we reinfused the withdrawn blood after the MAP had reached 50 mm Hg.
All the signals, i.e., at 465, 585, and 600 mm Hg, decreased to
levels of intensity below the prehemorrhage control levels. With
vital microscopy we observed hyperemia. The drop of intensity of
each signal and their reassociation demonstrates that the changes
produced by successive hemorrhages were not artifactual.
      (2) I am not familiar with the 'hunting' phenomenon. But the
oscillations suggest waves of local blood flow—perhaps as a result
of catecholamine release. Here I am referring to previous papers
in this symposium which demonstrated such an effect in perfused
organs.

Kovach: Did you try to bleed the animal for a long-lasting time
with some kind of standardized procedure to see what is happening,
because it is a little bit difficult to judge from these continuous
small bleedings what would happen?
      It is also not easy to compare it with the short models. Did

you check the hemodilution, because that can also be a factor, in
that you have some hemoglobin in red cells changing the rest of
volume in the tissue and that can change your fluorescence?

Rink: I agree. The plasma line expander was used only in the pO_2
measurements and for fluorescence measurements, we reinfused blood
and the values returned to below control levels because of evidently
a reactive hyperemia in this point, but the fluorescence decreased.
All signals decreased and became associated. The standardization
of bleeding does not relate to the procedures which are commonly
employed, a variation or a Wiggers-type of hemorrhagic shock, but
we have a beginning here now. The logical step would now be to
sustain or to bleed an animal to a certain blood pressure and then
record over a lengthened period of time.

DISCUSSION OF PAPER BY C. T. FITTS, H. I. BICHER AND
     D. R. YARBROUGH, III.

Messmer: I would like to refer you to the publications of Olson
et al., from Karolinska Institute in Stockholm concerning the "unknown" effects of protamine. Olson has shown that protamine induces
pulmonary hypertension associated with a decline in cardiac output
being mainly dependent upon the speed of injection of protamine.
(Europ. Surg. Res. 1971/72.)

Fitts: Yes, it is known that the rapid injection of protamine will
cause a drop in blood pressure, usually associated with bradycardia.
It does not suffice to say that it is "caused" by pulmonary hypertension, but decrease in cardiac output, however. It may indeed be
accompanied by a decrease in cardiac output and an increase in pulmonary pressure, but the mechanism by which it causes this effect
is unknown.

Kovach: I think that from 3 experiments were the control values
varied between 20 and 50 mm Hg pO_2, we cannot conclude anything
about the changes in hemorrhagic shock. In which regions of the
brain did you put the electrodes?

Fitts: One can always use more measurements and we believe, as you,
that these would be desirable. In three experiments, however, the
measurements were extremely stable throughout the experiment and
responded well to changes in respiratory gas mixtures in the predicted direction. The variability between 20 mm and 40 mm pO_2 between
electrodes is more than likely related to position, since even minute
differences in electrode position within the cerebral cortex are
known to be associated with differences in pO_2 levels of this
magnitude.

DISCUSSION OF PAPER BY D. F. J. HALMAGYI, J. LEIGH, A. H. GOODMAN
    AND D. VARGA

Kessler: I would like to make a short comment. In contrast to
your observation of oxygen uptake in the hind limb, we find a very
close relationship in liver between oxygen uptake and tissue oxygenation. We only see flow dependence on oxygen uptake when the blood
flow is below a critical value so that not enough tissue oxygenation
is provided.

Halmagyi: We have measured the mesenteric oxygen consumption in
dogs by the conventional catheter methods and we found a similar
relationship. We found the oxygen uptake of the mesenteric circuit
was also very closely related to flow. When the flow went down,
oxygen uptake went down and vice versa. I do not know to what
extent that is comparable.

Gelin: As I understand your data and conclusions, oxygen tension
in tissue depends on the permeability surface area (PS-value) as
defined by Rankin. Did you calibrate the PS values for different
flow values?

Halmagyi: Indeed, the Xenon technique would be suitable to examine
this hypothesis.

DISCUSSION OF PAPER BY C. E. SHIELDS, M. G. BURNS, A. ZEGNA,
    D. MEIXNER, J. BRATTON, D. BROOKS, L. O'MALEY AND G. PHILLIPS

Davidson: Don't you think that the oxygen transport changes shown
here after infusion of stored blood is due to impaired microcirculation, caused by platelet aggregation which gives microembolization
both in pulmonary circulation and in the artery. This platelet
aggregation which occurs in stored blood can be measured as screen
filtration pressure, according to Swank, and can be removed by using
a micropore filter when infusing blood.

Shields: This could very well be. The findings are in reference
to a considerable amount of information obtained on stored blood.
We did not actually measure the platelets. It is difficult to assess
the direct effect of platelets on the P_{50} at this point.

Sunder-Plassmann: I wonder if you could comment on the extraordi-
narily high control values of P_{50} in your dogs, which ranged from
30-34 mm Hg, which is in contrast to those values from a number of
other authors and our own findings. The P_{50} in the normal dog,
when corrected to pH 7.4, is 26.5 - 27.5 mm Hg.
    In addition, a response in P_{50} to hemorrhage within a time

period of 15 minutes is rather surprising. From our own studies, we have evidence that throughout a time period of at least 120 minutes of hemorrhagic hypotension, the 2,3-DPG concentration does not change.

Shields: The levels that we received on the experimental dogs may have been affected by the fact that our catheter and our electrode was changed by the manufacturer during the procedure. We do know what our levels were. We obtained the sample and had it run within the first 5 minutes. I have run across an article in which a study was done in which they did this immediately, and they received an average of 33.3 plus or minus .11. Our average is 33.3 plus or minus .13. So, we have one agreement for our results. One of our major questions is why would the body response be so prompt? 15 minutes is the most rapid change we have seen. Hypoxia, high altitude, and anemia certainly take a lot more time.

Subsession: HEART

Chairmen: Dr. Thomas K. Goldstick, Dr. David C. MacGregor

and Dr. Carl R. Honig

O_2 AND THE NUMBER AND ARRANGEMENT OF CORONARY CAPILLARIES: EFFECT ON CALCULATED TISSUE PO_2

Carl R. Honig and Jeannine Bourdeau-Martini

University of Rochester, Rochester, N.Y. USA, and

University of Paris at Orsay, Paris, France

O_2 transport in tissue depends largely on the abundance and arrangement of capillaries. To study these parameters in a tissue of high $\dot{V}O_2$ we devised a technique by which surface capillaries could be visualized in stop-motion ciné photomicrographs of rat heart beating in situ (1,2,6). In each rat under each experimental condition 100-900 individual measurements of intercapillary distance (ICD) were obtained. To date 65 rats have been so studied at various values of paO_2 obtained by adjusting pIO_2. Statistical analyses of ICD are based on the National Bureau of Standards Omnitab II computer program; technical details are provided in references 2 and 6.

Dual Effect of O_2
The relationship between paO_2, ICD, and capillary density is shown in Fig. 1. Each of the 68 data points represents mean ICD in 1 experiment in 1 rat. The line of positive slope extends about 100 mmHg above the tension at which hemoglobin is 90% saturated. This demonstrates that the mechanism which controls precapillary sphincters senses pO_2 rather than O_2 content (6). Note that ICD could be reduced from 17 μ, its mean value at normal paO_2, to 14 μ, by either lowering paO_2 to 30 or raising it to 630 mmHg. In both cases 800 capillaries/mm^2, or about 40% of the capillary reserve (2) become open and perfused.

If 2 independent processes underlie the dual effect of O_2, the data can be described by:

$$\overline{ICD} = 12.81 + 0.034\ paO_2, \text{ and}$$
$$\overline{ICD} = 19.60 - 0.009\ paO_2$$

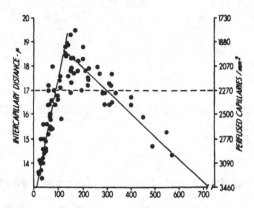

Fig. 1. Dual effect of O_2 on ICD and capillary density. Each data
point represents mean ICD in 1 rat.

If only 1 process is responsible, the data can be fitted by a
parabolic least squares regression:

$$\overline{ICD} = 14.85 + 0.025 \; paO_2 - 0.00005 \; paO_2^2$$

The correlation coefficients for these regressions range from 0.86
to 0.92, indicating that about 80% of the variance in $\overline{ICD}$ is at-
tributable to paO_2. Our conclusion that O_2 is the principal de-
terminant is supported by experiments which demonstrate that B.P.
pHa and $paCO_2$ do not affect coronary ICD significantly [1,2].

Degree of Order in Lateral Capillary Spacing

Distances between points on a line follow the Poisson distribution if they are randomly arranged [2]. Since ICD was measured
along a line oriented perpendicular to the long axis of the capillaries, if lateral spacing were random frequency distributions of
ICD should be exponential. All distributions, however, were roughly normal; see Fig. 2. This means that some degree of order exists in the lateral spacing, even though each precapillary sphincter functions independently of its neighbors. Though we made our
observations on 2-dimensional optical sections, the 3-dimensional
arrangement could not have been random if the 2-dimensional one
was non-random. The foregoing is consistent with the roughly hex-
agonal packing observed when all coronary capillaries are open.
Since about half the available capillaries were open at normal
paO_2, (2,6), the array at any moment should reflect the underlying
order. The available capillaries are not precisely spaced, however,
for if they were we should have observed peaks in the frequency
histograms of open capillaries corresponding to multiples of near-
est neighbor distances. Such peaks were not observed even for
small class intervals, indicating that the true state lies between
a fully random and perfectly ordered condition.

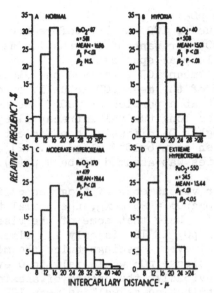

Fig. 2. Frequency distributions of individual ICD measurements in 4 rats, representing 4 ranges of paO_2

Effect of O_2 on lateral spacing.

The frequency distribution of individual ICD measurements was computed for experiments in each of 4 ranges of paO_2. Observations between 80 and 100 mmHg paO_2 characterize the normal animal, and those below 40 mmHg are typical of hypoxia. Observations in moderate hyperoxemia (between 120 and 200 mmHg) illustrate the range of tensions where O_2 promotes sphincter contraction and increases mean ICD. Data collected above 450 mmHg represent extreme hyperoxemia where O_2 favors sphincter muscle relaxation. All distributions tended to positive skewness, but this tendency was greatest, and was always statistically significant, in moderate hyperoxemia. All distributions in hypoxia and extreme hyperoxemia exhibited significant kurtosis.

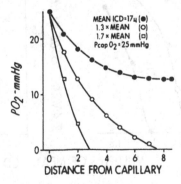

Fig. 3. Gradients in pO_2 for multiples of normal mean ICD.

Calculated Tissue pO_2

A unique value of ICD has heretofore been used in calculations of tissue pO_2 for want of information as to the actual distribution of the lateral spacings (4). To evaluate the impact of
the variance about mean ICD we solved the classical Krogh equation
(5) for multiples of the mean ICD actually encountered in a particular experiment at a particular paO_2. We assumed flow to be
co-current, and the longitudinal intracapillary gradient to be
exponential. Krogh's O_2 diffusion coefficient was used; $\dot{V}O_2$ for
rat heart was taken as 6.6×10^{-3} ml/g/sec. (2) and diameter of
coronary capillaries was assumed to be 4 μ (7).

Gradients for venous ends of Kroghian cylinders are shown in
Fig. 3, assuming $pcapO_2 = 25$ mmHg, the normal tension of rat coronary venous blood. Note that some of the tissue cylinder cross-
section is at zero pO_2 if ICD is only 1.3 times mean spacing. As
shown in Fig. 2, however, spacings twice the mean exist. For the
longest spacings, tissue pO_2 would fall to 0 even if $pcapO_2$ were
equal to paO_2! Obviously, the amount of anoxic tissue depends on
the frequency distribution as well as mean ICD.

To estimate the amount of anoxic tissue normally present, the
fraction of Kroghian cylinder cross-section which might have been
anoxic was determined from the intercepts on the abscissa in plots
like those in Fig. 3. End-capillary pO_2 was again 25 mmHg; pO_2
at the origin of the capillary was set at 50 mmHg to allow for
diffusion of O_2 from arterioles (3), and 35 mmHg was chosen as an
intermediate value. The anoxic fractions for multiples of mean
ICD are shown in Fig. 4A. The fractions were multiplied by the
observed frequency of spacings, as determined from ogive corresponding to the histogram in Fig. 2A. The product denotes the %

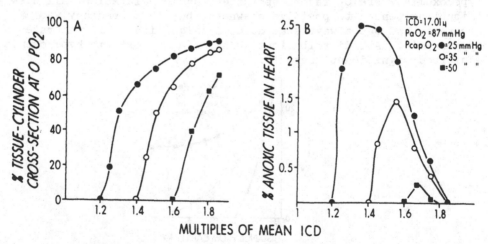

Fig. 4. Estimated amounts of anoxic tissue in rat myocardium.

anoxic tissue in bulk myocardium at a particular point in the longitudinal gradient. These products were plotted to generate Fig. 4B,
from which we estimate that only about 10% of tissue opposite the
venous ends of co-current capillaries would be anoxic. Opposite
the arterial end of a capillary tissue pO_2 would exceed 0 until
ICD exceeds 1.6 times mean ICD. Since only 2.5% of capillaries are
separated by more than 1.6 times mean ICD, almost no tissue would
be anoxic at the arterial end of the longitudinal gradient. Clearly, any factor which might minimize the longitudinal gradient,
such as counter-current blood flow, or diffusion from large vessels, could virtually eliminate anoxic regions if paO_2 were normal.
Any remaining anoxic regions would be "rotated" by precapillary
sphincters as described by Krogh (5). We conclude that rat subepicardium is nearly homogeneous with respect to oxidative metabolism.

To evaluate the effect of moderate hyperoxemia the above calculations were performed for the experiment shown in Fig. 2C
(paO_2 = 170 mmHg). Venous pO_2 would have been only about 3 mmHg
greater than normal if the increase in paO_2 did not change $\dot{V}O_2$ or
coronary blood flow. We therefore set end-capillary pO_2 at 28
mmHg. Calculated pO_2 fell to 0 at some point in the tissue at
spacings greater than 1.2 x mean ICD. Because the frequency distribution was skewed, 25% of spacings exceeded 1.2 x the mean, and
about 1/4 the myocardial tissue opposite the venous ends of capillaries would have been anoxic. Almost no anoxia would have ex-
isted at the origin of the capillary, had $pcapO_2$ at that point exceeded 60 mmHg. We previously showed that a precapillary sphincter obtains its O_2 chiefly from the surrounding tissue during the
contraction phase of its duty cycle (6). In effect a sphincter
"samples" pO_2 in its surround. It is therefore likely that diffusion of O_2 from the arteriolar lumen disrupts normal coupling
between tissue $\dot{V}O_2$ and diffusion distance and paradoxically decreases tissue pO_2, when paO_2 is moderately increased.

The apparent magnitude of this O_2-induced anoxia is, of course,
critically dependent on longitudinal gradients. Moderate hyperoxemia was well tolerated in rats, even though 25% of tissue at
the venous end of the gradient was calculated to have been anoxic.
This strongly suggests that at least some longitudinal gradients
are not exponential, as assumed in our calculation, presumably because of counter-current flow and/or diffusion from arterioles.
It seems unlikely, however, that these factors could completely
eliminate tissue anoxia at long ICD. We therefore suggest that
the therapeutic role of O_2 be carefully re-evaluated, particularly
in ischemic heart disease.

Calculation of the amount of anoxic tissue in hypoxemia and
extreme hyperoxemia (experiments like those in Figs. 2B and D) is
complicated by changes in $\dot{V}O_2$ and coronary blood flow. It is

nevertheless clear that in both conditions transport is greatly
facilitated by the kurtosis characteristic of the frequency distributions, as well as by the decrease in mean ICD.

Unknowns

The foregoing calculations, though extremely crude, illustrate
the importance of quantitative information about capillary anatomy.
It is unsettling to realize that our data on lateral spacing is
the only such information presently available. We emphasize that
the observations were made on 2-dimensional optical sections of
surface vessels. Consequently inferences about 3-dimensional arrangement are valid only to a depth equal to mean capillary
length. Nothing is presently known of the 3-dimensional arrangement of deep capillaries except that it is non-random. We are completely ignorant of the degree of order in alignment of arterial
and venous ends of capillaries, and of the influence of change in
capillary diameter with capillary length. The extent of capillary
branching is unknown, as is the orientation of the branches. In
addition to the foregoing anatomical uncertainties, $\dot{V}O_2$ is not
precisely known, and probably is non-uniform. Since the longitudinal intracapillary O_2 gradient has never been measured, we do not
know the effect of capillary branching, interaction of diffusion
fields, counter-current blood flow, or diffusion from large vessels. Doubtless many of the above factors change under different
physiological conditions, just as has been demonstrated for the
lateral spacing. The effect of error in any of the foregoing
factors will be greatest in organs like the heart in which $\dot{V}O_2$ is
high. We conclude that progress in O_2 transport is chiefly limited
by lack of knowledge of parameters. In view of advances in mathematical modelling techniques (4), it seems likely that exciting
new insights can be expected from theoreticians if experimental-
ists can provide the anatomical and physiological facts.

References:

1) Bourdeau-Martini, J. and C. R. Honig. Microvasc. Res.
   In press.
2) Bourdeau-Martini, J. and C. R. Honig. Am. J. Physiol.
   Submitted.
3) Duling, B. R. and R. Berne. Circ. Res. 27: 669, 1970.
4) Grunewald, E. K. Pflüger's Arch. 309: 266, 1969.
5) Krogh, A. J. Physiol. (London) 52: 457, 1919.
6) Martini, J. and C. R. Honig. Microvasc. Res. 1: 244, 1969.
7) Sobin, S. S. and H. M. Tremer. Microvasc. Res. 4: 330, 1972.

Acknowledgement:
  This research was supported by grant HE 03290, from the
National Institutes of Health.

RESPIRATORY GAS TRANSPORT IN HEART

Jürgen Grote and Gerhard Thews

Institute of Physiology, University of Mainz

The purpose of this paper is to describe an attempt to obtain a better understanding of the dynamics of the oxygen supply of the myocardium under physiological and pathophysiological conditions by examining the oxygen diffusion in the heart muscle tissue during systole and diastole. In comparison to other organs the oxygen supply of the myocardium is characterized by a number of specific features. The most important one is that the gas exchange in the myocardium is a nonsteady-state diffusion process.

BASIC CONCEPTIONS

Under normal conditions the oxygen uptake of the myocardium (MMR O_2) ranges between 9 and 10 mlO_2/100g min. Besides the basal metabolism of the heart and the energy need for activation as well as for external work the oxygen consumption rate of the heart muscle tissue is influenced by three major determinants. After Sonnenblick (23) these are: 1. the intramyocardial wall tension, which is mainly affected by the intraventricular volume, the ventricular pressure and the mass of the heart muscle; 2. the heart rate, which influences the times per minute the heart muscle is activated; and 3. the contractile state of the myocardium. Taking into account the different determinants, Bretschneider (2) presented an equation which allow a good approximation of the oxygen consumption rate of the myocardium for different conditions. During heavy exertion with an increase of stroke volume and heart rate the mean oxygen uptake of the heart muscle tissue increases above 20 mlO_2/100g min.

In consequence of the relatively high oxygen consumption rate the oxygen content and the oxygen tension in the blood decreases more during the capillary passage in the myocardium than in other tissues. According to Doll and coworkers (3,4) the AVD O_2 ranges between 10 and 12 mlO_2/100 ml blood while the oxygen tension of the venous blood leaving the myocardium ranges between 22 and 25 mmHg.

Under normal conditions mean blood flow values for the myocardium of 80 - 90 ml blood/100g min were measured in dogs, monkeys and humans (1). With regard to the rhythmical contraction of the heart coronary blood flow during cardiac cycle is nonhomogeneous (8). During systole the myocardial tissue pressure increases from epicardium to endocardium and in the deeper layers of the myocardium exeeds the blood pressure (13,14). It must be expected that, at least in the inner layer of the myocardium, capillary circulation can only take place in the diastole. Thus, oxygen supply is subjected to rhythmical alternations (8, 18, 20).

The oxygen release from capillary blood to tissue takes place by molecular diffusion. The diffusion process results from the existence of radial and axial gradients of oxygen concentration. Presently there is little information about the importance of convective oxygen transport from capillary blood to tissue (11). Inside the muscle cells a convective oxygen transport, especially as the consequence of cytoplasmic streaming, and a facilitated oxygen diffusion by MbO_2 diffusion are discussed (9,12,15,28).

In order to maintain a sufficient myocardial oxygen supply the supply area of a single capillary is relatively small. The average diameter of a normal heart muscle fiber is approximately 14 μm; each fiber is supplied by one capillary (8,10,17). During hypertrophy the muscle fibers increase in diameter and length, the muscle fiber/capillary ratio remains constant. At the critical heart weight of 500g average muscle fiber diameters of about 20 - 24 μm were measured (17,28).

The capillaries of the myocardium show parallel arrangement on the whole. According to the investigations of Fabel (5) and of Toborg (26) it must be expected that in adjacent capillaries there exists concurrent as well as countercurrent flow. The arterial influxes and the venous effluxes of the capillaries are mostly found at staggered locations. The radius of the cylindrical area supplied by a single capillary is under normal conditions approximately 14 μm and in hypertrophied hearts with the critical weight approximately 20 μm (8). As a result of theoretical and experimental investigations of Myers and Honig (19), which indicate that only a fraction of the available capillaries are perfused at rest, the supply area of a single capillary may be larger under resting conditions than we expect, taking into account anatomical data.

The rhythmical alternations of myocardial oxygen supply as a consequence of nonhomogeneous capillary blood flow in the inner layer of the heart muscle during cardiac cycle are damped by myoglobin (8,15). It is thought that myoglobin acts as a short-time oxygen store to tide the myocardium over situations of momentary fluctuations in oxygen supply. Recent studies of Reneau and coworkers (21) indicate that under conditions of capillary blood flow changings myoglobin has a stabilizing effect that would prevent instantaneous tissue oxygen tension fluctuations, particularly in hypoxia.

According to the photometric investigations of Fabel and Lübbers (6,18) it must be assumed that the oxygen uptake of the heart muscle remains constant throughout the cardiac cycle. The rhythmical ATP need of myofibrils probably is buffered completely by intracellular energy storages so that no changes occur in the redox-ratio of the cytochromes of the respiratory chain.

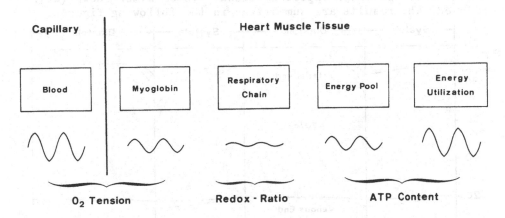

Fig. 1. Schematic representation of fluctuations in oxygen tension of capillary blood and myocardium and of fluctuations in the redox-ratio of cytochromes and in ATP content of myocardium during cardiac cycle according to Lübbers and Schuchardt (18,22).

OXYGEN DIFFUSION IN THE MYOCARDIUM

To investigate the dynamics of oxygen diffusion in heart muscle tissue during cardiac cycle we predicted spatial and transit distribution of oxygen tension in the idealized Krogh Capillary-tissue System (16) for different physiological and pathophysiological conditions.

The following assumptions were made:
The myocardial tissue is divided into cylindrical areas which are

supplied with oxygen from a central capillary. Oxygen is transported in the capillary by convection and molecular diffusion, and
in the tissue by molecular diffusion only (7). Within the capillaries
the oxygen tension decreases from 95 mmHg at the arterial end to
about 22 - 24 mmHg at the venous end. The heart muscle cells are
distributed homogeneously in the tissue cylinder. The oxygen consumption of the myocardium is constant during systole and diastole.
A periodic gas exchange results from the fluctuation of capillary
blood flow during the cardiac cycle. It is assumed that in large
areas of the heart the predominant portion of the capillary blood
supply takes place during diastole, whereas in the systole the
capillary blood flow stops or moves at a low rate.

Based on the assumptions and conditions which were outlined
above the spatial and transient distribution of oxygen tension in
the myocardium were predicted according to the laws of diffusion.
Solutions of the partial differential equations for the boundary
conditions of the Krogh Capillary-tissue System after Thews (24,25)
were used. The results are summarized in the following figures.

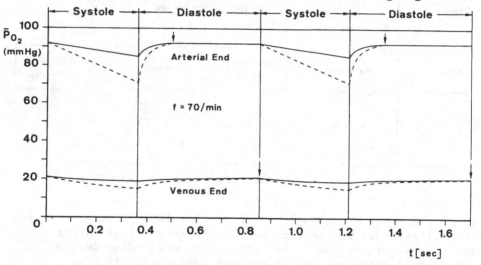

Fig. 2. Change of mean oxygen tension in myocardium during cardiac
cycle under resting conditions. Upper curve = $\bar{P}O_2$ at the end of
the tissue cylinder; lower curve = $\bar{P}O_2$ at the venous end of the
tissue cylinder. Solid lines = systolic stop of capillary blood
flow, oxygen diffusion from the capillaries; dotted lines =
systolic stop of capillary blood flow, no oxygen diffusion from the
capillaries.

Figure 2 shows the temporal changes of the mean oxygen tension
in the tissue cylinder during the cardiac cycle under resting
conditions (f = 70/min, MMR O_2= 10 mlO_2/100g min). The upper
curves give the mean oxygen tension values at the arterial end of

the tissue cylinder, the lower curves give the mean oxygen tension
at the venous end of the tissue cylinder. The calculations were
done for two different assumptions:
1. During systole capillary blood flow in the myocardium stops,
   but the erythrocytes remain inside the capillaries and a postdiffusion of oxygen from the capillary blood to the tissue
   takes place.
2. During systole capillary blood flow in the myocardium stops,
   but the erythrocytes are squeezed out of the capillaries and
   no oxygen diffusion from the capillaries to the tissue takes
   place.
The results of the first predictions are represented by solid lines;
the results of the second ones are represented by dotted lines.
Under the conditions in vivo we expect the mean oxygen tension
values of the myocardium to lie between the two extremes. As seen
in Figure 2 the mean oxygen tension at the venous end of the
tissue cylinder drops temporarily at the end of the systole to
15 - 19 mmHg. A complete resaturation of the tissue with oxygen
(98 % of the initial oxygen tension value) in the following
diastole, marked by arrows, is reached at the end of the cardiac
cycle.

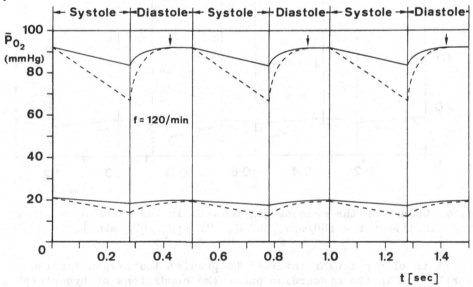

Fig. 3. Change of the mean oxygen tension in the myocardium during
medium exertion (f = 120/min, MMR O_2= 16 mlO_2/100g min).

     Under the conditions of medium exertion (f = 120/min,
MMR O_2= 16 mlO_2/100g min) the mean oxygen tension at the venous
end of the Krogh tissue cylinder decreases at the end of the
systole to 12 - 18 mmHg. The oxygen consumption rate of the heart
muscle tissue rises, but because the duration of the systole

decreases, the predicted mean oxygen tension values are in the
same range as under resting conditions. A complete resaturation
of the tissue with oxygen, however, is not possible so that a new
state of equilibrium on a lower level is reached after the next
cardiac cycle (Fig. 3).

During heavy exertion (f = 180/min, MMR O_2= 21 mlO_2/100g min)
the decrease of the mean oxygen tension in the different tissue
areas during systole is more pronounced. At the end of the systole
the mean oxygen tension value at the venous end of the tissue
cylinder falls between 6 and 13 mmHg as a result of the increase
in oxygen consumption rate and the shortening of the diastolic
recovery phase (Fig. 4).

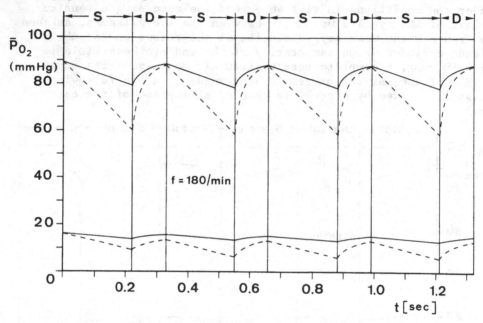

Fig. 4. Change of the mean oxygen tension in the myocardium during
heavy exertion (f = 180/min, MMR O_2= 21 mlO_2/100g min).

It is of particular interest to predict the oxygen tension
distribution in the myocardium under the conditions of hypertrophy.
In Figure 5 the results of a theoretical analysis of oxygen
diffusion in hypertrophied heart muscle under the assumptions:
heart weight = 500g, radius of the tissue cylinder = 20 /um,
f = 70/min, MMR O_2= 10 mlO_2/100g min, are given. In comparison to
normal heart muscle tissue, the mean oxygen tension values of the
hypertrophied myocardium decrease more during systole as a result
of the increasing diameter of the Krogh tissue cylinder. Under
resting conditions the mean oxygen tension values at the venous
end of the hypertrophied tissue cylinder are comparable with the

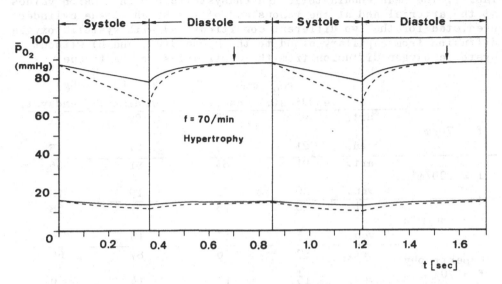

Fig. 5. Change of the mean oxygen tension in hypertrophied myocardium under resting conditions.

values predicted for the same tissue area in a normal heart for the conditions of medium exertion.

The results of the oxygen diffusion analyses for the different discussed cases are summarized in Table 1.

The mean oxygen tension values of the different parts of the Krogh tissue cylinder, calculated by integrating the local values of the same section, give no information about the spatial and transit distribution of oxygen tension in the myocardium. The regional oxygen tension distribution at the arterial and at the venous end of the tissue cylinder were therefore predicted for resting conditions as well as for the conditions of heavy exertion. (Fig. 6). The calculations were done first for the situation at the end of the diastole (upper curves) and second for the situation at the end of the systole (lower curves). The lower solid curves give the oxygen tension values which we predicted for the conditions of systolic oxygen diffusion from the capillary blood to the myocardium; the lower dotted curves give the oxygen tensions which are to be expected under the conditions of no systolic postdiffusion.

Tab. 1. The mean enddiastolic and endsystolic oxygen tension values at the arterial and at the venous end of the Krogh tissue cylinder predicted for the two different conditions: A) with systolic oxygen diffusion from capillary blood to the myocardium, and B) without systolic oxygen diffusion from the capillaries to the tissue.

		A $\bar{P}O_2$ (mmHg)		B $\bar{P}O_2$ (mmHg)	
		enddiast.	endsyst.	enddiast.	endsyst.
f = 70/min	art.	92	85	92	71
	ven.	21	19	21	15
f = 120/min	art.	91	83	91	66
	ven.	20	18	19	12
f = 180/min	art.	88	78	87	58
	ven.	15	13	13	6
Hypertrophy f = 70/min	art.	87	76	87	66
	ven.	15	13	14	9

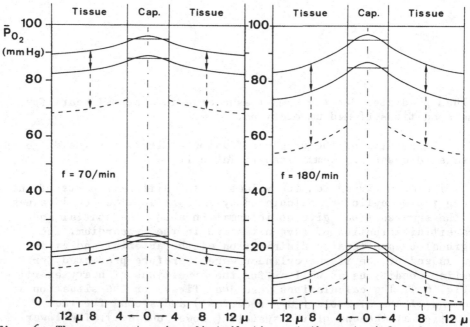

Fig. 6. The oxygen tension distribution at the arterial and at the venous end of the Krogh tissue cylinder in the myocardium. Upper solid curves = oxygen tension distribution at the end of the diastole; lower solid and dotted curves = oxygen tension distribution at the end of the systole.

It is to be seen in Figure 6 that in the least supplied areas of the tissue cylinder - the lethal corner - the oxygen tension decreases about 3 mmHg below the mean oxygen tension value of the same section at a heart rate of 70/min and about 6 mmHg during heavy exertion.

Under the conditions of heavy exertion the oxygen tension at the lethal corner may fall under unsufficient oxygen supply conditions below 1 mmHg. If we take into account an additional regional inhomogenity of myocardial blood flow, it is to be expected that the local oxygen tension may temporarily decrease below the critical value of the mitochondria.

Under the conditions of exertion the temporary tissue hypoxia at the lethal corner may be the reason for the increase of coronary blood flow. If one accepts this hypothesis it must be assumed that tissue hypoxia induces heart muscle hypertrophy during sport training. Obviously the alternation from heavy exercise with local tissue hypoxia to medium exertion with sufficient oxygen supply as in Interval Training seems to be the most effective stimulus for the hypertrophy of the athlete's heart.

REFERENCES

1. Bretschneider, H.J.: Verh. Dtsch. Ges. Kreisl.-Forsch. 27, 32 (1961).
2. Bretschneider, H.J.: In: Die therapeutische Anwendung β -sympathikolytischer Stoffe, p.45. Stuttgart: Schattauer 1972.
3. Doll, E., J.Keul, H.Steim, C.Maiwald and H.Reindell: Pflügers Arch. 282, 28 (1965).
4. Doll, E., J.Keul, H.Steim, C.Maiwald and H.Reindell: Z. Kreisl.-Forsch. 55,1076 (1966).
5. Fabel, H.: In: Oxygen Supply in Tissue, p.159. Stuttgart: Thieme 1968.
6. Fabel, H., and D.W.Lübbers: Verh. dtsch. Ges. inn. Med., p. 156 (1964).
7. Grote, J.: Pflügers Arch. 295, 245 (1967).
8. Grote, J., and G. Thews: Pflügers Arch. 276, 142 (1962).
9. Grote, J., W.Huhmann and W.Niesel: Pflügers Arch. 294, 256 (1967).
10. Hort, W.: Virchows Arch. path. Anat. 327, 560 (1955).
11. Hudson, J.A.,and D.B.Cater: Proc. roy. Soc. B, 161, 247 (1964).
12. Keller, K.H., and S.K.Friedländer: J. Gen. Physiol. 49, 663 (1966).
13. Kirk, E.S., and C.R.Honig: Am. J. Physiol. 207, 361 (1964).
14. Kirk, E.S., and C.R.Honig: Am. J. Physiol. 207, 661 (1964).
15. Kreuzer, F.: Respir. Physiol. 9, 1 (1970).
16. Krogh, A.: J. Physiol. 52, 409 (1918/19).

17. Linzbach, A.J.: In: Die Funktionsdiagnostik des Herzens, p.94.
    Berlin, Göttingen, Heidelberg: Springer 1958.
18. Lübbers, D.W.: In: Heart Failure, Pathophysiology and Clinical
    Aspects, p.287. Stuttgart: Thieme 1968.
19. Myers, W.W., and C.R.Honig: Am. J. Physiol. $\underline{207}$, 653 (1964).
20. Opitz, E., and G.Thews: Arch. Kreisl.-Forsch. $\underline{18}$, 137 (1952).
21. Reneau, D.D., E.J.Guilbeau and J.Grote: In press
22. Schuchardt, S.: In: Anaesthesiology and Resuscitation, vol.30,
    p.43. Berlin, Heidelberg, New York: Springer 1969.
23. Sonnenblick, E.H.: In: Heart Failure, Pathophysiology and
    Clinical Aspects, p.271. Stuttgart: Thieme 1968.
24. Thews, G.: Acta biotheor. (Leiden) $\underline{10}$, 106 (1953).
25. Thews, G.: Pflügers Arch. $\underline{276}$, 166 (1962).
26. Toborg, M.: Z. Zellforsch. $\underline{123}$, 369 (1972).
27. Wearn, J.T.: Johns Hopkins Hosp. Bull. $\underline{68}$, 363 (1941).
28. Wittenberg, J.B.: J. Gen. Physiol. $\underline{49}$, 57 (1965).

THE HISTOGRAM OF LOCAL OXYGEN PRESSURE (PO$_2$) IN THE DOG MYOCARDIUM AND THE PO$_2$ BEHAVIOR DURING TRANSITORY CHANGES OF OXYGEN ADMINISTRATION

B. Lösse, S. Schuchhardt, N. Niederle, and H. Benzing

Max-Planck-Institut für Systemphysiologie
Dortmund, West Germany   and
Physiologisches Institut I
Universität Tübingen, West Germany

The purpose of this study was to get information concerning the supply of oxygen to the canine heart under steady-state conditions and concerning the dynamic behavior of the myocardial Po$_2$ with sudden temporary changes of oxygen supply. Microelectrodes of the size generally used for Po$_2$ measurements in other organs proved to be too fragile for insertion into the beating heart. Therefore we had to employ electrodes with a tip diameter above 40 μ.

METHODS

The experiments were performed on 13 open chest mongrel dogs anesthetized with pentobarbital, relaxed with gallamine and artificially respired to maintain a mean arterial Po$_2$ of about 80 (S.D. 20.9) Torr. Po$_2$ was measured polarographically in the anterior wall of the left ventricle, in the arterial blood (continuously or by sampling) and in the coronary sinus blood (by sampling). Blood Po$_2$ measurements were made with Clark-type electrodes, tissue Po$_2$ measurements with recessed membranized obliquely ground platinum glass needle electrodes (Pt-diameter 15 μ, tip diameter 40-270 μ) of the riding type (Schuchhardt and Lösse 1973b). Many of these electrodes show a mechanical sensitivity, i.e. current changes independent of Po$_2$ when inserted into or moved within tissue (Schuchhardt and Lösse 1973a). For our measurements we used only electrodes whose mechanical sensitivity, tested in excised air-equilibrated heart tissue, was less than 5%. In connection with the systematic errors of the polarographic method (diffusion error, oxygen consumption of the electrode) we estimate that the measured Po$_2$ values lie about 5-10% below the true values. No correction of these errors was made.

Regional myocardial blood flow was determined qualitatively by heat clearance (for details see contribution of Benzing et al.)

Blood pressure and endexspiratory CO_2 were monitored simultaneously and amounted to 101 mmHg (mean value of mean pressure) and 3.5% CO_2, respectively.

The behavior of tissue Po_2 during and after transitory restriction of O_2 supply was studied by respiring the animal with pure nitrogen for 20 to 60 sec (41 cases) or 10% O_2 in N_2 for 6 to 20 minutes (8 cases).

RESULTS

The histogram of the tissue Po_2 consisting of 119 Po_2 values measured under steady state conditions in the anterior wall of the left ventricle showed a skewed distribution with a maximum in the lowest Po_2 class of 0 to 5 Torr (Fig.1). The median value was 13 Torr. 58 % of the values were below the mean coronary venous Po_2 of 17.25 (s.D. 4.95) Torr. The mean depth of insertion was 6 mm.

N_2 respiration for 20 to 60 sec induced - after a mean time delay of 11 (variation 1 to 30) sec - a decrease of tissue Po_2 from a mean value of 20.8 (variation 4.5 to 83) Torr to 8.6 (variation

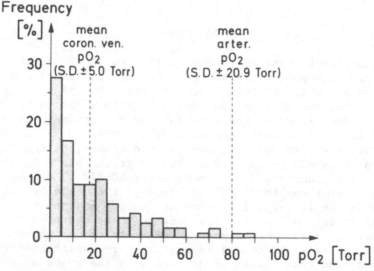

Fig. 1: Histogram of oxygen pressure (Po_2) in the anterior wall of the left ventricle of the dog heart.

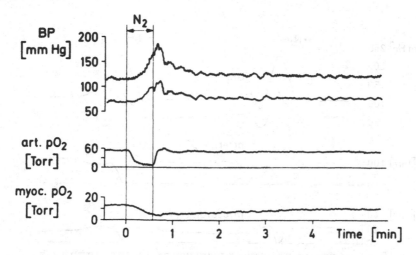

Fig. 2: Recording of Po₂ in the left ventricular myocardium and in
the thoracic aorta of the dog during temporary respiration
with nitrogen. BP: arterial blood pressure. Copy of the
original recording

0 to 41) Torr. In most cases Po₂ was still declining when the
respiration was switched back to the initial gas mixture (Fig.2-4).
Changes in arterial Po₂, regional myocardial blood flow, arterial
blood pressure and heart rate were rather uniform. Arterial Po₂
decreased in an approximately hyperbolic course. After switching
back to the initial gas mixture it showed a steep increase, frequently
a slight overshoot followed by a small counter wave and reestablished
the pre-nitrogen value after about one minute (Fig. 2 and 3). Blood
pressure rose by an average of 45 mmHg (Fig. 2 and 4), whereas heart
rate was lowered slightly. Both returned to constant values within
60 to 90 sec. The blood pressure behavior seen in Fig. 3 with a very
high increase and subsequent undershoot was exceptional. In the
myocardial blood flow course(Fig.4) frequently a slight undershoot
was seen in the post-hypoxic phase.

Behavior of tissue Po₂, on the other side,was quite inhomogeneous and showed no direct dependance on the parameters mentioned
above. Figures 2 to 4 serve as illustration of different kinds of
myocardial Po₂ changes during and after short N₂ administration.
Fig. 2: a slow decrease immediately beginning after arterial Po₂
decrease followed by a very slow linear increase during a few
minutes with no overshoot; Fig.3: steep decrease with a long delay
compared with the arterial Po₂, however a very short delay after
switching back, a steep increase, an overshoot with a subsequent
temporary undershoot; Fig. 4, upper Po₂ trace: a steep decrease,
then a steep increase straight to the pre-nitrogen value; Fig. 4,
lower Po₂ trace: insignificant or no definite reaction. The first

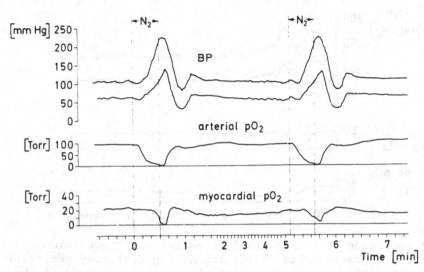

Fig. 3: Changes of Po_2 in the left ventricular myocardium and in the thoracic aorta of the dog during two administrations of nitrogen, one immediately following the other. BP: arterial blood pressure. Copy of the original recording.

three kinds of tissue Po_2 reaction - with many intergrades - were frequently seen, the last one very seldom.

In more than half the cases the rising Po_2 curve was rather linear, in the other cases it was more hyperbolic. In the initial rising phase, during the first minute after switching back to the initial gas mixture, the Po_2 only in 32 % of the cases exceeded and in further 12% reached the pre-nitrogen value (after a mean time of 26 sec). In 63% of the cases Po_2, after a certain period of increase, began to decrease again, and in 44% of the cases it showed fluctuations for 2 to 14 minutes, before it reached its final value. A constant final Po_2 was reached in 80% of the cases after a mean time of 5 1/2 minutes (variation 31 sec. to more than 30 min). At the end of observation time in 39% of the cases Po_2 lay 2 to 18 Torr above, also in 39% 2 to 38 Torr below, and in 22% equaled the pre-nitrogen Po_2 level.

In the 8 cases of hypoxic respiration for 6 to 20 min we made qualitatively very similar observations. Whereas arterial Po_2 fell from about 80 to 31 Torr, tissue Po_2 decreased from a mean value of 29.2 (variation 10 to 46) Torr to 13.3 (variation 5 to 22) Torr. In most cases a plateau was reached after a mean time of 5 (variation 2.5 to 9) min, but in 2 cases Po_2 began to rise again slightly in spite of continuous hypoxic respiration. Mean blood pressure rise averaged 36 mmHg. The observations after switching back to the

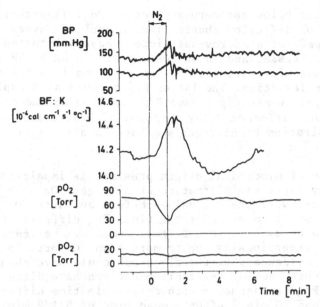

Fig. 4: Recording of myocardial Po_2 at two locations, myocardial
blood flow (BF, K: thermal conductivity) and arterial blood
pressure (BP) in the dog during administration of nitrogen
for 60 sec. Copy of the original recording.

original respiratory gas mixture were quite consistent with those
after N_2 respiration.

DISCUSSION

Employing electrodes with such tip dimensions we used and
especially in the few cases when there is no tissue Po_2 reaction on
N_2 administration as in fig. 4, an important question arises: how
much tissue is damaged, especially: how many vessels are obstructed?
We could not measure the distance between the electrode, once positioned in the myocardium, and the closest perfused blood vessels.
However, from the time needed by the electrode to indicate the Po_2
decrease after a sudden occlusion of the supplying coronary artery we
could estimate the distance roughly. Because this time was rather short
(3.9$\pm$2.6 sec) we conclude that the distance was sufficiently small.

In connection with the normal coronary venous Po_2, which is
quite consistent with that found by Schaper (1969) in more than
500 dogs, we consider the measured Po_2 histogram to be typical for
a normally supplied left ventricle as we have found it also in
rabbits (Schuchhardt and Lösse, 1973b).

The following possibilities may explain the surprisingly high

number of Po_2 values below the coronary venous Po_2: 1) arteriovenous shunts, 2) O_2 diffusion shunts, i.e. a part of oxygen diffuses
from an arterial part of a microvessel into a nearby situated venous
end of another microvessel and is so lost for the area to be supplied,
and 3) inhomogeneous microcirculation, i.e. some capillaries are
closed for more or less time. The latter point could also explain
the sometimes delayed or missing tissue Po_2 reaction on sudden change
of O_2 supply and the different delay compared with arterial Po_2 when
switching the respiration to nitrogen and back to air-oxygen mixture
(Fig. 3).

The regulation of myocardial oxygen pressure is impaired for
a prolonged time by short administration of nitrogen. Only in the
minority of our cases were the Po_2 values before and after O_2
restriction equal, but in most cases the final Po_2 differred from
the pre-nitrogen value by less than 5 Torr. Sometimes we found also
larger deviations, exceptionally up to more than 30 Torr. In all
cases there was no evidence that the electrode could have changed its
position. The Po_2 curve during reestablishment can have different
shapes. The final Po_2 is reached - with remarkable time differences
from 1/2 to more than 30 min - after a mean time of 5 1/2 min. Even
if the posthypoxic Po_2 is rising quickly, often there are fluctuations,
which delay the approaching of the initial value. The posthypoxic
tracing is influenced neither by the systemic blood pressure nor
by the arterial Po_2. There is no distinct relationship to the
regional blood flow. We therefore conclude that the reestablishment
of the myocardial oxygen pressure is determined for the most part
by the local circulation.

REFERENCES

Schuchhardt, S. and B. Lösse: Methodological problems when measuring
    with Po_2 needle electrodes in semisolid media. In: Oxygen Supply,
    ed. by M. Kessler, D.F. Bruley, L.C. Clark, Jr., D.W. Lübbers,
    I.A. Silver and J. Strauss, pp. 108-109 (Urban & Schwarzenberg,
    München-Berlin-Wien 1973a)

Schuchhardt, S. and B. Lösse: Static and dynamic behavior of local
    oxygen pressure in the myocardium. VII. Conf. Europ. Soc.
    Microcirculation, Aberdeen, August 1972 (Karger, Basel/New York
    1973, in press)

Xhonneux, R. and W. Schaper: The Po_2 in the coronary sinus.
    Correlation studies with other circulatory and respiratory
    parameters based on a population of 500 dogs.
    Progr. Resp. Res. 3, 89-93 (Karger, Basel/New York 1969)

SIMULTANEOUS MEASUREMENT OF REGIONAL BLOOD FLOW AND OXYGEN PRESSURE IN THE DOG MYOCARDIUM DURING CORONARY OCCLUSION OR HYPOXIC HYPOXIA [+])

H. Benzing, B. Lösse, S. Schuchhardt, N. Niederle

Physiol.Inst. I, University of Tübingen, and Max-

Planck-Inst. f. Arbeitsphysiologie, Dortmund, Germany

One of the problems of the oxygen supply to the heart is the importance of the local oxygen pressure (pO_2) for the regulation of the local myocardial blood flow. We studied the relation between the local pO_2 and the regional blood flow (RBF) under the conditions of temporary occlusion of the R. interventr. ant. of the left coronary artery (RIA) or during hypoxic hypoxia.

METHODS

The RBF was measured either qualitatively or quantitatively by means of two alternately heatable thermistors which were inserted about 4 mm into the anterior wall of the left ventricle. The temperature difference u between the heated and non-heated thermistor depends on the heat conduction (independent on the blood flow) and on the heat transport by the blood within the tissue. For a continuous evaluation of qualitative blood flow changes we recorded the temperature difference u and transformed it into K values by means of the equation (Golenhofen et al., 1963)

$$K = \frac{k \cdot I^2}{u}$$

(K: thermal conductivity [$cal \cdot cm^{-1} \cdot sec^{-1} \cdot {}^{\circ}C^{-1}$] ; k: constant of the probe; I: heat current (A)). Intermittent quantitative determination of RBF in a volume of about 50 – 100 mm^3 was obtained by means of the heat clearance technique

[+]) Supported by the Deutsche Forschungsgemeinschaft

(theoretical details s. Müller-Schauenburg, 1972) by separation of heat conduction and heat transport: when heating was
switched off (or on), the change of the temperature difference with time (du/dt) was determined in the perfused tissue
(du$_\Phi$/dt) and in the same tissue without blood flow (du$_o$/dt).
The relation is described by the following equation

$$du_\Phi/dt = du_o/dt \cdot e^{-\frac{\Phi}{\lambda} \cdot t}$$

Φ is the blood flow (ml $\cdot$ ml^{-1} tissue $\cdot$ min^{-1}), λ is the heat
partition coefficient between myocardium and blood (about
0.9) and t is the time in min. From one heat clearance curve
a series of 15-20 Φ-values was calculated using the equation above. The single values differed by 10-20 %. The assumption was made that the RBF does not change within the measuring time (0.5 - 0.6 min).

The local tissue pO_2 was measured polarographically by
means of glass-insulated Pt needle electrodes of the riding
type (theoretical details s. Schuchhardt, 1971). The tip diameter was between 40-250 μ. The electrodes were placed about
3-7 mm into the anterior wall of the left ventricle.

We further recorded the arterial blood pressure, heart
rate, endexpiratory CO_2 and intermittently the arterial pO_2.
The experiments were performed on 14 open-chest mongrel dogs
anesthetized with pentobarbital (25 mg/kg), relaxed with gallamine and artificially respired with 21-60 % O_2 in N_2. The
mean arterial pO_2 was 101 ± 29 Torr. The RIA was occluded
temporarily by an inflatable balloon constrictor placed 2 -
5 cm from the origin. The measured values are given as $\bar{x} \pm$ s.

RESULTS

RBF and Local pO_2 in the Normally Supplied Myocardium

The RBF in the anterior wall of the left ventricle was measured quantitatively at 19 points in 14 dogs. The mean value
was 0.82 ± 0.42 ml $\cdot$ ml^{-1} tissue $\cdot$ min^{-1}. When the thermistors were placed near a vessel we regularly found higher RBF
values. The RBF values at the same measuring point and under
the same experimental conditions differed by 5-15 %. The pO_2
histogram consisting of 87 pO_2 values measured at different
points was in good agreement with former results (Schuchhardt
and Lösse, 1973). The median was 12 Torr. The mean arterial
blood pressure amounted to 117 ± 23 mm Hg.

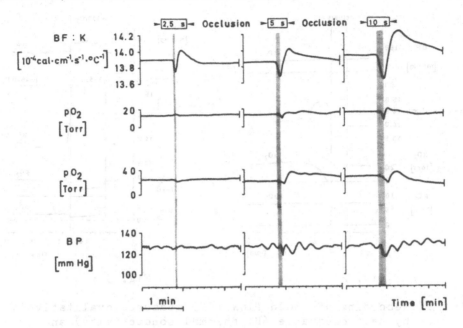

Fig. 1: Continuous recording of blood flow (BF) measured qualitatively by heat clearance (K: thermal conductivity) and oxygen pressure (pO_2) measured by 2 Pt needle
electrodes in the left ventricular anterior wall during occlusion of the R.interventr.ant. of the left
coronary artery.(Occlusion time: 2.5, 5 and 10 sec).
BP: mean arterial blood pressure. Copy of the original registration.

RBF and Local pO_2 during Temporary Occlusion of the RIA

Temporary occlusion (2.5 sec - 60 min) of the RIA was performed on 9 dogs in 45 experiments. Fig. 1 shows the time course
of 3 short occlusions (2.5, 5 and 10 sec). In these experiments there was a decrease in RBF (measured qualitatively)
followed by a reactive hyperemia after release of the occlusion. A clear reaction of both pO_2 electrodes (decrease and
following reactive hyperoxia) was seen only in the occlusions
lasting 5 and 10 sec.

RBF and pO_2 values dropped regularly and reached a constant level in most cases within 1 min (fig. 2). When an electrode was inserted into a normally supplied region or into
the border zone we saw only small or no changes in pO_2 (fig.
2, lower pO_2 tracing). The mean decrease in blood pressure
was about 5 mm Hg. Quantitative RBF values during occlusion

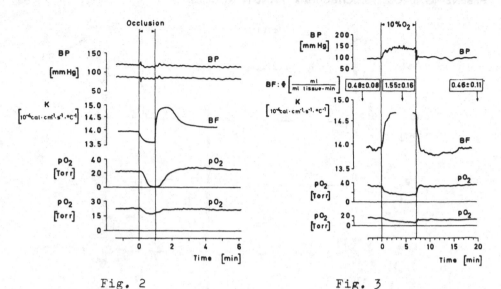

Fig. 2   Fig. 3

Fig. 2: Recording of blood flow (BF) measured qualitatively
        by heat clearance (K: thermal conductivity) and oxy-
        gen pressure (pO_2, upper tracing) in the left ventri-
        cular anterior wall of the dog heart during temporary
        occlusion of the R.interventr.ant. of the left coro-
        nary artery. Lower pO_2 tracing from an electrode in-
        serted into a region proximal to the occlusion. pO_2
        was measured by Pt needle electrodes. BP: blood pres-
        sure. Copy of the original registration.

Fig. 3: Recording of blood flow and pO_2 (measured by 2 Pt
        needle electrodes) in the dog myocardium during tem-
        porary hypoxia (1o % O_2 in N_2). Blood flow (BF) was
        determined by heat clearance either qualitatively
        (continuous recording, K: thermal conductivity) or
        quantitatively (Φ : evaluation of intermittent clea-
        rance curves). BP: mean arterial blood pressure. Co-
        py of the original registration.

could be calculated in 9 points on 8 dogs and ranged between
0.2-0.8 (mean value 0.45 $\pm$ 0.23)ml $\cdot$ ml^{-1} tissue $\cdot$ min^{-1}. The
pO_2 fell in 2/3 of the cases (occlusion time above 30 sec) to
values near 0 Torr. Sometimes the pO_2 began to re-increase
slightly after a few minutes in spite of the continuous occlusion.

    After release of the occlusion we observed a reactive
hyperemia (mean quantitative RBF value 3.2 $\pm$ 1.4 ml $\cdot$ ml^{-1}
tissue $\cdot$ min^{-1}; n = 4) and in 80 % of the cases a reactive
hyperoxia. The median pO_2 values (48 points, 39 experiments,

occlusion time more than 30 sec) were 22 Torr before, 2 Torr during, and 45 Torr (maximum of reactive hyperoxia) after the occlusion.

RBF and pO_2 during Hypoxic Hypoxia

In 11 experiments (8 dogs) 10 % O_2 in N_2 in the inspiratory gas was given for a period of 6 - 20 min. The arterial pO_2 fell to about 30 - 35 Torr. RBF and arterial blood pressure increased steeply (mean value of RBF 1.55 $\pm$ 0.49 ml $\cdot$ ml $^{-1}$ tissue $\cdot$ min^{-1}; increase in mean arterial blood pressure 24 $\pm$ 14 mm Hg). The myocardial pO_2 fell to an average of about the half the initial values (n = 16). Fig. 3 shows a single experiment.

After readjustment to normal ventilation RBF and the arterial blood pressure returned quickly in most experiments to almost the starting level. Sometimes an undershoot of several minutes duration occurred. The pO_2 behaviour in the posthypoxic period was not uniform. In 8 cases the initial value was reached within one minute. In 6 cases the recovery of the pO_2 was incomplete after the first minutes, and only in 2 cases we found a posthypoxic hyperoxia (compared to the initial pO_2).

Dipyridamole (0.4 mg/kg) injected during hypoxic hypoxia induced a further increase in RBF (mean quantitative value in 4 experiments 2.3 $\pm$ 1.0 ml $\cdot$ ml^{-1} tissue $\cdot$ min^{-1}). The blood pressure was decreased by 5 - 15 mm Hg. The pO_2 (8 measuring points) did not change (3 cases) or increased (5 cases).

DISCUSSION

Our method for quantitative blood flow measurement provides data about the blood flow in small regions of the myocardium, but not about the behaviour of the local microcirculation. The values are more uniform than the pO_2 values covering much smaller tissue volumes. The RBF measurements in the present investigation are in good agreement with previous findings (Benzing et al., 1973).

The pO_2 median and the pO_2 histogram in our experiments are also consistent with previous data from the myocardium (Schuchhardt and Lösse, 1973). The pO_2 median in the experiments with hypoxic hypoxia and local ischemia is higher because most of these experiments were performed when the electrodes recorded pO_2 values markedly above 0 Torr. The relatively high pO_2 median during the occlusion period is due to

this selection and furthermore to the short duration of the
occlusion in some experiments.

The RBF in the postocclusion period was considerably
higher than that in the hypoxemic period, though the systemic
blood pressure was increased during the low O_2 ventilation.
The hypoxic hyperemia could be enhanced further by dipyridamole. These findings indicate that the local pO_2 is not a very potent stimulus for the myocardial vasodilation. The conclusions drawn from the comparatively small increase in the
RBF during the hypoxic hypoxia may be criticized because of
the relatively high local pO_2 (compared to the values in the
ischemic myocardium). But if the local pO_2 itself is a deci-
sive factor in the adjustment of the vascular tone, our experiments with hypoxic hypoxia should cover the pO_2 range important for the physiological blood flow regulation.

REFERENCES

Benzing, H., S.H. Wahl, H.P. Bender and M. Rabe: Quantitative
    local blood flow changes in the insufficiently supplied
    dog myocardium measured by means of the heat clearance
    method. VII. Conf. Europ. Soc. Microcirculation, Aber-
    deen, August 1972 (Karger, Basel/New York 1973 (in press)).

Golenhofen, K., H. Hensel and G. Hildebrandt: Durchblutungs-
    messung mit Wärmeleitelementen. G. Thieme Verlag, Stutt-
    gart 1963.

Müller-Schauenburg, W.: Über einen Ansatz zur Trennung von
    Wärmeleitung und Wärmetransport durch das Blut - ein neu-
    es Verfahren zur quantitativen Messung der lokalen Ge-
    websdurchblutung. Med. Diss. Tübingen (1972).

Schuchhardt, S.: pO_2-Messung im Myocard des schlagenden Her-
    zens. Pflügers Arch. _322_, 83-94 (1971).

Schuchhardt, S. and B. Lösse: Static and dynamic behaviour of
    local oxygen pressure in the myocardium. VII. Conf. Eu-
    rop. Soc. Microcirculation, Aberdeen, August 1972 (Kar-
    ger, Basel/New York 1973 (in press)).

MASS SPECTROMETRY FOR MEASURING CHANGES IN INTRAMYOCARDIAL pO_2 AND pCO_2

G.J. Wilson, D.C. MacGregor, D.E. Holness, W. Lixfeld
and H. Yasui

Cardiovascular Lab., Banting Inst., Univ. of Toronto
and Defence and Civil Inst. of Environmental Med.,
Toronto, Ontario, Canada

Mass spectrometry provides an attractive alternative to polarography for the measurement of extracellular oxygen tension in the beating heart. This method also permits the simultaneous measurement of extracellular carbon dioxide tension which is not possible using polarographic techniques.

In this study, mass spectrometry has been applied to the measurement of intramyocardial pO_2 and pCO_2 during anoxic arrest of the heart of sufficient duration to produce a final equilibrium level of pCO_2. A technique for the correction of the inherent lag in response of the measurement system was developed to allow more accurate monitoring of rapidly changing gas tensions as exemplified by the reduction in intramyocardial pO_2 following cessation of coronary blood flow.

MATERIALS AND METHODS

The measurement system (Medspect® MSBR medical mass spectrometer) consists of an ionization chamber maintained at a near vacuum connected to a flexible stainless steel sampling catheter leading to a Teflon® diffusion membrane (Fig. 1). Gas molecules cross the membrane to enter the near vacuum environment in quantities determined by the partial pressure of each gas and the diffusion properties of the membrane itself. In this manner, the various components of a gas mixture may be quantitatively analysed.

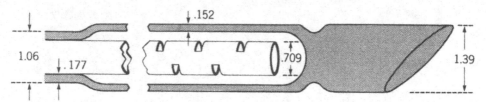

Figure 1.   The stainless steel sampling catheter and Teflon
            diffusion membrane. This produces a diffusion
            chamber through which diffused gases may enter
            the sampling catheter through both its end hole
            and wall slots. All measurements are in millimeters.

     Intramyocardial pO_2 and pCO_2 were continuously measured in a
series of 8 dogs subjected to prolonged periods of normothermic
anoxic arrest of the heart. Each dog was placed on total cardiopulmonary bypass and the left ventricle was vented. The sampling
catheter was gently inserted to a depth of 2 to 4 mm in the left
ventricular myocardium midway between the base and apex of the
heart and parallel to the left anterior descending coronary artery.
After allowing a minimum of 15 minutes for the recorded pO_2 and
pCO_2 values to stabilize, the ascending aorta was cross-clamped to
produce anoxic arrest of the heart by cessation of coronary blood
flow. The experiment was terminated when the pCO_2 had reached a
plateau as indicated by its remaining at a stable value for a
period of 200 seconds. Before and after each experiment the mass
spectrometer was calibrated by placing the sampling catheter in a
stirred, constant temperature water bath (37°C) into which a gas
mixture was bubbled, providing reference pO_2 and pCO_2 values of 90
and 40 mm Hg respectively.

OBSERVATIONS AND CALCULATIONS

     Following cross-clamping of the ascending aorta, a rapid fall
in intramyocardial pO_2 from 26 $\pm$ 10 (SD) to 12 $\pm$ 6 mm Hg was accompanied by a gradual, prolonged rise in pCO_2 from 37 $\pm$ 11 to 287
$\pm$ 60 mm Hg, the latter occurring over a period of 1 to 2 hours. A
typical pair of O_2 depletion and CO_2 accumulation curves are presented in Fig. 2.

     The measurement system was observed to produce a characteristic
lag in response to a step change in gas tension. In Fig. 3, the
response of the system to a step change in pO_2 at 37°C is presented.
The response consisted of a pure delay phase (35 seconds) during
which no change in pO_2 was recorded, followed by a phase of gradual
change which can be approximately described by a second order exponential function. The 90% response time of the system was 290
seconds. This lag was of quantitative significance during the

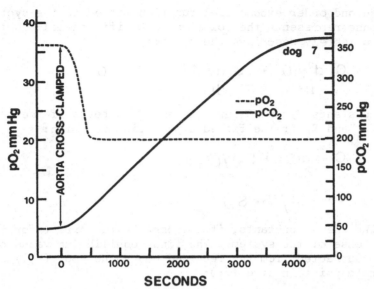

Figure 2.   A typical pair of myocardial O_2 depletion and CO_2 accumulation curves in a dog following cross-clamping of the ascending aorta. Note the rapid fall in pO_2 compared with the gradual, prolonged rise in pCO_2.

rapid change in intramyocardial pO_2 at the onset of anoxic arrest. Since the recorded time for 90% completion of the pO_2 change was 404 ± 58 seconds, only moderately in excess of the 90% response time of the system, the depletion of intramyocardial oxygen was actually much more rapid than recorded.

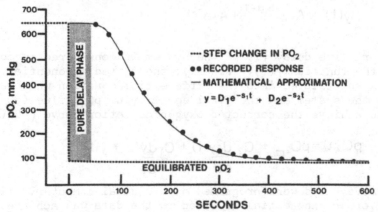

Figure 3.   The recorded response to a step change in pO_2 from 90 mm Hg to 640 mm Hg with its mathematical approximation. Note the pure delay phase followed by a phase of gradual change.

The second order exponential function fitted to the system step response represents the solution to a differential equation which approximately describes the system:

$$C_2 \frac{d^2y(t)}{dt^2} + C_1 \frac{dy(t)}{dt} + y(t) = 0$$

The constants C_1 and C_2 are expressed in terms of the known constants S_1 and S_2 of the fitted exponential function:

$$C_1 = (S_1 + S_2)\big/(S_1 S_2)$$

$$C_2 = 1\big/(S_1 S_2)$$

Knowing these constants, it is possible to correct for the lag in response of the system. The final equilibrium value of pO_2 (pO_{2_E}) is subtracted from the recorded pO_2 value ($pO_{2_R}(t_i)$) for each discrete point in time (t_i):

$$x(t_i) = pO_{2_R}(t_i) - pO_{2_E}$$

A second order exponential function is fitted to the set of values ($x(t_i)$):

$$x(t_i) \cong y(t), \qquad t = t_i$$

$$y(t) = A_1 e^{-b_1(t-T)} + A_2 e^{-b_2(t-T)}$$

The pure time delay (T) of the system is considered in constructing the function $y(t)$. Finally, the fitted exponential function is substituted into the differential equation which approximates the system and the final equilibrium pO_2 value (pO_{2_E}) is added to achieve the corrected oxygen depletion curve ($pO_2(t)$):

$$pO_2(t) = pO_{2_E} + C_2 \frac{d^2y(t)}{dt^2} + C_1 \frac{dy(t)}{dt} + y(t)$$

The above steps were programed on a digital computer. Fitting the second order exponential function to the data was achieved by a subroutine which obtained least squares estimates of the parameters entering into this nonlinear function. Fig. 4 illustrates a typical oxygen depletion curve which has been corrected by this method.

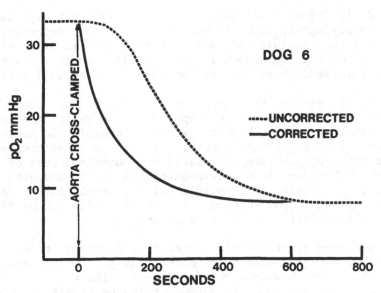

Figure 4. A typical oxygen depletion curve showing the uncorrected
and corrected measurements.

DISCUSSION

Mass spectrometry was first used by Woldring et al. (1966)
for the measurement of in vivo blood gases and more recently, Owens
(1969) reported monitoring of intracerebral pO_2 and pCO_2. Brantigan
(1972) has reported measurements of intramyocardial pO_2 following
coronary artery ligation and Gardner et al. (1971) have used mass
spectrometry to monitor intramyocardial gas tensions in the human
heart during coronary artery surgery.

Most attempts to measure tissue oxygen tension have involved
polarographic techniques. Both Moss (1968) and Winbury (1971) have
utilized bare tipped cathodes to measure intramyocardial pO_2. These
measurements may be influenced by other electroreducible substances
and are subject to problems in calibration due to the uncertainty
of the diffusion coefficient of oxygen in the biological medium
(Silver, 1967). Although mass spectrometry is not influenced by
these factors, both techniques share the common problem of tissue
damage associated with probe insertion.

In this study, gross bleeding at the site of catheter insertion was seldom observed and wide variations in arterial pO_2 (100
to 500 mm Hg) did not appreciably alter the recorded intramyocardial
pO_2. When gross bleeding was encountered, the intramyocardial pO_2
paralleled changes in arterial pO_2 and the catheter was resituated.

Myers and Honig (1964) have calculated myocardial mean capillary
pO_2 to be approximately 38 mm Hg and Whalen's (1971) determinations
of myocardial intracellular pO_2 have ranged from 0 to 31 mm Hg with
a mean of 6.9 mm Hg. Consequently, our results appear to represent
reasonable intermediate values between capillary and cell interior.

The lag in response to changes in pO_2 measured by mass spectrometry is an obvious disadvantage compared to the rapid response
times one can achieve with bare tipped polarographic electrodes.
However, we have been able to correct for the lag in system response
during the rapid pO_2 changes associated with anoxic arrest of the
heart. The method described does require the use of a digital computer but, in principle, it is sufficiently general that it can be
applied to any set of gas tension measurements which can be fitted
to some continuous differentiable function.

Although mass spectrometry is clearly not capable of measuring
intercapillary pO_2 gradients or intracellular pO_2, it is capable of
measuring pO_2 averaged over a volume of myocardium which is small
in relation to the total muscle volume of the heart without producing
sufficient damage to the microcirculation and cell function to prevent monitoring the marked changes in intramyocardial gas tensions
during anoxic arrest.

REFERENCES

BRANTIGAN, J.W., V.L. GOTT and M.N. MARTZ. 1972. J. Appl.
     Physiol., 32, 276.
GARDNER, T.J., J.W. BRANTIGAN, A.M. PERNA, H.W. BENDER,
     R.K. BRAWLEY and V.L. GOTT. 1971. J. Thorac. Cardiovasc.
     Surg., 62, 844.
MOSS, A.J. 1968. Cardiovasc. Res., 3, 314.
MYERS, W.W. and C.R. HONIG. 1964. Amer. J. Physiol., 207, 653.
OWENS, G., L. BELMUSTO and S. WOLDRING. 1969. J. Neurosurg.,
     30, 110.
SILVER, I.A. 1967. Phys. Med. Biol., 12, 285.
WHALEN, W.J. 1971. Physiologist, 14, 69.
WINBURY, M.M., B.R. HOWE and H.R. WEISS. 1971. J. Pharmacol.
     Exp. Ther., 176, 184.
WOLDRING, S., G. OWENS and D.C. WOOLFORD. 1966. Science, 153, 885.

ACKNOWLEDGEMENTS

The authors would like to express their appreciation to
Mr. A.J. Brock, Mr. W.K. Burley and Mr. R.R. Adams for their fine
technical assistance. This work was supported by the Ontario
Heart Foundation, Grant No. 1-29.

EFFECT OF INCREASING HEART RATE BY ATRIAL PACING ON MYOCARDIAL TISSUE OXYGEN TENSION

Harvey R. Weiss

Dept. of Physiology, College of Medicine and Dentistry

of N.J. – Rutgers Medical School, Piscataway, N.J. 08854

Measurement of tissue oxygen tension of heart muscle by polarography has been extensively performed by many investigators. It has been used to measure normal regional differences in the ventricular walls [6,7,15,17] the effects of various drugs [15,17], gases [8], and physiologic interventions [17]. These studies have shown a higher subepicardial tissue oxygen tension (Epi Po_2) then subendocardial tissue oxygen tension (Endo Po_2) in the left ventricular free wall [6,7]. Tissue oxygen tension is controlled by the balance between the oxygen supply and the tissue oxygen demand. The interaction of these two factors in the control of Epi Po_2 and Endo Po_2 with changes in heart rate are unknown and the rationale for the present study.

Increases in heart rate by pacing do not increase cardiac output, in fact, at higher heart rates, cardiac output may decline [9,11,12]. There are marked increases in metabolic demand as measured by increased oxygen consumption [1,13] even though cardiac output does not increase with pacing. Coronary blood flow was reported to increase during pacing [1,16]. Thus, both the supply to and the demand from the left ventricle for oxygen increases with a pacing induced increase in heart rate.

Atrial pacing has been used in clinical situations to test for the presence of coronary artery disease and angina pectoris [1,2,3]. There are usually electrocardiographic changes characteristic of ischemia, when angina pectoris is induced in this manner. This may indicate regional oxygen lack that can be measured by polarography.

Under various stressful conditions, it appears that the deeper, subendocardial region of the left ventricle suffers most [5,17]. With reduced flow there is a greater reduction in tissue oxygen tension and aerobic enzyme activity levels [4]. The proportion of blood reaching the subendocardium is also less. The possibility of an unequal distribution of coronary blood flow has been shown with several pharmacological agents [10]. Such an unequal distribution of flow may also occur with pacing induced tachycardia.

METHODS

Eighteen adult mongrel dogs were anesthetized with intravenous injections of either sodium pentobarbital, 30 mg/kg, or α-chloralose, 100 mg/kg. The femoral artery and vein were catheterized. Blood pressure was measured from the femoral artery catheter which was advanced into the aorta. Artificial respiration was instituted after tracheal intubation.

The chest was opened at the fifth interspace on the left side. The pericardium was incised and tied back. An electromagnetic flow probe was placed near the origin of the anterior descendant branch of the left coronary artery. An occluder was placed distal to the flow probe to determine zero flow. Calibration of the probe had been previously performed. An electrode which was used to pace the heart was sewn on the left atrium and connected to a stimulator. Parameters used were 10 to 20 volts, 3 msec. duration and appropriate frequency setting. The hearts were paced at 150, 175, 200, and 225 beats/min.

Two electrodes were placed at depths of 3 and 9 mm into the left ventricular free wall in an area supplied by the left anterior descending artery to record myocardial tissue Po_2. These platinum electrodes were 177μ in diameter with 0.2 - 0.3 mm cleared of the special teflon insulation. The electrodes were attached to each other by an electrically insulating material so that the tips were 6 mm apart. A diagram representing the position of these electrodes relative to the left ventricular wall is shown in Figure 1. A reference electrode was placed under a skin flap. Calibration of the electrodes after connection to the electrometer were performed in saline at 37°C equilibrated with various percentages of oxygen before and after each experiment. Only those electrodes that exhibited stable linear responses to changes in Po_2 were used. The electrodes, electrometer, and calibration procedure have been described previously [15,17].

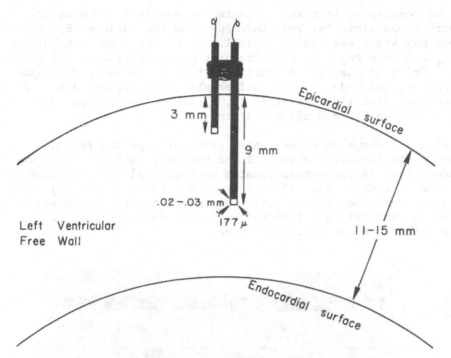

Fig. 1 - Diagram of size and placement relationships of tissue
oxygen - electrodes in left ventricular wall.

A prepacing control was obtained and when all parameters were
stable a period of pacing of five to ten minutes was instituted.
A recovery was recorded until the measured variables returned to
control. At least a half hour was allowed between each period of
atrial pacing. The Student T-test for paired means was used to
determine if changes from control were significant for blood
pressure, coronary blood flow, Epi Po_2, Endo Po_2 and the Epi
Po_2/Endo Po_2 ratio.

RESULTS AND DISCUSSION

Under unpaced control conditions, the mean heart rate was
141.8 beats/min. Thirteen dogs had resting heart rates below 150
beats/min.; these averaged 130.6 beats/min. Only these dogs were
paced at the lowest pacing rate. For all dogs, the mean Epi Po_2
averaged 26.4 mm Hg and the Endo Po_2 was 19.5 mm Hg. These values
are in close agreement with previously published reports [6,7,15,17].

The results of left atrial pacing on aortic blood pressure, coronary blood flow, Epi Po_2, Endo Po_2, and the ratio of Epi Po_2 to Endo Po_2 are presented in Table 1. It can be seen that both Epi Po_2 and Endo Po_2 fell significantly below control at all pacing rates. Using an analysis of variance it is possible to determine that Epi Po_2 and Endo Po_2 were different al all pacing rates. All changes were also significant ($P < .05$) except the change in Epi Po_2 between 150 and 175 beats/min.

Figure 2 shows an experimental trial at a pacing rate of 175 beats/min including a control and recovery period. There was a gradual fall in the oxygen tension of both regions. The levels stabilize at a new lower value after a few minutes. The Po_2 remains at these new levels until the end of pacing, up to ten minutes in many trials. Both Epi Po_2 and Endo Po_2 return to control after the cessation of pacing.

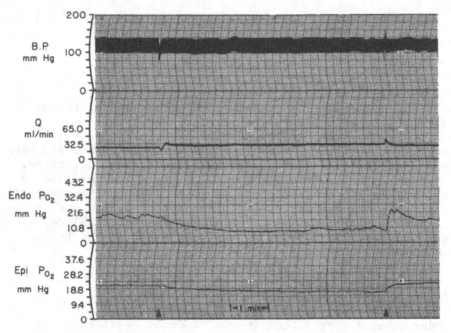

Fig. 2 - Effect of left atrial pacing. The heart was paced at 175 beats/min between the arrows.

There was a significant increase in the Epi Po_2/Endo Po_2 ratio except at the lowest pacing rate. This is caused by the greater proportional fall in the oxygen tension of the deeper, subendocardial region. Pacing markedly increased the disparity between the levels of oxygenation of the subepicardium and subendocardium. This can also be seen by considering the percentage decline in Po_2 with pacing. Epi Po_2 decreased from control 4.6%, 6.4%, 10.2% and 18.8% at 150, 175, 200 and 225 beats/min. The Endo Po_2 declined 8.0%, 14.3%, 24.4% and 34.2% at these same rates. Thus at all rates, the subendocardium appears to suffer a greater fall in tissue Po_2.

Tissue oxygen tension is controlled by both the supply and demand for oxygen. One important factor in oxygen supply is coronary blood flow which increased markedly at each pacing rate. Another factor in oxygen supply is arterial oxygen content. This was not measured although blood gas analysis was performed in eight dogs, indicating it was probably adequate. Pao_2 averaged 85.4 mm Hg, Pa_{CO_2} was 35.9 mm Hg and arterial pH was 7.409. These values did not change significantly during the course of the experiment. A third factor in O_2 supply is open capillary density. There are no reports in the literature on the effects of pacing on this parameter. Thus it is fairly safe to assume an increase in oxygen supply with pacing.

The alterations in cardiac function produced by atrial pacing do not increase cardiac output [9,11,12]. At high heart rates a decline in cardiac output has been reported. Nevertheless, there is a marked increase in myocardial oxygen consumption and metabolism with pacing in both externally working and non-working isolated hearts as in intact animals [13,14,16]. From the data presented in Table 1, it is apparent that pacing under the conditions imposed by the present experimental design must increase oxygen consumption to a greater extent than oxygen supply. This effect appears greater in the subendocardial region of the left ventricle.

Pacing has been used clinically in patients with coronary artery disease to induce attacks of angina pectoris [1,2,3]. The added work of pacing was thought to produce regional myocardial ischemia which led to the pain. The present study provides direct experimental evidence for reductions in tissue oxygenation. The differences in regional tissue Po_2 may make the subendocardium more susceptable to ischemia of angina [17]. It is also the most likely site for myocardial infarction [5]. Results of the present study also indicate a greater decline in Endo Po_2 with pacing.

In coronary artery disease and angina, tachycardia would seem likely to complicate the problem, if one could extrapolate from the present study to man. This relation seems to exist, since pacing has been used to induce angina pectoris. The present study also indicates that the subendocardial region is more likely to exhibit a decrease in oxygen tension. Thus, the polarographic evidence developed here is in substantial agreement with other studies indicating the vulnerability of the subendocardium.

TABLE 1 – EFFECTS OF ATRIAL PACING

	Syst. B.P. mm Hg	Δ** mm Hg	Diast. B.P. mm Hg	Δ mm Hg	Q ml/min	Δ ml/min	Epi Po2 mm Hg	Δ mm Hg	Endo Po2 mm Hg	Δ mm Hg	Epi Po2 / Endo Po2	Δ
Control	146*** ± 7		107 ± 5		34.8 ±2.5		25.6 ±2.5		21.3 ±2.2		1.30 ±0.13	
Pacing 150 BPM	147 ± 7	+1 ±1	108 ± 5	+1 ±1	38.4 ±2.4	+3.7* ±0.4	24.5 ±2.6	-1.2* ±0.5	19.4 ±2.0	-1.7* ±0.4	1.35 ±0.15	+0.05 ±0.04
Control	139 ± 6		99 ± 5		32.5 ±2.0		27.5 ±1.7		19.2 ±1.0		1.48 ±0.09	
Pacing 175 B.P.M.	138 ± 6	-1 ±1	100 ± 5	+1 ±1	37.7 ±2.2	+5.2* ±0.7	25.8 ±1.6	-1.8* ±0.4	16.5 ±1.1	-2.7* ±0.5	1.64 ±0.10	+0.16* ±0.05
Control	139 ± 5		102 ± 5		31.5 ±1.3		25.6 ±1.6		18.2 ±1.1		1.49 ±0.11	
Pacing 200 B.P.M.	135 ± 6	-4* ±1	99 ± 5	-3* ±1	39.2 ±1.5	+7.8* ±1.1	22.0 ±1.7	-3.6* ±0.6	13.7 ±1.1	-4.4* ±0.4	1.71 ±0.14	+0.23* ±0.04
Control	142 ± 5		103 ± 5		30.3 ±1.1		26.8 ±2.1		20.2 ±1.3		1.39 ±0.10	
Pacing 225 B.P.M.	135 ± 6	-6* ±1	99 ± 5	-4* ±1	44.5 ±3.7	+14.2* ±3.6	21.8 ±1.9	-5.0* ±0.9	13.3 ±1.2	-6.9* ±1.0	1.88 ±0.23	+0.49* ±0.16

* Significant at P < .05
** Paired mean differences
*** mean ± standard error

REFERENCES

1. Conti, C. R., B. Pitt, W. D. Gundel, G. C. Friesinger and
    R. S. Ross. 1970, Circulation 42:815.

2. Forrester, J. S., R. H. Helfant, A. Pasternac, E. A.
    Amsterdam, A. S. Most, H. G. Kemp and R. Gorlin. 1971,
    Am. J. Cardiol. 27:237.

3. Frick, M. H., R. Balcon, D. Cross and E. Sowton. 1968,
    Circulation 37:160.

4. Griggs, D. M., V. V. Tchokoev and C. Chen. 1972, Am. J.
    Physiol. 222:705.

5. Guy, C. and R. S. Eliot. 1970, Chest 58:555.

6. Kirk, E. S. and C. R. Honig. 1964, Am. J. Physiol. 207:661.

7. Moss, A. J. 1968, Cardiovasc. Res. 2:314.

8. Moss, A. J. and J. Johnson. 1970, Cardiovasc. Res. 4:436.

9. Ross, Jr. J., J. W. Linhart and E. Braunwald. 1968,
    Circulation 37:549.

10. Rowe, G. G. 1970, Circulation 42:193.

11. Rushmer, R. F. and O. A. Smith, Jr. 1959 Physiol. Rev. 39:41.

12. Sarnoff, S. J., E. Braunwald, G. H. Welch, Jr., R. B. Case,
    W. N. Stainsby and R. Macruz. 1958, Am. J. Physiol. 192:148.

13. Somani, P., A. R. Laddu, and H. F. Hardman. 1969, Life Sci.
    8:1151.

14. VanCitters, R. L., W. E. Ruth and K. R. Reissmann. 1957,
    Am. J. Physiol. 191:443.

15. Weiss, H. R. and M. M. Winbury. 1972. Microvasc. Res.
    4:273.

16. White, S., T. Patrick, C. B. Higgins, S. F. Vatner,
    D. Franklin and E. Braunwald. 1971, Am. J. Physiol. 221:1402.

17. Winbury, M. M., B. B. Howe and H. R. Weiss. 1971,
    J. Pharmacol. Exp. Ther. 176:184.

OXYGEN CONSUMPTION AND CONVECTIVE TRANSPORT DURING CARDIO-
PULMONARY BYPASS[1]

R. E. Safford, J. D. Whiffen, E. N. Lightfoot,
R. S. Tepper, and J. H. G. Rankin
Departments of Chemical Engineering, Surgery,
Physiology, and Gynecology and Obstetrics
University of Wisconsin, Madison, USA, 53706

INTRODUCTION

Described here are the progressive changes in blood-flow distribution that accompany four-hour heart-lung bypass in dogs and the effects of perfusion rate on flow distribution and oxygen consumption. The corresponding changes produced by anesthesia alone and by the thoracotomy needed for a bypass procedure are also shown for comparison purposes. These data indicate that the bypass procedure itself puts a very significant stress on the test animals and that perfusion rates in excess of resting cardiac output are required to prevent hypoxia induced irreversible tissue damage.

Control Studies. Sixteen experiments were made on 12-18 kg. dogs to evaluate the effects of α-chloralose anesthesia and thoracotomy.

In four animals, catheters were implanted in the left subclavian artery, the left atrium, the right atrium and then exteriorized. The following day, with the animal conscious and in the right lateral position, microspheres labelled with ^{141}Ce, ^{51}Cr, or ^{85}Sr were injected into the left atrium at five minute intervals and cardiac output was determined using indicator dilution by means of a continuous withdrawal via the left subclavian artery. Oxygen consumption was determined by measuring total oxygen contents of right atrial and left subclavian blood samples using a Lexicon oxygen meter. Blood flow to major organs was determined by counting aliquots of each in a three channel gamma spectrometer.

561

Catheters were implanted in seven other animals in the same
manner. The following day the animals were premedicated with
3 mg./kg. of morphine sulfate, anesthetized with 100 mg./kg. of
α-chloralose, intubated and ventilated. Microsphere injections
were made immediately, after 30 minutes, and after 4 hours. Cardiac
output and oxygen consumptions were determined as before.

Finally, in five animals the same catheterization procedure
was repeated except that the chest of each animal was left opened
and measurements started immediately. Thus, this was the sham
procedure for total heart-lung bypass.

Total Heart-Lung Bypass Experiments. Fifteen total bypass
experiments were made on 12-18 kg. dogs using a Cardiovascular
Electrodynamics polycarbonate disc oxygenator and American Optical
roller pump. The chest of each animal was opened through the left
third intercostal space and venous return and arterial infusion
cannulas were inserted into the right atrium (via the atrial
appendage) and the left subclavian artery, respectively. In
addition, the left ventricle was vented to prevent coronary blood
pooling. A Dextran-75-electrolyte solution having approximately
the same ionic composition and colloidal osmotic pressure as dog
plasma was used for priming and five perfusions each were made at
60, 100, and 140 ml./min./kg. Arterial O_2 and CO_2 tensions were
maintained at about 85-115 and 32 to 37 mmHg respectively.

RESULTS

Cardiac output in the control studies, Fig. 1a, shows an
immediate drop from the unanesthetized state (U) and a further slow
decrease over the total 4 hour period of observation. The drop is
less for a closed chest and here there is a slight and possibly
significant recovery during the first 30 minutes. It may be seen
from Fig. 1b that oxygen consumption drops sharply at onset of
anesthesia, much more than in proportion to cardiac output, but
holds nearly steady for both open and closed chests at about 5 ml.
O_2/min./kg. over the entire four hours observed. The above
results are in agreement with the prior literature.

Coronary flow is seen to stabilize satisfactorily at about
75% of the unanesthetized value for both open and closed chest
controls. Coronary flows on bypass were always higher than in the
controls (Fig. 2b) and increase with perfusion rate. The increase
over controls probably results from lack of systolic obstruction
of coronary arteries during bypass and indicates adequate coronary
perfusion in all experiments.

Brain flows decreased about 50% on anesthesia and held constant
at that value for 4 hours with the chest open. For the closed

chest procedure, brain flow showed a steady rise over the four hours to approximately 66% of the unanesthetized value (Fig. 2a), even though cardiac output continued to drop. Brain perfusion is probably adequate for all control experiments. During bypass, however, brain flow (Fig. 2b) was adequate only at the highest perfusion rate and dropped essentially to zero for all experiments at 60 ml./min./kg. This is the most important result of the study and strongly suggests the need for higher than basal blood flow during prolonged bypass.

Renal blood flows (Fig. 2c) appear to be satisfactory as long as the chest is closed but fall steadily after thoracotomy, to about one half the unanesthetized value after four hours. However, the fraction of the cardiac output remains constant at 25-30% with the chest open. Renal flows fall with time on bypass but remain at a nearly constant fraction of perfusion rate after 1/2 hour. Surprisingly fractional renal flows were normal (about 25%) at perfusion rates of 60 and 100 but only about half this value at 140 ml./min./kg.

Flows to the liver are very nearly normal over four hours with the chest closed but are initially very low following thoracotomy and during bypass. They do not fully recover in either of the latter cases and appear to be affected more by the thoracotomy than by bypass perfusion rates. There is, however, an apparent anomaly at 30 minutes for a perfusion rate of 60 ml./min./kg. The large and small bowel behaved similarly to the liver and are omitted here to conserve space.

Additional effects of bypass conditions are shown in Figs. 3 and 4. Blood pressure is seen to fall during bypass and most strongly for the lowest perfusion rates. Metabolic acids[2] accumulated in all bypass experiments but the rate of accumulation dropped strongly with increase in perfusion rate. This behavior is apparently paralleled by an increase in oxygen debt[3] with a decrease in perfusion rate. For the bypass experiments, our preliminary results with respect to oxygen debt are semiquantitative since oxygen consumptions were calculated via blood oxygen tensions and Kelman's algorithm.[4] It does appear that very serious oxygen debts accumulated in all experiments at 60 ml./min./kg. (Fig. 5) and that this situation improved markedly with increase in perfusion rate. Ambiguities due to errors in measurement are leading us to repeat these experiments with the direct measurement of oxygen content.

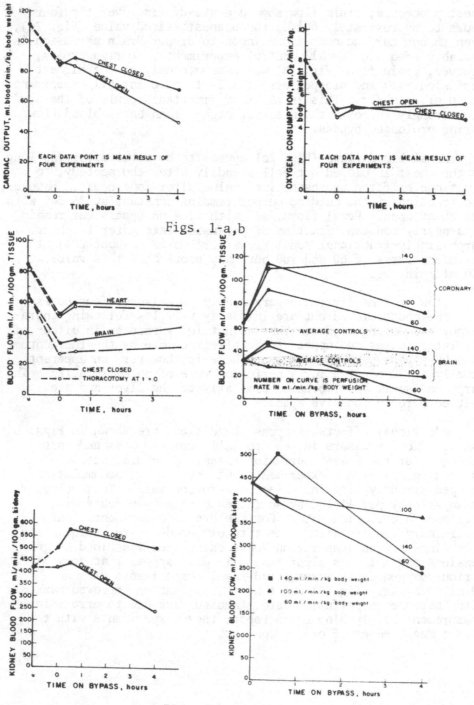

Figs. 1-a,b

Figs. 2-a,b,c,d

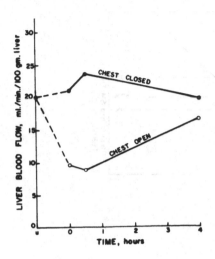

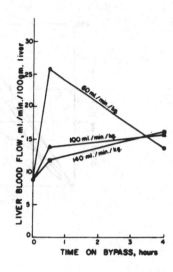

Figs. 2-e,f

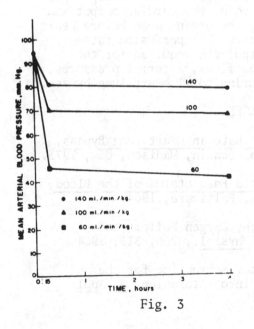

Fig. 3

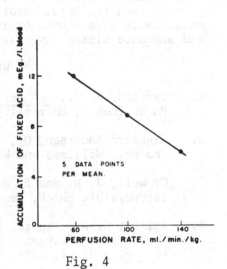

Fig. 4

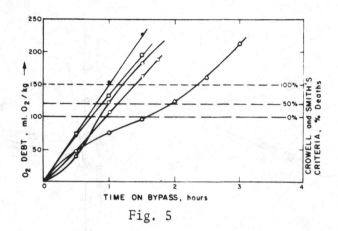

Fig. 5

CONCLUSION

We conclude that thoracotomy and even α-chloralose/morphine anesthesia result in major reduction of the cardiac output and redistribution of blood flow among the organs even before heart-lung bypass is initiated. It appears that perfusion rates greater than the basal cardiac output are required for the maintenance of adequate brain blood flows, arterial pressures, and adequate tissue oxygenation during total heart-lung bypass.

REFERENCES

1.   Safford, R. E., The Perfusion Rate in Heart-Lung Bypass, Ph.D. Thesis, University of Wisconsin, Madison, USA, 1973.

2.   Siggaard-Andersen, O., The Acid-Base Status of the Blood, 2nd ed., Williams and Wilkens, Baltimore, 1964.

3.   Crowell, J. W. and E. E. Smith, Oxygen Deficit and Irreversible Shock, Amer. J. Physiol., 206, 313, 1964.

4.   Kelman, G. R., Digital Computer Subroutine for the Conversion of Oxygen Tension into Saturation, J. Appl. Physiol., 21, 4, 1966.

RED CELL WASHOUT FROM THE CORONARY VESSELS OF ISOLATED FELINE HEARTS

S.H. Song

Biophysics Department, University of

Western Ontario, London, Ontario

In cases of ischemic heart disease, it has been generally accepted that collateral channels may develop to help supply blood to the myocardial region having occluded coronary vessels. However, an adequate theory has not been established yet to elucidate the mechanism of developing collaterals in the coronary circuit. Some difficulties arising from various characteristics of the vessels have discouraged investigation on this specific topic. These are: (1) The microscopic pathways for blood in the coronary system are much more complicated than expected from similar structures in any other organs (Wearn et al. 1933). (2) Direct communication between blood in the myocardial capillaries and blood in the ventricular chambers appears to play a significant role, depending on the phase of the cardiac cycle (Hammond & Moggio, 1971). (3) The intraventricular pressure always exceeds that in coronary arteries during systole due to the myocardial contraction.

In view of these features, the normal pattern of blood flow through the beating heart is difficult to assess. If we were to trace red cells traversing through the coronary system, we might expect to find different time courses of red cell clearance according to different routes where particular red cells have passed through. In other words, the red cells which travel via the direct pathway will appear first in the coronary sinus and eventually in the right auricle, and those cells which may have flowed through myocardial sinusoids or long capillaries will be cleared later from the coronary vessels. Thus the coronary circuit may not behave as a uniformly distributed system. If this be so, we may expect to find interesting kinetics of red cell washout from coronary vessels when the heart is perfused

with cell-free Ringer's solution. Therefore, this study is aimed
at establishing kinetics of red cell washout from normal,
isolated feline hearts.

METHODS

Ten healthy, adult cats were used in these experiments. Each
animal was anesthetized with sodium pentobarbital (40 mg/Kg,
intraperitoneally). To keep bleeding from major vessels to a
minimum, thermal cauterization was used. After left thoracotomy,
the heart was exposed and the animal was heparinized. The
pulmonary vessels and all the arterial branches arising from the
arch of aorta were tied off and two cannulae were inserted into
the right auricle and the aorta respectively. Both heart and
lungs were removed from the animal and placed in a lucite chamber
in which mineral oil was kept at 37°C. Before beginning the
perfusion, the residual blood in the right and left ventricular
lumens was sucked out.

The perfusate, which contained 100 mg % of glucose in modified
Ringer's solution, was prepared free of particles by filtration
through millipore filters (GSWP 04700, 0.22µ) three times before
use, and equilibrated with 5% CO_2 in O_2 during the experimental
period. The isolated heart was perfused constantly at a flow rate
of 5 ml/min by means of a sigmamotor pump through the aortic
cannula, and the venous outflow from the right auricle was
collected in a measuring cylinder. At prearranged time intervals,
the samples of the venous outflow were taken and the cellular
concentrations were determined by means of a Celloscope Counter
(Particle Data Inc.).

RESULTS AND DISCUSSION

All the isolated hearts showed a continuous beating throughout the perfusion, but heart rates ranged only from 80 to 40 per
minute. This relatively low rate was probably the result of
denervation of the heart. Infusion pressures recorded were
between 150 cm H_2O as the highest and 20 cm H_2O as the lowest
pressure, whilst each individual pressure tracing was always
steady during the whole experimental period.

The red cell concentrations in the outflow, determined at
various times of perfusion, were plotted on a semilogarithmic
scale against the volumes of Ringer's solution perfused (Fig.).
The initial concentrations were around 6.0×10^9 cells per ml.
During the first 10 ml perfusion, the concentrations dropped
rapidly to a range of 3.0×10^8 and 4.5×10^7 cells per ml. Over
the 10 ml to 100 ml perfusion period, a decrease by another order

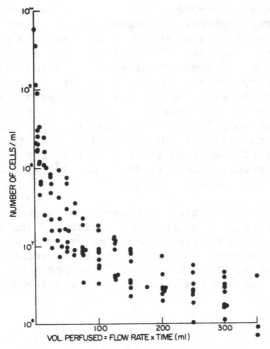

Fig. 1 - Red cell counts in the samples of venous outflow
         determined at various stages of perfusion.

of magnitude occurred and thereafter the counts decreased very
slowly. In fact, during perfusion from 150 ml to 400 ml, the cell
concentration decreased by less than an order of magnitude in all
experiments.

The overall picture of red cell washout from the coronary
circuit of isolated feline hearts suggested three different
phases; the first rapid washout, the second moderately fast, and
the last the slowest phase. If the red cells were stored in a
single direct pathway from arteries to veins we would expect only
the rapid phase of washout. In addition, the very slow phase
would not be expected unless there are cyclic pathways which may
delay washout (Thron, 1972), or unless certain sticky red cells
have a tendency to adhere to vessel walls. In order to prove that
the slowest component of washout did indeed consist of red cells,
the cell counts were determined again after hemolysis using one
drop of "redout" (Stromatolytic agent, Becton, Dickinson). Also,
smears of samples on microscopic slides stained with supravital
stains (B.S.B. or M.B.) were observed under a microscope. After
200 ml perfusion, reticulocytes were found to be a major constituent of cells in the venous outflow. Therefore, reticulocytes
were considered to be responsible for the slowest phase of the
washout and this agrees with similar findings from both spleen
(Song & Groom, 1972) and skeletal muscle (Groom & Song, 1972).

By applying a curve-peeling method, the washout curve can be resolved into three exponential components; the first with the slowest rate constant, the second with intermediate and the third with the fast rate constant. This analysis has led us to consider a model, consisting of three compartments, for red cells flowing through the coronary system. On the basis of this tentative model, the first compartment with the slowest rate constant (desaturation half volume $V_{1/2}$ = 170 ml) received only 0.1% of the total flow rate and contained only 1.3% of the total red cell content; the intermediate having $V_{1/2}$ = 11 ml received 4.5% of the total flow and contained 33% of the total red cells; the fast compartment with $V_{1/2}$ < 1 ml received most of the flow (95.5%) and contained more than 65% of the total red cells.

At present, morphological counterparts responsible for these three compartments may be suggested as follows: The fast (III) compartment may represent red cells in major branches of arteries and veins, the intermediate (II) the cells in myocardial sinusoids, or Thebesian vessels, while the slow (I) compartment corresponds to reticulocytes and abnormal red cells in the coronary circuit.

REFERENCES

1. Wearn, J.T. et al. 1933. Am. Heart J. P:143.
2. Hammond, G.L. and Moggio, R.A. 1971. Am. J. Physiol. 220:1463.
3. Thron, C.D. 1972. Bull. Math. Biophys. 34:277.
4. Song, S.H. & Groom, A.C. 1972. Can. J. Physiol. and Pharmacol. 50:400.
5. Groom, A.C. & Song, S.H. 1972. Microcirculatory Soc. 20th (Abstract).

(Senior Research Fellow of the Ontario Heart Foundation. This project is supported by the Ontario Heart Foundation Grant-in-Aid).

MEAN MYOGLOBIN OXYGEN TENSION IN SKELETAL AND CARDIAC MUSCLE

R.F. Coburn

Department of Physiology, School of Medicine

University of Pennsylvania, Philadelphia, Pa.

We have utilized the concept first developed by Millikan (1936, 1937) that myoglobin may be a useful indicator of intracellular oxygen tension. We have not made spectrophotometric measurements of oxymyoglobin % saturation, as did Millikan, since the presence of hemoglobin interferes with this measurement, but instead compute a mean myoglobin oxygen tension from measurements of carboxymyoglobin % saturation (MBCO). This method has been described previously (Coburn and Mayers, 1971; Coburn et al, 1973). The basis of the method is illustrated in Fig. 1. Binding of O_2 and CO to myoglobin is competitive, therefore, at a given partial pressure of CO, MBCO is a function of the oxygen tension in proximity to myoglobin molecules. This figure also illustrates that mean tissue Pco is equal to mean capillary Pco since CO is neither produced nor consumed at a significant rate.

The following equation shows the relationship of CO and O_2 tensions to MBCO and MBO_2 concentrations in terms of the equilibrium reaction of CO with MBO_2. Mmb is the equilibrium constant for this reaction which is approximately 25 in canine skeletal muscle at 37° C (Coburn, 1971); MBO_2 and MBCO are in the same units.

$$PmbO_2/MBO_2 = Mmb\ Pco/MBCO \qquad (1)$$

It is seen that in a given myoglobin molecule the ratio of PO_2 to O_2 binding is proportional to the ratio Pco to CO binding. Thus, if the ratio of Pco to MBCO is known, one can compute PO_2 from the ratio PO_2/MBO_2 since the oxymyoglobin dissociation curve is mono-tonic (Antonini, 1965). If we consider a living muscle where PO_2 may vary in different areas of the cell where myoglobin is present,

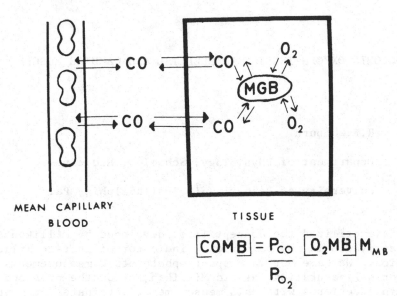

$$\boxed{COMB} = \frac{P_{CO}}{P_{O_2}} \boxed{O_2MB} M_{MB}$$

Fig. 1   Competition of CO and O_2 for myoglobin

if it is assumed that CO and O_2 are in kinetic equilibrium with myoglobin, ratios of Pco/MBCO in different myoglobin molecules can be summed allowing calculation of a mean value, which allows calculation of a mean myoglobin PO_2 (mPmbO$_2$).

Mean myoglobin PO_2 can also be computed using the following equation which is derived elsewhere (Coburn and Mayers, 1971)

$$mPmbO_2/MbO_2 = HBCO\ Mmb\ mPc_{O_2}\ /\ MBCO\ Mhb\ mHBO_2 \qquad (2)$$

where mPc_{O_2} and $mHBO_2$ are mean capillary values and Mhb the equilibrium constant for the reaction of CO and HBO_2. This equation states that the partition of CO between mean capillary blood and myoglobin is a function of mean capillary PO_2 and $mPmbO_2$; therefore it is possible to compute the relationship of $mPmbO_2$ to mPc_{O_2} from measurements of HBCO and MBCO.

Our experiments were performed on dogs anesthetized with pentobarbital or alpha chloralose and ventilated with a volume respirator. Our goal in these experiments was to measure COMB in skeletal muscle and myocardial apex at different steady state PaO_2 and to compute tissue Pco so that $mPmbO_2$ could be computed. In skeletal muscle experiments the left hind leg was skinned and hamstring muscles isolated. In cardiac experiments the chest was opened and pericardium removed. Thirty minutes prior to biopsy the inspired PO_2 was set to give a desired PaO_2. Just prior to biopsy blood gases and PH were determined in arterial blood and in blood draining skeletal muscle or blood from the coronary sinus. Muscle biopsies were performed by V clamping and dissection of 10 to 20 g of tissue which was cut into 1-2 g aliquots and stored in N_2.

CO tension in muscle at the time of biopsy is computed from blood HBCO and estimates of mean capillary PO_2 and HBO_2 (Douglas and Haldane, 1912) obtained from arterial and venous blood data using an integrative technique and assuming kinetic equilibrium of CO, O_2 and hemoglobin in mean capillary blood, an assumption which has experimental support (Coburn and Mayers, 1971). Fortunately blood Pco changes as a function of PO_2 are small due to the fact that HBCO remains nearly unchanged and that HBO_2 changes are in the same direction as PO_2 changes, thus it is not at all critical to determine mean capillary PO_2 precisely. Using venous PO_2 and HBO_2 values, instead of mean capillary data, causes a difference of less than 1 mm Hg in computed $mPmbO_2$ (Coburn and Mayers). Another implication of this is that tissue Pco is probably quite uniform even in the presence of nonuniform ratios $\dot{Q}/\dot{V}O_2$ and nonuniform PcO_2. MBCO is determined in biopsy specimens by determining total CO and subtracting CO bound to hemoglobin at the time of biopsy. Our methodology has been described previously (Coburn et al, 1973).

Fig 2 shows measured values of MBCO, given as the ratio MBCO/HBCO. Note that at $PaO_2 < 40$ mm Hg, MBCO /HBCO became elevated. Also that there is not an impressive difference between data obtained in resting skeletal muscle and myocardial apex.

Fig. 3 shows $mPmbO_2$ data computed from MBCO and Pco in the experiments shown in Fig. 2. Note the low $mPmbO_2$ values, 4 to 8 mm Hg at near normal PaO_2 in both hamstring muscle and myocardial apex. Also, there is a lack of a large decrease in $mPmbO_2$ as PaO_2 was decreased over a wide range to about 40 mm Hg. At steady state PaO_2 levels less than 40 mm Hg, $mPmbO_2$ decreased, in most of the experiments, to approximately 1 mm Hg. Other data have shown that resting skeletal muscle oxygen uptake decreases when PaO_2 is < 40 mm Hg.

In discussing these data we must consider the major assumptions. In analyzing biopsy specimens of MBCO we assume that intracellular CO is bound only to myoglobin. This probably is not a cause of significant error, at least in "red" skeletal muscle, due to the high concentration of myoglobin. For example, in rabbit skeletal muscle, myoglobin concentrations are 100-300 times larger than the concentration of cytochrome a_3 (Jobsis, 1963). Also CO affinity for myoglobin is much greater, at the same PO_2, than for cytochrome

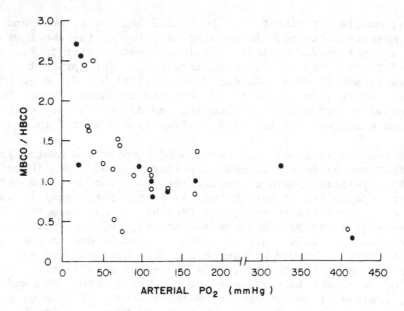

Fig. 2   Measurements of MBCO/HBCO in canine resting hamstring
muscle (open circles) and in canine myocardium (closed circles).
Data obtained under steady state conditions.

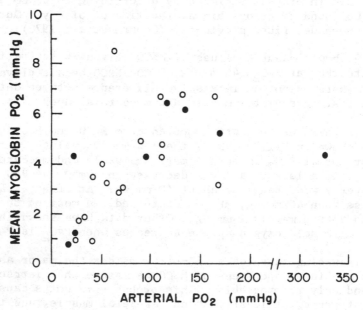

Fig. 3   Mean myoglobin PO_2 values computed from MBCO measurements
and calculated values for tissue P_{CO}. M_{MB} was 25. Hamstring muscle
(open circles); myocardial apex (closed circles).

a_3. Other hemoproteins are found in even smaller concentrations.
In the myocardium where cytochrome concentrations are larger, we
can not be as certain about this assumption.

The assumption that CO and O_2 are in kinetic equilibrium with
myoglobin is probably not a source of significant error under steady
state conditions where it is reasonable to assume that gas tensions
at a given point in the cell are not changing markedly. The dissociation velocity constant of MBCO is not fast enough for the method
to precisely detect rapid changes in $mPmbO_2$ and if there are rapid
changes in intracellular PO_2 our method will probably underestimate
mean values.

The concept "mean myoglobin" PO_2 is somewhat vague, especially
since the exact intracellular location or locations is still not
definitively known, although it is suspected that myoglobin is
physically dissolved and freely diffusible in cytoplasmic water
(Wittenberg, 1970; James, 1968). If myoglobin is widely dispersed
in the cell there may be a PO_2 gradient across a myoglobin "layer"
in the cell. This will result in a gradient of MBCO in the cell
as illustrated in Fig. 4. We, of course, can not put PO_2 boundaries
on this plot; this plot does suggest, however, that if myoglobin is

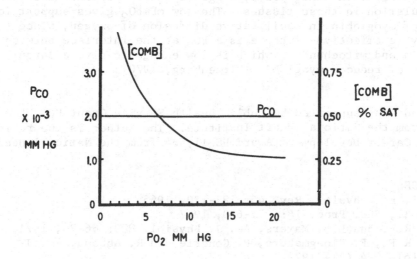

Fig. 4   Computed change of MBCO in a myoglobin solution at constant
          P_{CO}, as a function of PO_2.

uniformly distributed that a mean MBCO may be less than our calculated value since the relationship of MBCO and PO_2 is not linear. Even with rather extreme PO_2 values across the myoglobin layer, this will result in only about a 1 mm Hg overestimation in calculated $mPmbO_2$. If myoglobin is freely diffusible in cell water the possibility must be entertained that there is a MBCO and Pco shuttle, association of CO in myoglobin diffusing toward mitochondria and dissociation as MBCO diffuses toward the cell membrane or superficial boundary of the intracellular myoglobin layer.

There are data which indicate that myoglobin is a satisfactory oxygen tension indicator in that Mmb does not vary as a result of changes in pH, osmolarity, protein concentration, myoglobin concentration or the presence of reduced myoglobin (Antonini, 1965). It is clear that $mPmbO_2$ reflects muscle fibers containing myoglobin and is not directly influenced by white fibers. Our biopsy techniques are too gross for us to, at this time, demonstrate changes in endocardium versus epicardium. If there is variation in PO_2 in adjacent fibers we can not detect this since we are sampling a relatively large area of muscle.

The low $mPmbO_2$ suggest that intracellular PO_2 may be regulated so that the PO_2 adjacent to mitochondria is near the mitochondrial critical oxygen tension (Chance, 1957). The very small decrease in $mPmbO_2$ as PaO_2 is decreased over a wide range (above 40 mm Hg), which can not be convincingly shown in the data shown here but can be demonstrated in other plots, suggests finely controlled oxygen autoregulation in these tissues. The low $mPmbO_2$ gives support for a role of myoglobin in facilitative diffusion of oxygen, since this can only be effective if there is a PO_2 at the interface between myoglobin and mitochondria which is low enough to give a large fraction of reduced myoglobin (Wittenberg, 1970).

This study was supported by Public Health Service Grant R01 HL 10331 from the National Heart Institute. The author is the recipient of Career Development Award HE 11,564 from the National Heart Institute.

REFERENCES
Antonini, E., Physiol. Rev. 45: 123-170, 1965.
Chance, B., Fed. Proc. 16: 671-680, 1957.
Coburn, R.F. and L.B. Mayers, Am. J. Physiol. 220: 66-74, 1971.
Coburn, R.F., F. Ploegmakers, P. Gondrie and R. Abboud, Am. J. Physiol. 224 (4), 1973.
Douglas, C.C. and J.S. Haldane, J. Physiol. (Lond) 44: 305-354, 1912.
James, N.T., Nature 219: 1174-1175, 1968.
Jobsis, F.F., J. Gen. Physiol. 46: 905-928, 1963.
Millikan, G.A., Proc. Roy. Soc. London Ser. B 120: 366-388, 1936.

Millikan, G.A., Proc. Roy. Soc. London Ser B 123: 218-241, 1937.
Rossi-Fanelli, A. and E. Antonini, Arch. Bioch. Biophys. 77: 478-
    492, 1958.
Wittenberg, J.B., Physiol. Rev. 50: 559-636, 1970.

DISCUSSION OF SESSION II   SUBSESSION: HEART

Chairmen: Dr. Thomas K. Goldstick, Dr. David C. MacGregor and
           Dr. Carl R. Honig

DISCUSSION OF PAPER BY C. R. HONIG

Schuchhardt: (1) It is a surprising fact that there is a linear
relationship between arterial pO_2 and intercapillary distance; this
is not expected, because there is no linear relationship between
height of pO_2 and region of supplied tissue, especially not in the
range 100-150 Torr.
     (2) Did you have to prove the difference of myocardial blood
content between high and low levels of heart work, which has to
exist according to your results?

Honig: With respect to your first question, I think that we will
have to consider what the explanation can be, but I think that, as
an experimentalist, I can only say that is what exists. We will
have to try and account for it. The linear relationship is very
clear-cut. We have measured coronary blood volume or attempted to
measure it by studying the distribution of chromium 51, tagged
erythrocytes in hearts of dogs, but we have not done that in rat.
We would like very much to do it in order to correlate our results
with the direct distance measurements. There is a problem, however,
that one must eventually assign some fraction of the blood volume
to the capillaries and I rather think one can make the thing come
out depending on how you make that assignment. I do not think it
is really a very direct test, but I think this method is about as
direct as one can get it.

Lübbers: First, I would like to congratulate you for the beautiful
studies because you don't have much other material to do any calculations; so it is very nice to have some. We observed, in some vital
microscopic studies on the inside of the heart, that if you open it
up and then if you made a certain tension in rabbit heart, then it
starts as Rubuck has shown in a normal heart. We can see then,
that sometimes flow changes its direction.
     Have you also seen changing flow in the single capillaries?
We have seen that the single capillary has the tendency to close
and then to open up so really what you are measuring is a fluctuation of the capillary. Also, sometimes we have seen that there are
no red cells in the capillaries so that it is like plasma streaming.
Probably this would upset your measurement of capillary distance,
or can you also observe a capillary which has no red cells, only
plasma streaming in it?

Honig: We are defining an open capillary as a capillary which contains erythrocytes. The way in which we can identify a capillary is through the color contrast in ektachrome film between hemoglobin and myoglobin. If it does not contain an erythrocyte, we do not count it as an open capillary.

     With respect to your question about the opening and closing of capillaries, Dr. Bourdeau-Martini, in the blood-perfused rat heart, has, in fact, observed rhythmic opening and closing of coronary, precapillary sphincters, just as you have. We believe that this occurs in skeletal muscle, and we have seen it very clearly there. But the distributions which I have are averages with respect to time, and we are really measuring changes in the duty cycle of the precapillary sphincters.

Lübbers: There could be a possibility you could combine these photographic measurements by the hydrogen clearance method. We have now constructed a method for this.

Van Liew: I would like to ask how you explain the opening of capillaries at very high pO_2's?

Honig: Our present interpretation of that is that it is a toxic effect of oxygen on precapillary sphincters in smooth muscle. Presumably, the effect would be the same as hypoxia, where the ability of smooth-muscle mitochondria to conserve ATP would be impaired in both instances.

DISCUSSION OF PAPER BY J. GROTE AND G. THEWS

Barr: I would be interested to have a comment on the difference in the pO_2 in the tissue as a function of heart rate for different animals.

Grote: It is not proper to answer this question here today because our calculations were done for the condition in the human heart muscle. However, I think that the differences between the condition in the dog myocardium and the human nyocardium or in the monkey myocardium are not so great.

Song: If we dissect the ventrical muscle into three layers, which is supposed to have three different capillary distributions along the layers, and if there is a pressure gradient from endocardium to endocardium to epicardium, then do you expect any pO_2 difference by the layers?

Grote: I think this question should be better answered by Dr. Honig. Under this condition you will have a very sharp change in blood flow, and this means that we have to expect decreases in the mean oxygen tension in the inner layers of the myocardium.

Honig: I think that we still believe that there exists a transmural oxygen gradient, and I understand from Dr. MacGregor that this gradient has also been measured by mass spectrometry. We did it by use of oxygen electrodes. I would like to ask our speaker if he would comment on the effect of including oxygen diffusion from arterioles on the fraction of tissue which would be anoxic. Dr. Duling and his collaborators have shown that the oxygen tension in capillaries at the origin of the capillaries is substantially below the arterial level.

Grote: Under the special conditions of the simple model that we took as the basis for all the calculations, we could not put these special effects into our calculations but there are a lot of results which indicate the existence of these effects.

Whalen: I wish to confirm that we also found a pO_2 gradient higher in the epicardium than in the endocardium.

DISCUSSION OF PAPER BY B. LÖSSE, S. SCHUCHHARDT, N. NIEDERLE AND
     H. BENZING

Coburn: I thought it was a beautiful paper. I want to ask a very basic question. Can you make any guess as to what percentage of your penetrations actually are in the cell, vs. those that perhaps are in extracellular space? I am trying to relate intracellular pO_2 to the histogram that you get.

Schuchhardt: No, we cannot get it because our tips are larger than a myocardial cell.

Coburn: So you are probably not in a cell.

Schuchhardt: Normally we are not in a cell.

Coburn: Even though you get very low values, they are probably higher than a mean intracellular pO_2 that could be measured.

Schuchhardt: I think the distinction between extracellular and intracellular is not the dominant problem. If you have a gradient which goes through the capillary to the farthest point of tissue, there always is a gradient across the myocardial cell.

Coburn: This is one of the points I think none of us understands. We do not know what the gradients are. I would think that inside

of a cell, where oxygen is being consumed, that you would find a
big decrease with distance from the cell surface down to the center
of the cells, but you are going through a layer of mitochondria.

Schuchhardt: Exactly speaking, it is at the bands of mitochondria
which are arranged parallel to the myofibrils that oxygen is consumed, and these are the tanks of the oxygen.

Whalen: (With reference to the question of Dr. Coburn as to whether
Schuchhardt's measurements were intracellular, and that intracellular measurements would be lower.) Intracellular measurements we
have made do indicate lower values, many close to zero, especially
in the endocardium. These observations are consistent with the
observations of others that, following a coronary occlusion, reductions in the change of pressure with time are already apparent by
the third heartbeat. A comment: I think both intracellular and
regional measurements of pO_2, as done by Dr. Schuchhardt, are
important.

DISCUSSION OF PAPER BY H. BENZING, B. LÖSSE, S. SCHUCHHARDT AND
      N. NIEDERLE

Weiss, Harvey: What was the response time of the electrodes used
for measuring oxygen tension? What differences were observed in
oxygen tension with depth of insertion of the electrodes? Were
there any differences in absolute control values or in responses
and response time to hypoxia?

Benzing: The response time, determined by switching between different solutions of known pO_2, amounts to 11 sec (90% value of mean
steady state deflection). The response time determined in tissue,
by switching the breathing gas to a 10% O_2-concentration, for
instance, is superimposed on the effect of the different gas mixture
on the local blood flow. The mean time delay between switching to
the hypoxic gas mixture and the first decrease of time pO_2 amounted
to 10 sec.

Weiss, Harvey: Was there any difference in depth within the myocardium or were all these electrodes put in the same depth?

Benzing: The electrodes were about 3-7 millimeters in to the myocardium, for the pO_2 electrodes. The blood flow drops there in the
middle of the heart muscle by about 4 or 5 millimeters. From our
experiments, together with Dr. Schuchhardt, we have no clear relation; therefore, we cannot say we have a direct function with the
depth of the electrodes.

Schubert: (1) What was the size of your blood flow sensory thermistor?

(2) Do you have an estimate of the stability of the blood flow sensor in the myocardium? This could be stated alternately, what was the effect of altering the sequence of the experiment (occlusion then hypoxia vs. hypoxia then occlusion) on the % of regional blood flow change seen in each perturbation.

Benzing: (1) The probe consists of a thermistor (diameter 0.3 mm) surrounded by a Constantan heating coil. This configuration was implanted into a gold tube (5 mm in length and 1 mm in diameter).

(2) We did the experiment both ways and additionally we reversed the measuring points and found the results were within the repeatability described in the results. The reproducibility during hypoxia was somewhat better. The results from the occlusion experiment are dependent on probe location and on the amount of the collateral flow in this region.

Honig: Your last slide (Figure 3) showed that if inspired O_2 tension is half normal, tissue pO_2 does not go to zero. However, your electrodes certainly sampled many capillary domains. Our frequency distributions indicate that in some of these domains, tissue pO_2 would in fact have been zero.

Benzing: We agree. Our measurement does not allow statements about the pO_2 gradients or maybe anoxic regions in the dimensions of a few microns.

DISCUSSION OF PAPER BY G. J. WILSON, D. C. MACGREGOR, D. E. HOLNESS, W. LIXFELD AND H. YASUI

Halmagyi: You have shown that pCO_2 went up to 350 mm Hg. What happened to the nitrogen?

Wilson: During these studies we were not recording nitrogen.

Halmagyi: But how was there room for 350 mm Hg CO_2? I mean, there was nitrogen and oxygen. The oxygen fell to zero, well then, there is 120 mm Hg room for CO_2 because the rest was nitrogen in the tissues, was there not?

Wilson: Yes, I think there is some nitrogen in the tissues.

Halmagyi: I have never heard of a value like 350 mm Hg in a tissue unless you had an animal that was saturated with oxygen. There is no room for the CO_2.

Wilson: I think you are suggesting that the combined partial pressure of the carbon dioxide and the partial pressure of nitrogen in atmospheric air would add up to a total value which would exceed atmospheric pressure. I do not have a quick response to that question, but we are fairly certain that the carbon dioxide values that we are measuring are those which exist in the myocardium. The instrument does provide the capability to measure nitrogen so that I will be able to check out your question in future experiments. We are able to measure oxygen, carbon dioxide, and if we wish, we may measure nitrogen in the tissue as well.

Van Liew: Gases in solution can be quite different from gases in a bubble. The CO_2 can have any value in the solution.

Schuchhardt: (1) What is the influence of the vacuum induced by the sampling probe on the pO_2 gradients in the adjacent tissue?
        (2) Why does the tissue pO_2 not reach zero during ischemia?

Wilson: We are certainly concerned that the oxygen tension values did not move down to zero during anoxic arrest and our suspicion is that there may be some leakage of air down the length of the catheter through the insertion site. We are considering surrounding it with pure nitrogen gas and seeing if that makes any difference. Regarding the effect of gas flow through the catheter or the accuracy of the measurements, the figures which we were familiar with before attending this conference, those of Brantigan, indicate that the maximum error for oxygen tension would be about 18% and for carbon dioxide tension would be 1%, depending on the rate of fluid flow over the catheter.

Van Liew: What was the flow or stirring dependence of your calibrating system? In the measurements, there must have been a change from a reasonably well-stirred system (due to capillary perfusion) to an unstirred system (after blood flow was stopped).

Wilson: In the series of experiments we have reported, the assumption has been made that the myocardial interstitial space represents an unstirred environment. This seems a reasonable assumption after blood flow to the heart ceased, but may be questioned during coronary perfusion. The issue is the sensitivity of pO_2 and pCO_2 measurements to interstitial fluid flow over the catheter surface. Brantigan (J. Appl. Physiol, 1972) indicated maximum errors (zero to any linear flow velocity in excess of approximately 10 cm/sec) of 18% and less that 1% for oxygen and carbon dioxide tensions respectively. Nelson, at this symposium, has reported larger flow sensitivities. If one can estimate the tissue fluid flow rate over the catheter surface, some correction might be made. We are exploring this possibility. We are particularly interested in intramyocardial pCO_2 to assess myocardial metabolism during surgical cardiac arrest and it is reassuring to note that the pCO_2 measurements are much less sensitive to flow over the catheter than the pO_2 measurements.

DISCUSSION OF PAPER BY H. R. WEISS

Schuchhardt: We have had the experience that it is extremely difficult to measure with bare electrodes of this size. Did you observe an influence of mechanical oscillations on the electrodes induced by the heart beat?

Weiss: No, these electrodes were specially filtered so that mechanical and electrical motion were completely eliminated; however, if there was a gross movement of the electrodes in the heart, in other words, if the electrode did not remain steady in the heart, there was a sharp drop in pO_2 in both regions, and readings of this kind were eliminated.

Schuchhardt: You did observe the oscillations and you did eliminate them?

Weiss: No, with the filtering we have, which has a time constant of approximately 2 seconds, there is normally no motion of the electrodes. You will notice that most of my traces look fairly steady. This was fairly characteristic of the heart with the specific system we used which had this built-in time constant.

Schuchhardt: Yes, but I could imagine that the different pressure in the different layers of the myocardium have influenced your pO_2 measurement.

Beran: We have implanted coaxial electrodes in different areas of the myocardium and observed that artifact due to myocardial contractility immediately following the implantation were not frequent. Several days or weeks later they were non-existent.
    However, my question is related to a different aspect of your presentation. You have used bare wire Pt electrodes and your data are expressed in mm Hg tissue pO_2. I wonder how the reducing current uA was transferred into mm Hg pO_2.

Weiss: The electrodes used in the present study were calibrated and tested for linearity by placing them in saline equilibrated with different percentages of oxygen. The usual mixtures employed were 10% O_2, 5% O_2 and pure N_2. The pO_2 in mm Hg was then plotted against the current. When a straight line could be drawn through these points, the electrodes were considered linear and pO_2 in mm Hg could be obtained directly from this straight line function. There was always a small residual current even after bubbling for over an hour in N_2, which must be taken into account in constructing this function to obtain pO_2. The possibility of a difference between the in vitro and in vivo calibration must also be considered.

DISCUSSION OF PAPER BY R. E. SAFFORD, J. D. WHIFFEN, E. N. LIGHTFOOT
    R. S. TEPPER AND J. H. G. RANKIN

Shapiro: I am somewhat concerned about the effect of the microspheres themselves upon the microcirculation. A thirty-five micron
diameter is rather large when compared to capillary dimensions. I
would expect that, especially in pathologic low flow states, microcirculatory occlusion due to repeated microsphere embolization
episodes might occur. This could lead to a progressive systematic
error in your flow calculation.

Safford: I misspoke during the presentation. We used 25 micron
microspheres, not the 35 micron size as I stated from the podium.
Twenty-five micron spheres were selected because survey of the
literature revealed that they were the smallest spheres that would
not pass through A-V shunts in dogs to any appreciable degree[1].
    Also, it has been reported in the literature[2] that so long as
the total dose of microspheres given to a 20 kg dog does not exceed
20 mg, the microspheres themselves will have no measureable effect
on the circulation. The total dose in any experiment never exceeded 20 mg. in this study.
1. Safford, R. E., PhD Thesis, U. of Wisconsin, 1973.
2. Karhara et al., JAP, 27, 218, 1969.

Messmer: I wonder if you would not comment on the priming solution
in your machine because it is well established that the perfusion
rate and distribution of total flow rate are decidedly dependent
upon the degree of hemodilution achieved.

Safford: A Dextran-75-electrolyte solution having approximately
the same ionic composition and colloid osmotic pressure as dog
plasma was used as the hemodiluent in the prime solution for the
oxygenator.
    A 2300 cc. prime (57% blood, 43% Dextran-electrolyte solution)
was used. Thus, at the start of an experiment, for a 20 kg. animal
on bypass, the circulating blood was diluted about 23%.
    We performed an earlier series of experiments (not reported
here) in which whole blood primes were used. In every respect, the
experiments in which hemodilution was used were superior to the
earlier experiments.

Honig: It should be recognized that results with microspheres are
initially dependent on the size of the spheres, because of the
vagaries introduced by axial streaming. The results must therefore
be considered only semiquantitative, and characteristic of the
sphere size employed.

Safford: I know of no reference in the literature which shows that
the distribution of microspheres between major vessels is dependent
on the size of the microspheres. It is true that the size of the

microspheres does effect the distribution of the spheres within the microcirculation - i.e., within an organ - however, the distribution of blood flow among the organs has been shown to be independent of sphere size. Since this study did not involve intraorgan flow distributions, sphere size need not have been considered and the results are probably <u>not</u> characteristic of the microsphere size as suggested.

Some references for this topic are:

Karhara et al., <u>JAP</u>, <u>25</u>, 696, 1968.

Phibbs et al., <u>Nature</u>, <u>216</u>, 1339 (1967).

Rudolph & Heymann, <u>Circ</u>. <u>Res</u>, <u>21</u>, 163 (1967).

DISCUSSION OF PAPER BY S. H. SONG

<u>Cameron</u>: Are your three compartments essentially two anatomical compartments while the third (slow) compartment is not defined anatomically but by an erythrocyte class?

<u>Song</u>: Yes, I am suggesting that, but at present it is not confirmed yet.

<u>Coburn</u>: I wonder if your technique could be used to ask questions about effects of various perfusing solutions at non-pulsatile vs. pulsatile flow on distribution of blood flow? There are considerable published data on tissue pO_2 obtained in organs perfused with artificial solutions and non-pulsatile way and it is of interest to determine if distribution of flow is normal under this condition.

<u>Song</u>: Maybe there can be differences in RBC washout between two conditions.

DISCUSSION OF PAPER BY R. F. COBURN

<u>Cameron</u>: How do you correct for CO bound to the hemoglobin in the tissue biopsy?

<u>Coburn</u>: The major problem is to measure hemoglobin. If we can measure hemoglobin and measure blood carboxyhemoglobin at the time of biopsy, we can determine the amount of carbon monoxide that is in the biopsy specimen bound to hemoglobin. We do this two ways. We either break all the cells and measure it spectrophotometrically, or we, and this was the usual case, label hemoglobin with chromium 51 and measure the radioactivity of the sample. We get the same

values with both ways.

Duling: What do you think about the possibility that the myoglobin dissociation curve might be somewhat different intracellularly than the ones that have been determined?

Coburn: Myoglobin is such a stable molecule that changes in the environment in the cell compared to in a solution where most of the measurements are made are unlikely to have much of an effect, because it does not have confirmational changes with pH, osmolality, protein, myoglobin concentrations, and so forth. I think that is rather unlikely.

Subsession: VASCULAR CHEMORECEPTORS AND OXYGEN BARRIER

Chairmen: Dr. Thomas K. Goldstick, Dr. David C. MacGregor

and Dr. Carl R. Honig

MICROVASCULAR DIAMETER CHANGES DURING LOCAL BLOOD FLOW REGULATION: INDEPENDENCE OF CHANGES IN PO_2

Brian R. Duling

Dept. of Physiol., School of Medicine, University of

Virginia, Charlottesville, Virginia 22901

The flow of blood to tissues is largely regulated by the contractile activity of the vascular smooth muscle of the arterioles and precapillary sphincters in the microcirculation. It has long been recognized that there is a feedback mechanism between tissue and vessel which modulates vascular smooth muscle contraction. One of many substances which has been proposed as a mediator of this regulation is oxygen (1,2). It is apparent that oxygen might be a regulator either via its action, if any, directly on the smooth muscle cells themselves or alternately by an indirect mechanism which initially alters parenchymal cell function. It is usually assumed that oxygen acting via an indirect mechanism causes altered release of a vasodilator metabolite which then reduces the contraction of the vascular smooth muscle (1,2).

If oxygen is to operate in the regulatory process by a direct action, then vascular wall PO_2 must change as the relation between oxygen demand and supply changes and also the smooth muscle must show adequate reactivity to changes in PO_2. It was the purpose of the present experiments to assess the reactivity to oxygen of the smooth muscles of hamster cheek pouch arterioles and compare the reactivity with the effects of altered oxygen demand on this tissue.

METHODS

These experiments were performed on 21 male golden hamsters which were anesthetized with nembutal (60 mg/kg i.p.) supplemented with urethane. The trachea and a femoral vein were cannulated and the cheek pouches were prepared for microscopic viewing as a single layered preparation (3).

Luminal microvessel dimensions were obtained with a Vickers image splitting eyepiece at magnifications of 20X to 50X. The

oxygen tension of the tissue and vessels was measured using Wha-
len-type oxygen microelectrodes with tip diameters between 2 and
6 μ (4). Oxygen tension measurements on the vessels were made on
the external wall.

Perivascular PO_2 was changed in one of two ways: 1) locally
in a small region around a single arteriole by micropipette application of solutions equilibrated with either 95% O_2 (O_2 pipettes)
or solutions equilibrated with N_2 (N_2 pipettes), and 2) by elevating the PO_2 of the suffusion solution covering the cheek pouch
surface to 150 mm Hg (air suffusion). The suffusion solution temperature was maintained at 37.5°C and had the following composition in mM: NaCl, 119.9; KCl, 4.7; $CaCl_2$, 1.6; and $MgSO_4$, 1.2;
pH was maintained at 7.35 with 21 mM Tris buffer.

RESULTS

Table 1 shows the results of these experiments. As can be
seen in the first column, elevation of suffusion solution PO_2
from the control level, which averaged 14 mm Hg, to 150 mm Hg
caused a significant reduction in vascular diameter which was correlated with an elevation in mean perivascular PO_2 of 40 mm Hg.
However, when oxygen was elevated locally, through the use of the
oxygen pipettes, the perivascular PO_2 could be increased to much
higher levels and only a small and statistically insignificant
change in diameter was produced.

TABLE 1   CHANGES IN OXYGEN TENSION AND MICROVASCULAR DIAMETER
STIMULUS

	Air Suffusion	95% O_2 Pipette	N_2 Pipette
ΔOxygen Tension	40 ± 6.2* (14)	186 ± 34* (13)	-2.5 ± 0.6* (15)
ΔVascular Diameter	-7.3 ± 1.1* (14)	-1.3 ± 0.7 (13)	-1.8 ± 0.9 (15)

Suffusion solution PO_2 averaged 14 mm Hg during the control period and was elevated to 150 mm Hg during air suffusion. Values
are means ± standard errors. Numbers in parentheses are numbers
of observations. * indicates a significant difference at p<0.05.

If high flows were forced from the O_2 pipettes it was usually possible to induce constrictions but these occurred only in
conjunction with extremely high PO_2's. It should be pointed out
that in no case were constrictions induced by micropipettes at
PO_2 changes comparable to those associated with the large diameter reductions observed during air suffusion. Furthermore, the
vessel PO_2 in one instance was raised as high as 184 mm Hg

without any discernable effect on the vascular diameter.

The change in diameter of the vessels observed during micro-application of high PO_2 solutions might have been due to any of several effects. Mechanical stimulation due to the fluid jet hitting the vessels might induce constrictions. Also, if a vaso-dilator metabolite were present it might alter vascular diameter either by its effect on the arteriolar smooth muscle or by an in-direct effect on the parenchymal cells. For this reason, the vessels were also tested with the N_2 pipettes. The data shown in Table 1 indicate that N_2 and O_2 pipettes produced equivalent di-ameter responses but opposite changes in perivascular PO_2.

Additional efforts were made to differentiate between the effects of air suffusion on PO_2 and those on vascular diameter by combining a change in suffusion solution PO_2 with microapplica-tion of low oxygen solutions to the arterioles. Using this tech-nique in combination with air suffusion, it was possible to pro-duce a complete separation of the constrictor effect and the PO_2 change. An example of this is shown in Fig. 1. Vascular diameter in μ's is shown in the upper trace and PO_2 in the lower trace.

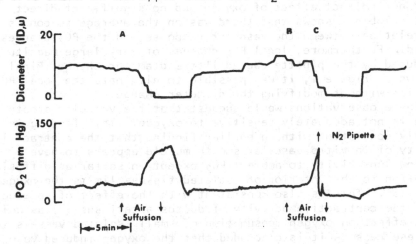

Figure 1. A comparison of the effect of elevated suffusion solu-tion PO_2 on microvascular diameter in the presence and absence of a change in perivascular PO_2. See text for description.

During the control period the suffusion solution was bubbled with N_2 and also an N_2 micropipette was positioned over the ves-sel. At A the suffusion solution was bubbled for four minutes with room air. This resulted in an increase in perivascular PO_2 and a decrease in vascular diameter. After return to baseline the suffusion solution was again bubbled with room air but at C, shor-tly after the perivascular PO_2 began to rise, the mercury column which pressurized the N_2 pipette was raised and the perivascular PO_2 was reduced to less than the baseline value. In spite of this the effect of elevated suffusion solution PO_2 was essentially

unaltered.   The order shown in part B and C of Figure 1 could be
reversed without affecting the diameter change. Experiments similar to those shown in Figure 1 were carried out repeatedly with
similar results. That is, vascular diameter changes showed a close
temporal relation to suffusion solution PO_2 but no consistent relation to perivascular PO_2.

DISCUSSION
     Elevation of suffusion solution PO_2, as was done in these
experiments, caused a vasoconstriction which was obviously the
result of a primary alteration in the pattern of oxygen supply
to the tissue. The increase in oxygen supplied by the solution
diminished the requirement for O_2 supply by the blood flow to
the pouch. Under these circumstances, we have shown previously
that there is a simultaneous elevation of both arteriolar PO_2 and
tissue PO_2 (5). The aim of the present experiments was to separate two possible effects; the direct effect of elevated oxygen
tension on the arteriolar smooth muscle and the indirect effect
of elevated tissue PO_2. The data presented argue strongly in favor of an indirect effect of oxygen and no significant direct
effect.   Table 1 shows that there was on the average no consistent relation between the vascular response and the PO_2 changes
induced.   Furthermore, local PO_2 changes of very large magnitude
as induced by the pipette caused little diameter change. Finally,
as shown in Figure 1, it was possible to eliminate the local PO_2
elevation without modifying the diameter change.
     These observations would suggest that the vascular smooth
muscle is not adequately sensitive to oxygen.   This finding is
entirely consistent with an earlier finding that the contractile
activity of in vitro vascular smooth muscle appears to have a
very low sensitivity to ambient PO_2 except in so far as diffusion
limitation to the interior of isolated tissues limits the oxygen
supply (6).   This is also consistent with the effect of reduced
PO_2 on the contractile activity of ductus arteriosus (7) as well
as the effect on oxygen consumption of small isolated vessels (8).
For these reasons it is concluded that the oxygen induced vasoconstriction is due to an initial effect on parenchymal cells and
a secondary one on vascular smooth muscle via a metabolically
linked feedback.

REFERENCES

1.   Johnson, P.C. (ed.): Symposium on autoregulation of blood
        flow. Circ. Res. 14 & 15 (Suppl. 1): I-1-I-291, 1964.
2.   Rodbard, S. (ed): Symposium on local regulation of blood
        flow. Circ. Res. 28 (Suppl. 1): I-1-I-58, 1971.
3.   Duling, B.R.: Preparation and use of the hamster cheek pouch.
        Microvasc. Res. 5: in press.
4.   Whalen, W.J., Riley, J., and Nair, P.: Microelectrodes for
        measuring intracellular PO2. J. Appl. Physiol. 23: 793-

801, 1967.

5. Duling, B.R.: Microvascular responses to alterations in oxygen tension. <u>Circ</u>. <u>Res</u>. 31: 481-489, 1972.

6. Pittman, R.N., and Duling, B.R.: Oxygen sensitivity of vascular smooth muscle. I. In vitro studies. <u>Microvasc</u>. <u>Res</u>. 5: in press.

7. Fay, F.S.: Guinea pig ductus arteriosus. I. Cellular and metabolic basis for oxygen sensitivity. <u>Am</u>. <u>J</u>. <u>Physiol</u>. 221: 470-479, 1971.

8. Howard, R.O., Richardson, D.W., Smith, M.H., and Patterson, J.L.: Oxygen consumption of arterioles and venules as studied in the Cartesian diver. <u>Circ</u>. <u>Res</u>. 16: 187-196, 1965.

ACTIVITY OF CHEMORECEPTOR FIBERS IN THE SINUS NERVE AND TISSUE PO$_2$ IN THE CAROTID BODY OF THE CAT

D. Bingmann, H. Acker and H. Schulze

Physiologisches Institut der Univ., Münster/Westf.

Max-Planck-Institut für Arbeitsphysiologie, Dortmund

Fed. Rep. Germany

ACKER, LÜBBERS and PURVES (1) found that tissue pO$_2$ (p$_T$O$_2$) in the carotid body of the cat is related to arterial oxygen pressure (p$_a$O$_2$) in a nearly linear function. In accordance with these results BISCOE et al. (3) described a close correlation between changes of the p$_a$O$_2$ and the activity of chemoreceptor units in the carotid body. In our own experiments, however, especially in few fiber preparations this close relation was often missing. In parallel with a stepwise lowering of the p$_a$O$_2$ from normoxic to hypoxic values of about 20 mmHg we observed a time course of receptor activity which frequently differed from the response found during the following reincrease in the p$_a$O$_2$ up to normal levels. As a whole, our experiments led to assume that the relation between the p$_a$O$_2$, the pO$_2$ in tissue and the chemoreceptor activity was altered, if the experimental variations of the p$_a$O$_2$ exceeded the physiological range either to hypoxic or to hyperoxic values. To test this hypothesis, simultaneous measurements of the p$_a$O$_2$, of pO$_2$ in tissue of the carotid body and recordings of the discharge rate in few fiber preparations of the sinus nerve were performed in anaesthetized, relaxed and artificially ventilated cats. These experiments have been carried out together with KELLER, CASPERS and LÜBBERS and will be reported elsewhere. In the following the relationship between the activity of nerve fibers and the tissue pO$_2$ will be especially discussed.

Preparation technique and recording methods were the same as in earlier experiments (2). To control the reactions of different chemoreceptor units, the sinus nerve was splitted to such an extent that single fiber potentials could be identified and evaluated by means of an electronical amplitude discrimination.

597

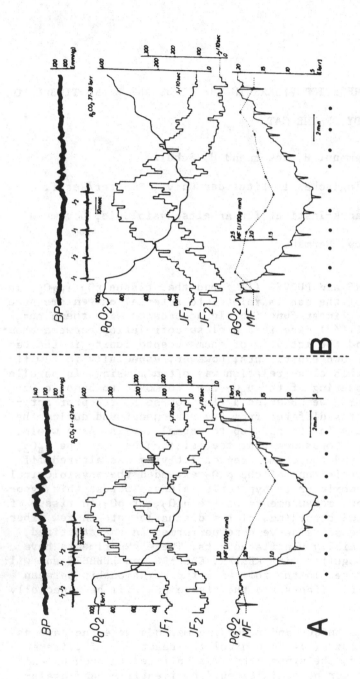

Fig. 1   Changes of the p_aO_2, of tissue pO_2 (p_GO_2) and of the discharge rate of two chemo-receptor fiber potentials J1 and J2 (displayed as frequency curves JF1 and JF2) induced by various O_2 contents in the inspired gas mixture (marked by points at the bottom of the figure). The arterial-blood pressure (BP) was monitored in the aorta abdominalis. Hydrogen clearances were used for measurements of the microflow (MF). B demonstrates the same experiment as in A half an hour later.

In a first series of experiments the relationship between the arterial pO_2, varied from normal levels to severe hypoxia, and the reaction of the pO_2 in the tissue of the carotid body was investigated. Simultaneously, the correlation of these parameters to the discharge rate in chemoreceptor fiber units was studied. A typical curve obtained in an anaesthetized and artificially ventilated cat is displayed in Fig. 1A. In this experiment, the p_aO_2 was reduced stepwise by lowering the O_2 concentration in the applied gas mixture. The tracing of tissue pO_2 followed the changes of p_aO_2 strictly down to the lowest value. The reincrease of the p_aO_2, however, was accompanied by a steeper rise of the p_TO_2 which finally exceeded its initial value for about 25%. In accordance to the reaction of the pO_2 in tissue the discharge rate in two receptor fiber units (J1 and J2) was found to change with greater steepness during the reenhancement of the p_aO_2 than in the phase of falling pO_2. This behavior of the receptor may be interpreted as adaptation. However, the parallel time course of the p_TO_2 suggests that this hysteresis in the relation between the p_aO_2 and the discharge frequency is caused by local changes of the p_aO_2 - p_TO_2 correlation.

The local mechanisms which seem to disturb locally this correlation to a varying extent are still unknown. Therefore, the pO_2 course at the receptor site, from which recordings are being taken, cannot be predicted if the arterial pO_2 is lowered to 20-30 mmHg. Even a repetition of the same experiment in the same animal can lead to another reaction of the p_TO_2 at various sites in the carotid body. The experiment subsiding in Fig. 1A was repeated half an hour later. The tracings are demonstrated in Fig. 1B. The position of the p_TO_2 microelectrode and the receptor fiber units which were recorded from had not been changed. Nevertheless, the responses of the p_TO_2 and of the discharge frequencies JF1 and JF2 to variations of the arterial pO_2 were markedly different from those found in Fig. 1A. The p_TO_2 now followed the p_aO_2 in an almost linear function and the overshoot of tissue pO_2 present in Fig. 1A was missing. The discharge rate of the fiber potential J1 corresponded to the pO_2 curves, whereas the frequency curves of the fiber potential J2 showed a steep decline in parallel with the first reincrease of the p_aO_2. The various shapes of these frequency curves suggest that the time course of tissue pO_2 at different receptor sites can vary to a considerable extent. This assumption could be confirmed in other experiments by simultaneous recordings of tissue pO_2 with two Pt- microelectrodes. These results allow to conclude that the linear relationship between p_aO_2 and p_TO_2 usually found under normoxic conditions shows considerable local variations in cases of severe hypoxia. In such instances the reactions of p_TO_2 at the receptor site are hard to predict.

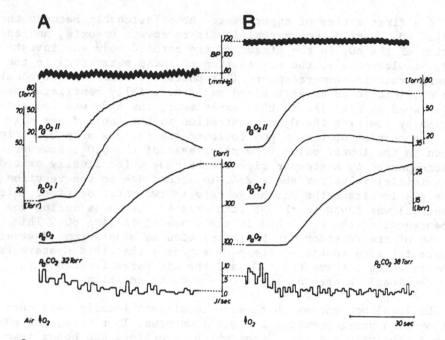

<u>Fig. 2</u>   A: Changes of tissue pO_2 (p_GO_2 I and p_GO_2 II measured simultaneously with two Pt-microelectrodes) and of chemoreceptor-activity (I/sec) induced by an increase of the arterial pO_2 from normal to hyperoxic values. B: Same experiment as in A, performed one hour later.

The same difficulty arises if the arterial pO_2 is shifted to hyperoxic values. With an enhancement of the p_aO_2, tissue pO_2 at first showed a corresponding increase. In the further course, however, p_aO_2 and p_TO_2 tended to change. Thus, tissue pO_2 reached a peak and declined when the p_aO_2 still progressed to its final level. As shown in Fig. 2, such dissociations varied to some extent. The experiments illustrated in parts A and B of Fig. 2, were performed with the Pt-microelectrodes left in the same position.

Nevertheless, increase of the p_aO_2 induced variable reactions of the p_TO_2 in subsequent recordings. The curves differed markedly in the slope of rise and fall.

In summary, the experiments have shown that the relations between p_aO_2 and p_TO_2 can vary to a considerable extent under hypoxic and hyperoxic conditions. In such cases neither measurements of p_aO_2 nor of $p_{T}O_2$ in the carotid body are suitable to receive exact data about the pO_2 behavior in the sensitive field of a single receptor unit, since the positions of chemoreceptors from which recordings are taken are usually unknown.

References

1) ACKER, H., LÜBBERS, D.W. and PURVES, M.J. Local oxygen tension field in the glomus caroticum of the cat and its change at changing arterial pO_2. Pflügers Arch., 1971, 329: 136-155.

2) ACKER, H., KELLER, H.-P., LÜBBERS, D.W., BINGMANN, D., SCHULZE, H. and CASPERS, H. The relationship between neuronal activity of chemoreceptor fibres and tissue pO_2 of the carotid body of the cat during change in arterial pO_2. (In preparation).

3) BISCOE, T.J., PURVES, M.J. and SAMPSON, S.R. The frequency of nerve impulses in single carotid body chemoreceptor afferent fibres recorded in vivo with intact circulation. J.Physiol. (Lond.), 1970, 208: 121-131.

ROLE OF THE CAROTID CHEMOREFLEXES IN THE REGULATION OF ARTERIAL OXYGEN PRESSURE

Heidrun Schöne, Wolfgang Wiemer* and Peter Kiwull

Arbeitsgruppe Regulationsphysiologie, Inst. Physiol.

Ruhr-Universität, 463 Bochum, Fed. Rep. Germany

As in other species also in the anaesthetized rabbit the ventilatory minute volume increases with decreasing arterial oxygen pressure, thereby counteracting the fall of PaO_2. The present paper describes how effectively the chemoreflex drive approaches, under various conditions, the arterial oxygen pressure to that of the inspiratory gas mixtures.

Methods

Experiments were performed on 43 rabbits anaesthetized with pentobarbital sodium, anaesthesia maintained as constant as possible by continuous infusion of 9.0 ± 0.4 mg/kg/h in Ringer solution. The animals inhaled successively 100 % O_2, air, 11.9 % O_2 in N_2 and 6.7 % O_2 in N_2. At every level of arterial oxygen pressure both vagi were reversibly cold blocked. After changing the inspiratory mixture respectively blocking or deblocking the vagi steady state conditions were awaited for about 10 min. Then the following variables were determined: Arterial oxygen pressure (measured continuously in the femoral artery with a Beckman microelectrode), endtidal CO_2-concentration (infrared absorption), tidal volume (pneumotachograph and integrator), respiratory rate (electronic counter connected to the integrator output) blood pressure (strain gauge), heart rate (counter connected to the gauge output). Oxygen saturation of the blood was estimated from

*Supported by grants Wi 165 and SFB 114 from the Deutsche Forschungsgemeinschaft

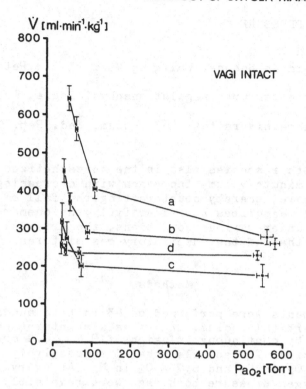

Fig. 1. Average minute volume of ventilation as function of the average arterial oxygen pressure. Four groups of rabbits with intact vagi, each breathing successively pure oxygen, air, 11.9 % O_2 in N_2 and 6.7 % O_2 in N_2, representing four different levels of chemoreflex drive: (a) both sinus nerves intact and PA_{CO_2} kept constant, n = 12; (b) both sinus nerves intact, PA_{CO_2} uncontrolled, n = 11; (c) one sinus nerve intact, n = 6; (d) both sinus nerves cut n = 14. Bars indicate standard errors of the mean $s_{\bar{x}}$.

the measured values of Pa_{O_2} and PA_{CO_2} using the O_2-dissociation curve for rabbit blood determined by Korner and Smith, 1954. Measurements before and after vagal inactivation were averaged and compared to those during the blockade. From the resulting values of the individual preparations under equivalent sinus nerve, vagal and inspiratory gas conditions, mean values, mean differences and the respective significances were computed by the usual methods. Measures of distribution refer to the standard error $s_{\bar{x}}$.

Experimental Condition

Inspiratory gas mixture	Variable	Both sinus nerves cut		One sinus nerve intact		Both sinus nerves intact, CO2 uncontrolled		Both sinus nerves intact, nerves intact, CO2 constant	
		n = 14 (*7,**4)		n = 6		n = 11		n = 12	
Air	PaO2	66.3 ± 2.9	(69.5 ± 3.6)	71.2 ± 5.4	(73.1 ± 6.5)	87.3 ± 4.5	(86.4 ± 4.3)	104.3 ± 4.5	(105.4 ± 5.0)
	$\Delta\dot{V}$	1.3 ± 4.5	(-9.2 ± 3.7)a	19.9 ± 5.0	(24.0 ± 8.9)	26.5 ± 6.0	(21.6 ± 8.2)	123.8 ± 25.9	(108.8 ± 27.9)
11.9 % O2 in N2	PaO2	30.7 ± 1.4	(33.4 ± 1.7)	34.4 ± 4.4	(35.4 ± 4.4)	40.7 ± 2.7	(41.4 ± 2.9)	56.3 ± 2.7	(57.6 ± 3.8)
	$\Delta\dot{V}$	9.3 ± 7.8	(-31.4 ± 8.4)a	93.9 ± 18.7	(93.0 ± 20.3)	106.6 ± 15.2	(107.6 ± 18.3)	281.0 ± 27.4	(206.1 ± 34.9)a
6.7 % O2 in N2	PaO2	*19.5 ± 2.0	(18.4 ± 0.6)	21.1 ± 3.4	(24.6 ± 4.4)	24.6 ± 1.6	(27.6 ± 2.2)a	37.7 ± 2.8	(40.2 ± 3.6)
	$\Delta\dot{V}$	**22.7 ± 25.8	**(-47.9 ± 25.6)a	138.6 ± 24.6	(147.8 ± 27.8)	188.7 ± 23.9	(166.8 ± 23.1)	361.2 ± 32.1	(231.6 ± 32.5)a

Table 1. Mean values and standard errors of the arterial oxygen pressure PaO2 [Torr] during inhalation of air, 11.9 % O2 in N2 and 6.7 % O2 in N2, and of the changes of ventilatory minute volume $\Delta\dot{V}$ [ml/min/kg] measured at these PaO2 values in reference to the respective initial ventilation during breathing of pure oxygen. Four different groups of rabbits at different levels of chemoreflex ventilatory drive with vagi intact (upper values) or inactivated by cold block (values in brackets). In the group with both sinus nerves cut, the severe hypoxic mixture was tolerated only by 7 animals with intact and by 4 with inactivated vagi. a) Significance of difference between vagi intact and inactivated p < 0.05.

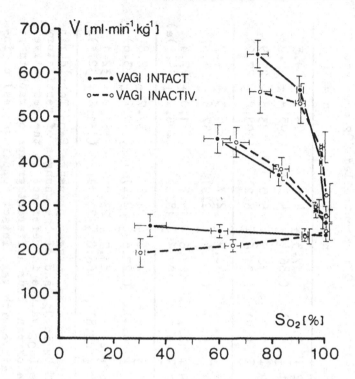

Fig. 2. Average minute volume of ventilation as function
of the average oxygen saturation of the blood (S_{O_2}-values
calculated from the measured Pa_{O_2} values according to Korner
and Smith, 1954). Same groups of rabbits as fig. 1/a, b, d,
each breathing successively pure oxygen, air, 11.9 % O_2 and
6.7 % in N_2, with both sinus nerves intact and Pa_{CO_2} kept
constant (upper pair of curves), both sinus nerves intact and
Pa_{CO_2} uncontrolled (middle), and both sinus nerves cut (lower). Solid lines: vagi intact, broken lines: vagi cold
blocked. Bars indicate standard errors of the mean $s_{\bar{x}}$.

In a first group of 14 rabbits both sinus nerves were
cut; in a second group (n = 6) one sinus nerve was cut, the
other left intact; in a third one (n = 11) both sinus nerves
were intact, the Pa_{CO_2} - as in the previous groups - remaining uncontrolled, and in a fourth group (n = 12) both sinus
nerves were also intact, but the Pa_{CO_2} was kept constant during the hypoxic hyperpnea at 30.7 ± 0.7 Torr by addition of
CO_2 to the inspiratory gas.

Results

1. During inhalation of pure oxygen neither the arterial oxygen pressure nor the ventilatory minute volume differed distinctly between the various preparations, the Pa_{O_2} ranging between 532 and 577 (mean 552.5 ± 7.0) Torr, the ventilation between 181 and 283 (mean 248.3 ± 10.2) ml/min/kg.

2. In the preparation with both sinus nerves cut ventilation was augmented only insignificantly, or even decreased, under hypoxic conditions. In the other preparations ventilation increased with falling Pa_{O_2}, the hyperpnea at each level of oxygenation increasing upon transition from the group with one sinus nerve intact to that with both these nerves functioning, and finally to the preparation with both sinus nerves intact and PA_{CO_2} kept constant. Concomitantly the Pa_{O_2} attained by these preparations under equal normoxic or hypoxic inspiratory O_2-concentrations increased. However, the absolute amount of the improvement in arterial oxygen pressure decreased with the Pa_{O_2}, although the chemoreflex-induced hyperpnea increased progressively, yielding the typical hyperbolic $\dot{V}/Pa_{O_2}$ response curve (fig. 1, table 1).

3. Since the oxygen content of the blood is not linearly related to the arterial oxygen pressure, the relatively small increases of the latter resulting from the hypoxic hyperpnea do not adequately reflect the actual improvement of the oxygen supply by the chemoreflex ventilatory drive. The ventilatory minute volume was therefore related to the arterial oxygen saturation instead of to the Pa_{O_2} (fig. 2). Similarly as before, at all normoxic and hypoxic levels of inspiration the arterial oxygen saturation improved with increasing ventilation. But contrary to fig. 1, on each of these levels the improvement of S_{O_2} produced by the respective chemoreflex drive increased with decreasing Pa_{O_2}: In the animals with bilaterally cut sinus nerves the mean S_{O_2} during respiration of air was 92.2 ± 1.1 %, during breathing of 11.9 % O_2 in N_2 60.3 ± 3.7 %, and during breathing of 6.7 % O_2 in N_2 34.0 ± 6.0 %. During inhalation of air the mean increase of S_{O_2} upon transition to the preparation with both vagi and one sinus nerve intact (not shown in the diagram) was 2.4 ± 1.8 %, to the preparation with both sinus nerves intact 4.6 ± 1.3 %, and to the intact preparation at constant PA_{CO_2} 6.1 ± 1.2 %. During breathing of 11.9 % O_2 in N_2 the respective values were 12.7 ± 6.9 %, 22.3 ± 5.0 % and 30.2 ± 4.1 %, and during breathing of 6.7 % O_2 in N_2 11.1 ± 10.6 %, 25.6 ± 8.2 % and 40.2 ± 9.8 %.

4. After inactivation of the vagi the results were principally the same. However, in the animals with one or both

sinus nerves intact the mean P_{aO_2} (and S_{O_2}) measured during
the inhalation of the normoxic and hypoxic mixtures was often
somewhat higher (although significantly only with both sinus
nerves intact during 6.7 % O_2) than with intact vagi, whereas
the corresponding increase of pulmonary ventilation above the
reference value during pure oxygen was not significantly greater, or even slightly smaller, than before vagal inactivation.
Thus the ventilatory efficiency of the chemoreflex drive as
expressed by the relation $\Delta P_{aO_2}/\Delta \dot{V}$ appeared increased. On the
other hand, in the group with both sinus nerves cut under
6.7 % O_2 in N_2 both the minute volume of ventilation and the
mean P_{aO_2} (respectively S_{O_2}) decreased after vagal inactivation (fig. 2, table 1).

Conclusion

The results indicate that in the rabbit, despite of
seemingly small changes of P_{aO_2}, the carotid chemoreflexes
play an essential role in maintaining the oxygen supply of
the organism during hypoxia.

Reference

P.I. Korner and I. Darian Smith: Cardiac output in normal unanaesthetized and anaesthetized rabbits. Australian
J. exp. Biol. 32, 499 - 510 (1954).

THE OXYGEN BARRIER IN THE CAROTID BODY OF

CAT AND RABBIT

H. Acker, D. W. Lübbers, H. Weigelt, D. Bingmann,
D. Schäfer, and E. Seidl

Max-Planck-Institut für Systemphysiologie, Dortmund, and
Physiologisches Institut der Universität Münster, Germany

After a careful preparation of the carotid body of the cat the surface Po_2 has been measured by means of a Pt needle electrode with a Pt diameter of $3\,u$ fixed within Araldite to increase the outer diameter to $700\,u.$ We found that the surface Po_2 almost reached the arterial Po_2.

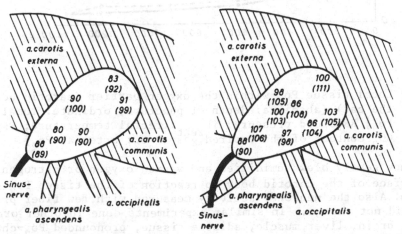

Fig.1: Po_2 measured in different locations at the Surface of the carotid body of the cat. The arterial Po_2 measured simultaneously is given in brackets.

In the first figure the surface Po_2 values are related to the corresponding arterial values (written in brackets). These values mean

that under normal conditions the carotid body of the cat is surrounded by a tissue which has a rather high oxygen tension.

   Puncturing the carotid body of the cat with the Pt needle electrode and inserting the electrode 30 - 70 micron into the tissue the
local oxygen tension dropped to very low values which lie in the
range of 0 - 10 Torr. Together with Purves (1) we succeeded in
puncturing the body in such a way, that the needle went almost
parallel to the surface and could be continuously observed during
the measurements. In this case as shown in Fig. 2 we measured approximately the same Po_2 along the path of the electrode.

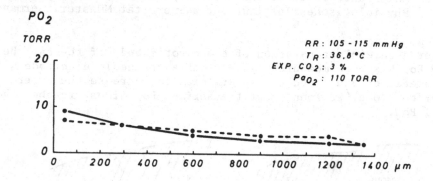

Fig. 2: Local tissue Po_2 within the oxygen barrier (carotid body of
   the cat) (abscissa: depth of puncture; ordinate: local tissue
   Po_2; RR blood pressure; TR_{rekt}: rectal temperature; Exp. CO_2:
   CO_2 content of the expired gas; P_aO_2: arterial Po_2).

If we now gently blew humidified and warmed oxygen or nitrogen over
the surface of the carotid body no reaction of the tissue Po_2 could
be seen. Also the neuronal activity measured with few fiber preparations did not change. In similar experiments done in other organs as
kidney, brain, liver, muscle, adipose tissue, pronounced Po_2-changes
always followed the corresponding gas application. Thus we have
concluded that in the carotid body of the cat there must exist an
oxygen-impermeable zone, - this name describes only the experimental
facts and does not express a possible mechanism. In order to investigate the physiological behavior of this zone we controlled the
reactions of the local Po_2 by two tests: 1. We rose or lowered the
arterial Po_2 by respiration of different gas mixtures, 2. we applied
different gases from the ouside to the surface of the carotid body.
   Applying these tests we were able to distinguish three different

zones: In the outer zone we observed in most cases a positive
reaction to changes of the arterial as well as of the outside Po_2.
In the next zone neither the change of arterial Po_2 nor of the
surrounding Po_2 had any effect on the local Po_2. This corresponds
to the oxygen impermeable zone, or perhaps better "non reactive"
zone. After penetrating this zone we reached a third zone, in which
the local Po_2 reacts to changes in arterial Po_2, but is not influenced by the outside Po_2. The non reactive zone could be destroyed
in different ways.
1) By local electrolysis. The local electrolysis was brought about
by a Pt-electrode with a diameter of 100 u. After the electrolysis
O_2 diffuses into the carotid body. Now in the third zone the locally
measured Po_2 is influenced from outside as well as by the arterial
Po_2.
2) By application of carbonmonoxide, cyanide, antimycine (1 mg
antimycine to 1 ml Ringer solution). Antimycine was applied into
an arterial loop.

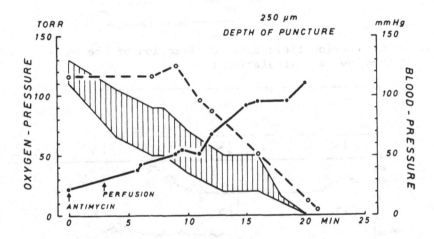

Fig. 3: Destruction of the oxygen barrier by antimycine (solid line:
        tissue oxygen pressure; broken line: arterial Po_2)

Fig. 3 shows the effect of antimycine: With decreasing arterial Po_2
(broken line) and blood pressure a continuous increase in tissue Po_2
(solid line) was observed. Thus later on the local Po_2 is far above
the arterial one.
3) By the death of the animal. About 20 minutes after the animal
being sacrificed diffusion of oxygen into the carotid tissue is
observed again. Fig. 4 shows the oxygen pressure fields as they were
found after this time in the cat's carotid body. The figure shows
measurements performed in four carotid bodies. We can see that there
are high values outside and low ones inside the carotid body corres-

ponding to the diffusion from outside. The depth of the punctures
was maximum 600/u.

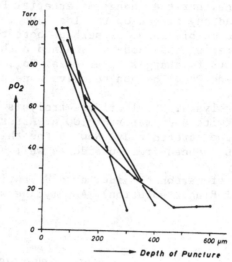

Fig. 4: Oxygen tension field after destruction of the oxygen barrier
by 20-minutes' circulation stop.

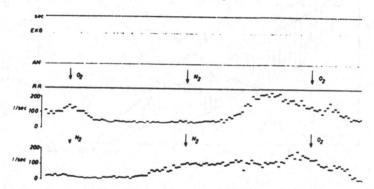

Fig.5: Influence of different gases applied from the outside of the
carotid body of the cat on the neuronal activity (few fiber
preparation) (EKG: electrocardiogram; arrow O_2: blowing of
oxygen onto the surface of the carotid body; arrow N_2: blowing
of nitrogen; I/sec: number of pulses per second)

Fig. 5 shows that, after this time, also the chemoreceptor activity
could be influenced from the ouside what was impossible before. Blood
pressure decreased to zero, ventilation was stopped. The EKG (electrocardiogram) reveals single discharges. The chemoreceptor can be
still active producing impulses at a rate of 100/sec. When adiminist-
ering oxygen or nitrogen from outside, the chemoreceptor activity
changes in a direction as was expected. It decreases with the

application of oxygen and increases with nitrogen. Electron microscopic photographs (Fig. 6a,b,c) showed in this area below the
outer fat cells (6a; F), looking empty because of the technique of
preparation, a zone containing blood vessels of different diameters
(a; B) and nerves (6a; N).

Fig. 6a,b,c: Electron micrograph from the oxygen barrier of the
    glomus caroticum of the cat. a) Low power electron micrograph.
    The drawn line marks the proceeding of the boundary zone (upper
    part) towards the centrally situated receptor cells (RF). (F =
    fat cell; B = blood vessel; N = nerve; arrows = type-I cell; E =
    elastic fibers; C = collagen fibers; CT = cells of connective
    tissue; /um bar: 10/um in 6a, c, and 5/um in 6b). [See next page]

This zone marked by a line proceeds into the central zone of the
carotid body containing receptor cells (6a, RF; type I cells marked
by arrows). Higher magnification of the boundary zone shows that it
contains fibers of collagen (6a; C) and elastic fibers (6b, c; E)
between which cells of connective tissue (6b, c; CT) are situated
with pseudopod-like processes. Around the larger arterial vessels
the fore-mentioned structures are more or less parallel arranged
(6c), but this arrangement was not found on the other places.

An oxygen barrier could also be found in the carotid body of the
rabbit. In this animal the oxygen barrier seems to be larger than
in the cat. Puncturing the carotid body of the rabbit (Fig.7) from
the surface one observes first tissue Po_2 value being within the
normal range which could be increased by blowing for 20 -30 seconds
oxygen onto the surface of the carotid body.

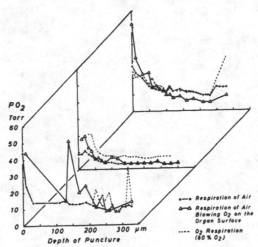

Fig. 7: Local tissue Po_2 of the carotid body of the rabbit (abscissa:
    depth of puncture in /um; ordinate: local tissue Po_2 in Torr.
    Three different punctures.

614

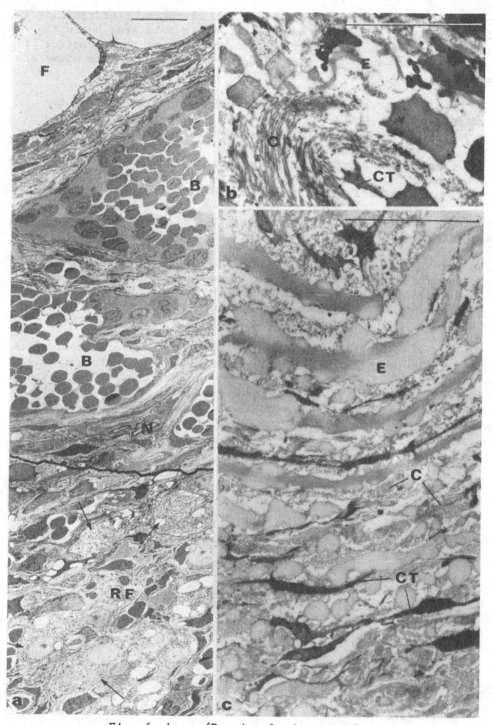

Fig. 6a,b,c: (Previously described).

The same reaction was obtained by applying oxygen or nitrogen-saturated Ringer solution. After deeper penetration this reaction stopped, sometimes in a range of only 10 um. Histological controls showed that the first reaction was found in a zone containing fat cells and connective tissue. The second reaction corresponded to a zone where specific glomus cells began to appear. In this area the oxygen barrier must be situated. After penetration of this second zone one reaches the third zone. In the third zone application of oxygen to the surface produced either no change or a decrease of local tissue Po_2. At the moment we have no explanation for the latter reaction. I may mention that an oxygen-impermeable zone was also found in the wall of the carotid artery (2).-In summary, our experiments have shown that the carotid body of the cat as well as the carotid body of the rabbit are isolated from the Po_2 of the surrounding tissue by a special zone which does not allow the oxygen to penetrate in to the inner part of the organ. We think, this is important for a correct function of the chemoreceptor which, being so small , otherwise would be influenced by the metabolism of the surrounding tissue. The mechanism of this oxygen-impermeable barrier is not understood. We think that probably a combination of oxidative processes with a structural change of the tissue, probably the collagen; could be involved .

REFERENCES

1) Acker, H., Lübbers, D.W., Purves, M.J.: O_2-Transfer in der Bindegewebskapsel des Glomus caroticum der Katze und seine funktionelle Bedeutung. Pflügers Arch. 316, R 30 (1970).

2) Acker, H., Lübbers, D.W.: Eine sauerstoffdurchlässige Zone in der Wand der Arteria. Experentia 27, 394 - 395 (1971).

ROLE OF THE CAROTID CHEMORECEPTORS IN THE ADJUSTMENT OF ARTERIAL BLOOD PRESSURE TO HYPOXIA

Wolfgang Wiemer*, Heidrun Schöne and Peter Kiwull

Arbeitsgruppe Regulationsphysiologie, Inst. Physiol.

Ruhr-Universität, 463 Bochum, Fed. Rep. Germany

Excitation of the arterial chemoreceptors has been shown to cause reflex vasoconstriction (Daly and Scott, 1962) modified secondarily by vagal inflation reflexes and baroreflexes (Korner, 1965; Daly and Robinson, 1968; Crocker et al., 1968). The following experiments dealt with the chemoreflex regulation of blood pressure under hypoxia in the rabbit.

Methods

Anesthesia and recording apparatus were the same as described in the previous presentation (Schöne et al., this publication). In a first series on 11 rabbits with intact and 14 with cut sinus nerves the animal breathed successively 100 % O_2, air, 11.9 % O_2 in N_2, and 6.7 % O_2 in N_2. In addition, in both types of preparation the vagi were reversibly inactivated under these conditions by cold blocking. In two further series on 6 respectively 10 rabbits with sectioned vagi both sinus nerves were temporarily cold blocked. In the former group this was done alternately during inhalation of 100 % oxygen and 10.5 % O_2 in N_2, with common carotid arteries clamped or unclamped under either condition. In the latter group the animal inhaled air, whereas the sinus nerves were blocked alternately at normal systemic blood pressure and after lowering this pressure to an average of (diastolic) 44.1 + 8.7 mm Hg by bleeding the animal from the femoral artery (Ott et al.,

---

*Supported by grants Wi 165 and SFB 114 from the Deutsche Forschungsgemeinschaft

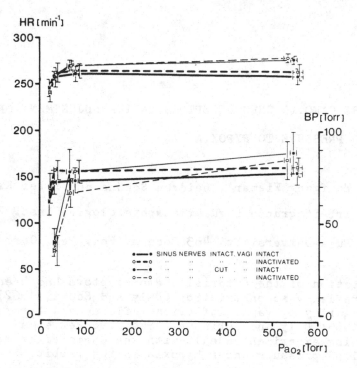

Fig. 1. Mean arterial blood pressure (lower curves) and
heart rate (upper curves) as function of the arterial Pa_{O_2}.
Average values and standard errors (bars) of six rabbits
breathing successively 100 % oxygen, air, 11.9 % O_2 in N_2 and
6.7 % O_2 in N_2 before (heavy lines) and after (thin lines)
section of both sinus nerves, with vagi intact (solid lines)
or inactivated by cold block (broken lines). Since after elimination of the sinus nerves the latter mixture was not tolerated by part of the animals, values are given for preparations
with intact sinus nerves only.

1971). These blockades were also performed with open as well
as clamped carotid arteries. In the fourth series on 7 rabbits
both sinus nerves were cut. The animal was given successively
pure oxygen, air, 11.9 % O_2 in N_2, and 6.7 % O_2 in N_2, and
the vagi were - as before - inactivated reversibly on each
level of oxygenation by cold blocking. Under every one of
these blood gas and vagal conditions one sinus nerve was then
stimulated electrically for about 40 s, the intensity of stimulation (square waves of 1 ms duration and 40 imp/s frequency;
voltage adjusted in every preparation for distinct, sub-maxi-
mal responses) remaining constant throughout the experiment.
Pa_{CO_2} remained uncontrolled in all experiments described in
this section.

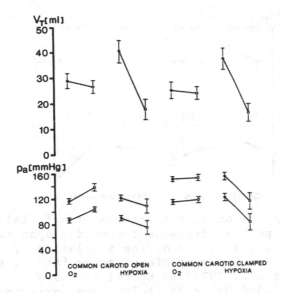

Fig. 2. Effects of cold blocking of both sinus nerves on
tidal volume (upper curves) and systolic respectively diastolic blood pressure (lower curves), before (left sections)
and after (right) bilateral clamping of the common carotid
artery. Under both these conditions blockades were performed
during inhalation of O_2 and of 10.5 % O_2 in N_2. Mean values
and standard errors from the same 6 rabbits before (dots)
and during (open circles) blockade.

Results

(1) Fig. 1 demonstrates the typical influence of lowering
the PaO_2 on mean blood pressure and heart rate in 6 rabbits
in which measurements could be obtained from the same animal
with intact as well as with cut sinus nerves: As long as the
latter nerves were intact, this influence was rather slight,
blood pressure and heart rate decreasing significantly only
during rather severe hypoxia. After section of the sinus
nerves both variables - although starting from slightly higher initial levels - decreased more distinctly with the PaO_2,
the reaction being dominated by a steep fall of blood pressure. Thus, elimination of the sinus nerves below 30 Torr
PaO_2 frequently resulted in circulatory and secondary respiratory failure. Inactivation of the vagi modified these reactions slightly but did not change them essentially.

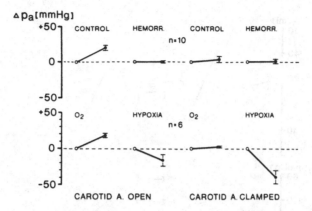

Fig. 3. Comparison of the changes of arterial blood pressure (increase upwards, decrease downwards) upon cold blocking
of both carotid sinus nerves during inhalation of air at normal ('control') or low systemic pressure (above, same experiments as Ott et al., 1971)and normal pressure during inhalation of O_2 or 10.5 % O_2 in N_2 (below, same experiments as fig.
2), the respective initial values before the blockades ser-
ving as reference. The upper diagram represents mean values
and standard errors of 10 rabbits, the lower diagram corresponding measurements in 6 rabbits, each before (left sections) and after (right) bilateral clamping of the common carotid artery.

(2) In animals with intact sinus nerves, the chemoreflex
drive on blood pressure was also modified by counterregula-
tion through carotid baroreflexes. Thus, the moderate decrease of blood pressure resulting from cold blocking the sinus nerves during hypoxia with open common carotid arteries
(chemo- and baroreflexes activated) appeared, grossly, as the
resultant of the increase observed upon blocking these nerves
during hyperoxia with open carotids (only baroreflexes activated) and the much greater decrease caused by the blockade
during hypoxia with these arteries clamped (only chemoreflexes
activated, cf. fig. 2).

(3) In the rabbit, excitation of the carotid chemoreceptors under these conditions was due primarily to hypoxia of
the blood, not to concomitant lowering of blood pressure.
This became apparent in the experiments with hemorrhage under
normoxia: Neither before nor after clamping of the common ca-
rotied arteries (causing the local pressure in the sinus region to decrease even below 40 mm Hg) blocking of the carotid
sinus nerves was followed by a decrease of blood pressure or

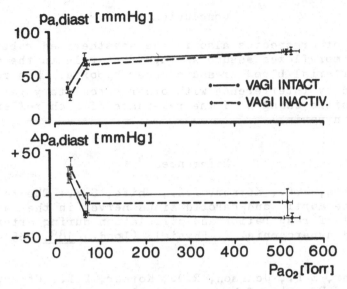

Fig. 4. Response of diastolic blood pressure to electrical stimulation of one cut carotid sinus nerve as function of
the Pa_{O_2}. Mean values and standard errors (bars) of the pressure before (upper diagram) stimulation, and of the change of
pressure upon (lower diagram) stimulation, obtained from 7
rabbits breathing successively 100 % oxygen, air, and 11.9 %
O_2 in N_2, with vagi intact (solid lines) or inactivated by
cold blocking (broken lines).

diminution of respiration which would have indicated a significant chemoreflex drive (fig. 3, above).

(4) Under normoxic conditions, electrical stimulation of
the sinus nerve usually caused - besides an increase of ventilation - a decrease of blood pressure. The latter evidently
resulted from concomitant excitation of baroreceptor fibres
overweighing the stimulator effects of the chemoreceptor component. However, under hypoxia this depressant effect reversed
into a distinct increase of blood pressure (fig. 4). This
seems to indicate that the chemoreflex support of blood pressure is not only due to the magnitude of hypoxic excitation
of the chemoreceptors, but also to an increase of efficacy of
this drive under low Pa_{O_2}. The mechanisms - which could, principally, involve central as well as effector components of
the reflexes involved - can, at present, only be conjectured.

Conclusion

As in other species also in the anesthetized rabbit the
carotid chemoreflexes assume an important role in the maintenance of arterial blood pressure under hypoxia. This role is
complicated by interference with other circulatory reflexes
and by possible changes of the relevance of such reflex factors under hypoxia.

References

Chalmers, I.P., Korner, P.I., White, S.W.: The relative
roles of the aortic and carotid sinus nerves in the rabbit in
the control of respiration and circulation during arterial
hypoxia and hypercapnia. J. Physiol. (Lond.) 188, 435 - 450
(1967).

Crocker, E.F., Johnson, R.O., Korner, P.I., Uther, J.B.,
Withe, S.W.: Effects of hyperventilation on the circulatory
response of the rabbit to arterial hypoxia. J. Physiol. (Lond.)
199, 267 - 282 (1968).

Daly, M. de B., Robinson, D.H.: An analysis of the reflex vasodilator response by lung inflation of the dog. J.
Physiol. (Lond.) 195, 387 - 406 (1968).

Daly, M. de B., Scott, M.J.: Analysis of the primary
cardiovascular reflex effects of stimulation of the carotid
body chemoreceptors in the dog. J. Physiol. (Lond.) 162,
555 - 573 (1962).

Korner, P.I.: The role of the arterial chemoreceptors
and baroreceptors in the circulatory response to hypoxia of
the rabbit. J. Physiol. (Lond.) 180, 279 - 303 (1965).

Ott, N., Kiwull, P., Wiemer, W.: Zur Bedeutung der Che-
moreflexe des Karotis- und Aortengebietes für die Atmungs-
und Blutdruckregulation bei herabgesetztem Blutdruck. Z.
Kreislaufforsch. 60, 648 - 660 (1971).

Wiemer, W., Schöne, H., Kiwull, P.: The influence of
PaO2 on the effects of sinus nerve stimulation with intact
and inactivated vagi. Pflügers Arch. (in press), 1973.

DISCUSSION OF SESSION II   SUBSESSION: VASCULAR CHEMORECEPTORS
                                                 AND OXYGEN BARRIER

Chairmen: Dr. Thomas K. Goldstick, Dr. David C. MacGregor and
           Dr. Carl R. Honig

DISCUSSION OF PAPER BY B. R. DULING

Goldstick: (1) The level of oxygen in the smooth muscle cells is
going to depend both on the intravascular and extravascular pO_2.
In the case of the pipette in the suffusion solution on the velocity
of the fluids involved, it wasn't clear to me what the relationship
is between your measurement of perivascular pO_2 and the average pO_2
in the muscle cell.
    (2) What kinds of vessels did you test?

Duling: (1) The vessels that were tested were all small and terminal arterioles. This was done on the basis of some previous work
that we had done which indicated that that was probably where any
regulation that did occur was taking place. Obviously, the geome-
tries of this thing are such that there are fairly large gradients
in pO_2. What I have presented are the most conservative estimates
of the changes on pO_2.
    (2) With regard to the problem of pO_2 across the wall, we have
measured previously, in vessels larger than this (by larger, I am
talking of 40 or 50 microns), intravascular vs. extravascular pO_2.
In those vessels, we found no more than a 5 mm Hg pressure difference
across the wall. Furthermore, you can calculate that it should not
be any more than that, and these vessels have substantially thinner
walls than that. I think that the pO_2 that I am measuring is very
close to the pO_2 of the smooth-muscle cell at that point and is the
lowest pO_2 when I am applying the oxygen solutions.

Goldstick: The experiments that you have described clearly eliminate the possibility that oxygen, per se, controls flow through
direct effect on arteriolar muscle. Some sort of feedback signal,
presumably humural is necessary. Your previous work on the transmural oxygen gradient in small vessels also clearly established
this idea. However, I think it should be recognized that there is
a danger in the use of the term 'vascular smooth muscle,' that vessels in organs of different metabolic rates behave in different
ways. The tissue that you have used has a relatively low oxygen
consumption, and the controls of both arterioles and precapillary
sphincters appear different in low and high oxygen consumption
tissues. Also, in the case of precapillary sphincters, I think
that oxygen does, in fact, control these particular vascular muscles.
It seems to me that the diffusion condition around the precapillary
sphincter is such that the sphincter could detect what is going on

in the tissue during the contraction phase of its duty cycle, and that, from the data I presented earlier, it seems that oxygen, per se, is, for this particular vascular effector, the controlling substance. I am suggesting that the role of oxygen in the control of blood flow is quite different from the role of oxygen in the control of diffusion distance. We have to clearly separate these two things. Different processes—different effectors.

Duling: One of the things that I think is reasonably important about the work that I have done is that it shows how you don't need to have different controls for different things. The vascular smooth muscle responds fairly uniformly, as far as I can see. The difference is in the geometrics of the system, not in the vascular smooth muscle. I think it is important to recognize that, as far as I am aware, nobody has any evidence that vascular smooth muscle, anywhere in high metabolic tissues or low metabolic tissues, responds to oxygen at levels that are in excess of a couple of mm Hg. As far as the interactions between the tissue and the smooth muscle, certainly there are differences in different tissues, and there are probably differences in precapillary sphincters.

Nicoll: I would like to raise a point about the role of oxygen in control of blood flow. I think the evidence that oxygen is not itself a stimulant to the activation of smooth muscle should not be taken as the final word that oxygen does not control the activity of controlling smooth muscles. In other words, you may have other situations which are the stimulants for smooth muscle activity, but it is the level of oxygen available at the precapillary sphincters that tends to regulate the duration of their constriction or the failure of their constriction, and hence, the amount of blood that will flow through the microvascular beds.

Lübbers: I would like to ask if, in the oxygen which you applied to the vessel, you had added some CO_2 or some other things, because it would probably wash out some of the CO_2 which was originally in the blood.

Duling: I think CO_2 is a very real possibility for the thing that was causing the constriction. I cannot distinguish CO_2 from hydrogen or adenosine or whatever you might want to propose.

Lübbers: But you controlled the pH?

Duling: The pH is controlled with trisk buffers so that I don't have problems with loss of CO_2 and uncontrolled pH.

Lübbers: It has been shown, at least in the brain vessel, that they are very sensitive against sodium bicarbonate concentration. There is a medium range between 12, as I remember, and 18. This basic concentration in the perivascular space influences, at least in the brain vessels, the tone and the reaction of two gases and CO_2. Probably the basic situation in your preparation would have changed if you had changed the CO_2 concentration and the bicarbonate concentration, even the response to oxygen.

Duling: It is a possibility, certainly. The feeling that I have on the matter is that it is generally accepted that, with one exception that I am aware of at least, the cytochrome oxidase system of tissues is not limited until the pO_2 falls to very low values. This was what put me on to this particular problem. I am simply assuming that the vascular smooth muscle behaves the same way and that is what I have attempted to demonstrate in vivo here. We have done other in vitro studies to show that it does.

Lübbers: But I think nobody knows if there are other oxygen-receptor nodes around the tissue because we don't know how they look. We cannot find them.

Duling: As a matter of fact, I suppose that the sum of my experiments would be a plea to look for other oxygen receptors than the cytochrome oxidase system or the smooth muscle cells themselves.

DISCUSSION OF PAPER BY D. BINGMANN, H. ACKER AND H. SCHULZE

Zielinski: (1) What was a situation with efferent innervation of carotid body in your experiments?

(2) Do you think there is any possibility that sustained sympathetic innervation can participate in discrepancies of the tissue and arterial pO_2 time course?

Bingmann: (1) In the experiments presented here, both sinus nerves were cut, whereas the sympathetic innervation was left as well intact as possible.

(2) Variations of sympathetic influence on the carotid body can certainly attribute to the discrepancy in the relation between the tissue pO_2 and the PaO_2 found in severe hypoxia, but our point was, first, to find out the general reactions.

DISCUSSION OF PAPER BY H. ACKER, D. W. LÜBBERS AND H. WEIGELT
     (Paper was presented by Dr. D. W. Lübbers.)

<u>Song</u>: I am interested and impressed by your beautiful electron
microscopic picture. I wonder whether you have observed any gland-
ular or secretory structures in the carotid body, such as erythro-
protein like granules?

<u>Lübbers</u>: We observed only the well-known structural elements in
the glomus cells. Thus I have no new information.

<u>Whalen</u>: As you know, we have made measurements of tissue pO_2 in the
same preparation you use and have obtained very few low values and
oppositely-directed profiles of pO_2. Our results, in one respect
do agree, however. That is, that when the cat is breathing air,
the pO_2 in the outer 100 μ of the cat carotid body is not notice-
ably affected by changes in the pO_2 of the solution flowing over
the body. Of course, our values there are near arterial. When the
cat has breathed low O_2 mixtures for some time, and has a low arterial pressure and presumeably slower flow in the carotid body, there
the external pO_2 has some affect on the intra-carotid body measurements. I think it is a question of the sizes of the sink and source
of O_2. Generally, the question I do not understand is, how the
impermeable layer works, is it a double membrane?

<u>Lübbers</u>: Since the meeting in Dortmund (1971), we have tried to
find out why our group in Dortmund and Muunster finds constantly
different results from Dr. Whalen. At the moment, the only reason
I could think of is, there are species differences. We have found
that the carotid body of the rabbit varies greatly in respect to
its structure. In some rabbits, it is very differentiated, but we
always found the "oxygen impermeable" zone. To settle this important
disagreement, we should try to do experiments together.

SUMMARY - SESSIONS I AND II

I. A. Silver

Department of Pathology

University of Bristol, England

Mr. Chairman, Ladies and Gentlemen, I have two alter-
natives, one is to read a list of contributors and their
titles, and the other is to give rein to my personal pre-
judices and naturally I shall indulge in the latter.

In the section on Instrumentation and Methods it is
clear that there is a cheerful rivalry between the people
who wield electrodes and those who hide behind mass spec-
trometers and those who illuminate their work with optical
probe techniques. In the field of oxygen electrodes there
is still some controversy over the question of whether
voltages should be applied as a D.C. potential or in
pulses. Although theoretically the pulsing system should
be superior the many practical difficulties still limit
its use to relatively few intrepid investigators.

The newest application of fluorescent probes both for
potentiometric investigation of membranes and for the
direct demonstration of oxygen tension with pyrene deriva-
tives opens up exciting possibilities for the study of
organ surfaces or tissue culture mono-layers with a relatively non-destructive system for examining cellular
states. The present trend appears to be to combine different techniques and to marry the chemical, physiological
and engineering approaches.

Mass spectrometry seems to be a useful tool in many
situations involving relatively gross work and is obviously an excellent clinical weapon. It has however a
relatively slow response and poor resolution. It will

surely   require considerable development before it can be
used to advance our understanding of tissue oxygen transport at the cellular level.   It is however clearly useful
for obtaining an integrated oxygen tension value in a
relatively small volume of tissue and is excellent in that
it combines oxygen, CO_2 and nitrogen measurements.

Techniques for continuous monitoring of arterial PO_2
are increasingly becoming more sophisticated both in terms
of trans-cutaneous measurements and of intra-arterial
catheters.   There still seems to be a conflict in the
assessment of the usefulness of superficial measurements
but it has been demonstrated that at least in young children, these are directly related to arterial PO_2. The
major problems with the intra-arterial probes are also not
yet solved;   these include drift and platelet adhesion.
There is as yet no long term intra-arterial system which
can be relied upon.   Intravascular mass-spectrometry also
has its problems and leakage still appears not to have
been overcome.

Of the other techniques now being developed, glucose
oxidase anodal electrodes which have been elegantly demonstrated by the Clarks, should considerably extend our
understanding of tissue metabolism.   Of course, this type
of electrode is not limited to investigations of glucose
and will undoubtedly give rise to a whole field of study
in the future.

The rapid increase in the utilisation of multiparameter methods indicates the degree of confidence in
techniques being used. One wonders whether this confidence is always entirely justified since it is dangerously
easy to become lulled into a sense of false security if
one accepts the infalibility of the technique without the
most rigorous checks. A few years ago the oxygen electrode
was regarded with the gravest of suspicion by many people
and it is still a tool which has to be treated as a form
of modified witchcraft, even though of course it can give
very useful information.   On the other hand if one is too
timid, no progress can be made, but I would like to empha-
sise that the ideal oxygen electrode has still to be found.
We have problems with insulation near the tips of microelectrodes and we also have problems with membranes and
stability.   The newer systems involving the deposition in
high vacuum of silicon dioxide as an insulator and the deposition of polymer membranes in ionising fields show that
improvements are being sought very actively.

With regard to oxygen transport to tissue, the factors involved in the release of oxygen from haemoglobin
and especially the role of 2,3,DPG and other phosphates
are very much a realm for active investigation. Together
with the question of release of oxygen from haemoglobin we
have had extensive discussions on how the body regulates
the blood reaching the tissue and on what happens to the
tissue that gets too much or too little oxygen. The
problems of auto-regulation of oxygen supply still provide a fertile field for experimentation and imagination.
This seems to be an area in which computer modeling has
the most to offer at present. The other area which excited much comment may be summarised as:-
"Having restricted or overdone the oxygen supply, what
happens in the tissue; what is the physiological limit of
hypoxia or hyperoxia and when does the system start to become pathological? How can we detect this pathophysiological borderline and at what point does the pathological
change become irreversible? Is the damage that results
from hypoxia or hyperoxia due directly to oxygen lack or
to some other factor such as pH or CO_2 or are the changes
due to failure of energy production?"

A very valuable aspect to the Sessions has been the
interchange between the people who think in terms of
enzymatic electron transfer, those who think in terms of
sub-cellular organelles and membranes, those who work at
whole cell level, those who consider only whole organs and
the unsophisticated among us who believe that what happens
to the whole organism is what ultimately matters. At
least we should all know now how to convert from micro-
moles of oxygen to PO_2. The serious aspect of this discussion was relevant to many pathological states and
especially conditions such as haemorrhagic shock, and
cerebro-vascular or coronary-arterial accidents.

Oxygen detectors in tissues, the presence of which
are indicated repeatedly by studies on the carotid body,
on microcirculation and in the intriguing observations of
Haim Bicher pose a most fascinating problem as to what is
the oxygen sensor? We seem to have accepted the idea of
oxygen sensors without too much discussion as to what they
actually are. The biochemists have shown us that cytochromes can act as sensors, but of course they can only do
so at very low oxygen tensions, yet it is clear that the
organism is very much more sensitive to changes of oxygen
tension higher up the scale than are the cytochromes.

The first two sessions here have done three things,
1) they have tested the resiliance of workers in the field

and observations suggest that working on oxygen transport
develops an unusual toughening of the moral fibre, 2) they
have indicated the areas which may be suitable for attack
in the biological and clinical context and 3) they have
produced fuel for mathematical analysis of what is really
going on in the tissues, and we are all looking forward to
learning from the sessions at Clemson that all our problems
will be solved by the computers.

Perhaps I should finish with a somewhat scurrilous
story about the definition of the surgeon, the physician
and the pathologist.   The surgeon is reputed to be a man
who knows nothing but is willing to undertake anything.
The physician on the other hand is a man who claims to
know everything, but is unwilling to do anything except
possibly to take a large fee.   The pathologist, of
course, is a man who not only knows everything but does
everything; unfortunately he always does it a day too
late.   This meeting will I hope, have stimulated surgeons
to think before they act and physicians to put their
thoughts into action.   Pathologists, I am afraid, are a
more difficult case; if we were to act earlier we would
soon work ourselves out of a job and that is not a
natural human response.

Finally I would like to congratulate the local
committee and particularly Haim Bicher.   We have all
been told that the greatest use of these congresses is
that we should make friends and it is a tribute to Haim
Bicher to say that not only have we made friends, but we
have even been able to smile at each other at 8 o'clock
in the morning.

GENERAL DISCUSSION OF SESSION II

Chairmen: Dr. Thomas K. Goldstick, Dr. David C. MacGregor and
Dr. Carl R. Honig

Ernest: I am interested in chronic preparation and would like to ask: Once the perfusion pressure has been lowered to a steady level and held, autoregulation has occurred and a new steady state takes place, is that new steady state, then, acceptable for the organism or will there, with time, be a breakdown?

Goldstick: It would seem to me that operating at a lower oxygen level would eventually lead to cell death, of some cells, at least. I guess that that should be apparent to a pathologist, and if there is one here who would care to comment, I would appreciate it.

Silver: I can't answer that particular question. I think that you do get areas of cell death when you get a resetting at the lower levels. The only place we have done any critical investigation has been in brain, where you find that certain areas of the brain seem to have set pO_2's, and that they will deviate from this, as a result of activity. My experience is that, if you record oxygen at a particular site and then drive the cell at that site, there will be about a 1.5-second lag, during which time the oxygen tension will fall. It will then, return to the original level during the time of maximal cellular activity. As soon as you stop driving the cell, there will be a pO_2 overshoot. It goes hyperoxygenated for, again, about 1.5 or 2 seconds and then the level will go back to the original one, but the level which is set in any one place is not the same as that which may be 10, 15, or 20 microns away.

Lübbers: Normally, at a little bit lower temperature, we could not find any change in the redox potential of the redox state of cytochrome-cytochrome A, which should have been affected. Even if the pO_2 is as low as 1 millimeter, it means we cannot exactly say it is zero or very close to it. The trouble is, that these photometric measurements integrate over an area of 3 millimeters square, or a diameter of 3 millimeters, so it could be that in this area it is a little bit smaller. It could be that in one part of the area, oxygen tension is lower, but at least we didn't see any reduction of cytochrome A_3.

Honig: Perhaps, Dr. Silver, a partial answer to your question might be that the same cells are not always the ones with exceedingly low oxygen tensions. Many years ago, Grote pointed out that in skeletal muscle, the anoxic regions are, so to speak, rotated. This has now been shown for heart, and presumably it would occur in brain as well, so that, perhaps, one cell is hypoxic for a short

time and another cell then becomes hypoxic when the first one
receives some oxygen.

Lübbers: This is very true for the brain. It can share very
quickly in one site. I don't have the cycle of rotation, but
this is exactly what we have seen.

Kessler: I would like to point out that hypoxia itself, for a
short time, is not as dangerous as ischemia. When we have hypoxia,
there is a kind of inhibition of metabolism, so the energy requirement is relatively low. From our measurements we know that under
these conditions, anaerobic glycolysis can provide the cell with
enough energy for a certain time. Of course, this is not possible
in an organ which has to do big work such as the heart, and I do
not know the situation in the brain, but they are certainly organs;
for instance, the liver and probably the skeletal muscle, where
short periods of anoxia do not harm the cells themselves. As soon
as we have ischemia then, of course, we get severe acidosis; this
severe acidosis depolarizes the cells, and then the sodium and
potassium pumps are activated. By this activation, we have a waste
of energy within a very short time, as we know. It is a little bit
different in the different organs, say in the brain, I think about
2 or 3 minutes, and in the liver, somewhat longer. This is a very
severe situation for tissue, indeed. What we need, is to prevent
ischemia in microcirculation, but anoxia for a short time is not
that dangerous.

MacGregor: I might make one comment myself, as a mass spectrometist
rather than a polarographer. We have had a tremendous exchange of
ideas in terms of the size of the probe and whether we are actually
measuring tissue, or damaged tissue, or intercellular, and so on.
The one thing that becomes evident to me with mass spectrometry is
that, although there may be a considerable degree of argument about
what some of the absolute values that we achieve are, certainly,
with any intervention, like marked hypoxia or anoxic arrest of the
heart when surgery is performed, the mass-spectrometric technique
certainly picks it up quite quickly. Also, we were able to demonstrate this gradient between the epicardium and endocardium, and
strangely enough, some of the values that we have, although the
range is quite wide, are pretty close to some of those found by
polarography in the various levels of tissue. We have found mass
spectrometry to be quite a reliable tool, particularly in the operating room where a rugged type of instrument is necessary.

Benzing: I agree with the opinion of Dr. Kessler. In experiments
performed together with Dr. Gebert (cf. G. Gebert, H. Benzing and
M. Strohm. Changes in the Interstitial pH of Dog Myocardium in
Response to local Ischemia, Hypoxia, Hyper- and Hypocapnia, Measured
Continuously by Means of Glass Microelectrodes, Pflügers Arch., 329:

72-81, 1971; H. Benzing, M. Strohm and G. Gebert. The Effect of
Local Ischemia on the Ionic Activity of Dog Myocardial Interstitium,
Vascular Smooth Muscle, edited by E. Betz, Springer-Verlag, Berlin,
Heidelberg, New York, 1972.) we investigated the changes on interstitial myocardial H^+, K^+ and Na^+ activity during hypoxic hypoxia
and during occlusion of the left descending artery. If the blood
flow was reduced by shortlasting occlusions, we found an increase
in H^+ and K^+ activity, and a decrease of Na^+ activity. After release of blood flow, all values returned to the starting level.
During hypoxic hypoxia, there was an increase in blood flow, a
small decrease in H^+ activity and no visible changes in K^+ and Na^+
activity in the interstitial tissue. This indicates that local
tissue hypoxia is tolerated relatively better than a decrease of
blood flow below a critical value, which leads to an interstitial
acidosis and leakage of intracellular potassium ions.

MacGregor: That is probably why we get so much benefit from washing out of the coronary circulation during anoxia.

Lübbers: Dr. Silver, you mentioned that you have the idea that
collagen could be changed by the application of temperature. We
applied temperature of 42 degrees to the surface of the skin to
get enough blood flow for measuring, in a good approximation, the
arterial blood gas tension. We have done this for 6 or 7 hours
without seeing any damage to the skin. Later, you can occasionally
see a pink spot on the skin, but it goes away completely. Have
you, as a pathologist, any experience that you could show, after
such local damage, any change in the skin histology?

Silver: Chemically, skin collagen starts to denature at 40 degrees,
you begin to get changes in the end terminals of the alpha chains
of collagen. However, I think the only physiological thing that
is likely to happen with heating to 43 degrees, has not really to
do with the denaturing of collagen which is going to be very slow,
but the development of low-grade inflammatory changes. Certainly,
if you heat the skin to this temperature and then inject, you do
get very slight changes in vessel permeability at really quite low
temperatures. If you sit in a hot bath long enough, the structure
of the superficial capillary bed does change very slightly. It is
a reversible change, but it does change, and I suspect that, although
I don't think it is significant, I think if you let it go on for
longer, you would get distinct pathological changes.

Clark, L. C.: Drs. Albert and Renate Huch will present their
research with the surface pO_2 electrode later. I have just seen
a demonstration of their skin electrode and I must say it was most
impressive. It was, indeed, an elegant performance. The electrode
works like a charm. It should find wide use in clinical medicine
especially in the monitoring of the newborn.

INDEX

Pages 1-636 will be found in Volume 37A, pages 637-1144 in Volume 37B.

Acid,
    ascorbic, 131
    lactic, 814, 815, 816, 849, 854, 1043
    pyruvic, 849
    see Lactate-pyruvic, 849
    see Lactate-pyruvate ratio

Acidosis,
    fetal, 1067, 1068, 1071
    skeletal muscle, 447

Action potential,
    measurement of, 215
    relation to PO_2, 217

Adair model, 199, 927

Adenyl-cyclase, 1052

Aggregation,
    blood cell, 89, 641, 647, 657, 735
    during pulmonary embolism, 638, 733
    platelet, 681

Alkalosis, 447, 1067, 1068, 1073

Alloxan, 173, 174

Anaphylaxis, 638

Anatomical parameters, 803
    see Modeling

liii

Anemia, 1075, 1077

Anesthesia, 71, 340
        effect on oxygen transport, 261

Anoxia, 216, 219, 522, 832, 849, 854, 895
        effect on liver, 371
        fetal, 1021, 1024

Anti-adhesive drugs, 657, 737

Arterial PO_2
        see PO_2

Arterial pressure, 21
        regulation, 617
        sinusoidal oscillation, 417
        see Blood pressure

Asphyxia, 1047, 1049, 1050, 1051

ATP, 814, 815
        effect of diabetes, 175
        effect of ischemia and anoxia, 371
        in perfused liver, 371

Autoregulation, 755, 820, 908
        blood flow, 417, 491
                effect of hypoglycemia, 221
                effect of hypoxia, 455
                effect of metabolism, 451
                effect of oxygen, 623
                effect of PO_2, 591
                in skeletal muscle, 452
                in spleen, 391
                model for, 420
        oxygen, 215
                definition, 441
                in skeletal muscle, 441
        perfusion, 258

Barbiturates, 116, 263, 266, 268

Blood,
        base excess, 305
        replacement, 687
        sludged, 641
        velocity measurement, 102
        volume measurement, 102
        see Aggregation, Flow, Red blood cell

Blood pressure,
        effect on chemoreceptors, 617
        see Arterial pressure

Bohr effect, 1056

Bolus, 830

Boundary layer, 867, 952, 961

Brain, 215-347, 752, 753, 754, 762, 771, 798, 849, 887
        effect of anesthetic drugs, 263
        effect of arterial PO_2, 251
        effect of cyanate, 321
        effect of hypercapnia, 246
        effect of hyperoxia, 299
        effect of hypoxia, 227, 245
        effect of NADH, 243
        fetal, 1047, 1048, 1050, 1051
        flow to 219
        neuronal activity, 218, 229, 245
        see PO_2, Modeling

Capillary
        diffusion distance, 804, 806
        intercapillary distance, 519, 579
        neurons, 808
        see Diffusion, Flow, Modeling

Carbon dioxide, 814, 816, 942, 943, 969, 970
              1070, 1071, 1072
        see PCO_2

Carbon monoxide, 951, 960, 997, 1055
    see PCO

Carbonic anhydrase, 969, 970, 1056

Carboxyhemoglobin, 1006
    fluorescence determination of, 94

Carotid body
    oxygen histograms, 19
    see Chemoreceptors, PO$_2$

Catecholamine metabolism, 313, 699

Catheter, 1043, 1090, 1095, 1104, 1107, 1111, 1113, 1117
    diffusion limitations of, 73, 121
    see Electrode, Mass spectrometry, Photometry

Cell membrane potential, 227, 229, 230

Central nervous system,
    effect of cyanate, 319
    effect of hyperoxia, 293
    effect of spinal cord injury, 311

Cerebral blood flow, 817, 821
    see flow

Cerebral cortex, 822
    see Brain

Chemoreceptors, 597, 625
    in carotid body, 603, 617

Chemotherapy, 641

Choriallantoic membrane, 1001, 1002

Circulation,
        coronary, 543, 975
        effect of histamine, 699
        effect of norepinephrine, 425, 428
        effect of spinal cord injury, 346
        effect of sympathetic nerve stimulation, 425, 428
        effect of catecholamine metabolism, 313, 315, 316, 318
        in salamander Desmognathus fuscus, 61
        intestinal, 423, 436
        rate, 102
        see Flow, Microcirculation

Consumption
        see Oxygen

Control, 755, 816, 859, 903

Cornea, 897

Cotyledon, 1028, 1029, 1030, 1041, 1043

Cyanate
        effect on brain metabolism, 321, 323
        effect on CNS, 319
        effect on oxygen dissociation curve, 319, 322
        effect on sickle cells, 319

Cyclic AMP, 1052

Cytochrome, 53

Dextran, 649, 669, 739

Diabetes, 163, 208
    effect on ATP, 175
    effect on blood PO_2, 175, 177
    effect on pH, 174
    ketoacidosis, 163, 173, 174, 176, 208, 209
    see DPG

Diffusion, 150, 151, 850, 929, 934
    carbon dioxide, 938, 969
    glucose, 729, 851
    inert gases, 59
    measurement, 74
    oxygen, 12, 65, 66, 118
        effect of plasma proteins, 730, 744
        in heart, 525, 527
        through skin, 115
    resistance, 836, 861, 1068
    semi-infinite film, 931

Dissociation curve, 762, 783, 844, 923, 926
                        998, 1056
    see Homoglobin, Kinetics, Oxygen, Oxyhemoglobin

DPG, 163-211
    effect on erythrocytes, 179, 188
    effect on hemoglobin, 163, 179, 187, 193
                        197, 199
    effect on myocardium, 188
    effect on oxygen dissociation curve, 182, 193, 194
                        195
    effect on oxygen transport, 210
    effect on pH, 179

  effect on P_{50}, 179, 188, 194, 207
  kinetic model of, 202
  pharmacological effects on, 693
  transfusion and hemorrhage, 449, 503
  see Diabetes, Metabolism, Phosphate, P_{50}

EEG, 233, 240

Electrode, 627, 1089, 1090, 1091, 1092, 1109, 1117, 1121, 1123
  antimony-in-glass, 7
  calibration, 25, 36, 142, 145
    in situ, 18, 116
    residual current, 10, 18, 33, 42, 147
  catheter, oxygen, 107, 152
  chamber, 35, 41
  construction, 18, 23, 30, 35, 225, 262
  dropping mercury, 115
  enzyme, 131
  glucose, 127, 131, 154, 628
    effect of PO_2, 154, 155
  gold, 30, 32
  intracellular, 9, 10, 11, 17, 225
  micro, 135, 138, 763, 903, 946, 947, 963
    oxygen, 115, 116, 224, 262
      biological problems, 10, 18, 141
      history, 7
      technical problems, 9, 13, 18, 23, 32, 142, 144
      versus mass spectrometer, 71
  multiwire, 35, 36, 40, 41, 470
  needle, 11, 23, 40, 41, 442
  non-invasive device, 117
  pH, 224
  plated steel needle, 8
  platinum, 35, 224
    in glass, 8, 23
    on glass, 9
  potassium, 224
  pulsed, 29, 35
  recessed, 7, 9, 18, 30
  reference, 9, 30, 42
  scalp, 1129
  skin, 1097
  transcutaneous, 115, 153, 154

Entrance region, 867, 868

Enzyme, 131
    catalase, 128
    glucose oxidase, 128
    polarography, 127

Epinephrine, 1051, 1052, 1063

Equilibrium, 1055, 1056

Exercise, 818

Facilitated transport, 951, 960, 969, 970

Farism, 1075, 1078, 1079, 1081

Fetus, 1007, 1010, 1011, 1012, 1017, 1061

Filtering, 918

Flow, 217, 219, 252, 253, 254, 551
    after hemorrhagic shock, 508
    effect of heart-lung bypass, 561
    effect on skin PO_2, 115, 116
    heart, 526, 527, 533, 541
    maternal, fetal, 1010, 1012, 1023, 1029, 1030, 1056, 1058,
            1062, 1063
    measurement, 541
    micro, 355
    placental, 1018, 1019
    skin, 115, 116, 117
    splenic, 433
    see Aggregation, Autoregulation, Cerebral

Fluorescence, 11, 57, 148, 472, 627
    micro, 278, 418
    NAD, 283
        effect of hemoglobin, 377
        in brain, 239
        in liver, 378, 432
    pyrenebutyric acid, 55
    Stern-Volmer relationship, 55

Frequency distribution, 761, 784, 790

Friction factor, 869, 870

Gas chromatography, 60

Gas transport
   effect of pH, 306
   respiratory, 59, 305, 345

Gibbs principle, 116

Glial cell, 229

Glucose, 814, 815, 851, 853, 854
   distribution, 130
   measurement, 127
   see Diffusion, Electrode, Enzyme

Glycolysis, 849, 850, 852

Heart, 777, 778, 860
   atrial pacing, 553
   bypass, 407
   cardio-pulmonary bypass, 561
   coronary red blood cell washout, 567
   myoglobin, 571
   physiological effects, 407, 435
   see Oxygen, PO_2

Heinz bodies, 1075, 1076, 1078, 1081
   see Hemoglobin

Hemochorial, 1027, 1030

Hemodilution, 395, 669, 739
   see Dextran

Hemoglobin, 45, 49, 84, 94, 99, 101, 152, 352, 470, 472, 794
             820, 824, 924, 931, 937, 938, 942, 951, 960, 963, 965,
             1050, 1075, 1076, 1079, 1080
   fluorescence determination of, 84, 94, 99, 326
   see Oxygen dissociation curve, P_{50}, shock

Hemorrhagic shock, 469–516
    after transfusion, 499
    effect on PO_2, 470, 477, 480, 485, 505, 513
    flow after, 508
    influence on hemoglobin, 470, 472
    oxygen consumption during, 491, 515
    oxygen transport after, 505, 515

High altitude preadaptation, 693

Histamine, 1099
    see Circulation

Histogram, 762, 769, 770, 777

Hyaline, 642

Hydrogen, 796
    clearance curve, 267
    ions, 816
    washout curve, 135, 136, 137, 138

Hypercapnia, 235, 335
    effect on metabolism, 236, 237
    effect on neurons, 246, 249, 337
    effect on PO_2, 237, 238
    in liver, 362, 369, 370

Hyperemia, 115, 116, 118, 1121

Hyperoxemia, 521, 523

Hyperoxia, 218, 220, 342, 1093, 1095
    effect on brain PO_2, 299
    effect on CNS, 293

Hypoglycemia, 220

Hypothermia, 361, 366, 370

Hypoxemia, 1117

Hypoxia
    fetal, 996, 1017, 1026, 1062, 1067, 1068, 1089, 1093
    physiolgoical effects, 227, 234, 245, 249, 334, 337
                        356, 362, 369, 404, 405, 455, 545, 617

Instrumentation, 903, 917, 927
    see Monitoring

Intercapillary distance, 519
    effect of PO_2, 579

Intervillous space, 1029

Intravascular catheter electrode, 152, 153

Intravascular photometry, 102

Ischemia
    liver, 371
    skin, 717

Ketamine, 265, 267, 268

Kidney
    see PO_2

Kinetics, 199, 955, 965, 966, 1055
    capillary-tissue exchange, 773
    carbon monoxide and oxygen, 997
    effect of light on carbon monoxide, 1004
    effect of silicon membrane, 1005
    of oxygen release, 820

Krogh cylinder, 137, 157, 528, 637, 751, 775, 780, 794
                    797, 804, 820, 827, 835, 843, 849, 911

Labor, 1007, 1017, 1018, 1022, 1041
    see Parturition

Lactate-pyruvate ratio, 166, 168, 170, 207

Lethal corner, 822, 823, 832

Liver, 774, 777, 813
    grafts, 383, 433
    histograms, PO_2, 351
    hypercapnia and hypoxia, 356, 362, 369, 370
    ischemia, 371
    NADH, 377

Mass spectrometer, 67, 121, 126, 547, 627
    see Catheter

Metabolism, 234, 827, 963, 1012, 1043, 1063
    cerebral effect of cyanate, 319
    see Catecholamine, DPG, Oxygen consumption

Microcirculation, 135, 140, 262, 311, 316, 317, 389, 592
                   639, 641
    see Flow, Fluorescence, Spectrophotometry

Modeling, 62, 73, 199, 257, 550, 747, 749, 813, 819
              852, 859, 868
    analytic, 835, 843
    geometric considerations, 761, 763, 765, 773, 779, 783
              786, 794, 797, 800, 803, 891
    hybrid techniques, 859, 862, 889
    Monte Carlo simulation, 794, 795, 796, 888, 889, 890
    stochastic, 793, 797

Monitoring, newborn, 1089, 1097, 1103, 1109, 1113, 1121, 1129
    See Electrode

Myocardium, 859, 860, 862
    see Heart

Myoglobin, 571, 815, 859, 860, 938

Muscle, 817, 860, 896
    capillary arrangement, 751, 911
    myoglobin, 571
    see Heart, PO_2

NAD,
    see Fluorescence

Necrosis, CNS, 294, 299

Neonatology, 991

Nicotinamide, 116

Norepinephrine, 425, 1063

Oximetry, 83

Oxygen,
    autoregulation, 215, 441
    barrier, 610
    consumption,
        after shock, 491, 515
        during heart-lung bypass, 561
        effect of dimethyl sulfoxide, 743
        in heart, 525, 529, 530
        in kidney, 412
        in sciatic nerve, 271
    dissociation curve, 163, 164, 166, 167, 168, 169, 171, 325
        after transfusion and hemorrhage, 499, 500, 503
        effect of cyanate, 319, 322
        effect of DPG, 182, 193, 194, 195
        measurement of, 326
    extraction,
        intestine, 423
        skeletal muscle, 451
    mitochondrial, 278
    saturation, measurement of, 83
    sensor, 216, 220, 221, 629
    transport, 64, 629, 637
        after transfusion and hemorrhage, 499, 505, 515
        during heart-lung bypass, 561
        effect of aggregation, 647
        effect of anesthetic drugs, 261
        effect of anti-adhesive drugs, 657
        effect of capillary arrangement, 519
        effect of DPG, 199, 210
        effect of hemodilution, 395, 669, 739
        effect of pharmacological agents, 713
        effect of plasma proteins, 729
        in brain, 339

in heart, 519, 525
in skeletal muscle, 451
see Diffusion, Electrode, Hemoglobin, Metabolism, PO_2

Oxyhemoglobin, 830
fluorescence determination of, 84, 94
see Hemoglobin

Parturition, 1043, 1044, 1045, 1133

PCO, 571

PCO_2, 70, 71, 118, 119
blood, 307
heart, 547
measurement by glass microprobe, 457, 462, 464
muscle, 459

Peclet number, 830

Perfusion, 116, 117, 135, 137, 138, 139, 140
after shock, 505, 513
perfluorinated compounds, 687, 741

Permeability, 895
see Diffusion

pH, 179, 224, 228, 229, 373

Phosphate, 163, 201, 693, 742
see DPG

Photolysis, 279

Photometry, 99
micro, 99, 326, 418, 997, 998
reflexim, 797, 798, 799
see Spectrophotometry

Placenta, 1000, 1007, 1010, 1055
blood flow, 1017, 1018, 1019, 1023
oxygen, 1020, 1024, 1025, 1026
see Diffusion, Flow

Platinum
    see Electrode

Polarography, 25, 31, 33, 36, 38, 40, 109, 147
    enzyme, 127
    pulse, 29, 35

Potassium
    electrode, 224
    leakage, 227

PO_2,
    abdominal viscera, 395
    after shock, 227, 505, 513
    arterial, 39, 110, 111, 115, 215, 477-778
    blood, 137, 175, 177, 307
    brain, 37, 38, 215
        effect of arterial PO_2, 251
    carotid body, 19, 597, 609
    CNS, 302
    heart, 37, 38, 535, 541, 547
        effect of atrial pacing, 553
    intestine, 423, 425, 436, 470
    intracellular, 55, 278
    kidney, 351, 411, 429, 485
    liver, 351, 361, 383, 398, 430, 433
    muscle, 20, 21, 143, 144, 398, 443, 459, 571
    regulation, 603
    sciatic nerve, 271
    skin, 45, 115
    spleen, 401
    tissue, 67, 479, 519, 579
        effect of anesthetic drugs, 261
    venous, 20

Pseudo-steady state, 829, 861

Pulmonary embolism, 638, 733

P_{50}, 93, 164, 173, 176, 177, 209, 320, 499, 501
    definition, 173
    effect of DPG, 179, 180, 188, 194, 207

Q-analysis, 49, 53, 148, 799
    see Spectrophotometry

Quantitative analysis, 51

Quasi-equilibrium, 942

Quasi-linearization, 972

Random variable, 919

Red blood cell, 946, 963, 964, 965, 997
    strain on, 946
    washout, 567
    see DPG

Redox potential tissue, 1051

Residual current
    see Electrode

Reoxygenation time, 658, 659, 660, 664

Respiration, 115, 116, 117, 118, 305, 345, 717, 897, 1061
                1092
    see Oxygen, Ventilation

Reynolds number, 868, 966

Shock
    see Hemorrhagic

Sickle cells, 319

Silicone, 1005

Sinusoids, 355

Spectrophotometry, 45, 55, 94
    see Q-analysis

Spectroscopy, 151

Spleen
    see Circulation, Flow, PO_2

State disturbances, 919

Sympathetic nervous control, 423

Thermodynamics, 946, 952

Tonometer, 93

Transport
    see Oxygen

Umbilical, 1041, 1043, 1045

Uterus, 1018, 1041, 1043, 1045, 1062
    blood flow, 1007, 1022
    contractions, 1050
    see Flow, Labor, Placenta

Van-Slyke method, 60, 326

Ventilation, 816

VO_2, 20, 95, 143, 144

Washout curve, 61, 135, 157, 778

Washout techniques, 59

Water, labelled, 773, 777